THIRD EDITION

Handbook of Liver Disease

Edited by

LAWRENCE S. FRIEDMAN, MD

Professor of Medicine, Harvard Medical School and Tufts University
    School of Medicine
Chair, Department of Medicine, Newton-Wellesley Hospital
Assistant Chief of Medicine, Massachusetts General Hospital
Boston, Massachusetts

EMMET B. KEEFFE, MD, MACP

Professor Emeritus, Medicine
Stanford University Medical Center
Stanford, California

Foreword by

JULES L. DIENSTAG, MD

Carl W. Walter Professor of Medicine
Dean for Medical Education
Harvard Medical School
Physician, Department of Medicine (Gastrointestinal Unit)
Massachusetts General Hospital
Boston, Massachusetts

ELSEVIER
SAUNDERS

ELSEVIER
SAUNDERS

1600 John F. Kennedy Blvd.
Ste 1800
Philadelphia, PA 19103-2899

HANDBOOK OF LIVER DISEASE ISBN: 978-1-4377-1725-9

Notices

Knowledge and best practice in this field are constantly changing. As new research and experience broaden our understanding, changes in research methods, professional practices, or medical treatment may become necessary.

Practitioners and researchers must always rely on their own experience and knowledge in evaluating and using any information, methods, compounds, or experiments described herein. In using such information or methods they should be mindful of their own safety and the safety of others, including parties for whom they have a professional responsibility.

With respect to any drug or pharmaceutical products identified, readers are advised to check the most current information provided (i) on procedures featured or (ii) by the manufacturer of each product to be administered, to verify the recommended dose or formula, the method and duration of administration, and contraindications. It is the responsibility of practitioners, relying on their own experience and knowledge of their patients, to make diagnoses, to determine dosages and the best treatment for each individual patient, and to take all appropriate safety precautions.

To the fullest extent of the law, neither the Publisher nor the authors, contributors, or editors, assume any liability for any injury and/or damage to persons or property as a matter of products liability, negligence or otherwise, or from any use or operation of any methods, products, instructions, or ideas contained in the material herein.

Library of Congress Cataloging-in-Publication Data
Handbook of liver disease / edited by Lawrence S. Friedman, Emmet B. Keeffe ; foreword by Jules Dienstag. -- 3rd ed.
    p. ; cm.
  Includes bibliographical references and index.
  ISBN 978-1-4377-1725-9 (pbk. : alk. paper) 1.
Liver--Diseases--Handbooks, manuals, etc. I. Friedman, Lawrence S. (Lawrence Samuel), 1953- II. Keeffe, Emmet B.
  [DNLM: 1. Liver Diseases--Handbooks. WI 39]
  RC845.H365 2012
  616.3'62--dc23   2011016970

Acquisitions Editor: Kate Dimock
Developmental Editor: Kate Crowley
Publishing Services Manager: Peggy Fagen
Project Manager: Srikumar Narayanan
Design Manager: Lou Forgione
Illustrations Manager: Kari Wszolek
Marketing Manager: Abby Swartz

Working together to grow
libraries in developing countries

www.elsevier.com | www.bookaid.org | www.sabre.org

ELSEVIER   BOOK AID International   Sabre Foundation

Printed in China
Last digit is the print number: 9 8 7 6 5 4 3 2 1

Handbook of Liver Disease

THIRD EDITION

CONTRIBUTORS

Jacob Alexander, MD
Fellow in Gastroenterology
University of Washington School of
    Medicine
Seattle, Washington

Armine Avanesyan, MD
Internal Medicine
Loma Linda University Medical Center
Loma Linda, California

**Helen M. Ayles, MBBS, MRCP,
DTM&H, PhD**
Senior Lecturer, Department of
    Clinical Research
London School of Hygiene and
    Tropical Medicine
London, England
Director, ZAMBART Project
University of Zambia
Lusaka, Zambia
Honorary Consultant, Physician
Brighton and Sussex University
NHS Trust
Brighton, England

Jay P. Babich, MD
Fellow, Division of Gastroenterology,
    Hepatology and Nutrition
Winthrop University Hospital
Mineola, New York

**Sarah Lou Bailey, BSc, MBChB,
MRCP**
Clinical Lecturer in Infectious
    Diseases and Global Health
Brighton and Sussex Medical School
Brighton, England

William F. Balistreri, MD
Dorothy M.M. Kersten Professor of
    Pediatrics
University of Cincinnati College of
    Medicine
Division of Gastroenterology,
    Hepatology and Nutrition
Cincinnati Children's Hospital
    Medical Center
Cincinnati, Ohio

Salvador Benlloch, MD
Consultant, Hepatology
Hepatology-Liver Transplantation Unit
CIBEREHD (National Network
    Center for Hepatology and
    Gastroenterology Research)
Hospital Universitario La Fe
Valencia, Spain

Marina Berenguer, MD
Associate Professor of Medicine
Consultant, Hepatology
Hepatology-Liver Transplantation Unit
CIBEREHD (National Network
    Center for Hepatology and
    Gastroenterology Research)
Hospital Universitario La Fe
Valencia, Spain

Martin Black, MD
Clinical Professor of Medicine
Chief, Hepatology Service
Associate Director, Solid Organ
    Transplant Program
Temple University School of Medicine
Philadelphia, Pennsylvania

Christopher L. Bowlus, MD
Professor of Medicine
Division of Gastroenterology and
  Hepatology
University of California Davis School
  of Medicine
Sacramento, California

**Catherine Petruff Cheney, MD,
AGAF**
Assistant Clinical Professor of Medicine
Harvard Medical School
Division of Gastroenterology
Beth Israel Deaconess Medical Center
Boston, Massachusetts

Sanjiv Chopra, MBBS, MACP
Professor of Medicine
Faculty Dean for Continuing Education
Harvard Medical School
Senior Consultant in Hepatology
Beth Israel Deaconess Medical Center
Boston, Massachusetts

Raymond T. Chung, MD
Director of Hepatology
Vice Chief, Gastroenterology
Massachusetts General Hospital
Associate Professor of Medicine
Harvard Medical School
Boston, Massachusetts

**Jeremy F.L. Cobbold, PhD,
MRCP**
Clinical Lecturer in Hepatology
Imperial College London
London, England

**Albert J. Czaja, MD, FACP,
FACG, AGAF**
Professor Emeritus of Medicine
Mayo Clinic College of Medicine
Rochester, Minnesota

**Adrian M. Di Bisceglie, MD,
FACP**
Professor of Internal Medicine
Chief of Hepatology
Chairman, Department of Internal
  Medicine
Saint Louis University School of
  Medicine
St. Louis, Missouri

Anna Mae Diehl, MD
Professor of Medicine
Chief, Division of Gastroenterology
Duke University Medical Center
Durham, North Carolina

Lawrence S. Friedman, MD
Professor of Medicine
Harvard Medical School and Tufts
  University School of Medicine
Chair, Department of Medicine
Newton-Wellesley Hospital
Assistant Chief of Medicine
Massachusetts General Hospital
Boston, Massachusetts

Wolfram Goessling, MD, PhD
Assistant Professor of Medicine
Assistant Professor of Health Sciences
  and Technology
Harvard Medical School
Harvard Stem Cell Institute
Genetics and Gastroenterology
  Divisions
Brigham and Women's Hospital
Gastrointestinal Cancer Center
Dana-Farber Cancer Institute
Boston, Massachusetts

Eric Mathew Goldberg, MD
Assistant Professor of Medicine
Director of Endoscopic Training and
  Research
University of Maryland School of
  Medicine
Baltimore, Maryland

John L. Gollan, MD, PhD, FRACP, FRCP, FACP
Dean, College of Medicine
University of Nebraska Medical
  Center
Omaha, Nebraska

Stevan A. Gonzalez, MD, MS
Division of General and Transplant
  Hepatology
Baylor Regional Transplant Institute
Baylor All Saints Medical Center
Fort Worth, Texas

Norman D. Grace, MD
Director of Clinical Hepatology
Brigham and Women's Hospital
Professor of Medicine
Tufts University School of Medicine
Lecturer in Medicine
Harvard Medical School
Boston, Massachusetts

Mónica Guevara, MD, PhD
Clinical Research Associate
Hospital Clinic de Barcelona
Institut d'Investigacions
Biomediques August Pi i Sonyer
  (INIBAPS)
Barcelona, Spain

E. Jenny Heathcote, MBBS, MD, FRCP, FRCP(C)
The Francis Family Chair in
  Hepatology Research
Professor of Medicine
University of Toronto
Head, Patient Based Clinical Research
Toronto Western Research Institute
Toronto Western Hospital
Toronto, Ontario, Canada

Alexander T. Hewlett, DO, MS
Assistant Professor of Medicine
Division of Gastroenterology
University of Nebraska Medical
  Center
Omaha, Nebraska

Gideon M. Hirschfield, MB, BChir, MRCP, PhD
Liver Centre
Toronto Western Hospital
Toronto, Ontario, Canada

Michael G. House, MD
Assistant Professor of Surgery
Department of Surgery
Indiana University School of Medicine
Indianapolis, Indiana

Ke-Qin Hu, MD
Associate Professor of Clinical
  Medicine
Director of Hepatology Services
Division of Gastroenterology
University of California Irvine
  Medical Center
Orange, California

Christine E. Waasdorp Hurtado, MD
Assistant Professor of Pediatrics
University of Colorado
Aurora, Colorado

Ira M. Jacobson, MD
Vincent Astor Professor of Clinical
  Medicine
Chief, Division of Gastroenterology
  and Hepatology
Weill Medical College of Cornell
  University
New York, New York

Janice H. Jou, MD
Division of Gastroenterology
Duke University
Durham, North Carolina

Emmet B. Keeffe, MD, MACP
Professor Emeritus, Medicine
Stanford University Medical Center
Stanford, California

Raymond S. Koff, MD
Clinical Professor of Medicine
University of Connecticut School of
   Medicine
Farmington, Connecticut

Kris V. Kowdley, MD, FACP
Director, Center for Liver Disease
Virginia Mason Medical Center
Clinical Professor of Medicine
University of Washington School of
   Medicine
Seattle, Washington

Michelle Lai, MD, MPH
Instructor in Medicine
Harvard Medical School
Department of Medicine
Beth Israel Deaconess Medical Center
Boston, Massachusetts

Jay H. Lefkowitch, MD
Professor of Clinical Pathology
Department of Pathology
College of Physicians and Surgeons
Columbia University
New York, New York

Keith D. Lillemoe, MD, FACS
Chairman, Department of Surgery
Surgeon-in-Chief
Massachusetts General Hospital
Professor of Surgery
Harvard Medical School
Boston, Massachusetts

Vincent Lo Re III, MD, MSCE
Assistant Professor of Medicine
   and Epidemiology
Division of Infectious Diseases
Department of Medicine
Center for Clinical Epidemiology
   and Biostatistics
University of Pennsylvania School
   of Medicine
Philadelphia, Pennsylvania

Peter F. Malet, MD
Director, Center for Liver Diseases
Division of Gastroenterology,
   Hepatology and Nutrition
Department of Medicine
Winthrop University Hospital
Mineola, New York

Paul Martin, MD, FRCP, FRCPI
Professor of Medicine
Chief, Division of Hepatology
University of Miami Miller School of
   Medicine
Miami, Florida

Mack C. Mitchell, Jr, MD
Professor of Medicine
Vice-Chairman of Internal Medicine
University of Texas Southwestern
   Medical School
Dallas, Texas

Kevin D. Mullen, MB, FRCPI
Professor of Medicine
Gastrointestinal Division
MetroHealth Medical Center
Cleveland, Ohio

**Santiago J. Muñoz, MD, FACP,
FACG**
Professor of Medicine
Director, Clinical Hepatology
Medical Director, Liver Transplant
   Program
Temple University School of Medicine
Temple University Hospital
Philadelphia, Pennsylvania

**Brent A. Neuschwander-Tetri,
MD**
Professor of Internal Medicine
Division of Gastroenterology and
   Hepatology
Saint Louis University School of
   Medicine
St. Louis, Missouri

Jacqueline G. O'Leary, MD, MPH
Medical Director of the Inpatient
    Liver and Transplant Unit
Baylor Simmons Transplant Institute
Baylor University Medical Center
Dallas, Texas

Vishal Patel, MD
Assistant Professor of Medicine
Temple University School of Medicine
Temple University Hospital
Philadelphia, Pennsylvania

Ravi K. Prakash, MD, MRCP (UK)
Division of Gastroenterology
MetroHealth Medical Center
Cleveland, Ohio

James Puleo, MD
Consultant
Albany Memorial Hospital
Albany, New York

Rania Rabie, MD, FRCP(C)
Hepatology Fellow
University of Toronto
Toronto, Ontario, Canada

K. Rajender Reddy, MD, FACP
Professor of Medicine
Director of Hepatology
Medical Director of Liver
    Transplantation
University of Pennsylvania
Philadelphia, Pennsylvania

Juan Rodés, MD, FRCP
Professor of Medicine
University of Barcelona
General Manager
Hospital Clinic de Barcelona
Barcelona, Spain

Hugo R. Rosen, MD, FACP
Waterman Endowed Chair in Liver
    Research
Professor of Medicine and
    Immunology
Division Head, Gastroenterology and
    Hepatology
University of Colorado School of
    Medicine
Aurora, Colorado

Bruce A. Runyon, MD
Professor of Medicine
Chief of Liver Service
Loma Linda University Medical
    Center
Loma Linda, California

Thomas D. Schiano, MD
Professor of Medicine
Medical Director, Adult Liver
    Transplantation
Director of Clinical Hepatology
Division of Liver Disease
The Mount Sinai Medical Center
New York, New York

Ronald J. Sokol, MD
Professor and Vice Chair of Pediatrics
Arnold Silverman MD Chair in
    Digestive Health
Director of Colorado Clinical and
    Translational Sciences Institute
Chief, Section of Pediatric
    Gastroenterology, Hepatology and
    Nutrition
University of Colorado School of
    Medicine and The Children's
    Hospital
Aurora, Colorado

Elena M. Stoffel, MD
Lecturer in Medicine
Division of Gastroenterology
University of Michigan Medical
    Center
Ann Arbor, Michigan

John A. Summerfield, MD, FRCP
Consultant in Gastroenterology
St. Mary's Hospital
London, England

Bernadette Vitola, MD
Assistant Professor of Pediatrics
Division of Pediatric Gastroenterology,
    Hepatology and Nutrition
Medical College of Wisconsin
Children's Hospital of Wisconsin
Milwaukee, Wisconsin

Douglas M. Weine, MD
Fellow in Gastroenterology and
    Hepatology
Weill Medical College of Cornell
    University
New York, New York

Jacqueline L. Wolf, MD
Associate Professor of Medicine
Harvard Medical School
Division of Gastroenterology
Beth Israel Deaconess Medical Center
Boston, Massachusetts

**Florence S. Wong, MD, FRACP,
FRCP(C)**
Professor of Medicine
University of Toronto
Staff Hepatologist
Toronto General Hospital
Toronto, Ontario, Canada

FOREWORD

In the 1970s, hepatology as a specialty was compared with neurology: both hepatologists and neurologists could name the "lesion," but neither could do anything about it. Physicians had access to a few heroic options (e.g., portosystemic shunt surgery) and therapy for a limited spectrum of liver diseases (e.g., corticosteroid therapy for autoimmune hepatitis, phlebotomy for hemochromatosis), but for most liver disorders, all they could do was watch with concern and consternation as diseases progressed inexorably. In the past three decades—in little more than a single human generation—advances in hepatology have been staggering.

In the 1970s, no therapy was available for chronic viral hepatitis (the use of corticosteroids was misguided), nor did salvage therapy exist for acute liver failure or end-stage liver disease. For the diagnosis of cholecystitis and hepatic mass lesions, we relied on radioisotope scintigraphy, an imaging approach that is now largely forgotten; we debated the value, now disproven, of corticosteroids for acute fulminant hepatitis and drug-induced liver injury (DILI); we considered whether splenorenal shunting was better than portacaval shunting (yes in Atlanta, no in Boston); we pursued medical dissolution therapy and, later, lithotripsy for gallstones; we debated whether asymptomatic primary biliary cirrhosis (PBC) shortened life spans (no in New Haven, yes in Rochester); we chased down many false leads to explain what was then called "non-A, non-B" hepatitis; and nonalcoholic fatty liver disease was not even on our radar screens.

Since wandering in the dark prior to the 1970s with the misperception that only two types of viral hepatitis existed, we have arrived at our present day elucidation of five distinct and well-characterized types of viral hepatitis. Fewer than 20 years elapsed between the discovery of the envelope protein of hepatitis B and the development of a hepatitis B vaccine (with the 1976 Nobel Prize to Baruch Blumberg along the way). Early dabbling with interferon to the availability of the current generation of highly potent oral drugs took fewer than 30 years. Today, although we cannot cure hepatitis B, we can treat it and prevent its complications. Who in the 1970s would have imagined the impact of therapy on the natural history of chronic hepatitis B—slowing of fibrosis and even reversal of cirrhosis, rescue therapy for and prevention of hepatic decompensation, and a 30% reduction in listing for liver transplantation—in the half decade after the introduction of oral antiviral agents?

Transfusion-associated hepatitis—most of which, in retrospect, was caused by hepatitis C—occurred in 30% of transfusion recipients prior to the 1970s; it declined to 10% in the early 1970s with the switch from commercial to volunteer blood donors, to under 5% when surrogate markers were introduced to screen blood, and to almost never (1 in 2.3 million transfusions) with sensitive nucleic acid amplification to test donor blood. Who could have predicted in the 1970s that hepatitis C was not primarily a transfusion-associated disease or that the annual incidence of acute hepatitis C would fall by almost 90% in the 1990s?

Although a vaccine remains elusive, we should celebrate the progress that took place in as little as 23 years, from the ultimate discovery of hepatitis C virus (HCV) in 1988 to a nearly 80% cure rate with protease inhibitor-pegylated interferon-ribavirin antiviral therapy in 2011 (and the 2000 Lasker Award to Michael Houghton and Harvey Alter along the way). Now that two hepatitis C protease inhibitors have been approved in the United States, attention is turning to the two dozen plus new protease inhibitors, polymerase inhibitors, NS5A inhibitors, and other agents in development and to the promise, even a first glimpse, of cures with all-oral regimens.

Perhaps the largest impact on the transformation of hepatology into an "activist" specialty was liver transplantation, which began haltingly as an experimental, last-ditch measure in the 1970s to become routine in little more than a decade; improvements in outcome followed better timing and more rational organ allocation, novel immunosuppressive drugs and strategies, and refinements in surgical technique. Currently, we are much better at navigating between levels of immunosuppression that prevent rejection but that limit predisposition to infection, and the frequency of recurrence of primary disease has been reduced in some disorders (e.g., hepatitis B) but not others (e.g., hepatitis C). Still vexing is the shortage of donor livers, barely touched by recent excursions into accepting living-donor allografts, split-liver allografts, and marginal donor livers. To address the donor shortage, we may have to rely in the future on xenotransplantation, artificial livers, and stem cells, which, today, remain a remote dream.

From old debates about the value of colchicine and methotrexate for PBC, now mostly discarded, we have moved on to an elucidation of the target antigen of mitochondrial antibodies and of the genetic underpinning of PBC. Now well established is the value of ursodeoxycholic acid (UDCA) and its long-term impact on the natural history of the disease, at least in patient subgroups, as reflected by the reduction in the rate of liver transplantation for PBC that paralleled the broad adoption of UDCA therapy.

Fatty liver has been transformed from an unappreciated curiosity to what is recognized now as one of the most common liver disorders; attention has been focused on its association with insulin resistance and the metabolic syndrome as well as on its supporting role in progressive hepatic fibrosis and its contribution to "cryptogenic" cirrhosis. Fatty liver is now recognized as a comorbid factor in hepatitis C and a negative predictor of hepatitis C treatment response. Indeed, the link between fatty liver and hepatitis C is intimate; HCV and lipids rely on the same low-density lipoprotein (LDL) assembly/secretion pathway. By masquerading as a lipoprotein and, essentially, hijacking this lipid metabolic pathway, HCV reduces its visibility to the host adaptive immune response, thereby contributing to its success as a human pathogen. An explanation for the mechanism of hepatic injury in fatty liver remains elusive, although the nontriglyceride-lipotoxicity hypothesis is gaining traction. Similarly elusive have been attempts to identify treatments for fatty liver disease.

Today, we have laparoscopic cholecystectomy, previously unimagined diagnostic and therapeutic endoscopic interventions for biliary tract disorders, and sophisticated digital hepatobiliary imaging. For variceal bleeding, non selective beta blockade is the cornerstone of prophylaxis; the combination of endoscopic ligation and pharmacologic therapy is the accepted approach to an acute bleed; endoscopic surveillance and ligation as well as beta blockade have an established role in preventing rebleeding after an initial bleed; and the transjugular intrahepatic portosystemic shunt (TIPS) has supplanted portosystemic shunt surgery for refractory bleeding (often as a bridge to liver transplantation). A role for TIPS has also been demonstrated in refractory ascites and hydrothorax, hepatorenal syndrome (HRS), and hepatic vein occlusion. Pharmacologic interventions are available now to treat HRS type 1 (terlipressin plus albumin), prevent (norfloxacin or trimethoprim-sulfamethoxazole) and treat (third-generation cephalosporins and intravenous albumin) spontaneous bacterial peritonitis (SBP), and manage hepatic encephalopathy (antimicrobials such as rifaximin, besides lactulose). The importance of intravascular volume expansion is recognized now as a mainstay of the management of refractory ascites and SBP.

For the treatment of hepatocellular carcinoma (HCC), which has been increasing in incidence each decade (in parallel with an aging cohort of patients who have chronic hepatitis C), we have evolved from occasional resection a generation ago to a contemporary menu that includes chemotherapy (recently approved sorafenib, an oral multikinase inhibitor that targets serine/threonine and tyrosine receptor kinases), surgical resection, angiographic chemoembolization, and percutaneous ablation.

All these advances are covered in succinct, well-documented, and clear chapters in this edition of the *Handbook of Liver Disease*. In addition, the current edition reflects recent advances in our understanding of the genetic bases for bilirubin conjugation and excretion disorders, familial intrahepatic cholestatic disorders, Wilson disease, hemochromatosis, alpha-1 antitrypsin deficiency, alcohol-metabolizing enzymes, responsiveness to interferon-based therapy for hepatitis C and susceptibility to ribavirin-associated hemolysis, acute fatty liver of pregnancy, and the risk of DILI. In addition, the *Handbook* includes detailed chapters summarizing other important liver diseases, including DILI; acute liver failure; autoimmune hepatitis, autoimmune biliary disorders, and overlap syndromes; acute and chronic alcoholic liver disease; the multisystem manifestations of end-stage liver disease; liver disorders of pregnancy; granulomatous disorders; infections of the liver besides viral hepatitis; vascular disorders affecting the liver; hepatic manifestations of systemic disease; the risk of surgery in patients with liver disease and postoperative jaundice; and disorders of the gallbladder and bile ducts. Coverage of liver disease in the early 21st century would be incomplete without a review of the protean hepatic manifestations of human immunodeficiency virus (HIV)/acquired immunodeficiency syndrome (AIDS) (including infiltrative opportunistic infections and malignancies, viral hepatitis, fatty liver, antiretroviral drug hepatotoxicity, and AIDS cholangiopathy), and this topic is well covered. The chapters are enhanced by instructive illustrations, useful tables, and suggested diagnostic and therapeutic algorithms. In addition, the anchoring of every topic to an understanding of pathophysiology as the foundation for diagnosis and management is one of the clear longitudinal themes threaded through all the chapters.

Whereas medical information in the 1970s was disseminated primarily through physical textbooks and journals, medical information today is available digitally from the vast reaches of cyberspace. At the touch of a button, physicians (and patients) can access a wealth of timely and updated information without ever touching a book. Why, then, publish a physical *Handbook of Liver Disease* in 2011? The answer is simple. Like a foundational lecture, the *Handbook* provides organizational perspective and a thoughtful overview of the field—thematically unified, scholarly, succinct, and evidence-based—an ideal starting point for the novice and the expert, for the generalist and the specialist. Some textbooks oversimplify, sacrificing accuracy and depth for easily digestible summaries. Others overwhelm readers with complexity and distracting detail. The *Handbook*, however, strikes an ideal balance between these extremes of depth and simplification. Of course, a physical text can be only as current as its publication date, and, given the accelerated pace of progress, both predictable and unpredicted advances will have occurred by the time the *Handbook* is published. If anything, this level of structural obsolescence is a metaphor for the rapidity of change and inspires us to imagine what hepatology will look like in another generation.

Jules L. Dienstag, MD

To our wives, children, and grandchildren

PREFACE TO THE THIRD EDITION

We are pleased to serve as editors of the third edition of *Handbook of Liver Disease*. The field of hepatology has continued to advance exponentially since publication of the second edition in 2004. We stand at the threshold of an exciting new era of therapy for chronic hepatitis C with the introduction of protease inhibitors and, in the near future, polymerase inhibitors to our armamentarium, which promises to expand rapidly in coming years. Treatment of chronic hepatitis B has also evolved with the introduction of entecavir and tenofovir, which have proved to be more potent and less likely to result in the development of resistance than older nucleoside and nucleotide analogs.

Pharmacogenetic testing has entered mainstream practice with the introduction of *IL28B* genotype testing for determination of responsiveness to pegylated interferon and the study of *ITPA* genotypes to predict the likelihood of anemia in patients treated with ribavirin. Genetic advances promise to inform other areas of hepatology, including prediction of hepatotoxicity from drugs as well as susceptibility to many metabolic liver diseases and gallstone formation. Our understanding of the pathogenic mechanisms involved in portal hypertension and associated complications has become more sophisticated, and approaches to enhance the reversibility of liver fibrosis, even when the underlying cause cannot be eliminated, loom on the horizon. Prognostication and determination of candidacy for liver transplantation have become more refined at the same time that surgical techniques have advanced. These are exciting times to study the liver and to care for patients with acute and chronic liver diseases.

The goal of this handbook remains the same as that for the first two editions—to provide a concise, accurate, up-to-date, and readily accessible reference for students of the liver and for busy practitioners. We continue to use an outline format, lists, tables, and figures in color to convey information efficiently, yet without losing the depth and richness of the field. State-of-the-art summaries are presented economically but without scrimping on necessary details of the scientific underpinnings needed for optimal decision-making in practice.

This edition has a new feature in the online version of the book, namely, board-review questions for each chapter prepared by the follows in the Division of Gastroenterology and Hepatology at Stanford University School of Medicine. We believe that these review questions will be of particular use to readers preparing for the certification and recertification examinations in gastroenterology and hepatology.

We have been fortunate to retain many of the renowned authors from the previous editions, all of whom are authorities in their respective fields. In this edition, we welcome two new senior authors—Drs. Marina Berenguer and Christopher Bowlus—and a number of new co-authors who have enhanced the diversity and currency of the book. We continue to believe that this handbook will serve as a useful and valuable reference for busy practicing gastroenterologists and hepatologists, internists, family practitioners, other specialists, and trainees in gastroenterology and hepatology or internal medicine.

Lawrence S. Friedman
Emmet B. Keeffe

ACKNOWLEDGMENTS

We are grateful to all the contributors for their expertise, careful writing and updating, and timeliness in submitting their chapters. We feel fortunate to learn from the foremost authorities in the field of hepatology. We particularly appreciate the support and counsel of Druanne Martin and Kate Dimock, our acquisitions editors, and Kate Crowley, our editorial assistant, at Elsevier Saunders, without whom this edition would not have been possible. We thank our friend and mentor, Jules Dienstag, for his eloquent foreword. We also appreciate the work of the fellows in gastroenterology and hepatology at Stanford University School of Medicine, who prepared review questions for this edition, and our assistants, Alison Sholock and Karen Ely, who helped keep us organized. Finally, we are eternally grateful to our families for their unfailing support during the preparation of this third edition.

CONTENTS

Handbook of Liver Disease

THIRD EDITION

CHAPTER 1

Assessment of liver function and diagnostic studies

Paul Martin, MD, FRCP, FRCPI ■ Lawrence S. Friedman, MD

KEY POINTS

1 Reflecting the liver's diverse functions, the colloquial term *liver function tests* (LFTs) includes true tests of hepatic synthetic function (e.g., serum albumin), tests of excretory function (e.g., serum bilirubin), and tests that reflect hepatic necroinflammatory activity (e.g., serum aminotransferases) or cholestasis (e.g., alkaline phosphatase).

2 Abnormal liver biochemistry test results are often the first clues to liver disease. The widespread inclusion of these tests in routine blood chemistry panels uncovers many patients with unrecognized hepatic dysfunction.

3 Normal or minimally abnormal liver biochemical test levels do not preclude significant liver disease, even cirrhosis.

4 Laboratory testing can assess the severity of liver disease and its prognosis; sequential testing may allow assessment of the effectiveness of therapy.

5 Liver biopsy remains the gold standard for assessing the severity of liver disease, as well as for confirming the diagnosis for some causes. Newer diagnostic noninvasive modalities including serum markers of fibrosis and transient elastography may complement the use of liver biopsy.

6 Various imaging studies are useful in detecting focal hepatic defects, the presence of portal hypertension, and abnormalities of the biliary tract.

Routine Liver Biochemical Tests

SERUM BILIRUBIN

1. Jaundice
   - Often the first evidence of liver disease
   - Clinically apparent when serum bilirubin exceeds 3 mg/dL; patient may notice dark urine or pale stool before conjunctival icterus
2. Metabolism
   - Bilirubin is a breakdown product of hemoglobin and, to a lesser extent, heme-containing enzymes; 95% of bilirubin is derived from senescent red blood cells.
   - Following red blood cell breakdown in the reticuloendothelial system, heme is degraded by the enzyme heme oxygenase in the endoplasmic reticulum.
   - Bilirubin is released into blood and tightly bound to albumin; free or unconjugated bilirubin is lipid soluble, is not filtered by the glomerulus, and does not appear in urine.

- **Unconjugated bilirubin** is taken up by the liver by a carrier-mediated process, attaches to intracellular storage proteins (ligands), and is **conjugated by the enzyme uridine diphosphate (UDP)–glucuronyl transferase** to form a diglucuronide and, to a lesser extent, a monoglucuronide.
- Conjugated bilirubin is water soluble and thus appears in urine.
- When serum bilirubin glucuronides are elevated, some binding to albumin occurs (delta bilirubin), leading to absence of bilirubinuria despite conjugated hyperbilirubinemia; this phenomenon explains delayed resolution of jaundice during recovery from acute liver disease until catabolism of albumin-bound bilirubin occurs.
- Conjugated bilirubin is excreted by active transport across the canalicular membrane into bile.
- Bilirubin in bile enters the small intestine; in the distal ileum and colon, bilirubin is hydrolyzed by beta-glucuronidases to form unconjugated bilirubin, which is then reduced by gut bacteria to colorless urobilinogens; a small amount of urobilinogen is reabsorbed by the enterohepatic circulation and mostly excreted in the bile, with a smaller proportion undergoing urinary excretion.
- Urobilinogens or their colored derivatives urobilins are excreted in feces.

3. Measurement of serum bilirubin
   a. van den Bergh reaction
      - **Total serum bilirubin** represents all bilirubin that reacts within 30 minutes in the presence of alcohol (an accelerating agent).
      - **Direct serum bilirubin** is the fraction that reacts with the diazo reagent in an aqueous medium within 1 minute and corresponds to **conjugated bilirubin.**
      - **Indirect serum bilirubin** represents **unconjugated bilirubin** and is determined by subtracting the direct reacting fraction from the total bilirubin level.
   b. More specific methods (e.g., high-pressure liquid chromatography) demonstrate that the van den Bergh reaction often overestimates the amount of conjugated bilirubin; however, the van den Bergh method remains the standard test.

4. Classification of hyperbilirubinemia
   a. **Unconjugated** (bilirubin nearly always less than 7 mg/dL)
      - Overproduction (presentation to liver of bilirubin load that exceeds hepatic capacity for uptake and conjugation): hemolysis, ineffective erythropoiesis, resorption of hematoma
      - Defective uptake and storage of bilirubin: Gilbert's syndrome (idiopathic unconjugated hyperbilirubinemia)
   b. **Conjugated**
      - Hereditary: Dubin–Johnson and Rotor's syndromes, bile transport protein defects
      - Cholestasis (bilirubin is not a sensitive test of hepatic dysfunction)
        - Intrahepatic: cirrhosis, hepatitis, primary biliary cirrhosis, drug-induced
        - Extrahepatic biliary obstruction: choledocholithiasis, stricture, neoplasm, biliary atresia, sclerosing cholangitis
   c. **Very high bilirubin levels**
      - Higher than 30 mg/dL: usually signifies hemolysis plus parenchymal liver disease or biliary obstruction; urinary excretion of conjugated bilirubin may help prevent even higher levels of hyperbilirubinemia; renal failure contributes to hyperbilirubinemia
      - Higher than 60 mg/dL: seen in patients with hemoglobinopathies (e.g., sickle cell anemia) who develop obstructive jaundice or acute hepatitis

5. Urine bilirubin and urobilinogen
   - Bilirubinuria indicates an increase in serum conjugated (direct) bilirubin.

- Urinary urobilinogen (rarely measured now) is found in patients with hemolysis (increased production of bilirubin), gastrointestinal hemorrhage, or hepatocellular disease (impaired removal of urobilinogen from blood).
- Absence of urobilinogen from urine suggests interruption of enterohepatic circulation of bile pigments, as in complete bile duct obstruction.
- Urobilinogen detection and quantification add little diagnostic information to evaluation of hepatic dysfunction.

SERUM AMINOTRANSFERASES (Table 1.1)

1. These intracellular enzymes are released from injured hepatocytes and are the most useful marker of hepatic injury (inflammation or cell necrosis).
   a. **Aspartate aminotransferase** (AST, SGOT [serum glutamic oxaloacetic transaminase])
      - Found in cytosol and mitochondria
      - Found in liver as well as skeletal muscle, heart, kidney, brain, and pancreas
   b. **Alanine aminotransferase** (ALT, SGPT [serum glutamic pyruvic transaminase])
      - Found in cytosol
      - Highest concentration in liver (more sensitive and specific than AST for liver inflammation and hepatocyte necrosis)

TABLE 1.1 ■ **Causes of elevated serum aminotransferase levels***

Mild elevation (<5× normal)	Marked elevation (>15× normal)
Hepatic: ALT predominant	Acute viral hepatitis (A–E, herpes)
Chronic viral hepatitis	DILI
Acute viral hepatitis (A–E, EBV, CMV)	Ischemic hepatitis
NAFLD	Autoimmune hepatitis
Hemochromatosis	Wilson disease
DILI	Acute bile duct obstruction
Autoimmune hepatitis	Acute Budd–Chiari syndrome
Alpha-1 antitrypsin deficiency	Hepatic artery ligation
Wilson disease	
Celiac disease	
Hepatic: AST predominant	
Alcohol-related liver injury (AST:ALT >2:1)	
Cirrhosis	
Nonhepatic	
Strenuous exercise	
Hemolysis	
Myopathy	
Thyroid disease	
Macro-AST	

*Almost any liver disease may be associated with ALT levels 5 times to 15 times normal.

ALT, alanine aminotransferase; AST, aspartate aminotransferase; CMV, cytomegalovirus; DILI, drug-induced liver injury; EBV, Epstein-Barr virus; NAFLD, nonalcoholic fatty liver disease.

2. Clinical usefulness
   - **Normal levels of ALT are up to 30 U/L in men and up to 19 U/L in women.**
   - Levels increase with body mass index and may correlate with the risk of coronary artery disease and mortality.
   - Levels may rise acutely with a high caloric meal or ingestion of acetaminophen 4 g/day; coffee appears to lower levels.
   - Aminotransferase elevations are often the first biochemical abnormalities detected in patients with viral, autoimmune, or drug-induced hepatitis; the degree of elevation may correlate with the extent of hepatic injury but is generally not of prognostic significance.
   - In alcoholic hepatitis, the serum AST is usually no more than 2 to 10 times the upper limit of normal, and the ALT is normal or nearly normal with an AST:ALT ratio greater than 2; relatively low ALT levels may result from a deficiency of pyridoxal 5-phosphate, a necessary cofactor for hepatic synthesis of ALT. In contrast, in nonalcoholic fatty liver disease, ALT is typically higher than AST until cirrhosis develops.
   - Aminotransferase levels may be higher than 3000 U/L in acute or chronic viral hepatitis or drug-induced liver injury; in acute liver failure or ischemic hepatitis (shock liver), even higher values (higher than 5000 U/L) may be found.
   - Mild to moderate elevations of aminotransferase levels are typical of chronic viral hepatitis, autoimmune hepatitis, hemochromatosis, alpha-1 antitrypsin deficiency, Wilson disease, and celiac disease.
   - In obstructive jaundice, aminotransferase values are usually lower than 500 U/L; rarely, values may reach 1000 U/L in acute choledocholithiasis or 3000 U/L in acute cholecystitis, followed by a rapid decline to normal.
3. Approach to the patient with an elevated ALT is shown in Fig. 1.1.
4. Approach to the patient with mild diffuse liver test abnormalities is shown in Fig. 1.2.
5. Abnormally low aminotransferase levels have been associated with uremia and chronic hemodialysis; chronic viral hepatitis in this population may not result in aminotransferase elevation.

SERUM ALKALINE PHOSPHATASE

1. Hepatic alkaline phosphatase is one of several alkaline phosphatase isoenzymes found in humans and is bound to hepatic canalicular membrane; various laboratory methods are available for its measurement, and thus comparison of results obtained by different techniques may be misleading.
2. **This test is sensitive for detection of biliary tract obstruction** (a normal value is highly unusual in significant biliary obstruction); interference with bile flow may be intrahepatic or extrahepatic.
   - An increase in serum alkaline phosphatase results from increased hepatic synthesis of the enzyme, rather than leakage from bile duct cells or failure to clear circulating alkaline phosphatase; because it is synthesized in response to biliary obstruction, the alkaline phosphatase level may be normal early in the course of acute suppurative cholangitis when the serum aminotransferases are already elevated.
   - Increased bile acid concentrations may promote the synthesis of alkaline phosphatase.
   - Serum alkaline phosphatase has a half-life of 17 days; levels may remain elevated up to 1 week after relief of biliary obstruction and return of the serum bilirubin level to normal.

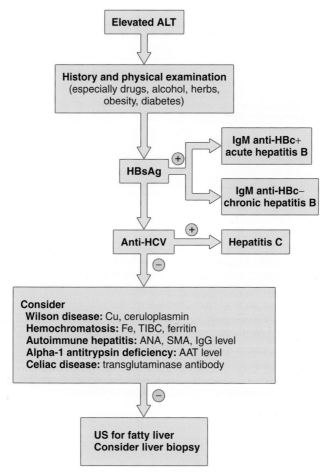

Fig. 1.1 Approach to patients with an elevated serum alanine aminotransferase (ALT) level. AAT, alpha-1 antitrypsin; ANA, antinuclear antibodies; anti-HBc, antibody to hepatitis B core antigen; anti-HCV, antibody to hepatitis C virus; CT, computed tomography; HBsAg, hepatitis B surface antigen; IgG, immunoglobulin; SMA, smooth muscle antibodies; TIBC, total iron binding capacity; US, ultrasonography.

3. **Isolated elevation of alkaline phosphatase**
   - This may indicate infiltrative liver disease: tumor, abscess, granulomas, or amyloidosis.
   - High levels are associated with biliary obstruction, sclerosing cholangitis, primary biliary cirrhosis, sepsis, acquired immunodeficiency syndrome, cholestatic drug reactions, and other causes of vanishing bile duct syndrome; in critically ill patients, high levels may indicate secondary sclerosing cholangitis with rapid progression to cirrhosis.
   - Nonhepatic sources of alkaline phosphatase are bone, intestine, kidney, and placenta (different isoenzymes); striking elevations are seen in Paget's disease of the bone, osteoblastic bone metastases, small bowel obstruction, and normal pregnancy.

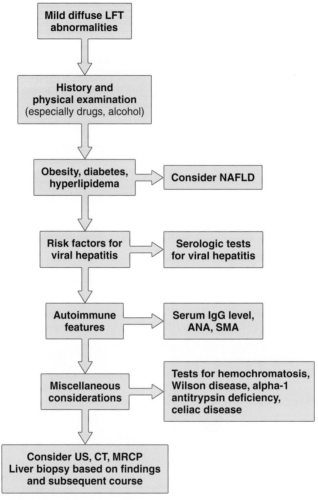

Fig. 1.2 Approach to a patient with mild diffuse liver biochemical test abnormalities. ANA, antinuclear antibodies; CT, computed tomography; LFT, liver function test; IgG, immunoglobulin; MRCP, magnetic resonance cholangiopancreatography; NAFLD, nonalcoholic fatty liver disease; SMA, smooth muscle antibodies; US, ultrasonography.

- ■ **Hepatic origin of an elevated alkaline phosphatase level is suggested by simultaneous elevation of either serum gamma glutamyltranspeptidase (GGTP) or 5'-nucleotidase (5NT).**
- ■ Hepatic alkaline phosphatase is more heat stable than bony alkaline phosphatase. The degree of overlap makes this test less useful than GGTP or 5NT.
- ■ The diagnostic approach is shown in Fig. 1.3.
4. Mild elevations of serum alkaline phosphatase are often seen in hepatitis and cirrhosis.
5. Low serum levels of alkaline phosphatase may occur in hypothyroidism, pernicious anemia, zinc deficiency, congenital hypophosphatasia, and fulminant Wilson disease.

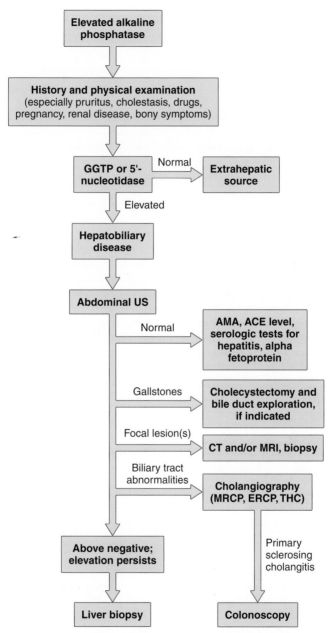

Fig. 1.3 Approach to a patient with isolated serum alkaline phosphatase elevation. ACE, angiotensin-converting enzyme; AMA, antimitochondrial antibodies; CT, computed tomography; ERCP, endoscopic retrograde cholangiopancreatography; GGTP, gamma glutamyltranspeptidase; MRCP, magnetic resonance cholangiopancreatography; MRI, magnetic resonance imaging; THC, transhepatic cholangiography; US, ultrasonography.

GAMMA GLUTAMYLTRANSPEPTIDASE (GGTP)

1. Although present in many different organs, GGTP is found in particularly high concentrations in the epithelial cells lining biliary ductules.
2. It is a very sensitive indicator of hepatobiliary disease but is not specific. Levels are elevated in other conditions, including renal failure, myocardial infarction, pancreatic disease, and diabetes mellitus.
3. **GGTP is inducible, and thus levels may be elevated by ingestion of phenytoin or alcohol** in the absence of other clinical evidence of liver disease.
4. Because of its long half-life of 26 days, GGTP is limited as a marker of surreptitious alcohol consumption.
5. Its major clinical use is to exclude a bony source of an elevated serum alkaline phosphatase level.
6. Many patients with isolated serum GGTP elevation have no other evidence of liver disease; an extensive evaluation is usually not warranted. Patients should be retested after avoiding alcohol and other hepatotoxins for several weeks.

5'-NUCLEOTIDASE (5NT)

1. 5NT is found in the liver in association with canalicular and sinusoidal plasma membranes.
2. Although 5NT is distributed in other organs, serum levels are believed to reflect hepatobiliary release by the detergent action of bile salts on plasma membranes.
3. Serum 5NT levels correlate well with serum alkaline phosphatase levels; **elevated 5NT in association with elevated alkaline phosphatase is specific for hepatobiliary dysfunction and is superior to GGTP in this regard.**

LACTATE DEHYDROGENASE (LDH)

Measurement of LDH and the more specific isoenzyme LDH5 adds little to the evaluation of suspected hepatic dysfunction. High levels of LDH are seen in hepatocellular necrosis, shock liver, cancer, and hemolysis. **The ALT:LDH ratio may help differentiate acute viral hepatitis (1.5 or higher) from shock liver and acetaminophen toxicity (less than 1.5)**

SERUM PROTEINS

Most proteins circulating in plasma are synthesized by the liver and reflect the synthetic capability of the liver.

1. Albumin
    - This accounts for 65% of serum proteins.
    - The half-life is approximately 3 weeks.
    - Concentration in blood depends on the albumin synthetic rate (normal, 12 g/day) and plasma volume.
    - **Hypoalbuminemia** may result from expanded plasma volume or decreased albumin synthesis. It is frequently associated with ascites and expansion of the extravascular albumin pool at the expense of intravascular albumin pool. Hypoalbuminemia is common in chronic liver disease (an indicator of severity); it is less common in acute liver disease. It is not specific for liver disease and may also reflect glomerular or gastrointestinal losses.

2. Globulins
   a. They are often nonspecifically increased in chronic liver disease.
   b. The pattern of elevation may suggest the cause of the underlying liver disease:
      - Elevated immunoglobulin G (IgG): autoimmune hepatitis
      - Elevated IgM: primary biliary cirrhosis
      - Elevated IgA: alcoholic liver disease
3. Coagulation factors
   a. **Most coagulation factors are synthesized by the liver,** including factors I (fibrinogen), II (prothrombin), V, VII, IX, and X and have much shorter half-lives than that of albumin.
      - Factor VII decreases first because of its shortest half-life, followed by factors X and IX.
      - Factor V is not vitamin K dependent, and its measurement can help distinguish vitamin K deficiency from hepatocellular dysfunction in a patient with a prolonged prothrombin time. Serial measurement of factor V levels has been used to assess prognosis in acute liver failure; a value less than 20% of normal portends a poor outcome without liver transplantation.
      - Measurement of factor II (des-gamma-carboxyprothrombin) has also been used to assess liver function. Elevated levels are found in cirrhosis and hepatocellular carcinoma and in patients taking sodium warfarin, a vitamin K antagonist. Administration of vitamin K results in normalization of des-gamma-carboxyprothrombin in patients taking warfarin but not in those with cirrhosis.
   b. **Prothrombin time is useful in assessing the severity and prognosis of acute liver disease.** The one-stage prothrombin time described by Quick measures the rate of conversion of prothrombin to thrombin after activation of the extrinsic coagulation pathway in the presence of a tissue extract (thromboplastin) and calcium (Ca^{++}) ions. Deficiency of one or more of the liver-produced factors results in a prolonged prothrombin time.
   c. **Prolongation of the prothrombin time in cholestatic liver disease may result from vitamin K deficiency.**
      - Other explanations for a prolonged prothrombin time apart from hepatocellular disease or vitamin K deficiency include consumptive coagulopathies, inherited deficiencies of a coagulation factor, or medications that antagonize the prothrombin complex.
      - Vitamin K deficiency as the cause of a prolonged prothrombin time can be excluded by administration of vitamin K 10 mg; intravenous administration can cause severe reactions, and the oral route is preferable, if possible. Correction or improvement of the prothrombin time by at least 30% within 24 hours implies that hepatic synthetic function is intact.
      - The international normalized ratio (INR) is used to standardize prothrombin time determinations performed in different laboratories; however, the results are less consistent in patients with liver disease than in those taking warfarin unless liver-disease controls are used.
      - The prothrombin time (and INR) correlates with the severity of liver disease but not with the risk of bleeding because of counterbalancing decreases in levels of anticoagulant factors (e.g., protein C and S, antithrombin) and enhanced fibrinolysis in patients with liver disease.

Assessment of Hepatic Metabolic Capacity

Various drugs that undergo purely hepatic metabolism and have predictable bioavailability have been used to assess hepatic metabolic capacity. Typically, a metabolite is measured in plasma, urine, or breath following intravenous or oral administration of the parent compound. These tests are not widely used in practice.

ANTIPYRINE CLEARANCE

1. Antipyrine is metabolized by cytochrome P-450 oxygenase with good absorption after oral administration and elimination entirely by the liver.
2. In chronic liver disease, good correlation exists between prolongation of the antipyrine half-life and disease severity as assessed by the Child–Turcotte–Pugh score (see Chapter 10).
3. Clearance of antipyrine is less impaired in acute liver disease and obstructive jaundice.
4. Disadvantages of this test include its long half-life in serum, which requires multiple blood sampling, poor correlation with in vitro assessment of hepatic microsomal capacity, and alteration of antipyrine metabolism by increased age, diet, alcohol, smoking, and environmental exposure.

AMINOPYRINE BREATH TEST

1. This test is based on detection of $[^{14}C]O_2$ in breath 2 hours after an oral dose of $[^{14}C]$ dimethyl aminoantipyrine (aminopyrine), which undergoes hepatic metabolism.
2. Excretion is diminished in patients with cirrhosis as well as in acute liver disease.
3. The test has been used to assess prognosis in patients with alcoholic hepatitis and in cirrhotic patients who are undergoing surgery.
4. A limitation of the aminopyrine breath test is its lack of sensitivity in hepatic dysfunction resulting from cholestasis or extrahepatic obstruction.

CAFFEINE CLEARANCE

1. Caffeine clearance after oral ingestion can be assessed by measuring levels in either saliva or serum; the accuracy appears similar to the $[^{14}C]$aminopyrine breath test, without the need for a radioisotope.
2. Results are clearly abnormal in clinically severe liver disease, but the test is insensitive in mild hepatic dysfunction.
3. Caffeine clearance decreases with age or cimetidine use and increases with cigarette smoking.

GALACTOSE ELIMINATION CAPACITY

1. Galactose clearance from blood as a result of hepatic phosphorylation can be determined following either intravenous or oral administration; serial serum levels of galactose are obtained 20 to 50 minutes after an intravenous bolus, with correction for urinary galactose excretion.
2. At plasma concentrations higher than 50 mg/dL, removal of galactose reflects hepatic functional mass, whereas at concentrations lower than this plasma level, clearance reflects hepatic blood flow.
3. $[^{14}C]$Galactose is distributed in extracellular water and is affected by changes in volume.
4. Galactose clearance is impaired in acute and chronic liver disease as well as in patients with metastatic hepatic neoplasms but is typically unaffected in obstructive jaundice.
5. The oral galactose tolerance test incorporates $[^{14}C]$galactose with measurement of breath $[^{14}C]O_2$; the results of this breath test correlate with $[^{14}C]$aminopyrine testing.
6. $[^{14}C]$galactose testing is no more accurate than standard liver biochemical tests in assessing prognosis in patients with chronic liver disease.

LIDOCAINE METABOLITE

1. Monoethylglycinexylidide (MEGX), a product of hepatic lidocaine metabolism, is easily measured by a fluorescence polarization immune assay 15 minutes after an intravenous dose of lidocaine.
2. The test may offer prognostic information about the likelihood of life-threatening complications in cirrhotic patients.
3. The test has also been used to assess the viability of donor liver allografts.
4. The test is easy to perform and has few adverse reactions, although it may be unsuitable for some cardiac patients. Test results may be affected by simultaneous use of certain drugs metabolized by cytochrome P-450 3A4 and high bilirubin levels; test results are affected by age and body mass and are higher in men than in women.

Other Tests of Liver Function

SERUM BILE ACIDS

1. Bile acids are synthesized from cholesterol in the liver, conjugated to glycine or taurine, and excreted in the bile. Bile acids facilitate fat digestion and absorption within the small intestine. They recycle through the enterohepatic circulation; secondary bile acids form by the action of intestinal bacteria.
2. Detection of elevated serum bile acid levels is a sensitive marker of hepatobiliary dysfunction.
3. Various methods are available to assay individual and total bile acids; assaying an individual bile acid is probably as useful as measuring total bile acid concentration.
4. Numerous different bile acid tests have been described, including fasting and postprandial levels and determination of levels after a bile acid load, either oral or intravenous.
5. Normal bile acid levels in the presence of hyperbilirubinemia suggest hemolysis or Gilbert's syndrome.

UREA SYNTHESIS

1. Hepatic metabolism of nitrogen from protein results in urea production. Urea is distributed in total body water and is excreted in urine or diffuses into the intestine, where urease-producing bacteria hydrolyze it to CO_2 and ammonia.
2. The rate of urea synthesis can be calculated from the urinary urea excretion and blood urea nitrogen after estimation of body water, with correction for gastrointestinal hydrolysis of urea.
3. The rate of urea synthesis is significantly reduced in cirrhosis and correlates with the Child–Turcotte–Pugh score, although it is insensitive for detection of well-compensated cirrhosis.

BROMSULPHALEIN (BSP)

Clearance of bromsulphalein (BSP) after an intravenous bolus was formerly used to measure hepatic function. The most accurate information was obtained by the 45-minute retention test and initial fractional rate of disappearance. BSP testing fell out of favor because of reports of severe allergic reactions, lack of accuracy in distinguishing hepatocellular from obstructive jaundice, and the availability of simpler tests of liver function.

INDOCYANINE GREEN

This dye is removed by the liver after intravenous injection. A blood level is obtained 20 minutes after administration. Compared with BSP, the hepatic clearance of indocyanine green is more efficient, and it is nontoxic. Its accuracy in assessing liver dysfunction is no better than standard Child–Turcotte–Pugh scoring. Its major role had been as a measure of hepatic blood flow.

NONINVASIVE SERUM MARKERS OF FIBROSIS

Various tests have been described to determine the extent of fibrosis in patients with chronic liver disease, to avoid the need for liver biopsy.

Direct Markers

These markers include serum hyaluronate, procollagen III n-peptide, and matrix metallo-proteinases.
- They are generally accurate in confirming cirrhosis and excluding severe liver disease in patients with minimal fibrosis.

Indirect Markers

Various formulas have been described that incorporate serum markers of fibrosis or routine laboratory tests, such as platelet count, INR, and serum aminotransferases.
- Examples include FibroSure, Fibrospect, and AST-to-platelet ratio (APRI).
- **FibroSure is used most commonly in the United States** and includes α_2-macroglobulin, haptoglobin, apolipoprotein A1, bilirubin, and GGTP; it is most useful for excluding fibrosis (low score) or suggesting cirrhosis (high score); intermediate scores can reflect a varying degree of severity of fibrosis.

Liver Biopsy

Despite advances in serologic testing and imaging, liver biopsy remains the definitive test for the following: to confirm the diagnosis of specific liver diseases such as Wilson disease, small duct primary sclerosing cholangitis, and nonalcoholic fatty liver disease; to assess prognosis in most forms of parenchymal liver disease, such as chronic viral hepatitis; and to evaluate allograft dysfunction in liver transplant recipients.

INDICATIONS

Indications for liver biopsy are shown in Table 1.2.

CONTRAINDICATIONS

Contraindications to liver biopsy are shown in Table 1.3. In patients with renal insufficiency, uremic platelet dysfunction should be corrected by infusion of arginine vasopressin (DDAVP) (0.3 µg/kg in 50 mL N saline intravenously) immediately before biopsy. Aspirin and nonsteroidal anti-inflammatory drugs, which may also produce platelet dysfunction, are prohibited for 7 to 10 days before elective liver biopsy.

TABLE 1.2 ■ Indications for liver biopsy

Evaluation of abnormal liver biochemical test levels and hepatomegaly

Evaluation and staging of chronic hepatitis

Identification and staging of alcoholic liver disease

Recognition of systemic inflammatory or granulomatous disorders

Evaluation of fever of unknown origin

Evaluation of the pattern and extent of drug-induced liver injury

Identification and determination of the nature of intrahepatic masses

Diagnosis of multisystem infiltrative disorders

Evaluation and staging of cholestatic liver disease (primary biliary cirrhosis, primary sclerosing cholangitis)

Screening of relatives of patients with familial diseases

Obtaining tissue to culture infectious agents (e.g., mycobacteria)

Evaluation of effectiveness of therapies for liver diseases (e.g., Wilson disease, hemochromatosis, autoimmune hepatitis, chronic viral hepatitis)

Evaluation of liver biochemical test abnormalities following transplantation

TABLE 1.3 ■ Contraindications to liver biopsy

Absolute	Relative
History of unexplained bleeding	Ascites
Prothrombin time >3–4 sec over control	Infections in right pleural cavity
Platelets <60,000/mm^3	Infection below right diaphragm
Prolonged bleeding time (>10 min)	Suspected echinococcal disease
Unavailability of blood transfusion support	Morbid obesity
Suspected hemangioma	
Uncooperative patient	

TECHNIQUE

1. Liver biopsy can be performed safely on an outpatient basis if none of the contraindications noted in Table 1.2 are present and the patient can be adequately observed for at least 3 hours following the procedure, with access to hospitalization if necessary (required in up to 5% of patients).
2. A local anesthetic is infiltrated subcutaneously and into the intercostal muscle and peritoneum. A short-acting sedative may be given to allay anxiety. Percussion at the bedside identifies the point of maximal hepatic dullness.
3. The routine use of ultrasonography to mark the biopsy site or guide the biopsy needle has become frequent. In diffuse liver disease, ultrasound-guided liver biopsy may be associated with a higher yield and lower rate of complications than blind biopsy.
4. A transthoracic approach is standard; a subcostal approach should be attempted only with ultrasound guidance.

5. The biopsy is performed at end-expiration; various needles (cutting [Tru-Cut, Vim-Silverman] or suction [Menghini, Klatskin, Jamshidi]) are used, including a biopsy "gun."
6. The biopsy site is tamponaded by having the patient lie on the right side.
7. When the standard approach is contraindicated (e.g., coagulopathy or ascites), **transjugular biopsy** may be performed. This technique also allows determination of the hepatic venous wedge pressure gradiant (see Chapter 10) to confirm portal hypertension, assess reponse to beta-blocker therapy, and determine prognosis.
8. Focal hepatic lesions are best sampled for biopsy under radiologic guidance.
9. An adequate specimen for histologic interpretation is at least 1.5 cm long and contains at least six portal triads.

COMPLICATIONS

1. Postbiopsy pain with or without radiation to the right shoulder occurs in up to one third of patients. Vasovagal reactions are also common. Serious complications are uncommon (less than 3%) and usually manifest within several hours of the biopsy. The fatality rate is 0.03% to 0.32%.
2. Intraperitoneal bleeding is the most serious complication. Increasing age, the presence of hepatic malignancy, and the number of passes made are predictors of the likelihood of bleeding, as is the use of a cutting needle rather than a suction needle.
3. Patients who have clinical evidence of hemodynamically significant bleeding, persistent pain unrelieved by analgesia, or other evidence of a serious complication require hospital admission. Pneumothorax may require a chest tube, whereas serious bleeding may be controlled by selective embolization at angiography or, if necessary, ligation of the right hepatic artery or hepatic resection.
4. Biopsy of a malignant neoplasm carries a 1% to 3% risk of seeding of the biopsy tract with tumor.

Hepatic Imaging

Several imaging modalities are available to assess the hepatic parenchyma, vasculature, and biliary tree: computed tomography (CT), magnetic resonance imaging (MRI) with cholangiopancreatography (MRCP), and endoscopic ultrasonography (EUS). A logical sequence of initial and subsequent studies should be determined by the clinical circumstances (Table 1.4). The ready availability of abdominal imaging for unrelated complaints such as vague abdominal pain has led to the frequent detection of hepatic masses that are nearly always benign and incidental to the patient's complaint but that require evaluation.

PLAIN ABDOMINAL X-RAY STUDIES AND BARIUM STUDIES

1. Plain abdominal x-ray studies add little to the evaluation of liver disease. On occasion, calcifications, usually resulting from gallstones, echinococcal cysts, or old lesions of tuberculosis or histoplasmosis, are detected. Tumors or vascular lesions may also be calcified.
2. A barium swallow is significantly less sensitive than endoscopy for detecting esophageal varices.
3. Wireless video capsule endoscopy has been used also to screen for esophageal varices.

TABLE 1.4 ■ **Approach to use of imaging studies**

Clinical problem	Initial imaging	Supplemental imaging studies (if necessary)
Jaundice	US	CT, if dilated ducts, to detect obstructing lesion or, if suspicion of a mass in the pancreas or porta hepatis; MRCP to determine site and cause of dilated ducts
Hepatic parenchymal disease	US CT MRI	Doppler US, color Doppler US, or MRI with flow sequences if a vascular abnormality is suspected and in some instances of portal hypertension
Screening for liver mass	US	CT, MRI
Characterizing known liver mass	CT, MRI	
Suspected malignancy	US- or CT-directed biopsy	CT portogram, intraoperative US
Suspected benign lesion	US, CT, or MRI; nuclear medicine scan (e.g., ^{99m}Tc-labeled red blood cell scan) for suspected hemangioma	US- or CT-directed biopsy
Suspected abscess	US or CT US- or CT-directed aspiration	Nuclear medicine abscess scan (gallium or ^{111}In-labeled white blood cell scan)
Suspected biliary duct abnormalities	US to detect dilatation, biliary stones, or mass MRCP, ERCP, or THC to define ductal anatomy	CT or endoscopic US to detect stones or cause of extrinsic compression

CT, computed tomography; ERCP, endoscopic retrograde cholangiopancreatography; MRCP, magnetic resonance cholangiopancreatography; MRI, magnetic resonance imaging; THC, transhepatic cholangiography; US, ultrasonography.

ULTRASONOGRAPHY

This is the initial radiologic study of choice for many hepatobiliary disorders. It is relatively inexpensive, does not require ionizing radiation, and can be used at the bedside. Ultrasound depicts interfaces in tissue of different acoustic properties. Contrast agents have been introduced to enhance the accuracy of ultrasonography; these include a micro-bubble technique for detection of discrete lesions and galactose-based contrast agents to assess vascularity.

1. Ultrasound cannot penetrate gas or bone, a characteristic that may preclude adequate examination of the viscera. Furthermore, increased resolution is generally at the expense of decreased tissue penetration.
2. "Real-time" ultrasonography demonstrates physiologic events such as arterial pulsation.
3. Ultrasonography is better at detecting focal lesions than parenchymal disease and is the initial test of choice to detect biliary dilatation.
4. Hepatic masses as small as 1 cm may be detected by ultrasonography, and cystic lesions may be distinguished from solid ones.
5. Ultrasonography can also facilitate percutaneous biopsy of solid hepatic masses, drainage of hepatic abscesses, or paracentesis of loculated ascites.
6. Ultrasonography with the Doppler technique is used to assess the patency of hepatic and portal vasculature in liver transplant candidates and recipients.

COMPUTED TOMOGRAPHY (CT)

1. CT scanning is generally more accurate than ultrasonography in defining hepatic anatomy, normal and pathologic.
2. Oral contrast defines the bowel lumen and intravenous contrast enhances vascular structures increase anatomic definition.
3. Spiral, or helical, CT is a refinement that allows faster imaging at the peak of intravenous contrast enhancement. A more recent advance is multidetector CT, which permits imaging in a single breath-hold and three-dimensional reconstruction of the hepatic vasculature and biliary tree.
4. **CT with intravenous contrast is an excellent way to identify and characterize hepatic masses**. Cystic and solid masses can be distinguished, as can abscesses. Contrast enhancement after an intravenous bolus may be accurate enough to identify cavernous hemangiomas, which have a characteristic appearance. Neoplastic vascular invasion may also be identified. Hepatocellular carcinoma exhibits rapid arterial enhancement (Fig. 1.4) and venous "washout" from the blood supply from the arterial rather than the portal system.
5. CT portography with intravenous contrast administered through a catheter in the superior mesenteric artery enhances the sensitivity of lesion detection within the liver.
6. Lipiodol is preferentially taken up and retained by hepatocellular carcinoma and can be used as a contrast agent to detect small (up to 5 mm) neoplastic lesions.
7. CT can also suggest the presence of cirrhosis and portal hypertension, as well as changes consistent with fatty liver or hemochromatosis.
8. Limitations of CT are cost, radiation exposure, and lack of portability.

MAGNETIC RESONANCE IMAGING (MRI)

1. MRI can provide images in numerous planes and provides excellent resolution between tissues containing differing amounts of fat and water. Ultrafast sequencing obviates motion artifacts. Unlike CT, MRI does not require ionizing radiation, but concern is increasing about the syndrome of nephrogenic systemic fibrosis in patients with impaired renal function after the use of gadolinium contrast.
2. MRI is an excellent method for evaluating blood flow and can detect hepatic iron overload.
3. MRI is not portable, remains expensive, and has a slow imaging time, so physiologic events such as peristalsis can result in blurred images. The magnetic field used precludes imaging in patients with pacemakers or other metallic devices. Claustrophobic patients find the enclosed space in the scanner unpleasant and many require sedation.
4. **MRI is the imaging study of choice in confirming the presence of vascular lesions, notably hemangiomas** (Fig. 1.5). It is also useful in differentiating regenerating nodules from hepatocellular carcinoma; on a T2-weighted image, the signal intensity of a regenerating nodule is equivalent to that of normal hepatic parenchyma, whereas that of a carcinoma is higher.
5. MRCP is an alternative to diagnostic endoscopic cholangiopancreatography.
6. Gadolinium administration accentuates the differences in signal intensity between normal and neoplastic tissue.
7. Magnetic resonance angiography has become a useful method to assess the hepatic vasculature before hepatic resection.
8. Use of liver-specific contrast media further enhances the accuracy of assessing hepatic mass characteristics by MRI.

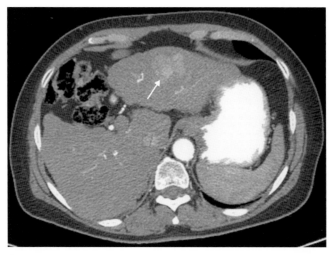

Fig. 1.4 Computed tomography scan showing a hepatocellular carcinoma.

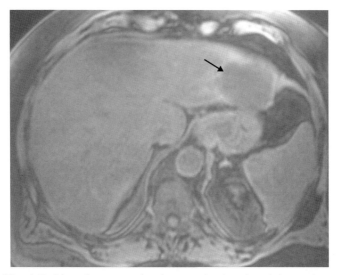

Fig. 1.5 Magnetic resonance imaging scan showing a hepatic hemangioma.

RADIOISOTOPE SCANNING

1. Specific isotopes used are preferentially taken up by hepatocytes, Kupffer cells, or neoplastic or inflammatory cells. Radioisotope scanning is particularly helpful in the assessment of suspected acute cholecystitis, although for parenchymal and focal liver disease, ultrasonography and CT have largely superseded nuclear medicine studies.
2. Technetium-99m (^{99m}Tc)–labeled sulfur colloid is used for anatomic evaluation of the liver and is taken up by Kupffer cells. Any process such as a neoplasm, cyst, or abscess that replaces those cells results in a "cold" area. Lesions greater than 2 cm in diameter can usually be detected.

3. Diffuse hepatic disease that leads to disrupted hepatic blood flow and reduced reticuloendo-thelial function results in diminished hepatic radioisotope uptake with diversion of isotope to bone marrow and spleen.
4. The caudate lobe of the liver, because of its independent venous drainage, may be unaffected by obstruction of the hepatic vein in Budd–Chiari syndrome and thus may have preferential uptake of isotope.
5. Indium-labeled colloid is also taken up by Kupffer cells but involves more radiation exposure than technetium. Additional techniques include single photon emission computed tomography (SPECT), which allows visualization of the cross-sectional distribution of a radioisotope, and positron emission tomography (PET) (see later), which provides information about blood flow and tissue metabolism.

POSITRON EMISSION TOMOGRAPHY (PET)

Positron emission tomography (PET) detects increased glucose metabolism characteristic of hepatic neoplasm.
1. Clinical applications include detection and staging of primary hepatic malignant diseases, evaluation of metastatic disease, and differentiation of benign from malignant hepatic tumors.
2. The accuracy of PET in hepatocellular carcinoma is limited by poor uptake of the most commonly used radiopharmaceutical ([18F]-fluoro-2-deoxyglucose [FDG]) by well-differentiated tumors.

TRANSIENT ELASTOGRAPHY

This technique incorporates an ultrasound transducer probe mounted on a vibrator to induce an elastic shear wave to measure hepatic stiffness, which reflects fibrosis, in a cylinder 1 cm wide and 4 cm long. The results are expressed in kilopascals (kPa) and range from 2.5 to 75 kPa, with normal values approximately 5.5 kPa.
1. It is most accurate for detecting advanced fibrosis and cirrhosis; considerable overlap exists between stages when fibrosis is less extensive.
2. It is technically difficult in obese patients or if ascites is present.
3. It may complement rather than replace liver biopsy.
4. Magnetic elastography uses magnetic resonance to measure liver stiffness.

FURTHER READING

Castéra L, Foucher J, Bernard PH, et al. Pitfalls of liver stiffness measurement: a 5-year prospective study of 13,369 examinations. *Hepatology* 2009; 51:828–835.
Castéra L. Transient elastography and other noninvasive tests to assess hepatic fibrosis in patients with viral hepatitis. *J Viral Hep* 2009; 16:300–314.
Chand N, Sanyal AJ. Sepsis-induced cholestasis. *Hepatology* 2007; 45:230–241.
Friedman LS. Controversies in liver biopsy: who, where, when, how, why? *Curr Gastroenterol Rep* 2004; 6:30–36.
Goessling W, Friedman LS. Increased liver chemistry in an asymptomatic patient. *Clin Gastroenterol Hepatol* 2005; 3:852–858.
Green RM, Flamm S. AGA technical review on the evaluation of liver chemistry tests. *Gastroenterology* 2002; 123:1367–1384.
Jang HJ, Yu H, Kim TK. Imaging of focal liver lesions. *Semin Roentgenol* 2009; 44:266–282.

Kechagias S, Ernersson A, Dahlqvist O, et al. Fast-food-based hyper-alimentation can induce rapid and profound elevation of serum alanine aminotransferase in healthy subjects. *Gut* 2008; 57:649–654.

Kim WR, Flamm SL, Di Bisceglie AM, et al. Serum activity of alanine aminotransferase (ALT) as an indicator of health and disease. *Hepatology* 2008; 47:1363–1370.

Rockey DC, Caldwell SH, Goodman ZD, et al. Liver biopsy. *Hepatology* 2009; 49:1017–1044.

Ruhl CE, Everhart JE. Elevated serum alanine aminotransferase and γ-glutamyltransferase and mortality in the United States population. *Gastroenterology* 2009; 136:477–485.

Shaked O, Reddy KR. Approach to a liver mass. *Clin Liver Dis* 2009; 13:193–210.

Tripodi A, Caldwell SH, Hoffman M, et al. Review article: the prothrombin time test as a measure of bleeding risk and prognosis in liver disease. *Aliment Pharmacol Ther* 2007; 26:141–148.

Tripodi A, Chantarangkul V, Primignani M, et al. The international normalized ratio calibrated for cirrhosis (INRliver) normalizes prothrombin time results for model for end-stage liver disease calculation. *Hepatology* 2007; 46:520–527.

Watkins PB, Kaplowitz N, Slattery JT, et al. Aminotransferase elevations in healthy adults receiving 4 grams of acetaminophen daily: a randomized controlled trial. *JAMA* 2006; 296:87–93.

CHAPTER 2

Acute liver failure

Stevan A. Gonzalez, MD, MS ■ Emmet B. Keeffe, MD, MACP

KEY POINTS

1 Acute liver failure is a syndrome of rapidly progressive hepatic dysfunction associated with a high risk of mortality.

2 The defining features of acute liver failure are hepatic encephalopathy, coagulopathy, and jaundice in patients without underlying liver disease.

3 Acetaminophen hepatotoxicity is the leading cause of acute liver failure in the United States; approximately one half of cases are unintentional.

4 Treatment strategies for acute liver failure include intensive care unit monitoring, implementation of specific therapies based on cause, and aggressive treatment of complications, including infection, renal failure, metabolic disorders, and cerebral edema.

5 The cause of acute liver failure is the strongest predictor of survival; prognostic criteria are important in identifying patients with a low probability of spontaneous recovery and potential candidacy for liver transplantation.

6 Liver transplantation is associated with a significant survival benefit in patients with acute liver failure and a high mortality risk.

Definitions

ACUTE LIVER FAILURE

Acute liver failure (ALF) is a syndrome characterized by a rapid decline in hepatic synthetic function and a significant risk of mortality. ALF is defined by the onset of jaundice, hepatic encephalopathy, and coagulopathy (international normalized ratio [INR] of prothrombin time greater than 1.5) in patients with no prior history of liver disease. Several classification systems have been developed based on the time interval from onset of hepatic illness or jaundice to hepatic encephalopathy.

FULMINANT HEPATIC FAILURE (FHF)

1. The earliest classification, introduced by Trey and Davidson, defined fulminant hepatic failure (FHF) by the interval from the onset of an acute hepatic illness to the development of hepatic encephalopathy:

   ■ Interval less than 8 weeks
   ■ No prior history of liver disease

2. An alternative classification, described by Bernuau et al, defined FHF by a shorter interval from the onset of jaundice to the development of hepatic encephalopathy:

- Interval less than 2 weeks
- No prior history of liver disease

SUBFULMINANT HEPATIC FAILURE

1. This designation refers to a prolonged course of ALF, characterized by a longer interval between the onset of illness or jaundice and the development of hepatic encephalopathy.
2. Different definitions of subfulminant hepatic failure have been introduced:
   a. **Late-onset hepatic failure**, proposed by Gimson et al, defined by an interval from the onset of hepatic illness to the development of hepatic encephalopathy between 8 and 26 weeks
   b. **Subfulminant liver failure**, introduced by Bernuau et al, defined by an interval from the onset of jaundice to the development of hepatic encephalopathy between 2 and 12 weeks
      - Subfulminant hepatic failure is more likely associated with
        - drug-induced liver injury or an indeterminate origin
        - worse prognosis
        - decreased incidence of cerebral edema
        - increased prevalence of features associated with portal hypertension

ACUTE LIVER FAILURE

1. O'Grady et al further classified ALF into categories based on the interval from the onset of jaundice to encephalopathy:

   - Hyperacute liver failure: interval less than 7 days
   - ALF: interval from 8 to 28 days
   - Subacute liver failure: interval from 29 days to 12 weeks

2. A hyperacute presentation is associated with
   - acetaminophen hepatotoxicity or fulminant hepatitis A or B
   - better prognosis
   - increased incidence of cerebral edema
   - absence of clinical jaundice

Epidemiology

1. The incidence of ALF in the United States is approximately 2000 cases per year; ALF accounts for 3.5 deaths per million and 31.2 hospitalizations per million.
2. Although ALF is rare, it is associated with a high mortality; ALF accounts for up to 6% of all liver-related deaths and 6% of liver transplants.
3. Outcomes of ALF have improved since 2000 in the United States, possibly because of shifting trends in etiology (Table 2.1); prospective data from the U.S. Acute Liver Failure Study Group found a rate of spontaneous recovery without liver transplantation of 45% and an overall mortality rate of 30%; approximately 25% of patients underwent liver transplantation.

TABLE 2.1 ■ **Most common causes of acute liver failure**

Cause	Frequency (%)
Acetaminophen overdose	46
Indeterminate	14
Idiosyncratic drug-induced liver injury	11
Hepatitis B	8
Autoimmune hepatitis	6
Ischemic hepatitis	4
Hepatitis A	3
Wilson disease	2
Budd–Chiari syndrome	1
Pregnancy*	1
Other	5

*Pregnancy-related acute liver failure includes acute fatty liver of pregnancy and the hemolysis, elevated liver enzymes, and low platelets (HELLP) syndrome.

Adapted from Lee WM. Etiologies of acute liver failure. *Semin Liver Dis* 2008; 28:142–152; based on 1213 cases of acute liver failure prospectively enrolled in the U.S. Acute Liver Failure Study Group (1998–2007).

Causes

The most common identifiable causes of ALF are drug-induced liver injury and acute viral hepatitis; substantial numbers of cases are considered indeterminate.

1. Based on prospective data from more than 1000 patients enrolled in the U.S. Acute Liver Failure Study Group from 1998 to 2007, acetaminophen overdose was the most common cause of ALF, followed by indeterminate cause, idiosyncratic drug-induced liver injury, acute hepatitis B, and autoimmune hepatitis (see Table 2.1); other causes of ALF are shown in Table 2.2.

2. Since 2000, the proportion of cases of ALF resulting from acetaminophen overdose in the United States has increased, whereas the percentage of cases caused by acute viral hepatitis has decreased.

Pathophysiology

1. Most cases of ALF are characterized by massive hepatocyte necrosis resulting in liver failure; ALF without histologic evidence of hepatocellular necrosis can also be seen, as in acute fatty liver of pregnancy and Reye's syndrome.

2. Hepatocyte necrosis and apoptosis may coexist in the setting of ALF; hepatocyte necrosis occurs through adenosine triphosphate (ATP) depletion followed by cellular swelling and cell membrane disruption; apoptosis is a process of programmed cell death triggered by extrinsic or intrinsic mechanisms and resulting in caspase activation, degradation of genetic material, and cell shrinkage.

TABLE 2.2 ■ **Causes of acute liver failure**

Viral hepatitis	Hepatitis A, B, C, D, and E viruses
	Herpes viruses 1, 2, and 6
	Varicella zoster virus
	Adenovirus
	Epstein–Barr virus
	Cytomegalovirus
	Parvovirus B19
Drug-induced liver injury	Acetaminophen overdose
	Idiosyncratic drug reactions
	Cocaine
	Ecstasy (methylenedioxymethamphetamine [MDMA])
Toxins	*Amanita* or *Galerina* mushroom poisoning (*Amanita phalloides* most common)
	Organic solvents
	Phosphorus
Metabolic disorders	Acute fatty liver of pregnancy
	Reye's syndrome
Vascular events	Acute circulatory failure, ischemic hepatitis
	Budd–Chiari syndrome
	Sinusoidal obstructive syndrome
	HELLP syndrome
	Heat stroke
Miscellaneous causes	Wilson disease
	Autoimmune hepatitis
	Giant cell hepatitis
	Malignancy with liver infiltration
	Liver transplantation with primary graft nonfunction

HELLP, hemolysis, elevated liver enzymes, and low platelets.

Adapted from Keeffe EB. Acute liver failure. In: McQuaid KR, Friedman SL, Grendell JH, eds. *Current Diagnosis and Treatment in Gastroenterology,* 2nd edn. New York: Lange Medical Books/McGraw-Hill; 2003:536–545.

Clinical Features

DRUG OR TOXIN-INDUCED ALF

ALF resulting from drug-induced liver injury may occur as an idiosyncratic reaction or in a dose-dependent manner; **more than one half of all ALF cases in the United States can be attributed to drug-induced liver injury, with acetaminophen the most common agent.**

1. Acetaminophen (see also Chapter 8)
    a. Acetaminophen hepatotoxicity is dose related, and a massive ingestion of at least 15 to 20 g is typically required for development of ALF.
    b. ALF secondary to acetaminophen hepatotoxicity frequently occurs in the setting of a suicide attempt (Table 2.3), and some individuals may be at increased risk of a severe or fatal outcome (Table 2.4).
    c. Acetaminophen is predominantly metabolized in the liver by glucuronidation and sulfation; a minority of the drug is metabolized by the cytochrome P-450 system. *N*-acetyl-*p*-benzoquinone imine (NAPQI) is a toxic intermediate generated by the cytochrome P-450 pathway during acetaminophen metabolism. Clearance of NAPQI requires

TABLE 2.3 ■ **Clinical syndrome of acetaminophen overdose**

Phases of acetaminophen hepatotoxicity

Initial phase (0–24 hr):
  Anorexia, nausea, vomiting

Latent phase (24–48 hr):
  Resolution of gastrointestinal symptoms
  Elevated serum aminotransferase levels

Overt hepatocellular necrosis phase (>48 hr):
  Coagulopathy, jaundice, encephalopathy
  Acidemia
  Renal failure

TABLE 2.4 ■ **Risk factors for acetaminophen hepatotoxicity**

Factors associated with increased risk

Alcohol abuse
Barbiturate abuse
Poor nutritional status
Chronic pain requiring multiple analgesics or narcotics
Age >40 yr
Concomitant viral hepatitis
Use of antidepressant medication
History of suicide attempt

conjugation by glutathione; however, glutathione stores can become depleted in the setting of an overdose, thus leading to direct hepatocyte injury mediated by NAPQI.
  ■ Induction of cytochrome P-450 metabolism through long-term alcohol use or barbiturates is associated with a greater risk of acetaminophen hepatotoxicity and ALF.
  ■ Alcohol abuse is more commonly associated with unintentional acetaminophen toxicity ("therapeutic misadventure"); lower doses of acetaminophen (less than 4 g per day) can be associated with development of ALF.
  ■ Depletion of glutathione stores associated with nutritional deficiency may result in an increased risk of acetaminophen hepatotoxicity.
2. Other drugs and toxins
    a. Antibiotics, antifungal, and antituberculosis drugs including isoniazid, pyrazinamide, tetracyclines, nitrofurantoin, ketoconazole, and sulfa-containing agents
    b. Anticonvulsants such as phenytoin, valproic acid, and carbamazepine
    c. Mushroom poisoning from *Amanita* or *Galerina* species
      ■ Amatoxins are cyclic octapeptides that inhibit RNA polymerase II and lead to hepatocyte necrosis as well as renal tubular injury.
      ■ Phallotoxins are cyclic heptapeptides that inhibit actin polymerization and depolymerization, with resulting cell membrane dysfunction.
    d. Organic solvents that contain chlorinated hydrocarbons, in which the severity of hepatotoxicity is related to the proximity and duration of exposure
    e. Herbal supplements in various forms

f. Illicit drugs including cocaine and methylenedioxymethamphetamine (MDMA), also known as ecstasy, that cause ALF possibly as a result of ischemic hepatic injury

g. Other drugs (partial list): propylthiouracil (PTU), disulfiram, nonsteroidal anti-inflammatory drugs (NSAIDs), dapsone, troglitazone, halothane, amiodarone, flutamide, imipramine, lisinopril, and niacin

VIRAL HEPATITIS (see also Chapter 3)

1. **Hepatitis A virus (HAV)**
   - The virus is transmitted through fecal–oral route and is diagnosed by detection of immunoglobulin M (IgM) antibody to hepatitis A virus (anti-HAV) in the serum.
   - The incidence of acute symptomatic cases in the United States is approximately 1 in 100,000, and the case-fatality rate is 0.3%.
   - Persons at risk of ALF include those with underlying chronic liver disease, injection drug users, and the elderly.
   - Hepatitis A is preventable with vaccination; the incidence of hepatitis A in the United States has decreased by as much as 92% since vaccination became available in 1995.
2. **Hepatitis B virus (HBV)**
   - The virus is transmitted through parenteral routes, mucosal contact, or perinatal exposure.
   - Most cases of acute infection with hepatitis B are asymptomatic; the incidence of reported cases of acute infection in the United States is 1.5 in 100,000, with a case-fatality rate of 0.5% to 1.0%.
   - Hepatitis B surface antigen (HBsAg) and IgM antibodies to the hepatitis B core antigen (anti-HBc) may be present in serum in the setting of acute infection; detection of serum HBV DNA is the most reliable test in ALF.
   - Risk factors for ALF include age greater than 60 years, coinfection with hepatitis C virus (HCV), and coinfection with hepatitis D virus (HDV).
   - Initiation of antiviral therapy with an oral nucleoside or nucleotide analogue may be considered in the setting of fulminant hepatitis B, although data to support this treatment are limited.
   - Inactive HBsAg carriers who undergo cancer chemotherapy or immunosuppressive therapy are at risk of reactivation of hepatitis B, including a fulminant course; antiviral prophylaxis in these patients is recommended.
   - Hepatitis B is preventable with vaccination; the incidence of new infections with hepatitis B in the United States has declined by approximately 82% since 1991.
3. **Hepatitis C virus (HCV)**
   - The virus is transmitted primarily through parenteral exposure.
   - Acute hepatitis C infection is rarely identified because most cases are asymptomatic.
   - Although rare, acute hepatitis C infection may potentially result in ALF.
   - The diagnosis of acute hepatitis C infection requires detection in serum of HCV RNA.
   - Persons with chronic hepatitis C may be at increased risk of ALF secondary to other causes, such as acute HAV superinfection or acetaminophen hepatotoxicity.
4. **Hepatitis D virus (HDV)**
   - Also known as hepatitis delta, hepatitis D is a defective virus that requires hepatitis B infection and the presence of HBsAg for assembly of virions and infectivity.
   - Transmission occurs primarily through parenteral routes or mucosal contact.
   - Infection may occur in the form of acute coinfection with HBV or as a superinfection in the setting of preexisting chronic hepatitis B, both of which are associated with a risk of ALF.

- The diagnosis can be made by detection of hepatitis D antigen (HDAg) and antibodies against HDAg (anti-HD) in the serum.
- Nucleoside and nucleotide analogues are not effective for hepatitis D.

5. **Hepatitis E virus (HEV)**
   - The virus is transmitted through the fecal–oral route and is a major cause of ALF in endemic regions, although HEV may also occur in developed countries.
   - **The incidence of acute HEV infection is increased among pregnant women, in whom the risks of ALF and mortality are increased**; the incidence of ALF in pregnant women with acute hepatitis E has been reported to be as high as 69% in some populations, with a mortality rate up to 20% in women infected during the third trimester.

6. **Herpes viruses**
   - Infection with herpes simplex or varicella zoster virus may result in ALF; immunosuppressed persons are at particularly increased risk of a fulminant course; cutaneous lesions and disseminated intravascular coagulation may be present.
   - Liver biopsy may be helpful in suspected cases; characteristic viral inclusions can be identified in the specimen; therapy with intravenous acyclovir should be started immediately once the diagnosis is established.

7. **Cytomegalovirus (CMV)**
   - CMV is a major cause of morbidity in liver transplant recipients (see also Chapter 31).
   - The risk of fulminant CMV hepatitis is greatest in CMV-seronegative transplant recipients of organs from CMV-seropositive donors. Strategies involving antiviral prophylaxis as well as preemptive therapy have been described. Immediate therapy with intravenous ganciclovir is indicated once the diagnosis is established.

8. **Other viruses** including parvovirus B19, Epstein–Barr virus (EBV), and adenovirus can result in ALF in the setting of acute infection. Parvovirus B19 infection is often associated with aplastic anemia; ALF is the leading cause of mortality in acute EBV infection. Severe adenovirus hepatitis with ALF is more likely to occur in immunocompromised persons.

AUTOIMMUNE HEPATITIS (see Chapter 5)

1. Serologic markers such as antinuclear antibodies (ANA), smooth muscle antibodies (SMA), and quantitative immunoglobulins (especially IgG), as well as examination of a liver biopsy specimen, may be useful in establishing the diagnosis.
2. ALF secondary to autoimmune hepatitis may also coincide with the presence of acute autoimmune hemolytic anemia.
3. Corticosteroid therapy may be considered in fulminant autoimmune hepatitis; some data suggest an increased rate of recovery with corticosteroid therapy.

WILSON DISEASE (see Chapter 17)

1. Fulminant Wilson disease may manifest with modest elevations in aminotransferase levels, characterized by a ratio of aspartate aminotransferase (AST) to alanine aminotransferase (ALT) greater than 2.2 and a ratio of alkaline phosphatase to bilirubin less than 4; these combined laboratory features are highly sensitive and specific for the diagnosis of ALF secondary to Wilson disease.
2. Other laboratory studies suggestive of Wilson disease include a low serum ceruloplasmin level (less than 5 mg/dL), elevated serum copper (greater than 200 μg/dL), and elevated 24-hour quantitative urine copper (greater than 40 μg/24 hours and typically higher than

125 μg/24 hours in ALF); increased quantitative hepatic copper content measured in a liver biopsy specimen (at least 250 μg/g dry weight) supports the diagnosis of Wilson disease.

3. Slit lamp ophthalmologic evaluation may be done to assess for the presence of Kayser–Fleischer rings; however, this finding may be absent in up to 50% of patients with ALF.

4. Coombs-negative hemolytic anemia and acute renal failure occur frequently in patients with fulminant Wilson disease as a result of elevated serum copper levels.

5. ALF arising from Wilson disease is associated with a high mortality rate; measures to decrease serum copper are ineffective, whereas chelation therapy may be associated with hypersensitivity. Therefore, emergency liver transplantation is indicated once the diagnosis is established.

BUDD–CHIARI SYNDROME AND SINUSOIDAL OBSTRUCTION SYNDROME (see Chapter 19)

1. Budd–Chiari syndrome occurs as a result of acute hepatic vein outflow obstruction secondary to thrombotic disease and may lead to ALF; all patients presenting with Budd–Chiari syndrome should be assessed for an underlying hypercoagulable disorder or myeloproliferative disease.
   - Anticoagulation therapy should be initiated in all patients.
   - Hepatic vein angioplasty, stent placement, or transjugular intrahepatic portosystemic shunt (TIPS) placement may be considered, particularly if patients do not respond to anticoagulation.

2. Sinusoidal obstruction syndrome, or veno-occlusive disease, is a known complication of high-dose chemotherapy in patients undergoing hematopoietic stem cell transplantation; this syndrome is associated with painful hepatomegaly.

ISCHEMIC HEPATITIS (see Chapter 20)

1. Also known as shock liver, this condition is most frequently associated with cardiovascular collapse arising in the setting of hypotension, hypovolemia, or cardiogenic shock; hepatic ischemia may frequently occur in the presence of heart failure, valvular heart disease, or pericardial disease.

2. Ischemic hepatitis rarely causes ALF; mortality is related to the underlying heart disease.

REYE'S SYNDROME

Reye's syndrome is a rare cause of ALF and occurs most frequently in children. Patients typically present with a recent viral illness, often treated with aspirin, followed by severe vomiting and rapidly progressive liver disease characterized by acute microvesicular steatosis and a high risk of cerebral edema with intracranial hypertension.

PREGNANCY-RELATED ACUTE LIVER FAILURE (see Chapter 21)

1. Acute viral hepatitis, acute fatty liver of pregnancy, and the hemolysis, elevated liver enzymes, and low platelets (HELLP) syndrome may occur during pregnancy and result in ALF.

2. Acute fatty liver of pregnancy and the HELLP syndrome occur most commonly during the third trimester.

3. A serum beta-human chorionic gonadotropin (hCG) level should be obtained in all women of childbearing age who present with ALF.

ACUTE LIVER FAILURE OF INDETERMINATE CAUSE

Up to 14% of ALF cases are considered indeterminate; studies in which serum acetaminophen-protein adducts were measured in patients with ALF suggest that acetaminophen may be a cause of many indeterminate cases.

Complications

INFECTION

1. A frequent complication; up to 80% of patients may develop bacterial infections, and up to 30% may develop fungal infections.
2. Surveillance cultures of blood, sputum, and urine should be obtained in patients with ALF.
3. Antimicrobial prophylaxis may not have an impact on clinical outcome in all patients, although empiric therapy should be initiated in any of the following circumstances:
   - A positive surveillance culture or fever
   - Grade 3 to 4 encephalopathy
   - Hemodynamic instability or the onset of systemic inflammatory response syndrome (SIRS)
   - Patients listed for liver transplantation

RENAL FAILURE

1. This is a key early prognostic indicator, particularly in patients with acetaminophen hepato-toxicity, in which renal failure or the presence of acidosis is highly predictive of mortality.
2. It may occur as a result of hypovolemia, acute tubular necrosis, or hepatorenal syndrome.
3. Use of vasopressor therapy with norepinephrine or dopamine should be initiated in the setting of circulatory dysfunction with severe hypotension.
4. Renal replacement therapy with continuous venovenous hemodialysis (CVVHD) is preferred once renal or circulatory dysfunction develops.

METABOLIC DISORDERS

Electrolyte and metabolic derangements contribute to progressive hepatic encephalopathy and an increased risk of cerebral edema; therefore, they must be corrected promptly.
1. **Hypoglycemia** may result from decreased hepatic glycogen production and impaired gluconeogenesis. Blood glucose levels must be measured at frequent intervals, and continuous infusions of 10% to 20% glucose should be given if hypoglycemia is present.
2. **Hypophosphatemia** may be seen in ALF as a result of ATP consumption in the setting of rapid hepatocyte regeneration, which has been reported to be associated with a more favorable prognosis. Life-threatening hypophosphatemia can occur, and phosphorus levels should be monitored frequently and repleted promptly.
3. **Acidosis** is one of the most important predictors of mortality; **metabolic acidosis with a pH lower than 7.3 may be associated with a mortality rate of up to 95% in patients with acetaminophen overdose in the absence of liver transplantation.**
4. **Alkalosis** may be present in ALF; hyperventilation is common.
5. **Hypoxemia** may result from acute respiratory distress syndrome (ARDS), aspiration, or pulmonary hemorrhage; patients with grade 3 to 4 encephalopathy should undergo endotracheal intubation.

COAGULOPATHY

Coagulopathy is a key feature of ALF and is an important prognostic indicator; although coagulopathy can be profound, serious bleeding events are uncommon.

1. Proton pump inhibitors or H_2-receptor blockers should be administered to all patients because of the potential for gastrointestinal bleeding with progressive coagulopathy and the risk of peptic ulcer associated with mechanical ventilation.
2. Platelet transfusions, plasma, and cryoprecipitate may be given to reduce the bleeding risk associated with invasive procedures; correction of coagulopathy is otherwise not recommended unless clinically significant bleeding occurs. Administration of recombinant factor VIIa may be considered, although it may be associated with an increased risk of thrombosis.
3. Vitamin K may be given if nutritional deficiency is suspected.

ENCEPHALOPATHY

Encephalopathy is the defining feature of ALF and may progress rapidly, leading to increased risks of cerebral edema, intracranial hypertension, and death.

1. The risk of **cerebral edema** increases with the severity of encephalopathy; up to 35% and 75% of patients develop cerebral edema at encephalopathy grades 3 and 4, respectively.
2. Computed tomography of the head should be considered in the presence of grades 3 or 4 encephalopathy to assess for cerebral edema or intracranial bleeding.
3. Lactulose therapy does not appear to have a significant impact on outcome in ALF, particularly with an advanced grade of encephalopathy.

CEREBRAL EDEMA

Cerebral edema with intracranial hypertension is the **most common cause of mortality** in ALF.

1. Persons who present with a hyperacute course are at greater risk of developing cerebral edema.
2. Elevated arterial ammonia levels higher than 200 μmol/L may predict an increased risk of developing intracranial hypertension.
3. Factors contributing to cerebral edema in ALF include hypoxia, systemic hypotension, decreased cerebral perfusion pressure (CPP), and swelling of astrocytes as a result of elevated blood ammonia levels and increased glutamine production within the brain; cerebral edema may ultimately lead to increased intracranial pressure (ICP), ischemic brain injury, and herniation.
4. Findings on physical examination such as abnormal papillary reflexes, muscular rigidity, or decerebrate posturing may suggest the development of intracranial hypertension.
5. Management of cerebral edema involves taking measures to minimize elevations in ICP, consideration of ICP monitoring device placement, and maintaining ICP at less than 25 mm Hg and CPP at more than 50 mm Hg (Table 2.5).

Treatment

Early recognition of ALF, establishment of the time course and exposure risks, implementation of specific therapies when indicated, and aggressive intensive care monitoring are critical to effective management; **liver transplantation should be considered in all patients, and contact should be made with a liver transplant center early during the clinical course.**

TABLE 2.5 ■ **Management of cerebral edema**

General

Reduction of surrounding stimuli to a minimum
Elevation of head of bed to 30 degrees
Endotracheal intubation and sedation at grade 3 encephalopathy
Initiation of vasopressor therapy and CVVHD if circulatory dysfunction or renal failure

Specific

Consider placement of ICP monitor
    Goal ICP <25 mm Hg and CPP >50 mm Hg
Initiation of hyperventilation-induced hypocapnea to promote cerebral vasoconstriction
    Goal Pco_2 30 to 40 mm Hg
Intravenous mannitol
    0.25 to 0.5 g/kg bolus for ICP ≥25 mm Hg for >10 min
    Repeat infusions for persistent ICP elevations
    Maintain serum osmolality <320 mOsm/L

CVVHD, continuous venovenous hemodialysis; CPP, cerebral perfusion pressure; ICP, intracranial pressure.

INITIAL ASSESSMENT AND TREATMENT

1. Historical information may suggest potential causes of ALF including exposure risks, a history of depression or suicidal ideation, illicit drug or alcohol abuse, or ingestion of hepatotoxic agents.
2. Diagnostic studies should include toxicology screening, viral serologic tests, autoimmune markers, and hepatic imaging (Table 2.6); abdominal ultasonography may reveal hepatic surface nodularity associated with parenchymal collapse and regenerative nodule formation.
3. Liver biopsy findings rarely influence clinical management and have no impact on prognosis, except in suspected autoimmune hepatitis, acute herpes simplex hepatitis, or malignant disease; if a liver biopsy is obtained, a transjugular approach is preferred.
4. **Patients should be transferred to an intensive care unit once the presence of encephalopathy is established** (Table 2.7); intensive care monitoring is critical to the prevention and management of complications such as shock, sepsis, renal failure, and cerebral edema.

DISEASE-SPECIFIC THERAPY

1. Establishing the potential cause of ALF guides the utilization of specific therapies, some of which may have a significant impact on outcome (Table 2.8).
2. **Prospective data have demonstrated that administration of *N*-acetylcysteine (NAC) may provide a survival benefit in cases of non–acetaminophen-associated ALF with grade 1 or 2 encephalopathy; therefore, NAC is recommended for all patients with mild to moderate hepatic encephalopathy, regardless of cause, until there is evidence of improved hepatic function.**
3. In acetaminophen hepatotoxicity, restoration of hepatocyte glutathione synthesis depends on cysteine, which may be administered in the form of NAC; **NAC should be given in all cases of suspected acetaminophen overdose regardless of serum acetaminophen level.**

LIVER TRANSPLANTATION (see also Chapter 31)

1. Liver transplantation has a major impact on survival, with an overall 3-year survival rate of up to 78%; evaluation for liver transplantation should be considered in all patients presenting with ALF.

TABLE 2.6 ■ Initial laboratory and imaging assessment of acute liver failure

Complete metabolic profile, PT/INR, CBC; amylase, lipase, ceruloplasmin, factor V level, pregnancy test, urinalysis, blood type and screen, surveillance cultures

Arterial blood gas; arterial blood lactate, arterial ammonia levels

Urine toxicology screen, acetaminophen level

Autoimmune hepatitis markers: ANA, SMA, quantitative immunoglobulins

Viral serologic tests: IgM anti-HAV, IgM anti-HBc, HBsAg, anti-HCV, IgM anti-HEV, IgM anti-HSV 1 and 2, IgM anti-VZV, HIV test

Imaging: abdominal ultrasonography with Doppler, chest radiography, CT scan of the head (if grade 3 to 4 encephalopathy)

Additional studies:
Viral hepatitis PCR: HBV DNA, HSV DNA, HCV RNA, EBV DNA, CMV DNA, VZV DNA, adenovirus DNA
Serum copper, 24-hr urine copper levels

ANA, antinuclear antibodies; anti-HBc, antibody to hepatitis B core antigen; CBC, complete blood count; CMV, cytomegalovirus; CT, computed tomography; EBV, Epstein–Barr virus; HAV, hepatitis A virus; HBsAg, hepatitis B surface antigen; HBV, hepatitis B virus; HCV, hepatitis C virus; HEV, hepatitis E virus; HIV, human immunodeficiency virus; HSV, herpes simplex virus; Ig, immunoglobulin; INR, international normalized ratio; PCR, polymerase chain reaction; PT, prothrombin time; SMA, smooth muscle antibodies; VZV, varicella zoster virus.

TABLE 2.7 ■ Intensive care management of acute liver failure

Hemodynamic monitoring (arterial line, central venous and pulmonary artery catheters)

Endotracheal intubation (grade 3 to 4 encephalopathy)

Renal replacement therapy (CVVHD)

Neurologic monitoring

Glucose monitoring for hypoglycemia

Laboratory parameter assessment at frequent intervals, correction of metabolic derangements

Enteral nutrition

Periodic surveillance bacterial and fungal cultures (blood, sputum, urine)

Medications:
Proton pump inhibitor or H_2-receptor blocker
Empiric antimicrobial therapy with infection risk
10%–20% glucose infusions if hypoglycemia present
Vasopressor management for circulatory dysfunction

Management of cerebral edema and consideration of ICP monitoring (see Table 2.5)

CVVHD, continuous venovenous hemodialysis; ICP, intracranial pressure.

2. Several prognostic criteria have been proposed to assess the likelihood of spontaneous recovery versus progressive hepatic dysfunction with a high mortality risk.

   a. Many studies have consistently demonstrated that the most important prognostic indicator in ALF is cause; acetaminophen hepatotoxicity and acute hepatitis A are associated with the most favorable rates of spontaneous recovery, approximately 68% and 65%, respectively.

   b. The most widely studied criteria for ALF are the **King's College criteria** (Table 2.9); these criteria are characterized by a high specificity for mortality; however, failure to fulfill the criteria does not ensure survival.

TABLE 2.8 ■ **Specific therapy according to cause of acute liver failure**

Cause	Treatment
Acetaminophen hepatotoxicity or Any cause of ALF with mild to moderate encephalopathy	N-acetylcysteine Intravenous (preferred): loading dose 150 mg/kg in 5% dextrose over 1 hr, then 12.5 mg/kg/hr over 4 hr, then 6.25 mg/kg/hr Oral: loading dose 140 mg/kg, then 70 mg/kg every 4 hr
Amanita phalloides poisoning	Gastric lavage and administration of activated charcoal Intravenous penicillin G 1g/kg/day
Herpes simplex hepatitis	Intravenous acyclovir 30 mg/kg/day
Cytomegalovirus infection	Intravenous ganciclovir 5 mg/kg every 12 hr
Acute hepatitis B	Oral nucleoside or nucleotide analogue (entecavir 0.5 mg/day or tenofovir 300 mg/day preferred)
Autoimmune hepatitis	Intravenous methylprednisolone 60 mg/day
Acute fatty liver of pregnancy or HELLP syndrome	Delivery of the fetus
Budd–Chiari syndrome	Anticoagulation therapy and consideration of TIPS placement

ALF, acute liver failure; HELLP, hemolysis, elevated liver enzymes, and low platelets; TIPS, transjugular intrahepatic portosystemic shunt.

TABLE 2.9 ■ **Assessment of prognosis in acute liver failure (King's College criteria)**

ALF secondary to acetaminophen overdose	ALF not associated with acetaminophen

pH <7.30
or
INR >6.5 (PT >100 sec) and serum creatinine >3.4 mg/dL (>300 µmol/L) in patients with grade 3 or 4 encephalopathy
	INR >6.5 (PT >100 sec)
	or
	Any 3 of the following:
	  Age <10 and >40 yr
	  Cause non-A, non-B hepatitis or idiosyncratic drug reaction
	  Duration of jaundice before encephalopathy >7 days
	  INR >3.5 (PT >50 sec)
	  Serum bilirubin >17.6 mg/dL (>300 µmol/L)

ALF, acute liver failure; INR, international normalized ratio; PT, prothrombin time.

Adapted from O'Grady JG, Alexander GJ, Hayllar KM, Williams R. Early indicators of prognosis in fulminant hepatic failure. *Gastroenterology* 1989; 97:439–445.

c. Other prognostic criteria predictive of mortality in ALF include
   ■ The presence of hepatic encephalopathy and a factor V level lower than 20% of normal in patients less than 30 years old or lower than 30% of normal in patients 30 years old or older (Clichy criteria)
   ■ Model for End-stage Liver Disease (MELD) score of at least 30 (see Chapter 10)
   ■ Acute Physiology and Chronic Health Evaluation (APACHE) II score higher than 15 to 20

3. Patients with ALF who are at high risk of mortality and who fulfill listing criteria defined by the United Network for Organ Sharing (UNOS) may be assigned to category Status 1A and receive top priority for liver transplantation allocation; patients with fulminant Wilson disease also may be given Status 1A priority because of the high mortality rate associated with this diagnosis.

4. Contraindications to liver transplantation in ALF
   a. Severe cardiopulmonary disease or multiorgan failure
   b. Septic shock
   c. Extrahepatic malignant disease
   d. Extensive thrombotic disease
   e. Irreversible brain injury or brain death
      ■ CPP lower than 40 mm Hg for more than 2 hours
      ■ Sustained ICP higher than 50 mm Hg
   f. Active substance abuse, repeated suicide attempts, or inadequate social support may preclude transplant candidacy

FUTURE THERAPIES

Extracorporeal hepatic assist devices, auxiliary liver transplantation, and hepatocyte culture systems have been studied in an effort to improve clinical outcomes in ALF; although some improvements in physiologic parameters have been shown, these methods have not demonstrated any significant impact on survival. Further study of bioartificial or nonbiologic hepatic assist devices, such as the Molecular Adsorbents Recirculating System (MARS), and the development of hepatocyte culture systems through tissue engineering may identify effective means of supporting patients with ALF through recovery or may act as a bridge to liver transplantation.

FURTHER READING

Keeffe EB. Acute liver failure. In: McQuaid KR, Friedman SL, Grendell JH, eds. *Current Diagnosis and Treatment in Gastroenterology*, 2nd edn. New York: Lange Medical Books/McGraw-Hill, 2003:536–545.

Larsen FS, Wendon J. Prevention and management of brain edema in patients with acute liver failure. *Liver Transpl* 2008; 14(Suppl 2):S90–S96.

Larson AM, Polson J, Fontana RJ, et al. Acetaminophen-induced acute liver failure: results of a United States multicenter, prospective study. *Hepatology* 2005; 42:1364–1372.

Lee WM, Hynan LS, Rossaro L, et al. Intravenous N-acetylcysteine improves transplant-free survival in early stage non-acetaminophen acute liver failure. *Gastroenterology* 2009; 137:856–864.

Lee WM, Squires Jr RH, Nyberg SL, et al. Acute liver failure: summary of a workshop. *Hepatology* 2008; 47:1401–1415.

Lee WM. Etiologies of acute liver failure. *Semin Liver Dis* 2008; 28:142–152.

Liou IW, Larson AM. Role of liver transplantation in acute liver failure. *Semin Liver Dis* 2008; 28:201–209.

O'Grady JG, Alexander GJ, Hayllar KM, et al. Early indicators of prognosis in fulminant hepatic failure. *Gastroenterology* 1989; 97:439–445.

O'Grady JG, Schalm SW, Williams R. Acute liver failure: redefining the syndromes. *Lancet* 1993; 342:273–275.

Polson J. Assessment of prognosis in acute liver failure. *Semin Liver Dis* 2008; 28:218–225.

Polson J, Lee WM. AASLD position paper: the management of acute liver failure. *Hepatology* 2005; 41:1179–1197.

Rutherford A, Chung RT. Acute liver failure: mechanisms of hepatocyte injury and regeneration. *Semin Liver Dis* 2008; 28:167–174.

Stravitz RT, Kramer AH, Davern T, et al. Intensive care of patients with acute liver failure: recommendations of the U.S. Acute Liver Failure Study Group. *Crit Care Med* 2007; 35:2498–2508.

CHAPTER 3

Acute viral hepatitis

Raymond S. Koff, MD

KEY POINTS

1 Viral hepatitis is the most common cause of liver disease in the world; acute infections with their sequelae are responsible for 1 to 2 million deaths annually.

2 The nonenveloped, enterically transmitted hepatitis viruses (HAV and HEV), in general, are self-limited infections, but severe hepatitis may develop in some cases; rarely, chronic hepatitis E has been reported in organ-transplant recipients. The blood-borne hepatitis viruses (HBV, HDV, and HCV) are enveloped agents frequently associated with persistent infection, prolonged viremia, and the development of chronic liver disease and its sequelae.

3 A wide spectrum of clinical illness is well documented, ranging from asymptomatic, anicteric infection to acute liver failure (fulminant hepatitis); with the exception of acute hepatitis C, no specific or effective treatment of acute viral hepatitis is available; liver transplantation is indicated in acute liver failure when recovery seems unlikely.

4 Highly effective and safe vaccines are available for preexposure immunoprophylaxis of HAV and HBV infection; for postexposure immunoprophylaxis of HAV, HAV vaccine is preferred but immune globulin may be used, whereas for postexposure immunoprophylaxis of HBV, both hepatitis B immune globulin (HBIG) and HBV vaccine are used.

5 Immune globulin preparations are not available for the prevention of HEV or HCV infection. No vaccine for the prevention of HCV infection exists. An effective HEV vaccine is not yet commercially available but remains in development. HBV vaccination prevents HDV infection, but for persons with established HBV infection, vaccines to prevent HDV superinfection are not available.

Importance

1. Viral hepatitis is the most common cause of liver disease worldwide.
2. As many as 7% of the global population is chronically infected by the hepatitis B virus (HBV), and 3% are infected by the hepatitis C virus (HCV).
3. Many episodes of hepatitis are anicteric, inapparent, subclinical, and unrecognized.
4. Other episodes of hepatitis are severe and may result in acute liver failure.
5. Globally, viral hepatitis is the major cause of persistent viremia.
6. The sequelae of chronic infection include cirrhosis, end-stage liver disease, hepatocellular carcinoma, and premature death.
7. With its sequelae, viral hepatitis is responsible for 1 to 2 million deaths annually.

Agents

The agents of acute viral hepatitis can be broadly classified into two groups: the enterically transmitted agents and the blood-borne agents.

ENTERICALLY TRANSMITTED AGENTS

These agents, namely, hepatitis A virus (HAV) and hepatitis E virus (HEV)
- are nonenveloped viruses
- survive intact when exposed to bile/detergents
- are shed in feces
- do not result in a prolonged viremic or intestinal carrier state
- only HEV has been linked rarely to chronic liver disease.
- A third enterically transmitted hepatitis virus may exist, is transmissible to chimpanzees,
- replicates in the liver, and induces immune responses but remains unidentified.

1. **HAV**
   a. Classified as a picornavirus, subclassified as a hepatovirus
   b. 27 to 28 nm in diameter with cubic symmetry
   c. Single-stranded, linear RNA molecule, 7.4 kb in one open reading frame
   d. One serotype in human beings; three or more genotypes
   e. Containing a single immunodominant neutralization site
   f. Containing four major virion polypeptides in capsomere
   g. Replication in cytoplasm of infected hepatocyte through RNA-dependent RNA polymerase; no definitive evidence of replication in intestine
   h. High degree of chemical and thermal resistance to inactivation
   i. Propagated in nonhuman primate and human cell lines
2. **HEV**
   a. Classified with Hepeviridae, subclassified as a hepevirus
   b. 27 to 34 nm in diameter
   c. Linear RNA molecule, 7.2 to 7.4 kb
   d. RNA genome with three overlapping open reading frames encoding structural proteins and nonstructural proteins involved in HEV replication:
      - RNA-dependent RNA polymerase (RNA replicase)
      - Helicase
      - Cysteine protease
      - Methyltransferase
   e. Only one serotype identified in human beings; four major genotypes
   f. Immunodominant neutralization site on structural protein encoded by second open reading frame
   g. Can be propagated in transfected human hepatocellular carcinoma cell lines and in human embryo lung diploid cells
3. Other enterically transmitted agents
   - Occasional outbreaks of other enterically transmitted hepatitis, without serologic markers of HAV or HEV; infection appears transmissible to chimpanzees, with replication in liver

BLOOD-BORNE AGENTS

These agents, namely, HBV, hepatitis D virus (HDV), and HCV, are
- enveloped viruses
- disrupted by exposure to bile/detergents
- not shed in feces
- linked to chronic liver disease
- associated with persistent viremia

1. **HBV**
   a. Human-infecting member of hepatotropic DNA-containing viruses, the Hepadnaviridae
   b. Eight genotypes (A through H): genotype C appears to be associated with more severe chronic disease, and genotype D is less responsive to interferon-based therapy
   c. 42-nm spherical particle with
      - A 27-nm diameter, electron-dense, nucleocapsid core
      - A 7-nm thick outer lipoprotein envelope
   d. HBV core containing circular, partially double-stranded DNA (3.2 kb in length) and
      - DNA polymerase protein with reverse transcriptase activity
      - Hepatitis B core antigen (HBcAg), a structural protein of the nucleocapsid
      - Hepatitis B e antigen (HBeAg), a nonstructural, secretory protein that correlates imperfectly with active HBV replication
      - Hepatitis B x protein, a transcriptional activator, linked to hepatocarcinogenesis.
   e. HBV outer lipoprotein envelope containing
      - Hepatitis B surface antigen (HBsAg), with three envelope proteins: major, large, and middle proteins
      - Minor lipid and carbohydrate components
      - HBsAg present in 22-nm spherical or tubular noninfectious particles, in excess of intact HBV particles
   f. One major serotype; many subtypes based on HBsAg protein diversity
   g. HBV mutant viruses as a consequence of poor proofreading ability of reverse transcriptase or emergence of resistance; examples:
      - HBeAg-negative precore or core promoter mutant
      - HBV vaccine-induced escape mutant (rare)
      - Nucleos(t)ide-induced resistant mutant
   h. Replication occurring through reverse transcription of pregenomic RNA
   i. Liver major but not only site of HBV replication
   j. Limited replication in vitro in primary adult and fetal human hepatocytes
2. **HDV**
   a. A defective RNA satellite virus (viroid-like) requiring helper function of HBV for its expression and pathogenicity but not for its replication
   b. Only one serotype recognized, eight genotypes
   c. 35- to 37-nm spherical particle, enveloped by HBV lipoprotein coat (HBsAg)
      - 19-nm corelike structure
   d. Containing an antigenic nuclear phosphoprotein (HDV antigen)
      - Binds RNA
      - Exists in two isoforms: smaller 195 amino acid and larger 214 amino acid proteins
      - Smaller HDV antigen transports RNA into the nucleus: essential for HDV replication
      - Larger HDV antigen prenylated: inhibits HDV RNA replication and participates in HDV assembly

e. HDV RNA, 1.7 kb, single stranded, covalently closed, and circular

f. HDV antigenome, a genome complementary, circular RNA found in infected hepatocyte and, to a much lesser extent, in purified HDV particles

g. HDV RNA the smallest RNA genome among the animal viruses; HDV resembling plant satellite viruses

h. RNA genome can form an unbranched rodlike structure by folding on itself through intramolecular base pairing

i. Replication limited to hepatocytes

j. Primary chimpanzee, woodchuck, and human hepatocellular carcinoma cell lines transfected with HDV cDNA constructs expressing HDV RNA and HDV antigens

3. **HCV**

a. A glycoprotein enveloped, single-stranded RNA virus

b. 55- to 60-nm spherical particle; 33-nm nucleocapsid core

c. Classified among the Flaviviridae, in the *hepacivirus* genus

d. HCV genome comprises approximately 9.4 to 9.6 kb, encoding a large polyprotein of approximately 3000 amino acid residues

- One third of the polyprotein consisting of a series of structural proteins (an internal nucleocapsid or core [C] protein and two glycosylated envelope proteins, termed E1 and E2, present in the lipid-containing envelope of the virus)
- Envelope proteins possibly generating neutralizing antibodies
- A hypervariable region localized in E2
- Remaining two thirds of the polyprotein consisting of nonstructural proteins (termed NS2, NS3, NS4A, NS4B, NS5A, and NS5B) involved in HCV replication: a zinc-dependent metalloproteinase in NS2/3, a nucleotide triphosphatase/helicase in NS3, a chymotrypsin-like serine protease in NS3-4A, RNA-dependent RNA polymerase in NS5B, an interferon sensitivity region in NS5A, and an ion channel, P7

e. Only one HCV serotype identified; six major HCV genotypes with multiple subtypes; genotypes variably distributed throughout the world

f. Genotypes correlated with likelihood of response of chronic infection to antiviral therapy and duration of therapy

Epidemiology and Risk Factors

HAV

1. Incubation period: 15 to 50 days (average, 30 days)
2. Worldwide distribution; highly endemic in developing countries
3. HAV excreted in stools of infected persons for 1 to 2 weeks before and for at least 1 week after onset of illness
4. Viremia short-lived, usually no longer than 3 weeks; occasionally up to 90 days in protracted or relapsing infection
5. Prolonged fecal excretion (months) reported in infected neonates; frequency, level of virus in stool, and epidemiologic importance uncertain
6. Enteric (fecal–oral) transmission predominantly by person-to-person household spread; occasional outbreaks linked to common-source vehicles:
   - Contaminated food, bivalve mollusks, water
7. Other risk factors including exposure:
   - In day care centers for infants, diapered children

- In institutions for developmentally disadvantaged
- Through international travel to developing countries (most common risk factor in U.S.)
- Through oral–anal homosexual behavior or multiple sexual contacts
- Through shared equipment/drugs by injection drug users

8. No evidence for maternal–neonatal transmission
9. Prevalence correlated with sanitary standards and large household size
10. Transmission by blood transfusion or blood products: very rare
11. No risk factor identified in 30% to 40% of cases in the United States
11. Overall seroprevalence in the United States: less than 30% and declining rapidly with expanded vaccine use
12. Increased disease severity in individuals with preexisting liver disease or age 40 years or older

HEV

1. Incubation period: approximately 40 days (range, 15 to 65 days)
2. Widely distributed; epidemic and endemic forms but symptomatic infections rare in the United States; nonetheless, seroprevalence in U.S. population of approximately 21%
3. HEV RNA in serum and stool during acute phase
4. Most common form of sporadic hepatitis in young adults in the developing world
5. Largely water-borne outbreaks in Asia, Africa, and Central America
6. Intrafamilial, secondary cases uncommon
7. Maternal–neonatal transmission documented
8. In the United States, imported cases in returning travelers, in recent immigrants from endemic regions; sporadic, rare cases of transmission through undercooked pork products, liver or other organ meats, shellfish, or venison or by transfusion
9. Prolonged viremia or fecal shedding unusual; continued viral shedding possible in rare cases in organ transplant recipients in whom chronic hepatitis develops
10. Genotypes 1 and 2 isolated from sporadic human cases and water-borne outbreaks; genotypes 3 and 4 in swine and other animals and apparently transmitted zoonotically

HBV

1. Incubation period: 15 to 180 days (average, 60 to 90 days)
2. HBV viremia lasting for weeks to months after acute infection
3. 1% to 5% of adults, 90% of infected neonates, and 50% of infants developing chronic infection and persistent viremia
4. Persistent infection linked to chronic hepatitis, cirrhosis, hepatocellular carcinoma, and premature mortality
5. Persistent infection linked to acute necrotizing vasculitis, membranous glomerulonephritis
6. Worldwide distribution: HBV carrier prevalence less than 1% in the United States, 5% to 15% in Asia and sub-Saharan Africa; declining incidence in areas where vaccine use has expanded
7. HBV present in blood, semen, cervicovaginal secretions, saliva, and other body fluids
8. Risk of HBV infection highly correlated with HBV DNA level and presence of HBeAg
9. Increased disease severity in individuals with preexisting liver disease
10. Modes of transmission:
    a. Blood-borne transmission
       - Transfusion of blood/blood products
       - Injecting drug users

- Hemodialysis recipients
- Health care and other workers exposed to blood

   b. Sexual transmission: responsible for 50% of acute cases in the United States
   c. Tissue penetrations (percutaneous) or permucosal transfer
- Needlestick accidents
- Reuse of contaminated medical equipment
- Shared razor blades
- Tattoos
- Acupuncture, body piercing
- Shared toothbrushes

   d. Maternal–neonatal, maternal–infant transmission
   e. No evidence for fecal–oral spread
   f. No risk factor identified in 25% of cases

HDV

1. Incubation period: estimated to be 4 to 7 weeks
2. Endemic in Mediterranean basin, Balkan peninsula, Central Europe, parts of Africa, Middle East, and Amazon basin
3. Declining incidence with increasing use of HBV vaccine
4. HDV infection in 2% to 5% of patients with chronic hepatitis B in the United States
5. Viremia short-lived (acute infection) or prolonged (chronic infection)
6. HDV infections occurring solely in individuals at risk for HBV infection (coinfections or superinfections)
7. Modes of transmission
   a. Blood-borne transmission
- Injection drug use the predominant mode of spread in the United States
- Recipients of high-risk blood products

   b. Sexual transmission
- Homosexual or bisexual adolescents and men
- Sexual partners

   c. Maternal–neonatal spread, but frequency uncertain

HCV

1. Incubation period: 15 to 160 days (major peak at approximately 50 days)
2. Prolonged viremia and persistent infection common (55% to 85%); wide geographic distribution
3. Persistent infection etiologically linked to chronic hepatitis, cirrhosis, hepatocellular carcinoma and premature death
4. Seroprevalence of past/present infection 1.3% in the United States, approaching 20% in some communities in Italy and Japan, and up to 40% in some villages in the Nile delta of Egypt
5. Modes of transmission
   a. Blood-borne transmission (the predominant mode)
- Injecting drug use accounting for 85% of new cases in the United States
- Recipients of blood/blood products (exceedingly rare in the United States, with estimated risk now 1 per 2,000,000 transfused units)
- Hemodialysis recipients
- Tattoos; body piercing

- Health care association from inadequate aseptic techniques or other breaks in infection control
- Cocaine snorting
b. Sexual transmission: low efficiency, low frequency
c. Maternal–neonatal transmission: low efficiency, low frequency
d. No evidence of fecal–oral transmission
e. No recognized risk factor in 10% of cases

Pathophysiology

1. Cell-mediated immune mechanisms largely responsible for hepatocyte injury including hepatocyte degeneration and apoptosis
   - CD8$^+$ and CD4$^+$ T-cell responses
   - Production of cytokines in liver and systemically
2. Direct viral cytopathic effect
   - Postulated in immunosuppressed patients with exceedingly high levels of viral replication, but no direct evidence

Clinical Features

SELF-LIMITED DISEASE

1. The spectrum of severity ranges from asymptomatic, inapparent infection to fatal acute liver failure; severity is increased in those with preexisting liver disease or 40 years of age or older.
2. Similar clinical syndromes are caused by all agents, beginning with nonspecific constitutional and gastrointestinal symptoms:
   - Malaise, anorexia, nausea, and vomiting
   - Flulike symptoms of pharyngitis, cough, coryza, photophobia, headache, and myalgias
3. Onset of symptoms tends to be abrupt for HAV and HEV; in the others, onset is usually insidious.
4. Fever is uncommon except in HAV infection.
5. A syndrome that is immune complex mediated and resembles serum sickness occurs in less than 10% of patients with HBV infection (rarely in others); it includes polyarthritis, polyarthralgias, angioedema, urticaria, maculopapular eruptions, purpura, petechiae, and more rarely hematuria and proteinuria or cutaneous or systemic vasculitis.
6. Prodromal symptoms abate or disappear with onset of jaundice, although anorexia, malaise, and weakness may persist.
7. Jaundice (the icteric phase) is heralded by the appearance of dark urine and lightening of stool color; pruritus (usually mild and transient) may occur as jaundice increases.
8. The icteric phase lasts for 1 to 3 weeks, followed by a convalescent phase that may last for months in which jaundice and symptoms abate and HBsAg, HBeAg, and HBV DNA disappear.
9. Physical examination reveals mild enlargement and slight tenderness of the liver.
10. Mild splenomegaly and posterior cervical lymphadenopathy are noted in 15% to 20% of patients.

ACUTE LIVER FAILURE (see Chapter 2)

1. Characterized by changes in mental status (encephalopathy)
   - Lethargy, drowsiness, coma
   - Reversal of sleep patterns
   - Personality changes
2. Cerebral edema (usually without papilledema)
3. Coagulopathy (prolonged prothrombin time; international normalized ratio [INR] 1.5 or more)
4. Multiple organ failure
   - Acute respiratory distress syndrome
   - Cardiac arrhythmias
   - Hepatorenal syndrome
   - Metabolic acidosis
   - Sepsis
   - Gastrointestinal bleeding
   - Hypotension
5. Development of ascites and anasarca
6. Case fatality rate approximately 60% to 80% without liver transplantation; 1-year survival rate with liver transplantation approximately 65% to 75%
7. Serial physical examination showing shrinking liver and progressive jaundice
8. Extraordinarily high frequency, approaching 10% to 20%, in pregnant women with hepatitis E, particularly during the third trimester; high maternal and fetal mortality

CHOLESTATIC HEPATITIS

1. Most commonly seen in HAV infection
2. Pruritus possibly prominent
3. Persistent anorexia and diarrhea in a few patients
4. Jaundice possibly striking and persistent for several months before complete resolution
5. Excellent prognosis for complete resolution without specific therapy

RELAPSING HEPATITIS

1. Symptoms and liver test abnormalities recur weeks to months after improvement or apparent recovery.
2. This is most commonly seen in HAV infection; IgM anti-HAV may remain positive, and HAV may once again be shed in stool.
3. Arthritis, vasculitis, and cryoglobulinemia may be seen.
4. Prognosis is excellent for complete recovery even after multiple relapses (particularly common in children).

Laboratory Features

SELF-LIMITED DISEASE

1. Most prominent biochemical feature: marked elevation of serum alanine and aspartate aminotransferase levels (alanine aminotransferase [ALT] and aspartate aminotransferase [AST], respectively)

2. Peak aminotransferase (ALT and AST) levels varying from 500 to 5000 U/L; ALT levels generally higher than AST levels
3. Serum bilirubin level uncommonly higher than 10 mg/dL, except in severe disease, acute liver failure, and cholestatic hepatitis (see later)
4. Serum alkaline phosphatase normal or mildly elevated
5. Prothrombin time normal or increased by 1 to 3 seconds
6. Serum albumin normal or minimally depressed
7. Peripheral blood counts: normal or mild leukopenia with or without relative lymphocytosis

ACUTE LIVER FAILURE (see Chapter 2)

1. Striking coagulopathy with prolonged prothrombin time (INR 1.5 or more)
2. Leukocytosis, hyponatremia, and hypokalemia common
3. Hypoglycemia
4. Marked elevations of serum bilirubin and aminotransferase levels, but the latter may decline toward normal despite disease progression
5. Mild to moderate hypoalbuminemia

CHOLESTATIC DISEASE

1. Serum bilirubin levels possibly exceeding 20 mg/dL
2. Serum aminotransferase levels possibly declining toward normal despite cholestasis
3. Variable elevation of serum alkaline phosphatase
4. Normal or nearly normal serum albumin
5. Prolonged prothrombin time, if present, responsive to vitamin K administration

RELAPSING HEPATITIS

1. After apparent normalization or near-normalization of serum aminotransferase and bilirubin levels during convalescence, both may rise again.
2. Infrequently, peak levels may exceed those of the initial bout.

Histology

Liver biopsy is rarely performed in acute self-limited viral hepatitis.

SELF-LIMITED DISEASE

1. Major hepatocyte injury
   ■ Focal hepatocyte necrosis
   ■ Loss of hepatocytes (cell dropout)
   ■ Ballooning degeneration
   ■ Apoptosis with Councilman-like bodies (mummified, hyalinized, necrotic hepatocytes, extruded into a hepatic sinusoid)
2. Endophlebitis, affecting the central vein
3. Diffuse mononuclear cell (CD8+ and natural killer cell) infiltrate
   ■ Within widened portal tracts
   ■ Segmental erosion of the limiting plate

- Within hepatic parenchyma
- Kupffer cells enlarged, hyperplastic, with lipofuscin pigment and debris; remnants of injured hepatocytes

ACUTE LIVER FAILURE

1. Liver biopsy usually precluded by coagulopathy
2. Extensive confluent hepatocyte dropout (disappearance)
3. Collapse of reticulin framework
4. Lobular inflammation
5. Variable cholestasis

CHOLESTATIC DISEASE

1. Hepatocyte degeneration and inflammation as in self-limited hepatitis
2. Prominence of bile plugs in dilated hepatocyte canaliculi and bilirubin staining of hepatocytes
3. Hepatocytes forming multiple, scattered, ductlike structures (pseudoglandular transformation)

RELAPSING HEPATITIS

Changes are similar to those in self-limited disease.

Diagnosis

DIFFERENTIAL DIAGNOSIS

1. Drug- and toxin-induced liver disease (see Chapter 8)
2. Ischemic hepatitis (see Chapter 20)
3. Autoimmune hepatitis (see Chapter 5)
4. Alcoholic hepatitis (see Chapter 6)
5. Acute biliary tract obstruction (see Chapter 33)
6. Reactivation of chronic hepatitis B or C (see Chapter 4)

SEROLOGIC DIAGNOSIS

For serologic diagnosis, see Table 3.1.
1. Enterically transmitted infections
   a. **HAV** (Fig. 3.1)
      - **IgM antibody to HAV (IgM anti-HAV) is detected during the acute phase and for 3 to 6 months thereafter** and rarely for as long as 24 months.
      - The presence of anti-HAV of the IgG class without IgM anti-HAV indicates past infection.
   b. **HEV**
      - No Food and Drug Administration (FDA)–approved commercial serologic assays are currently available.
      - **IgM and IgG antibodies to HEV (anti-HEV) are detected early by research assays.**
      - IgA anti-HEV may be useful for the diagnosis of acute HEV infection in patients who test negative for IgM anti-HEV.

TABLE 3.1 ■ **Serologic patterns in the diagnosis of acute viral hepatitis**

Agent	Acute phase	Convalescence
HAV	Total anti-HAV positive	Development of IgG anti-HAV
	IgM anti-HAV positive	Disappearance of IgM anti-HAV
HEV	IgM anti-HEV positive and/or HEV RNA (in stool or serum)	Loss of HEV RNA; development of IgG anti-HEV
	IgG anti-HEV may be present	Loss of IgM anti-HEV
HBV	HBsAg positive and IgM anti-HBc positive	Loss of HBsAg; later loss of IgM anti-HBc; development of IgG anti-HBc; late development of anti-HBs
HDV	HDV RNA positive or IgM anti-HDV positive in HBsAg-positive patient	Loss of HDV RNA; development of IgG anti-HDV or loss of anti-HDV
	HDV/HBV coinfection: IgM anti-HBc positive	Above plus usual loss of HBsAg
	HDV/HBV superinfection: IgG anti-HBc positive	Above usually without loss of HBsAg
HCV	Early presence of HCV RNA; presence of or development of anti-HCV	Loss of HCV RNA (in a minority of patients); anti-HCV persistence for decades

HAV, hepatitis A virus; HBc, hepatitis B core [antigen]; HBsAg, hepatitis B surface antigen; HBV, hepatitis B virus; HCV, hepatitis C virus; HDV, hepatitis D virus; HEV, hepatitis E virus; Ig, immunoglobulin.

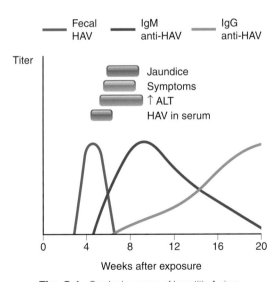

Fig. 3.1 Serologic course of hepatitis A virus.

- IgM anti-HEV may persist for at least 6 weeks after the peak of illness.
- IgG anti-HEV may remain detectable for as long as 20 months in self-limited infections.
- The presence of HEV RNA in stools or serum is confirmatory but usually unnecessary unless chronic hepatitis E is suspected on follow-up.

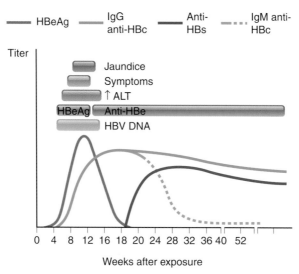

Fig. 3.2 Serologic course of hepatitis B virus.

2. Blood-borne infections
   a. **HBV** (Fig. 3.2)
      - **Serologic diagnosis is established by detection of the presence of IgM antibody to HBcAg (IgM anti-HBc) and HBsAg:**
        - Both are usually present at the onset of symptoms.
        - IgM anti-HBc is usually preceded by HBsAg.
        - HBsAg is the first routinely measured serologic marker of HBV infection to appear.
        - HBsAg may disappear, usually within several weeks to months after appearance, before the loss of IgM anti-HBc.
      - HBeAg and HBV DNA:
        - HBV DNA in serum is the first detectable marker of HBV infection but is not routinely measured.
        - HBeAg is usually detectable after the appearance of HBsAg.
        - Both markers disappear after weeks to months in self-limited infection; corresponding antibodies anti-HBs and anti-HBe persist.
        - It is not necessary for routine diagnosis.
      - IgG anti-HBc
        - replaces IgM anti-HBc in resolving infection
        - indicates past or continuing infection
        - is not induced by HBV vaccine
      - Antibody to HBsAg (anti-HBs)
        - is the last antibody to appear
        - is a neutralizing antibody
        - generally indicates recovery and immunity to reinfection
        - is elicited by HBV vaccine
   b. **HDV**
      - An HBsAg-positive individual:
        - **Antibody to HDV (anti-HDV) or circulating HDV RNA** (assays are not approved in the United States) is detected.
        - IgM anti-HDV may be present transiently.

- HBV/HDV acute coinfection:
  - HBsAg positivity
  - IgM anti-HBc-positivity
  - anti-HDV and/or HDV RNA detectable
- HDV superinfection of HBV carrier:
  - HBsAg positivity
  - IgG anti-HBc positivity
  - anti-HDV and/or HDV RNA detectable
- Anti-HDV titers decline to undetectable levels with resolution of infection.
c. **HCV** (Fig. 3.3)
  - Serologic diagnosis is established by the following:
    - Antibodies to recombinant HCV antigens (anti-HCV) from structural and non-structural regions are detected.
    - Anti-HCV is detected in approximately 60% of patients during the acute phase of illness; anti-HCV appears weeks to months later in most of the remainder.
    - Less than 5% of infected patients do not develop anti-HCV (a higher percentage of HIV-infected patients will not develop anti-HCV).
    - Assays for IgM anti-HCV are under development.
    - Anti-HCV generally persists for prolonged periods following acute infection in both self-limited and chronic HCV infections.
  - HCV RNA:
    - The earliest marker of acute HCV infection
    - Appears within a few weeks of exposure
    - Expensive; not routinely used for diagnosis except when HCV suspected in an anti-HCV negative individual
    - Useful in identifying neonatal infection
    - Present in chronic HCV infection

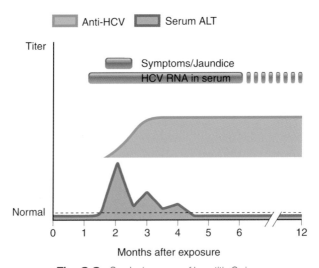

Fig. 3.3 Serologic course of hepatitis C virus.

Natural History and Outcome

ENTERICALLY TRANSMITTED INFECTIONS

1. Complete clinical, histologic, and biochemical recovery within 3 to 6 months; rare cases of chronic HEV infection in immunosuppressed organ transplant recipients
2. Occasional instances of acute liver failure
   - Age-dependent fatalities in HAV infection (increased risk after age 40 years)
   - Increased risk in pregnant women with HEV infection
   - Increased risk in those with preexisting liver disease
3. No chronic HAV-associated liver disease or prolonged carriage of virus

BLOOD-BORNE INFECTIONS

1. **HBV**
   a. Risk of persistent infection: age dependent and declining progressively with increasing age:
      - 90% of infected neonates becoming carriers
      - 1% to 5% of adult patients developing chronic HBV infection
   b. Acute liver failure in ≤ 1% of acute infections
   c. Persistent infection (HBsAg positive with or without active HBV replication)
      - Asymptomatic, inactive carrier with normal or nonspecific liver histologic changes
      - Chronic hepatitis, cirrhosis, hepatocellular carcinoma
      - Associated with membranous glomerulonephritis, polyarteritis nodosa, and, less certainly, mixed cryoglobulinemia
2. **HDV**
   - **HDV/HBV acute coinfections usually self-limited and resolved without sequelae**
   - Acute liver failure more common in HDV superinfection of HBV-infected individuals than in coinfection
   - HDV superinfection of HBV-infected individuals possibly leading to chronic HDV infection superimposed on chronic HBV infection with development of severe chronic hepatitis and cirrhosis
3. **HCV**
   a. Self-limited infections in 15% to 45% (higher number in infected children); spontaneous resolution more frequent in symptomatic cases and in persons with cc genotype *(IL28B)*
   b. Very rarely associated with acute liver failure
   c. **Persistent HCV infections with prolonged viremia and elevated, fluctuating, or normal serum aminotransferase levels common**
   d. Histology in persistent HCV infection
      - Chronic hepatitis: mild, moderate, or severe inflammation
      - Portal, periportal, bridging fibrosis, or cirrhosis
   e. Risk of hepatocellular carcinoma limited to those with bridging fibrosis and cirrhosis
   f. Associated with
      - mixed cryoglobulinemia
      - cutaneous vasculitis
      - membranoproliferative glomerulonephritis
      - porphyria cutanea tarda

- B-cell non-Hodgkin's lymphoma
- diabetes mellitus type 2

Treatment

SELF-LIMITED INFECTION

1. Outpatient care unless persistent vomiting or severe anorexia leads to dehydration
2. Maintenance of adequate caloric and fluid intake
   - No specific dietary recommendations
   - Large breakfast possibly the best-tolerated meal
   - Prohibition of alcohol during the acute phase
3. Vigorous or prolonged physical activity to be avoided
4. Limitation of daily activities and rest periods determined by severity of fatigue and malaise
5. No specific drug treatment for hepatitis A, E, D; peginterferon alfa with or without ribavirin in acute hepatitis C may reduce risk of chronic infection in those who fail to clear HCV RNA by week 12 to 16 after onset; no role of oral nucleos(t)ides in uncomplicated acute hepatitis B
6. All nonessential drugs discontinued

ACUTE LIVER FAILURE (see Chapter 2)

1. Hospitalization required
   - As soon as diagnosis made or suspected
   - Management best undertaken in a center with a liver transplantation program
2. Intravenous *N*-acetylcysteine apparently beneficial if given early after presentation; corticosteroids of no value
3. Treatment of acute liver failure from HBV with rapidly acting nucleos(t)ides (tenofovir, entecavir, and lamivudine) may be tried but efficacy uncertain
4. Goals
   - Maintenance of vital functions
   - Continuous monitoring and supportive measures while awaiting spontaneous resolution of infection and restoration of hepatic function
   - Early recognition and treatment of life-threatening complications
   - Preparation for liver transplantation if recovery appears unlikely
5. Survival rates of approximately 65% to 75% achieved by early referral for liver transplantation

CHOLESTATIC HEPATITIS

1. The course may be shortened by short-term treatment with prednisone or ursodeoxycholic acid, but no clinical trials of efficacy are available.
2. Pruritus may be controlled with cholestyramine.

RELAPSING HEPATITIS

Management is identical to that of self-limited infection.

Prevention

HAV

Immunoprophylaxis is the cornerstone of preventive efforts.

1. Preexposure immunoprophylaxis
   a. **Inactivated HAV vaccine**
      - **Highly effective (protective efficacy rate, 95% to 100%)**
      - Highly immunogenic (nearly 100% in healthy subjects)
      - Protective antibodies induced in 15 days after first dose in 85% to 90%
      - Safe, well tolerated
      - Estimated duration of protection 20 to 50 years, possibly lifelong
      - Injection site soreness the major adverse event
   b. Inactivated HAV vaccine (HAVRIX and VAQTA) doses and schedules
      - Adults 19 years of age or older: two-dose (1440 ELISA U) regimen of HAVRIX (Glaxo-SmithKline), with the second dose at 6 to 12 months after the first
      - Children more than 12 months of age: two-dose regimen of HAVRIX (720 ELISA U)
      - With second dose 6 to 12 months after the first
      - Adults 19 years of age or older: two-dose (50 U) regimen of VAQTA (Merck) with the second dose at 6 to 18 months after the first
      - Children more than 12 months of age: two-dose (25 U) regimen of VAQTA with the second dose 6 to18 months after the first
   c. Indications for inactivated HAV vaccine
      - All children beginning at age 12 to 23 months
      - Travelers to high-risk areas (for those leaving immediately, immune globulin may be given simultaneously, at a different site, although vaccine alone may be sufficient)
      - Homosexual and bisexual men and adolescents
      - Injecting drug users
      - Native peoples of the Americas and Alaska
      - Children and young adults in communities experiencing community-wide outbreaks
      - Children in regions, counties, and states with HAV attack rates higher than the national average
      - Susceptible patients with chronic liver disease
      - Laboratory workers handling HAV
      - Food handlers when vaccination is deemed cost-effective by local health officials
      - Household contacts of adoptees from endemic regions
      - Staff in day care centers and sewage and waste water treatment workers
2. Postexposure immunoprophylaxis
      - HAV vaccine in the postexposure setting is as efficacious as immune globulin if given within 2 weeks of the onset of exposure for individuals between ages 2 and 40 years; it is presumably also effective in younger and older subjects but has not been studied.
      - Vaccine-induced immunity is longer-lasting and therefore vaccine is favored over immune globulin.
      - The second vaccine dose should be given 6 to 18 months later to provide extended protection.
      - The efficacy of immune globulin is well established but availability is limited, and it provides only short-term protection.

Immune globulin schedule and dose
– 0.02 mL/kg body weight, deltoid injection, as early as possible after exposure

– well tolerated, injection site soreness
– indications: household and intimate contacts of individuals with acute HAV infection who refuse or cannot have HAV vaccine

HEV

IgG anti-HEV may be protective, but the efficacy of immune globulin containing anti-HEV is uncertain.

■ **An HEV vaccine has been reported to be highly effective in a phase II clinical trial** in an endemic area, but FDA approval has yet to be sought.

■ Development of high-titer, hyperimmune globulin

HBV

The cornerstone of immunoprophylaxis is the preexposure administration of HBV vaccine.

1. Preexposure immunoprophylaxis with HBV vaccine
   a. **Recombinant yeast-derived vaccines**
      ■ Contain HBsAg as the immunogen
      ■ **Are highly immunogenic, inducing protective levels of anti-HBs in more than 95% of healthy young (less than 40 years of age) recipients** after all three doses
      ■ Are 85% to 95% effective in preventing HBV infection or clinical hepatitis B
      ■ Have principal side effects of
         – transient pain at the injection site in 10% to 25%
         – short-lived, mild fever in less than 3%
      ■ Should not have boosters even as long as 20 years after initial immunization (may provide lifelong protection)
      ■ Should have boosters only for immunocompromised individuals if the anti-HBs titer is less than 10 mU/mL on annual testing
      ■ Have no proved immunotherapeutic value in the individual with established HBV infection
   b. HBV vaccine doses and schedules
      ■ Intramuscular (deltoid) injection of Engerix-B (GlaxoSmithKline) is given in a dose of 20 μg of HBsAg protein for adults; infants and children through age 19 years receive 10-μg doses, repeated 1 and 6 months later; for patients undergoing hemodialysis, a-40 μg dose (double dose of the 20-μg preparation) is given at 0, 1, 2, and 6 months.
      ■ Intramuscular (deltoid) injection of Recombivax HB (Merck) is given in a dose of 10 μg of HBsAg protein for adults and 5-μg doses for children up to age 19 years, repeated 1 and 6 months later; children between ages 11 and 15 years may receive 10 μg of Recombivax HB initially with a single booster at 4 to 6 months; for patients undergoing hemodialysis, a 40-μg three-dose schedule is available.
   c. Indications
      ■ Universal infant immunization is recommended shortly after birth.
      ■ Catch-up vaccination of adolescents through 19 years of age (if not previously vaccinated) is recommended.
      ■ Targeted high-risk groups
         – Household and spouse contacts of HBV carriers
         – Native Alaskans, Pacific Islanders, and Native Americans

- Health care and other workers exposed to blood (includes first responders)
- Injecting drug users
- Homosexual and bisexual men and adolescents
- Individuals with multiple sexual partners
- Workers in institutions for the developmentally disadvantaged
- Recipients of high-risk blood products
- Maintenance hemodialysis patients and staff
- Inmates of prisons (in which injecting drug use and homosexual behavior may occur)
- Household contacts of adoptees from endemic regions
- Individuals with preexisting liver disease (e.g., chronic hepatitis C)

2. Postexposure immunoprophylaxis with HBV vaccine and HBIG (a preparation of immune globulin containing high titers of anti-HBs)

   a. Indications
   - Susceptible sexual contacts of acutely HBV-infected individuals

     - 0.04 to 0.07 mL/kg HBIG as early as possible after exposure
     - First of three HBV vaccine doses given at another site (deltoid) at the same time or within days
     - Second and third vaccine doses given 1 and 6 months later

   - Neonates of HBsAg-positive mothers identified during pregnancy

     - A dose of 0.5 mL of HBIG given within 12 hours of birth into the anterolateral muscle of the thigh
     - HBV vaccine, in doses of 5 to 10 µg, given within 12 hours of birth (at another site in the anterolateral muscle), repeated at 1 and 6 months

     - Protective efficacy greater than 95%

   b. HDV
   - Neither specific high-titer anti-HDV–containing immune globulin nor HDV vaccine is available.
   - HDV immunoprophylaxis depends on the prevention of HBV by use of HBV vaccine.

   c. HCV
   - Immunoprophylaxis of HCV infection is not available, although neutralizing antibodies have been identified; work on an HCV vaccine is in progress.
   - Anti-HCV screening and nucleic acid testing for HCV RNA of blood and improved donor selection have reduced the risk of transfusion-associated hepatitis C dramatically in the United States (less than 1 per 2,000,000 U transfused).
   - Safe sexual practice for contacts of HCV-infected individuals with more than one partner may be appropriate.
   - Needle-exchange programs may reduce the risk in injection drug users.

Combined HAV and HBV Vaccine

A combination vaccine (Twinrix, GlaxoSmithKline) containing 20 µg of HBsAg protein (Engerix-B) and more than 720 ELISA U of inactivated hepatitis A virus (Havrix) provides dual protection with three injections spaced at 0, 1, and 6 months. **For more rapid protection, an accelerated schedule with three injections at 0, 7, 21 to 30 days and a booster at 1 year is also available.**

- This is indicated for susceptible individuals at risk of both HAV and HBV infections.
- The accelerated schedule provides earlier protection.
- Approved for adults only.

FURTHER READING

Armstrong GL, Wasley A, Simard EP, et al. The prevalence of hepatitis C virus infection in the United States, 1999 through 2002. *Ann Intern Med* 2006; 144:705–714.

Centers for Disease Control and Prevention. Update: Prevention of hepatitis A after exposure to hepatitis A virus and in international travelers: updated recommendations of the Advisory Committee on Immunization Practices (ACIP). *MMWR Morbid Mortal Wkly Rep* 2007; 56:1080–1084.

Centers for Disease Control and Prevention. A comprehensive immunization strategy to eliminate transmission of hepatitis B virus infection in the United States: recommendations of the Advisory Committee on Immunization Practices (ACIP). Part II: immunization of adults. *MMWR Recomm Rep* 2006; 55:1–25.

Centers for Disease Control and Prevention. A comprehensive immunization strategy to eliminate transmission of hepatitis B virus infection in the United States: recommendations of the Advisory Committee on Immunization Practices (ACIP). Part 1: immunization of infants, children, and adolescents. *MMWR Recomm Rep* 2005; 54:1–23.

FitzSimons D, Hendrickx G, Vorsters A, Van Damme P. Hepatitis A and E: update on prevention and epidemiology. *Vaccine* 2010; 28:583–588.

Khuroo MS, Khuroo MS. Hepatitis E virus. *Curr Opin Infect Dis* 2008; 21:539–543.

Liang JT. Hepatitis B: the virus and disease. *Hepatology* 2009; 49(Suppl):S13–S21.

Shih HH, Jeng KS, Syu WJ, et al. Hepatitis B surface antigen levels and sequences of natural hepatitis B virus variants influence the assembly and secretion of hepatitis D virus. *J Virol* 2008; 82:2250–2264.

Tang H, Grise H. Cellular and molecular biology of HCV infection and hepatitis. *Clin Sci* 2009; 117:49–65.

Victor JC, Monto AS, Surdina TY, et al. Hepatitis A vaccine versus immune globulin for post-exposure prophylaxis. *N Engl J Med* 2007; 357:1685–1694.

Vogt TM, Wise ME, Bell BP, Finelli L. Declining hepatitis A mortality in the United States during the era of hepatitis A vaccination. *J Infect Dis* 2008; 197:1282–1288.

CHAPTER 4

Chronic viral hepatitis

Salvador Benlloch, MD ■ Marina Berenguer, MD

KEY POINTS

1. Hepatitis B virus and hepatitis C virus are the major viral agents causing chronic hepatitis.

2. Long-term complications of chronic hepatitis include cirrhosis, liver failure, portal hypertension, and hepatocellular carcinoma.

3. Until recently, peginterferon plus ribavirin was the only approved treatment for chronic hepatitis C; overall more than 50% of patients treated with this dual therapy did not achieve viral eradication.

4. The direct-acting antiviral agents boceprevir and telaprevir were approved in May 2011 by the US Food and Drug Administration for the treatment of chronic hepatitis C genotype 1 infection in combination with peginterferon and ribavirin; the sustained virologic reponse rates up to 66% and 79%, respectively, with the addition of one of these two protease inhibitors to peginterferon plus ribavirin. In addition, approximately half to two-thirds of patients can achieve these high rates of viral eradication with only 24 to 28 weeks of therapy.

5. Seven drugs are approved for the treatment of chronic hepatitis B: interferon and peginterferon, three nucleoside analogues (lamivudine, telbivudine, entecavir), and two nucleotide analogues (adefovir and tenofovir); entecavir and tenofovir are the current first-line agents.

6. Hepatitis B virus mutates in response to antiviral drug treatment, which may lead to drug resistance, cross-drug resistance, and multidrug resistance; long-term treatment is required in these patients.

7. End-stage liver disease resulting from chronic viral hepatitis is a major indication for liver transplantation.

Overview

1. Chronic hepatitis is a condition characterized by persistent liver inflammation for more than 6 months after initial exposure or diagnosis of liver disease.
2. Causes of chronic viral hepatitis are hepatitis B virus (HBV), hepatitis C virus (HCV), hepatitis D virus (HDV), and, in some circumstances, hepatitis E virus (HEV).
3. Complications of chronic hepatitis include cirrhosis, portal hypertension, hepatic failure, and hepatocellular carcinoma.

Chronic Hepatitis B

CLINICAL FEATURES AND NATURAL HISTORY

1. Symptoms of chronic hepatitis range from none, to nonspecific complaints (fatigue, right upper quadrant pain), to complications of cirrhosis.

TABLE 4.1 ■ **Phases of HBV chronic infection**

	HBsAg	Anti-HBs	Anti-HBc	HBeAg	Anti-HBe	ALT	Liver biopsy	Treatment candidate	HBV DNA (IU/mL)
Immune tolerance phase	+	−	+	+	−	Normal	Normal or minimal inflammation	No	$2 \times 10^{8\text{-}11}$
Immune active (HBeAg+ CHB)	+	−	+	+	−	Elevated	Active inflammation	Yes	$2 \times 10^{4\text{-}10}$
Reactivation (HBeAg− CHB)	+	−	+	−	+	Elevated	Active inflammation	Yes	$2 \times 10^{3\text{-}8}$
Inactive carrier	+	−	+	−	+	Normal	Normal or minimal inflammation	No	<2000

ALT, alanine aminotransferase; CHB, chronic hepatitis B; HBeAg, hepatitis B e antigen; HBsAg, hepatitis B surface antigen; HBV, hepatitis B virus

2. Extrahepatic manifestations occur in up to 20% of patients with chronic hepatitis B and include arthralgias, polyarteritis nodosa, glomerulonephritis, mixed essential cryoglobulinemia, and a few other rare syndromes.

3. The risk of chronicity depends on the age and immune function when a person is infected; chronic infection occurs in
   ■ 90% of infants infected during the first year of life
   ■ 30% to 50% of children infected between one to four years of age
   ■ approximately 5% of healthy adults
   ■ more than 50% of immune compromised adults

4. Approximately 25% of adults who become chronically infected during childhood will die at some point in their lifetime of HBV-related liver cancer or cirrhosis.

5. The four phases of HBV chronic infection are summarized in Table 4.1.

6. The prevalence of hepatitis B e antigen (HBeAg) declines with age, with spontaneous loss of HBeAg in 7% to 20% of patients per year.

7. Spontaneous loss of hepatitis B surface antigen (HBsAg) occurs infrequently (0.5% to 1% per year); with most patients developing anti-HBs.

8. The natural history of chronic hepatitis B is outlined in Fig. 4.1.

9. Factors associated with progression of chronic hepatitis B include
   ■ older age (longer duration of infection), HBV genotype C, alcohol abuse, high levels of HBV DNA, concurrent infection with other viruses (human immunodeficiency virus [HIV], HCV, HDV), environmental factors (smoking, aflatoxin), obesity, and diabetes mellitus

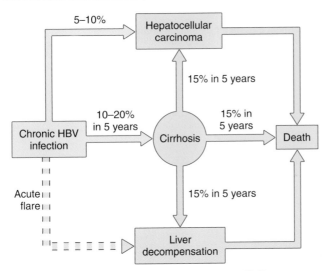

Fig. 4.1 Natural history of chronic hepatitis B.

SEROLOGIC AND VIROLOGIC TESTS (see Chapter 3)

1. The diagnosis of HBV infection relies largely on detection of HBsAg.
2. When HBsAg is detectable, further laboratory testing to assess disease status and need for treatment is indicated:
   - Quantitative HBV DNA by a sensitive assay: fluctuating levels dictate serial monitoring.
   - Alanine aminotransferase (ALT): levels can fluctuate; test ALT every 3 to 6 months if ALT is persistently normal and more often when elevated.
   - HBeAg and anti-HBe: define the type of chronic hepatitis B (i.e., HBeAg positive or HBeAg negative) and the end point of therapy (i.e., loss of HBeAg in HBeAg-positive patients).
   - Tests of liver disease severity: these include platelet count, total bilirubin, albumin, and prothrombin time/international normalized ratio (INR).
   - Liver biopsy: this is optional but is helpful to determine the histologic grade and stage of disease and to identify coexistent liver diseases such as steatohepatitis, iron overload, or autoimmune hepatitis; more studies are needed to assess the role of noninvasive tests of fibrosis, such as serum fibrosis markers and transient elastography.

PATHOLOGY AND PATHOGENESIS

1. HBV is a hepatotropic virus; most liver damage from HBV is caused by host immune responses with a cell-mediated response directed against cellular hepatitis B core antigen (HBcAg).
2. Cytotoxic T lymphocytes (CTLs) are the effector cells that mediate cell damage.
3. Non–antigen-specific immune responses, such as those mediated by inflammatory cytokines (tumor necrosis factor alpha, gamma interferon), may be more important for viral clearance than CTL-mediated mechanisms.
4. A hyperactive host response may lead to fulminant hepatitis, whereas a reduced host response increases the risk of chronic infection.

TABLE 4.2 ■ **Treatment criteria for chronic hepatitis B**

Guideline*	HBeAg-Positive		HBeAg-Negative	
	HBV DNA, IU/mL	ALT	HBV DNA, IU/mL	ALT
EASL 2009	>2,000	>ULN†	>2,000	>ULN†
APASL 2008	≥20,000	>2 × ULN†	≥2,000	>2 × ULN†
AASLD 2009	>20,000	>2 × ULN‡ or abnormal biopsy	≥20,000§	≥2 × ULN‡ or abnormal biopsy

*Although ALT and HBV DNA are primary tests used to determine treatment candidacy, investigators do not universally agree on the level of elevation that warrants consideration of treatment.

†Normal for laboratory.

‡30 U/L for men and 19 U/L for women.

§In patients older than 40 years of age, 2000 IU/mL should be considered as the minimum cutoff for treatment.

AASLD, American Association for the Study of Liver Diseases; ALT, alanine aminotransferase; APASL, Asian Pacific Association for the Study of the Liver; EASL, European Association for the Study of the Liver; HBeAg, hepatitis B e antigen; ULN, upper limit of normal.

Data from European Association for the Study of the Liver. EASL clinical practice guidelines: management of chronic hepatitis B. *J Hepatol* 2009; 50:227–242; Liaw YF, Leung N, Kao JH, *et al.* Asian-Pacific consensus statement on the management of chronic hepatitis B: a 2008 update. *Hepatol Int* 2008; 2:263–283; and Lok ASF, McMahon BJ. Chronic hepatitis B: update 2009. *Hepatology* 2009; 50:661–662.

5. In patients who fail to clear virus, both CD4+ and CD8+ T cells are markedly reduced.
6. Nonspecific histologic findings include a predominantly lymphocytic infiltrate, which may or may not be confined to the portal tracts.
7. Characteristic histologic findings of chronic hepatitis B: these include ground-glass hepatocytes in which the cytoplasm is stained pink with hematoxylin-eosin in response to massive production of HBsAg; HBcAg can be demonstrated in the hepatocyte nuclei, within the cytoplasm and on the cell membrane.
8. Grading and staging of chronic hepatitis B: numerous grading systems are available for assessing the severity of necroinflammation (grade) and the degree of fibrosis (stage); fibrosis stage is the most relevant histologic prognostic factor.

TREATMENT

1. **Goals of treatment**
   - Prevention of long-term complications (cirrhosis, hepatocellular carcinoma) and mortality by durable suppression of serum HBV DNA
   - Primary treatment end point: sustained decrease in serum HBV DNA level to low or undetectable (less than 10 to 15 IU/mL)
   - Secondary treatment end points: decreased or normalized serum ALT, improved liver histology, induced HBeAg loss or seroconversion, induced HBsAg loss or seroconversion, and prevention of secondary spread of infection

2. **Treatment criteria for chronic hepatitis B (Table 4.2)**
Clinical and laboratory parameters do not show a consistent correlation with liver histology, and current management guidelines recommend liver biopsies only in select patients based on age, HBV DNA levels, and HBeAg status.

3. **Treatment candidates and indications for HBV treatment (Table 4.3)**

TABLE 4.3 ■ **Indications for HBV treatment**

Evidence of benefit: treatment indicated	Treatment not indicated
Decompensated cirrhotic patients	Immune tolerance phase
HBV DNA–positive cirrhotic patient	Inactive chronic carrier
Fulminant liver failure	Acute hepatitis B
HBsAg-positive patient who is going to be immunosuppressed	
Chronic hepatitis B with elevated ALT levels and HBV DNA >2000 UI/mL	

ALT, alanine aminotransferase; HBsAg, hepatitis B surface antigen; HBV, hepatitis B virus.

TABLE 4.4 ■ **Rates of response to HBV antiviral therapy in noncomparative randomized clinical trials**

		Peg-IFN (%)	LAM (%)	ADV (%)	ETV (%)	LdT (%)	TDF (%)
HBeAg positive	HBeAg seroconversion	30	22	24	22	26	21
	Undetectable HBV DNA	24	39	21	67	60	74
	Normal ALT level	39	66	48	68	77	69
HBeAg negative	Undetectable HBV DNA	63	72	51	90	88	91
	Normal ALT level	38	74	72	78	74	77

ADV, adefovir dipivoxil; ALT, alanine aminotransferase; ETV, entecavir; HBeAg, hepatitis B e antigen; HBV, hepatitis B virus; LAM, lamivudine; LdT, telbivudine; Peg-IFN, peginterferon; TDF, tenofovir.

Data from European Association for the Study of the Liver. EASL clinical practice guidelines: management of chronic hepatitis B. *J Hepatol* 2009; 50:227–242.

4. **Drugs**
   a. Current first line therapies
      ■ Peginterferon alfa-2a (exceptions: pregnancy, chemotherapy prophylaxis, decompensated cirrhosis)
      ■ Entecavir
      ■ Tenofovir
   b. The first decision is selection of either a nucleos(t)ide analogue or peginterferon.
   c. Predictors of HBeAg response are the same for peginterferon and nucleos(t)ide analogues.
   d. Rates of HBeAg seroconversion, undetectable HBV DNA, and normal ALT at 1 year of therapy are shown in Table 4.4.
   e. Specific drugs
      ■ **Peginterferon**: Consider in young, noncirrhotic patients with low HBV DNA levels, high ALT levels, and a favorable genotype (better in genotype A > B > C > D). Treatment consists of 180 μg/week subcutaneously for 48 weeks.

- Advantages: finite treatment; absence of resistance; seroconversion in up to 32% of HBeAg-positive patients at 48 weeks of treatment; clearance of HBsAg in 6% of patients
- Drawbacks: many adverse effects; subcutaneous injections; frequent contraindications
- **Nucleos(t)ide analogues**: despite their high antiviral potency (greater than that of interferon), these drugs are not able to eradicate HBV, but they can maintain the sustained suppression of replication.
- Advantages: potent; negligible adverse effects; oral administration; safe and effective at all ages; suitable for cirrhotic and HIV-coinfected patients
- Disadvantages: lower rates of HBeAg and HBsAg seroconversion; prolonged treatment required, leading to an increasing risk of antiviral drug resistance
- **Lamivudine** (nucleoside analogue): dose, 100 mg daily; potent, with low genetic barrier and high rate of resistance. The most common mutation leading to lamivudine resistance is a specific point mutation in the conserved YMDD motif of the HBV polymerase.
- **Adefovir dipivoxil** (nucleotide analogue): less potent, but with higher genetic barrier and lower rate of resistance; dose, 10 mg daily; potentially nephrotoxic
- **Entecavir** (nucleoside analogue): potent antiviral activity with high genetic barrier and low rate of resistance; dose, 0.5 to 1 mg daily
- **Telbivudine** (nucleoside analogue); potency similar to that of entecavir, but with a resistance rate of 22% the second year of treatment; telbivudine-resistant mutations cross-resistant with lamivudine; dose regimen: 600 mg/daily; very infrequently can cause myopathy and peripheral neuropathy
- **Tenofovir** (nucleotide analogue); potent, with high genetic barrier and low rates of resistance; less nephrotoxic than adefovir; dose, 300 mg daily; adverse events including Fanconi syndrome (rare) and decrease in bone density

5. **Duration of HBV therapy with nucleos(t)ide analogues**
   - HBeAg positive: treat until HBeAg seroconversion, and stop after consolidation period 6 to 12 months after HBeAg seroconversion.
   - HBeAg negative: treat indefinitely because relapse is common after cessation of therapy.

6. **Resistance to antiviral drugs**
   a. Diagnosis of resistance
      - Viral rebound by at least 1.0 $\log_{10}$ compared with nadir; confirmed with repeat HBV DNA testing
      - Exclusion of non-HBV–related causes of failure (i.e., poor adherence)
      - Confirmation of genotypic resistance with HBV mutant detection, if available
      - Genotypic resistance; detection of HBV polymerase mutation(s) associated with resistance
      - Phenotypic resistance; decreased in vitro susceptibility to an antiviral agent in compliant patients
   b. Cumulative incidence of antiviral drug resistance (Table 4.5)
   c. Monitoring for drug resistance
      - Repeated ALT and serum HBV DNA measurements
      - Use of sensitive HBV DNA assay and the same assay over time
      - Frequency of assessments adapted according to disease severity (mild liver disease: at least six monthly; advanced disease or cirrhosis: three monthly)
   d. Management of resistance (Table 4.6); **roadmap** for management of patients receiving oral antivirals for chronic hepatitis B (Fig. 4.2)

TABLE 4.5 ■ **Cumulative incidence of HBV antiviral drug resistance**

Year of Treatment	LAM (%)	ADV (%)	ETV (%)	LdT (%)	TDF (%)
1st	24	0	0.2	4	0
2nd	38	3	0.5	22	0
3rd	49	11	1.2	—	0
4th	67	18	1.2	—	0
5th	70	29	1.2	—	—

ADV, adefovir dipivoxil; ETV, entecavir; HBV, hepatitis B virus; LAM, lamivudine; LdT, telbivudine; Peg-IFN, peginterferon; TDF, tenofovir.

TABLE 4.6 ■ **Management of resistance to HBV antiviral drugs**

Resistance	Rescue Therapy
Lamivudine	Add adefovir or tenofovir[*] Switch to entecavir (increased risk of entecavir resistance) Switch to emtricitabine/tenofovir[†]
Adefovir	Add lamivudine or telbivudine Switch to or add entecavir (if no previous resistance to lamivudine) Switch to emtricitabine/tenofovir[†]
Entecavir	Add or switch to adefovir or tenofovir[*] Switch to emtricitabine/tenofovir[†]
Telbivudine	Add adefovir or tenofovir[*] Switch to entecavir (increased risk of entecavir resistance) Switch to emtricitabine/tenofovir[†]

[*]Tenofovir preferred, if available.

[†]Truvada.

HBV, hepatitis B virus

Data updated from: Lok ASF, McMahon BJ. Chronic hepatitis B: update 2009. *Hepatology* 2009; 50: 661–662; Keeffe EB, Dieterich DT, Han SH, et al. A treatment algorithm for the management of chronic hepatitis B virus infection in the United States: 2008 update. *Clin Gastroenterol Hepatol* 2008; 6: 1315–1341; and European Association for the Study of the Liver. EASL clinical practice guidelines: management of chronic hepatitis B. J *Hepatol* 2009; 50: 227–242.

PREVENTION (see Chapter 3)

1. A vaccine against hepatitis B has been available since 1982; HBV vaccine is 95% effective in preventing HBV infection and its long-term consequences, and it is the first vaccine against a major human cancer.
2. Universal vaccination is the recommend strategy.
3. Protection lasts at least 15 years; a booster may be indicated in immunosuppressed patients with anti-HBs titer lower than 10 UI/mL.

LIVER TRANSPLANTATION (see Chapter 31)

1. This is the treatment of choice in patients with end-stage chronic liver disease.
2. Without prophylactic measures, HBV recurrence is universal, and post-transplant survival is reduced.

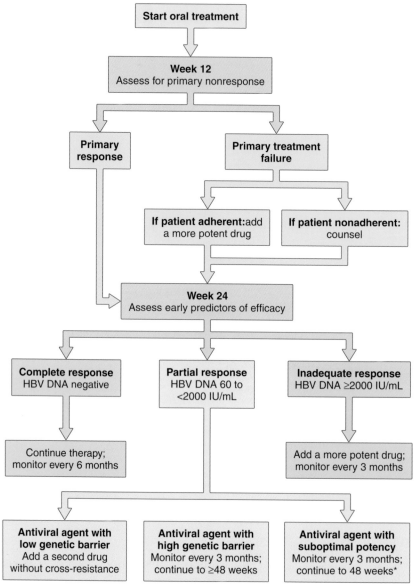

Fig. 4.2 Algorithm for management of patients receiving oral therapy for chronic hepatitis B. HBV, hepatitis B virus

3. Perioperative and postoperative hepatitis B immune globulin (HBIG) reduces recurrence and improves survival.

4. Nucleos(t)ide analogues have been given preemptively (before and after transplantation) as well as for post-transplantation recurrence.

5. The prophylactic strategy most commonly accepted is the combination of HBIG with an oral antiviral (preferably one with high barrier to resistance); this regimen has reduced the risk of recurrent hepatitis B in the graft to less than 10%.

Chronic Hepatitis C

CLINICAL FEATURES AND NATURAL HISTORY

1. Most patients with chronic hepatitis C have persistent or intermittent elevation of ALT levels, although ALT remains normal in one third of cases.
2. Most patients are asymptomatic; when symptoms are present, the most common is fatigue; other symptoms include musculoskeletal pain, pruritus, sicca syndrome, depression, anorexia, abdominal discomfort, difficulty with concentration, reduction in quality of life; the intensity of symptoms is not related to the severity of liver disease.
3. Once cirrhosis is established, patients are predisposed to complications of portal hypertension; jaundice is rare until hepatic decompensation occurs.
4. Extrahepatic manifestations: up to 40% to 74% of patients develop at least one extrahepatic manifestation during the course of their disease; rheumatologic and cutaneous manifestations are the most common.
5. Natural history
   - Disease progression is typically silent.
   - Only a few patients have severe outcomes during the first 2 decades of infection; at least 20 to 30 years of infection are required to develop clinically significant disease.
   - Once cirrhosis develops, actuarial survival is 83% to 91% at 5 years and 79% after 10 years in the absence of clinical decompensation.
   - Survival decreases to 50% at 5 years among those who develop clinical decompensation; the cumulative probability of developing an episode of decompensation is only 4% to 5% at 1 year, and it increases to 30% at 10 years.
   - The risk of developing hepatocellular carcinoma is 1% to 4% per year once cirrhosis is established.
   - Factors associated with progression of chronic hepatitis C include male gender, infection after age 40 years, use of alcohol greater than 50 g/day, immunosuppression, elevated ALT levels, significant necroinflammation and fibrosis on biopsy, and insulin resistance with obesity or diabetes mellitus.

SEROLOGIC AND MOLECULAR TESTS (see Chapter 3)

1. **Serologic assays**
   - Detectable anti-HCV indicates exposure but does not confirm active infection, because anti-HCV persists indefinitely after spontaneous or therapeutic resolution.
   - Anti-HCV sensitivity is 97% to 100%; the positive predictive value is 50% to 95%; false-negative results are more likely in immunosuppressed patients, HIV-positive patients, or patients with chronic renal failure who are undergoing dialysis.
2. **Molecular assays** are used to confirm active infection; two viral replication markers commonly used in clinical practice are the presence of viral RNA and core antigen in peripheral blood; HCV RNA testing should be performed in
   - All patients with a positive anti-HCV assay
   - Patients for whom antiviral treatment is being considered (quantitative assay)
   - Patients with unexplained liver disease whose anti-HCV result is negative if they are immunocompromised or suspected of having acute hepatitis C
3. Tests such as the real-time polymerase chain reaction–based assays have wide linear ranges for the quantification of HCV and similar sensitivity to qualitative tests; these tests are preferred to follow up a positive anti-HCV assay.

TABLE 4.7 ■ Indications for liver biopsy in patients with chronic hepatitis C

Indicated	Not indicated
Genotypes 1, 4, 5, 6 (recommended) onresponse or relapse after previous therapy	Patient's desire for treatment even if no fibrosis Contraindications to therapy Genotypes 2 or 3 High suspicion of cirrhosis

SCREENING AND COUNSELING

1. Universal testing is not currently recommended.
2. Screening for risk factors involves identifying persons who are at the highest risk of HCV infection (see Chapter 3).
3. Once a patient is determined to be at risk, HCV testing should be performed.
4. Persons infected with HCV should be counseled on how to avoid HCV transmission:
   ■ Avoid sharing dental or shaving equipment.
   ■ Cover bleeding wounds to prevent contact with others.
   ■ Discontinue illicit injection drugs.
   ■ Do not donate blood, organs, tissue, or semen.
   ■ Be aware that barrier protection is not needed in monogamous relationships.
   ■ Avoid alcohol intake.
   ■ For susceptible individuals, obtain hepatitis A and B vaccination.

PATHOGENESIS, LIVER BIOPSY, AND NONINVASIVE TESTS

1. Three mechanisms of pathogenesis of HCV-related liver injury have been proposed: direct cytopathic damage, immune-directed hepatocyte destruction, and viral-induced autoimmunity; the weight of evidence suggests that immune-mediated mechanisms predominate, with destruction of hepatocytes by sensitized T cells.
2. Pathologic features range from minimal periportal lymphocytic inflammation to active hepatitis with bridging fibrosis, hepatocyte necrosis, and cirrhosis; steatosis, lymphoid aggregates, and bile duct damage are frequent; these findings are common with other viral and nonviral causes of liver disease.
3. Value of liver biopsy
   ■ Assessment of the severity of liver damage (grade of hepatic necroinflammation and stage of fibrosis)
   ■ Detection of other potential coexisting diseases such as hemochromatosis, alcohol-induced injury, and nonalcoholic steatohepatitis
   ■ Determination of the rate of disease progression in patients with a known date of infection or prior liver biopsy
4. Noninvasive approach to the assessment of the extent of liver fibrosis: several noninvasive tests are based on direct or indirect markers of liver fibrosis (alone or in combination); transient elastography (FibroScan) measures liver stiffness and predicts significant fibrosis and cirrhosis accurately; currently noninvasive tests and techniques should not systematically replace liver biopsy in routine clinical practice.
5. Indications for liver biopsy are shown in Table 4.7.

TABLE 4.8 ■ **Contraindications to antiviral therapy in chronic hepatitis C**

	Absolute	Relative
Peginterferon	Major uncontrolled psychiatric disorder (especially depressive illness). Noncompensated hepatic cirrhosis (unless liver transplantation is being considered) Solid organ transplantation other than liver Cardiac arrhythmia Active autoimmune disease	Poorly controlled diabetes mellitus Pancytopenia Chronic obstructive pulmonary disease Active alcohol or intravenous drug abuse Age ≥75 yr Uncontrolled seizure disorder
Ribavirin	Renal failure Anemia (hemoglobin <10 mg/dL) Significant coronary heart disease Pregnancy risk Breast-feeding	Severe hypertension

TREATMENT

Treatment can interrupt disease progression and reduce complications of HCV-related cirrhosis.

1. **Goals of therapy**
   - The primary goal of therapy is to eradicate infection early in the course of disease to prevent progression to end-stage liver disease and hepatocellular carcinoma; sustained biochemical and virologic responses, which are often accompanied by histologic improvement, are the current standard therapeutic end points.
   - Additional goals are to prevent transmission of virus, reduce extrahepatic manifestations, and enhance quality of life.
2. **Indications**
   - All patients with chronic hepatitis C with detectable serum HCV RNA and persistent elevation of ALT levels considered potential candidates for antiviral therapy
   - In genotypes 1 and 4: moderate or severe necroinflammatory activity or more than portal fibrosis
   - Symptomatic mixed cryoglobulinemia
   - Controversial: patients with histologically mild chronic hepatitis
3. **Contraindications** (Table 4.8)
4. **Available drugs**
   These include peginterferon alfa-2a (180 μg once weekly) or peginterferon alfa-2b (1.5 μg/kg) combined with weight-based ribavirin (800 to 1400 mg/day, based on body weight with peginterferon alfa-2b, and 1000 to 1200 mg/day for body weight less than 75 kg or more than 75 kg with peginterferon alfa-2a) for genotype 1 infection and a fixed dose of 800 mg/day for genotypes 2 and 3 infection.
5. **Definitions of response to treatment**
   - **Rapid virologic response (RVR):** HCV RNA undetectable by week 4
   - **Early virologic response (EVR):** 2 log or greater decline in HCV RNA by week 12
   - **End of treatment (EOT) response:** undetectable HCV RNA at the end of treatment
   - **Partial virologic response:** 2 log or greater decline in HCV RNA by week 12, but HCV RNA detectable at week 24
   - **Sustained virologic response (SVR):** HCV RNA negativity 12 to 24 weeks after the end of treatment

TABLE 4.9 ■ **Factors associated with therapeutic outcomes in chronic hepatitis C**

Factor	Favourable therapeutic response	Impaired therapeutic response
Age	<40 yr	≥40 yr
Pretreatment HCV RNA level	<800,000 IU/mL	≥800,000 IU/mL
Gender	Female	Male
ALT	++	+
Genotype	2, 3	1
Fibrosis in liver biopsy	Mild	Advanced
Steatosis in liver biopsy sample	Absent	Present
Race	White	African American
BMI	Normal	>30
IL28B polymorphism	CC genotype	TT / CT genotype

ALT, alanine aminotransferase; BMI, body mass index; HCV, hepatitis C virus.

- **Nonresponse:** failure to achieve HCV RNA negativity at any time point during therapy
- **Relapse:** end of treatment response followed by return of HCV RNA after treatment discontinuation

6. **Duration of therapy**
   a. **Genotype 1**: 48 weeks
      - Week 12 stopping rule: patients without EVR unlikely to achieve SVR
      - Shorter treatment duration (24 weeks) possible in genotype 1 patients with RVR and low viral load (less than 600,000 IU/mL); more data needed
      - Longer treatment duration (72 weeks) possibly beneficial for slow responders
   b. **Genotypes 2, 3**: 24 weeks
      - Shorter treatment (12 to 16 weeks) possible in genotype 2/3 patients achieving RVR; more data needed

7. **Efficacy**
   - Genotype 1, 4: overall SVR: 42% to 52%
   - Genotypes 2, 3: overall SVR: 75% to 82%
   - Features associated with therapeutic response (Table 4.9)

8. **Adverse effects of treatment**
   - Common categories of side effects include influenza-like symptoms, psychiatric disorders, myelosuppression, and hemolytic anemia.

9. **Long-term follow-up**
   - Noncirrhotic patients achieving SVR: serum ALT levels at yearly intervals
   - Cirrhotic patients achieving SVR: complete blood count and liver biochemical tests and hepatic ultrasound every 6 months
   - Patients without SVR: complete laboratory tests and hepatic ultrasound at yearly intervals if no cirrhosis and every 6 months if cirrhosis

10. **Liver transplantation** (see Chapter 31)
    - Chronic hepatitis C is the most common indication for liver transplantation.
    - Post-transplant recurrence of HCV RNA is universal.
    - Histologic evidence of liver injury is present in approximately 50% of patients after transplant at 1 year, and the proportion increases with follow-up.

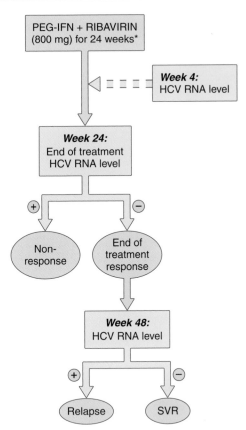

Fig. 4.3 Hepatitis C virus treatment algorithm genotypes 2 and 3. * Liver biopsy considered optional for genotype 2 and 3 infection. PEG-IFN peginterferon; HCV, hepatitis C virus; SVR, sustained virologic response.

- Serologic assays underestimate the frequency of post-transplantation HCV infection, and virologic tests are required for diagnosis.
- Histologic findings typical of post-transplant HCV infection include fatty infiltration, portal and parenchymal mononuclear infiltrates, and hepatocyte swelling and necrosis.
- Short-term survival is similar to that in patients who undergo liver transplantation for nonviral liver disease, but long-term survival is probably reduced by recurrent hepatitis C.
- Interferon-based therapy with and without ribavirin has been used to treat post-transplant HCV recurrence; transient reductions in serum HCV RNA levels have been observed, but sustained biochemical and virologic responses are uncommon (one-third or less).

11. HCV treatment algorithms (Figs. 4.3 and 4.4)
12. Potential future therapy of chronic hepatitis C
- A number of novel drugs that include protease inhibitors, polymerase inhibitors, cyclophilin inhibitors, immune modulators, and molecules with other mechanisms of action are undergoing study as a third drug added to the standard of care, with the goal of increasing the SVR rate in HCV genotype 1 infection.

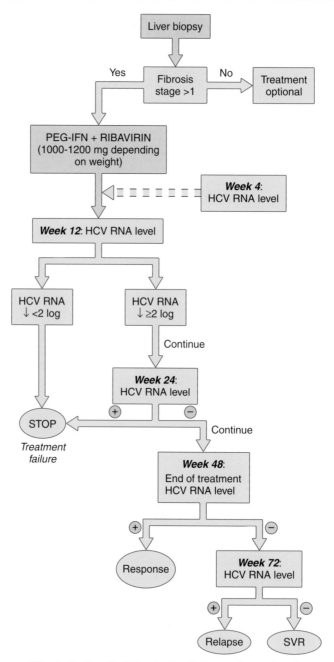

Fig. 4.4 Hepatitis C virus treatment algorithm for genotype 1.

■ Two direct-acting antiviral agents were approved in May 2011 by the U.S. Food and Drug Administration for the treatment of chronic hepatitis C genotype 1 infection. These new drugs, boceprevir and telaprevir, are NS3/4A protease inhibitors. Approval by European and other regulatory authorities is expected by the end of 2011.

a. **Telaprevir**
  ■ In phase 3 studies of telaprevir in combination with peginterferon alfa-2a plus ribavirin, SVR was achieved overall in 72% to 75% of naïve patients in two studies. A substantial percentage of patients required only 24 weeks of total therapy, which represents an additional importance advance in therapy.
  ■ In a study of patients who failed prior therapy, the SVR rates with telaprevir plus peginterferon and ribavirin were 86% in relapsers, 57% in partial nonresponders, and 31% in null responders.
  ■ In the naïve and nonresponder phase 3 studies, telaprevir was administered for 12 weeks in combination with peginterferon alfa-2a and ribavirin for either 24 or 48 weeks in different treatment arms.
  ■ The use of telaprevir was associated with incremental side effects, with the most prominent being rash and anemia, and higher dropout rates compared with the control arms receiving the standard of care.

b. **Boceprevir**
  ■ In phase 3 studies, the SVR rate with boceprevir in combination with peginterferon alfa-2b plus ribavirin was 66% in naïve patients and also 66% in patients who had failed prior peginterferon plus ribavirin therapy.
  ■ SVR rates were 69% and 53%, respectively, in non-African Americans versus African Americans.
  ■ Boceprevir is administered for 44 weeks in combination with peginterferon alfa-2b and ribavirin after a 4-week lead-in with peginterferon and ribavirin alone, except in patients receiving response-guided therapy who were able to stop all treatment at 28 weeks (naïve patients) or 36 weeks (prior nonresponders).
  ■ The use of boceprevir was also associated with incremental side effects, with the most prominent being anemia.

A wide range of questions will need to be resolved, such as which naïve patients warrant triple therapy using a protease inhibitor versus standard peginterferon plus ribavirin; will practicing physicians be able to adequately manage the incremental side effects to avoid premature discontinuation of therapy with lower SVR rates; will antiviral drug resistance to these agents surface as a problem; can patients in real life adhere to a regimen requiring dosing telaprevir or boceprevir three times a day; and how will patients and health care systems manage the expected high cost of telaprevir and boceprevir.

Hepatitis D Virus (HDV)

CLINICAL FEATURES AND NATURAL HISTORY

1. Symptoms of HDV infection are nonspecific.
2. HDV infection should be suspected in the following:
   ■ Fulminant HBV infection
   ■ Acute HBV infection that improves but subsequently relapses
   ■ Progressive chronic HBV in the absence of active HBV replication

3. Coinfection with HDV and HBV
   - More severe acute illness than HBV infection alone
   - Increased risk of fulminant hepatic failure
   - Rate of chronicity similar to that for HBV infection alone (less than 5%)
4. Superinfection with HDV in a patient with chronic HBV infection accelerates the natural history of chronic hepatitis B.
5. A negative association exists between HDV and HCC (mechanisms unknown).

SEROLOGIC AND VIROLOGIC TESTS (see Chapter 3)

1. Currently available tests are both enzyme-linked assay (EIA) and radioimmune assay (RIA) for the detection of total and immunoglobulin M (IgM) anti-HDV.
2. Persistence of IgM anti-HDV or a titer of anti-HDV IgG greater than 1:1000 correlates well with the presence of ongoing viral replication.
3. Detection of HDV RNA is available only on a research basis, but it has utility in distinguishing ongoing from prior infection.
4. Distinction between coinfection and superinfection is made by the presence or absence of anti-HBc IgM.
5. Detection of HDV antigen (HDVAg) by immunohistochemical analysis of liver tissue is considered the gold standard for diagnosis of persistent HDV infection; however, HDVAg staining is available only in research laboratories.

PATHOLOGY AND PATHOGENESIS

1. Necroinflammatory activity is often severe, but histologic features are not specific for chronic HDV infection.
2. HDVAg is readily demonstrated in nuclei and to a lesser extent in the cytoplasm of infected hepatocytes.
3. HDVAg and HDV RNA appear to be directly cytopathic; the other mechanism of cell injury is immune mediated; several autoantibodies have been described in association with chronic HDV infection.

TREATMENT

1. **Drugs**
   - High-dose interferon alpha (9 MU three times a week) and peginterferon alpha for 1 year are the only approved treatments for chronic hepatitis D.
   - The efficacy of interferon alpha therapy should be assessed at 24 weeks by measuring HDV RNA levels.
   - More than 1 year of therapy may be necessary but is of unproven efficacy.
   - Some patients become HDV RNA negative or even HBsAg negative, with accompanying improvement in histologic features.
   - Nucleos(t)ide analogues do not appear to affect HDV replication and related disease.
2. **Liver transplantation** (see Chapter 31)
   - Patients with chronic HDV infection are at lower risk for HBV recurrence than are those with chronic HBV infection alone.
   - HDV recurrence can be detected before signs of HBV reactivation.
   - Decreased recurrence rates and improved survival in HDV cirrhosis may result from the inhibitory effects of HDV on HBV replication.

■ No convincing treatments are available for preventing post-transplant recurrence of HDV, but it seems prudent to give combination therapy with lamivudine plus HBIG as for patients with HBV disease alone.

Chronic Hepatitis E

1. HEV is a single positive-stranded RNA virus that is a spherical nonenveloped virus 32 to 34 nm in size.
2. It is classified into four genotypes (1 to 4).
3. HEV is endemic in developing countries.
4. It is transmitted by the fecal–oral route.
5. HEV infection is self-limiting, although in pregnant women the illness is particularly severe and carries a high case fatality rate.
6. HEV has been responsible for acute hepatitis that does not progress to chronic hepatitis.
7. Several reports have appeared of chronic hepatitis E in the United States and Europe, mainly in immunosuppressed patients such as solid organ transplant recipients (most of whom had infection with genotype 3 HEV).
8. Treatment with ribavirin may be of benefit, but more data are needed.

FURTHER READING

Aggarwal R. Hepatitis E: does it cause chronic hepatitis? *Hepatology* 2008; 48:1328–1330.

Berg T, von Wagner M, Nasser S, et al. Extended treatment duration for hepatitis C virus type 1: comparing 48 versus 72 weeks of peginterferon-alfa-2a plus ribavirin. *Gastroenterology* 2006; 130:1086–1097.

Centers for Disease Control and Prevention. Hepatitis C information for health professionals. Accessed March 1, 2010 at www.cdc.gov/hepatitis/HCV/.

Dienstag JL, McHutchison JG. American Gastroenterological Association technical review on the management of hepatitis C. *Gastroenterology* 2006; 130:231–264.

European Association for the Study of the Liver. EASL clinical practice guidelines: management of chronic hepatitis B. *J Hepatol* 2009; 50:227–242.

Ghany MG, Strader DB, Thomas DL, et al. Diagnosis, management, and treatment of hepatitis C: an update. *Hepatology* 2009; 49:1335–1374.

Goodman ZD. Grading and staging systems for inflammation and fibrosis in chronic liver diseases. *J Hepatol* 2007; 47:598–607.

Kamar N, Rostaing L, Abravanel F, et al. Pegylated interferon-alpha for treating chronic hepatitis E virus infection after liver transplantation. *Clin Infect Dis* 2010; 50:e30–e33.

Keeffe EB, Dieterich DT, Han SH, et al. A treatment algorithm for the management of chronic hepatitis B virus infection in the United States: 2008 update. *Clin Gastroenterol Hepatol* 2008; 6:1315–1341.

Liaw YF, Leung N, Kao JH, et al. Asian-Pacific consensus statement on the management of chronic hepatitis B: a 2008 update. *Hepatol Int* 2008; 2:263–283.

Lok AS, McMahon BJ. Chronic hepatitis B: update 2009. *Hepatology* 2009; 50:661–662.

Mangia A, Santoro R, Minerva N, et al. Peginterferon alfa-2b and ribavirin for 12 vs. 24 weeks in HCV genotype 2 or 3. *N Engl J Med* 2005; 352:2609–2617.

Meng XJ. Recent advances in hepatitis E virus. *J Viral Hepat* 2010; 17(3):153–161.

Sorrell MF, Belongia EA, Costa J, et al. National Institutes of Health consensus development conference statement: management of hepatitis B. *Ann Intern Med* 2009; 150:104–110.

Veldt BJ, Heathcote EJ, Wedemeyer H, et al. Sustained virologic response and clinical outcomes in patients with chronic hepatitis C and advanced fibrosis. *Ann Intern Med* 2007; 147:677–684.

CHAPTER 5

Autoimmune hepatitis

Albert J. Czaja, MD, FACP, FACG, AGAF

KEY POINTS

1 Criteria for the diagnosis of autoimmune hepatitis have been codified, and two diagnostic scoring systems exist for difficult cases.

2 Two subtypes of autoimmune hepatitis are based on distinctive serologic markers.

3 Disease spectrum ranges from acute severe (fulminant) to asymptomatic mild presentations.

4 *DRB1*0301* and *DRB1*0401* are alleles that affect susceptibility, clinical phenotype, and treatment outcome in white North American and northern European patients.

5 Outcomes are improved by treatment in patients with normal liver tests and histologic features, by early identification of problematic patients, and by institution of maintenance azathioprine therapy after the first relapse.

6 Variant forms of autoimmune hepatitis are common, and treatment is empirically directed against the predominant features.

7 Recurrent and de novo autoimmune hepatitis must be excluded in all patients with graft dysfunction after liver transplantation.

Definition

1. Self-perpetuating hepatic inflammation of unknown cause characterized by interface hepatitis, hypergammaglobulinemia, and liver-associated autoantibodies
2. Exclusion of other conditions that have similar features, including Wilson disease, chronic viral hepatitis, alpha-1 antitrypsin deficiency, hereditary hemochromatosis, drug-induced liver disease (most commonly, minocycline toxicity), celiac disease, nonalcoholic steatohepatitis, primary biliary cirrhosis (PBC), and primary sclerosing cholangitis (PSC) (Table 5.1)

NOMENCLATURE

1. The designation *autoimmune hepatitis* replaces terms such as autoimmune liver disease and autoimmune chronic active hepatitis.
2. Type 1 and type 2 autoimmune hepatitis are defined by their principal autoantibody reactivity.

TABLE 5.1 ■ **Autoimmune hepatitis: Basic diagnostic tests**

Diagnostic tests	Clinical value
Serum AST and ALT, bilirubin, alkaline phosphatase, and γ-globulin levels	Estimate severity of inflammatory activity; characterize pattern of liver injury
Serum albumin level and INR	Estimate impairment of hepatic synthetic function
ANA, SMA, anti-LKM1, and AMA	Document presence and nature of immune activity
Serum immunoglobulin levels	Confirm mainly serum IgG elevation
Liver tissue examination	Document that histologic changes support diagnosis Exclude findings suggestive of other diagnoses
HBsAg, anti-HBc, IgM anti-HAV, and anti-HCV	Document absence of concurrent viral infection
Ceruloplasmin level	Exclude Wilson disease
Alpha-1 antitrypsin phenotype	Exclude alpha-1 antitrypsin deficiency
Serum iron, transferrin, iron saturation and ferritin levels	Exclude hereditary hemochromatosis

AMA, antimitochondrial antibodies; ANA, antinuclear antibodies; anti-HAV, antibody to hepatitis A virus; anti-HBc, antibody to hepatitis B core antigen; anti-HCV, antibody to hepatitis C virus; anti-LKM1, antibodies to liver kidney microsome type 1; AST, aspartate aminotransferase; ALT, alanine aminotransferase; HBsAg, hepatitis B surface antigen; IgG, immunoglobulin G; INR, international normalized ratio; SMA, smooth muscle antibodies.

Diagnosis

1. Criteria for *definite* and *probable* diagnoses are established by consensus of an international panel (Table 5.2).
2. **The requirement for 6 months of disease to establish chronicity is waived, and an acute, rarely severe (fulminant) form, is possible.**
3. Interface hepatitis (Fig. 5.1) is required for the diagnosis, but lobular (panacinar) hepatitis (Fig. 5.2) in conjunction with interface hepatitis is within the histologic spectrum.
4. Plasma cell infiltration (Fig. 5.3) is characteristic but not specific or essential for the diagnosis.
5. Centrilobular necrosis is rare and may be an early or acute histologic stage.
6. **Prominent cholestatic changes (bile duct injury, ductopenia) or histologic features suggestive of other disease (fat, granulomas, copper or iron) exclude the diagnosis.**
7. Conventional serologic markers of autoimmune hepatitis are antinuclear antibodies (ANA), smooth muscle antibodies (SMA), and antibodies to liver kidney microsome type 1 (anti-LKM1).
8. Other nonstandard serologic markers are antibodies to soluble liver antigen (anti-SLA), antibodies to liver cytosol type 1 (anti-LC1), and atypical perinuclear antineutrophil cytoplasmic antibodies (pANCA); they support a *probable* diagnosis of autoimmune hepatitis if conventional markers are absent.
9. Two scoring systems are used for the diagnosis of difficult cases: (1) the **revised original scoring system** of the International Autoimmune Hepatitis Group (IAIHG), which is most useful in patients with few or atypical symptoms (Table 5.3); and (2) the **simplified scoring system** of the IAIHG, which is most useful in patients with other diseases and concurrent autoimmune features (Table 5.4).
10. Gold standard assays for serologic markers of autoimmune hepatitis are based on indirect immunofluorescence (IIF); clinical correlations made by IIF have not been validated against results of enzyme-linked immunosorbent assays (ELISAs) based on recombinant antigens.

TABLE 5.2 ■ **International criteria for definite or probable diagnosis of autoimmune hepatitis**

Diagnostic features	Definite diagnosis	Probable diagnosis
Exclusion of risk factors for other diseases	Daily alcohol <25 g/day No recent hepatotoxic drugs Normal alpha-1 AT phenotype Normal ceruloplasmin level Normal iron and ferritin levels No active hepatitis A, B, and/or C	Daily alcohol <50 g/day No recent hepatotoxic drugs Heterozygous alpha-1 AT deficiency Abnormal copper or ceruloplasmin level but Wilson disease excluded Nonspecific iron and/or ferritin abnormalities No active hepatitis A, B, and/or C
Inflammatory indices	Serum AST/ALT elevation Minimal-mild cholestatic changes	Serum AST/ALT elevation Minimal-mild cholestatic changes
Autoantibodies	ANA, SMA, or anti-LKM1 >1:80 in adults and >1:20 in children; no AMA	ANA, SMA or anti-LKM1>1:40 in adults; other autoantibodies
Immunoglobulins	Globulin, γ-globulin, or IgG level >1.5 times normal	Hypergammaglobulinemia of any degree
Histologic findings	Interface hepatitis, moderate to severe No biliary lesions, granulomas or prominent changes suggestive of another disease	Interface hepatitis, moderate to severe No biliary lesions, granulomas or prominent changes suggestive of another disease

AMA, antimitochondrial antibodies; ANA, antinuclear antibodies; AT, antitrypsin; anti-LKM1, antibodies to liver kidney microsome type 1; AST, aspartate aminotransferase; ALT, alanine aminotransferase; IgG, immunoglobulin G; SMA, smooth muscle antibodies.

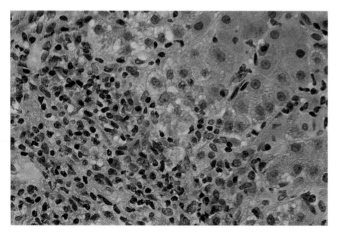

Fig. 5.1 Histopathalogy of interface hepatitis in autoimmune hepatitis. Disruption of the limiting plate of the portal tract by mononuclear inflammatory infiltrate that extends into the acinus is shown (hematoxylin and eosin, ×400).

Pathogenesis

PRINCIPAL HYPOTHESES

1. The **autoantigen-driven cell-mediated hypothesis** requires the following:
   - A triggering viral, drug, toxic, or environmental agent that resembles a self-antigen (molecular mimicry)

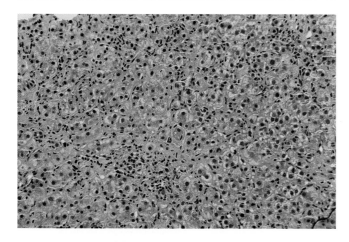

Fig. 5.2 Histopathology of panacinar hepatitis in autoimmune hepatitis. Mononuclear inflammatory cells line the sinusoidal spaces in association with liver cell degenerative and regenerative changes (hematoxylin and eosin, ×100).

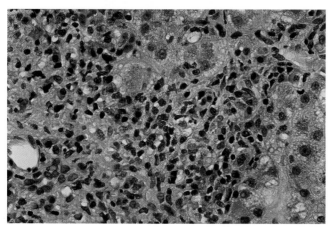

Fig. 5.3 Histopathalogy of plasma cell infiltration in autoimmune hepatitis. Plasma cells typified by perinuclear cytoplasmic haloes contribute to mononuclear inflammatory infiltrate within the portal tract (hematoxylin and eosin, ×400).

TABLE 5.3 ■ **Revised original international scoring system for the diagnosis of autoimmune hepatitis**

Factor		Score	Factor	Score
Female gender		+2	Alcohol use <25 g/day	+2
Alkaline phosphatase:	>3	−2	>60 g/day	−2
AST/ALT ratio:	<1.5	+2	HLA DRB1*03 or DRB1*04	+1
γ-globulin or IgG levels	>2 normal	+3	Concurrent immune disease	+2
	1.5–2 normal	+2	Other liver-related autoantibody	+2
	1–1.4 normal	+1	Interface hepatitis	+3
ANA, SMA, or anti-LKM1	>1:80	+3	Plasmacytic infiltrate	+1
	1:80	+2	Rosettes	+1
	1:40	+1	No characteristic features	−5
	<1:40	0	Biliary changes	−3

Continued

TABLE 5.3 ■ **Revised original international scoring system for the diagnosis of autoimmune hepatitis—*cont'd***

Factor		Score	Factor	Score
Antimitochondrial antibodies		+4	Other features (fat, granulomas)	−3
Viral markers	Positive	−3	Treatment response complete	+2
	Negative	+3	Relapse	+3
Hepatotoxic drugs	Yes	−4		
	No	+1		
Pretreatment score:	Definite diagnosis >15 Probable diagnosis 10–15		**Post-treatment score:**	Definite diagnosis >17 Probable diagnosis 12–17

ANA, antinuclear antibodies; AT, antitrypsin; anti-LKM1, antibodies to liver kidney microsome type 1; AST, aspartate aminotransferase; ALT, alanine aminotransferase; HLA, human leukocyte antigen; IgG, immunoglobulin G; SMA, smooth muscle antibodies.

TABLE 5.4 ■ **Simplified international scoring system for the diagnosis of autoimmune hepatitis**

Variable	Result	Points
Autoantibodies		
ANA or SMA	≥1:40	+1
ANA or SMA	≥1:80	+2
anti-LKM1	≥1:40	+2
anti-SLA	Positive	+2
Immunoglobulin level		
Immunoglobulin G	>ULN	+1
	>1.1 ULN	+2
Histologic findings		
Morphologic features	Compatible	+1
	Typical	+2
Viral disease markers		
No viral hepatitis	No viral markers	+2
Pretreatment aggregate score:		
Definite diagnosis		≥7
Probable diagnosis		6

ANA, antinuclear antibodies; anti-LKM1, antibodies to liver kidney microsome type 1; anti-SLA, antibodies to soluble liver antigen; SMA, smooth muscle antibodies; ULN, upper limit of normal.

■ Presentation of antigenic peptide by the human leukocyte antigen (HLA) DR molecule encoded by susceptibility alleles (*DRB1*0301* and/or *DRB1*0401* in white North Americans and northern Europeans)
■ **A six amino acid motif within an antigen binding groove, encoded as LLEQKR (leucine-leucine-glutamic acid-glutamine-lysine-arginine) in positions 67 to 72 of the**

DRβ polypeptide chain, that optimizes autoantigen display in white North American and northern European patients

■ Lysine at position DRβ71 that facilitates contact among the HLA DR molecule, antigenic peptide, and T-cell antigen receptor of CD4 cell and that promotes susceptibility

■ **Other autoimmune promoter genes in synergy (epistasis) with principal susceptibility alleles, including polymorphisms for** *cytotoxic T- lymphocyte antigen 4,* **tumor necrosis factor** *alpha,* **and** *Fas (tumor necrosis factor receptor superfamily-6)* **genes**

■ Activation of CD4 lymphocytes within the type 1 cytokine milieu (interleukin-12 [IL-12], IL-2, tumor necrosis factor alpha) and clonal proliferation of autoantigen-sensitized cytotoxic T lymphocytes

■ **Deficiencies in number and function of T-regulatory cells (CD4⁺CD25⁺ cells), which impair suppression of CD8⁺ T-cell proliferation and facilitate liver injury**

■ Liver cell destruction by tissue-infiltrating cytotoxic T lymphocytes

2. The **antibody-dependent cell-mediated cytotoxicity hypothesis** requires the following:

■ A triggering viral, drug, toxic, or environmental agent that resembles a self-antigen (molecular mimicry)

■ Activation of CD4 lymphocytes within the type 2 cytokine milieu (IL-4, IL-10)

■ A defect in suppressor activity or dysregulated cytokine homeostasis (e.g., increased constitutive or inducible amount or function of IL-10) favoring B-cell production of immunoglobulin G (IgG)

■ IgG directed against normal hepatocyte membrane constituents

■ Antigen–antibody complexes on the hepatocyte surface targeted by natural killer cells with Fc receptors

■ Ligation of natural killer cells to antigen–antibody complexes triggering cytolysis

■ HLA A1-B8-*DRB1*03* associated with a defect in suppressor activity

ANCILLARY HYPOTHESES

1. **Shared motif hypothesis**

■ Different susceptibility alleles encode the same or similar six amino acid motif within the antigen binding groove of the HLA DR molecule between positions 67 and 72 of the DRβ polypeptide chain and thereby affect susceptibility similarly.

■ *DRB1*0301* and *DRB1*0401* (white North American and northern European patients), *DRB1*0404* (Mexican Mestizo patients), and *DRB1*0405* (Japanese, mainland Chinese, and adult Argentine patients) encode either LLEQKR or LLEQRR at positions DRβ67 to 72.

■ *DRB1*0302, *0303, *0409, *0413, *0416, *1303* and *DRB3*0101, *0201, *0202, *0301* encode lysine at DRβ71 and contribute to susceptibility by increasing the "dose" of lysine.

2. **Autoimmune promoter hypothesis**

■ Polymorphisms of genes inside and outside the major histocompatibility complex act in synergy with each other or the principal susceptibility alleles in a non–disease-specific fashion to promote susceptibility ("permissive gene pool").

■ Polymorphisms of the *tumor necrosis factor alpha* gene (*TNFA-308*), *cytotoxic T-lymphocyte antigen 4* gene (*CTLA4*G*), and *tumor necrosis factor receptor superfamily-6* gene (*TNFRSF6*G,G* or *A,G*) affect disease occurrence in white North American and northern European patients.

■ Multiple similar promoters exist, and interactive constellations of polymorphic genes contribute to disease occurrence, susceptibility, and outcome.

3. **Molecular "footprint" hypothesis**

■ Region- or ethnicity-specific susceptibility genes favor infection with or reactivity to indigenous etiologic agents, and the susceptibility allele is a "footprint" of the triggering agent.

- *DRB*1301* is the susceptibility allele for autoimmune hepatitis in Argentina and Brazil, especially among children, and it encodes a six amino acid sequence at positions DRβ67 to 72 (ILEDER) in which the substitution of glutamic acid (E) for lysine at DRβ71 defeats the shared motif hypothesis.
- *DRB*1301* is associated with protracted hepatitis A virus, and prolonged exposure to this viral antigen may predispose to autoimmune hepatitis in this geographic region.
- Other indigenous agents may trigger the disease in other regions by selecting genetically susceptible individuals.

Subclassifications

TYPES

1. **Type 1 autoimmune hepatitis**
   a. Characterized by SMA and/or ANA
   b. Ancillary markers (i.e., atypical pANCA [frequently present] and anti-SLA [16%])
   c. **Most common type in the United States and affecting all ages, including infants**
   d. Most (78%) patients women (female-to-male ratio, 3.6:1)
   e. Concurrent extrahepatic immune diseases in 38%, including the following:
      - Autoimmune thyroiditis (12%)
      - Graves' disease (6%)
      - Ulcerative colitis (6%)
      - Rheumatoid arthritis (1%)
      - Pernicious anemia (1%)
      - Systemic sclerosis (1%)
      - Coombs-positive hemolytic anemia (1%)
      - Idiopathic thrombocytopenic purpura (1%)
      - Leukocytoclastic vasculitis (1%)
      - Nephritis (1%)
      - Erythema nodosum (1%)
      - Fibrosing alveolitis (1%)
   f. Concurrent ulcerative colitis cholangiography to exclude PSC
   g. Acute onset in 40% and rarely, acute severe (fulminant) presentation
   h. Implicated HLA: *DRB1*0301* (northern European), *DRB1*0401* (northern European), *DRB1*0404* (Mexican), *DRB1*0405* (Japanese), *DRB*1301* (South American), *DRB1*1501* (protective)
   i. Implicated polymorphic autoimmune promoters (all North American): *TNFA-308*A*, *CTLA4*G*, *TNFRSF6*G*, *MICA*008*
   j. Target autoantigen unknown
   k. ***DRB1*0301* (principal susceptibility allele) and *DRB1*0401* (secondary but independent susceptibility allele) in white North American and northern European patients**
   l. Cirrhosis at presentation in 25% indicating subclinical aggressive stage
2. **Type 2 autoimmune hepatitis**
   - Characterized by anti-LKM1
   - Ancillary marker (i.e., anti-LC1 [32%]); no atypical pANCA
   - Affects mainly children (age range, 2 to 14 years)
   - Of Europeans with type 2 autoimmune hepatitis, adults comprising 20%
   - Anti-LKM1 in only 4% of North American adult patients

- Commonly associated with concurrent immune diseases, including vitiligo, insulin-dependent diabetes mellitus, and autoimmune thyroiditis
- Frequent organ-specific autoantibodies (antibodies to parietal cells, thyroid, or islets of Langerhans)
- Acute or acute severe (fulminant) presentation possible
- **_DQB1*02_01 principal genetic risk factor in strong linkage disequilibrium with _DRB1*07_ and _DRB1*03_**
- **Cytochrome monooxygenase, CYP2D6, the target autoantigen**
- Five antigenic sites located within recombinant CYP2D6; amino acid sequence between positions 193 and 212 main epitope of anti-LKM1
- Homologies between recombinant CYP2D6 and genome of hepatitis C virus, cytomegalovirus, and herpes simplex virus type 1
- Anti-LKM1 in 10% with chronic hepatitis C in Europe but rare in United States
- **Equally responsive to corticosteroid therapy as type 1 autoimmune hepatitis**

VARIANTS

1. **Overlap syndrome with PBC**
   - Defined by features of autoimmune hepatitis, antimitochondrial antibodies (AMA), and histologic findings of bile duct injury or loss
   - Most (88%) patients with AMA titers up to 1:160; seropositivity for antibodies to M2 autoantigens rare (8%) (see Chapter 14)
   - AMA reactivity possibly false because of confusion with anti-LKM1 by IIF
   - Empiric treatment (3 to 6 months) with prednisone alone (20 mg daily) or prednisone (10 mg daily) plus azathioprine (50 mg daily) effective if autoimmune features predominant and alkaline phosphatase level less than twice the upper limit of normal (ULN)
   - Prednisone (20 mg daily) combined with ursodeoxycholic acid (13 to 15 mg/kg daily) if PBC features predominant, alkaline phosphatase level more than twice the ULN, and/or florid duct lesions on histologic examination
2. **Overlap syndrome with PSC**
   - Defined by features of autoimmune hepatitis, cholestatic biochemical changes, histologic evidence of cholestasis including bile duct injury or loss, and abnormal bile ducts by endoscopic retrograde cholangiography (ERC) or magnetic resonance cholangiography (MRC)
   - Cholangiography required for diagnosis if inflammatory bowel disease present
   - Histologic features of bile duct injury, portal edema, and/or ductopenia and normal cholangiogram compatible with small duct PSC
   - Clues to diagnosis: inflammatory bowel disease, suboptimal response to corticosteroid therapy, and/or rising serum alkaline phosphatase level
   - Empirical therapy with prednisone (20 mg daily) and ursodeoxycholic acid (13 to 15 mg/kg daily) justified
   - Children with autoimmune hepatitis and abnormal cholangiograms in the absence of inflammatory bowel disease ("autoimmune sclerosing cholangitis") typically respond to corticosteroid therapy but have shorter transplant-free survival than patients with normal bile ducts
   - Biliary changes by MRC in 8% of adults with classic autoimmune hepatitis, but similar frequency by MRC in non-autoimmune liver diseases and may incorrectly implicate PSC
3. **Autoimmune hepatitis and chronic viral hepatitis**
   a. Concurrence of active viral hepatitis, high-titer autoantibodies, and histologic features of interface hepatitis with or without portal plasma cell infiltration

b. *Definite* or *probable* autoimmune hepatitis by diagnostic scoring systems defining autoimmune predominant disease with background coincidental viremia

c. *Nondiagnostic* autoimmune features by diagnostic scoring systems with active viremia defining viral predominant disease with coincidental autoimmune findings

d. Immune manifestations common in chronic viral hepatitis, including SMA in 11%, ANA in 28%, diverse autoantibodies in 62%, and concurrent immune disease in 23%
   - SMA and ANA titers typically low in chronic viral hepatitis (up to 1:80 in 89%, 1:160 or higher in 11%; 1:320 or higher rarely)
   - Concurrent positivity for SMA and ANA in only 4% of patients with chronic viral hepatitis
   - Median serum titers of SMA and ANA in classical autoimmune hepatitis of 1:160 and 1:320, respectively; 60% with concurrent SMA and ANA; and only 6% with isolated titers up to 1:80

e. Liver tissue evaluation essential in discriminating predominantly autoimmune from predominantly viral hepatitis
   - Moderate to severe portal plasma cell infiltration (66% versus 21%), acinar (lobular) inflammation (47% versus 16%), and interface hepatitis (23% versus 0%) more common in autoimmune-predominant disease
   - Portal lymphoid aggregates (49% versus 10%), steatosis (72% versus 19%), and bile duct damage or loss (91% versus 20%) more frequent in viral-predominant (chronic hepatitis C) disease (Fig. 5.4)

f. Treatment administered according to the prevailing condition: corticosteroids for autoimmune-predominant disease and peginterferon and ribavirin for viral-predominant disease (chronic hepatitis C)

g. Treatment results assessed at 3 months, and therapy changed if response poor

4. **Autoimmune hepatitis with cholestatic syndrome**
   - Heterogeneous syndrome with composite features of autoimmune hepatitis and AMA-negative PBC or small duct PSC
   - ANA and/or SMA typically present in women with cholestatic biochemical changes, normal cholangiogram, absent AMA, and/or histologic findings of bile duct injury or loss
   - Possible resemblance to mainly PBC or autoimmune hepatitis
   - Variable response to empirical therapy with corticosteroids, ursodeoxycholic acid, or both

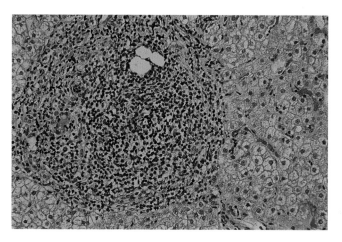

Fig. 5.4 Histopathology of portal lymphoid aggregate in chronic hepatitis C. Dense mononuclear lymphoid aggregate in the portal tract distinguishes chronic hepatitis C from autoimmune hepatitis (hematoxylin and eosin, ×200).

■ Possible therapy-induced improvements in clinical and laboratory findings but not in histologic changes

5. **Cryptogenic (autoantibody-negative) chronic hepatitis**
   ■ Satisfies international criteria for diagnosis of autoimmune hepatitis but lacks conventional autoantibodies (SMA, ANA, anti-LKM1)
   ■ Similarities in age, female predominance, frequency of concurrent immune diseases, histologic features, occurrence of HLA B8, DRB1*03 and A1-B8-DRB1*03, and laboratory findings to classic autoimmune hepatitis
   ■ As responsive to corticosteroid treatment as in autoantibody-positive patients
   ■ Possibly representing a form that has escaped detection by conventional serologic markers
   ■ Conventional autoantibodies possibly appearing late, or possible presence of nonstandard autoantibodies (atypical pANCA, anti-SLA)
   ■ Must be distinguished from inactive cryptogenic cirrhosis and liver disease associated with celiac disease (i.e., negative for IgA antibodies to tissue transglutaminase or endomysium)
   ■ Should be considered "autoantibody-negative autoimmune hepatitis" and treated with conventional corticosteroid regimens

Epidemialogy

1. The mean annual incidence of type 1 autoimmune hepatitis is 1 to 1.9 cases per 100,000 per year in Western Europe (and ethnically similar populations), and the point prevalence is 11 to 16.9 per 100,000.
2. Type 2 autoimmune hepatitis is rare, with an estimated prevalence of 3 cases per 1,000,000 and an annual incidence of 0.16 per 1,000,000. It affects only 4% of adults in the United States.
3. Autoimmune hepatitis accounts for 11% to 23% of cases of chronic hepatitis and affects 100,000 to 200,000 persons in the Unites States.
4. Autoimmune hepatitis accounts for 2.6% of liver transplants in Europe and 5.9% in the United States.
5. The prevalence is greatest among white populations of northern Europe, North America, and Australia, with a high frequency of HLA *DRB1*03* and *DRB1*04*.
6. **Diverse ethnic groups are afflicted, and global distribution is likely, with occurrences in African Americans, Native Alaskans, Japanese persons, mainland Chinese persons, Hispanics, Subcontinental Indians, Turks, and Arabs.**

Prognosis

SEVERITY OF INFLAMMATION

1. **Laboratory indices**
   ■ **Serum aspartate aminotransferase (AST), alanine aminotransferase (ALT), and γ-globulin levels are most useful in assessing the severity of inflammatory activity.**
   ■ The estimated 3-year mortality is 50% and the 10-year mortality is 90% if the serum AST/ALT level is at least 10-fold greater than the ULN or at least 5-fold greater than the ULN and the serum γ-globulin level is at least twice the ULN.
   ■ The 10-year mortality rate is 10% and the frequency of cirrhosis is low (49% after 15 years) if laboratory abnormalities are less severe at presentation.

- Spontaneous resolution occurs in 13% to 20% regardless of disease activity.
- Untreated patients with severe disease who survive the first 2 years of illness survive long term but commonly have inactive cirrhosis (41%).
- Laboratory indices of inflammatory activity can fluctuate spontaneously from mild to severe.
- Cytopenia at presentation, especially thrombocytopenia, is indicative of cirrhosis.

2. **Histologic indices**
   - Interface hepatitis is associated with excellent 5-year survival and a 17% frequency of progression to cirrhosis.
   - **Bridging necrosis or multilobular (confluent) necrosis is associated with a 5-year mortality of 45% and a frequency of cirrhosis of 82% at 5 years.**
   - Cirrhosis at presentation is associated with a 5-year mortality of 58%.
   - Esophageal varices develop in 54% of patients with cirrhosis, and death from hemorrhage occurs in 20% of patients with varices.
   - Histologic patterns of inflammatory activity can undergo spontaneous transitions from portal hepatitis to confluent necrosis, with no "safe" stable pattern of mild disease.
   - Centrilobular necrosis is an unusual acute severe manifestation that can transition to interface hepatitis.
   - Isolated bile duct changes are probably coincidental with exuberant inflammatory activity and are typically transient, without diagnostic or therapeutic relevance.

3. **Clinical indices**
   - Ascites or hepatic encephalopathy at presentation indicates advanced severe disease and a poor prognosis.
   - An **acute severe (fulminant) presentation is possible and life-threatening if the disease is not diagnosed and treated promptly with corticosteroids.**
   - At presentation, 25% to 34% of patients are asymptomatic, but later symptoms in 26% to 70% and the initial asymptomatic state do not preclude aggressive disease.
   - Physical examination is normal in 25% and does not exclude cirrhosis or severe disease.
   - A Model of End-stage Liver Disease (MELD) score of at least 12 points at presentation identifies 97% of patients in whom corticosteroid therapy will fail and has 68% specificity for treatment failure.
   - Concurrent inflammatory bowel disease is associated with cholangiographic changes of PSC in 41% and a poor response to corticosteroids.
   - "Autoimmune sclerosing cholangitis" in 50% of children is associated with shortened transplant-free survival despite treatment.

GENETIC STATUS

1. **HLA *DRB1*03* in white North American and northern European patients are associated with early age of onset, severe inflammatory activity, less responsiveness to therapy, and greater frequency of liver transplantation than in patients with HLA *DRB1*04*.**
2. **HLA *DRB1*04* in white North American and northern European patients is associated with late age of onset, female predominance, frequent concurrent immune diseases, and better response to therapy than in patients with HLA *DRB1*03*.**
3. *DRB1*0301* (86% versus 45%) and *DRB1*0301–DRB3*0101* (79% versus 42%) are more common in white North American and northern European patients in whom corticosteroid treatment fails.
4. *DRB1*0401* and *DRB1*0401–DRB4*0103* are associated with a lower frequency of death from liver failure or need for transplantation than other alleles (0% versus 37%) in white North American and northern European patients.

5. Non-*DRB1*0401 DRB1*04* alleles occur more commonly in women than in men with type 1 autoimmune hepatitis (15% versus 0%), a finding suggesting that women react to greater diversity of autoantigens than men.
6. Null allotypes at the complement *C4A* and *C4B* locus are present in 90% of patients with early-onset disease.

GENDER EFFECTS

1. Women have greater susceptibility to autoimmune hepatitis than do men (3.6:1).
2. Women with autoimmune hepatitis have higher frequencies of concurrent immune disease (34% versus 17%) and HLA *DRB1*04* (49% versus 24%) than do men.
3. **Men and women respond similarly to therapy and have the same long-term outcome.**
4. Treatment failure occurs more commonly in men only if they have HLA *DRB1*03* and in women who have HLA *DRB1*04* (25% versus 4%).
5. Women develop a type 1 cytokine response to an infectious agent or antigen more commonly than do men, and this response may increase women's propensity for autoimmune disease.
6. Women with autoimmune liver disease may have an acquired preferential X chromosome loss that weakens their ability to maintain self-tolerance because genes crucial for immune tolerance are located on the X chromosome (as described in PBC).

AGE EFFECTS

1. Of adults with autoimmune hepatitis, 20% develop the disease at age 60 years or more.
2. Patients aged 60 years or more have a greater degree of hepatic fibrosis at presentation than do adults up to 30 years of age, a higher frequency of ascites, and more cirrhosis (33% versus 10%).
3. An advanced stage at presentation suggests that elderly patients have indolent and unsuspected aggressive disease and "underdiagnosis."
4. HLA *DRB1*04* is more frequent in white North American and northern European patients aged 60 years or more than in patients aged up to 30 years (47% versus 13%), and HLA *DRB1*03* is more common in adult patients aged up to 30 years than in those 60 years old or older (58% versus 23%).
5. Elderly patients aged 60 years or more respond more quickly to corticosteroid therapy than do adults less than 40 years old because 18% enter remission within 6 months (versus 2%) and 94% within 24 months (versus 64%).
6. Genetic susceptibilities to different antigenic triggers may distinguish elderly from young adult patients.
7. Differences in the vigor of the immune response ("immunosenescence" in the elderly) may affect the response to treatment.
8. **Treatment responses are similar between elderly and young adults, and advanced age does not limit treatment or preclude successful liver transplantation.**

Clinical Features

1. Easy fatigability most common symptom (85%); weight loss unusual; intense pruritus against diagnosis
2. Hepatomegaly (78%) and jaundice (69%) most common physical findings of severe or advanced disease
3. Hyperbilirubinemia in 83%, but serum level usually less than threefold ULN (54%)

4. Serum alkaline phosphatase level frequently increased (81%), but usually less than twofold ULN (67%); values higher than fourfold ULN unusual (10%) and suggestive of alternative or variant diagnosis
5. Polyclonal hypergammaglobulinemia typical, with predominance of IgG fraction
6. Acute severe (fulminant) onset possible as part of new-onset disease or spontaneous exacerbation of previously unrecognized chronic disease
7. Diverse nonspecific serologic findings common, including antibodies to bacteria (*Escherichia coli, Bacteroides,* and *Salmonella*) and viruses (measles, rubella, and cytomegalovirus)
8. Concurrent immune diseases frequent (38%), especially autoimmune thyroiditis, synovitis, and ulcerative colitis
9. SMA, ANA, and anti-LKM1 required for the diagnosis, but other autoantibodies possible

PROMISING NEW AUTOANTIBODIES

1. **Antibodies to soluble liver antigen (anti-SLA)**
   - Highly specific for autoimmune hepatitis (99%), but limited sensitivity
   - Global distribution (Japan, Brazil, Germany, and United States)
   - **Possible surrogate markers for genetic propensity for severe disease and relapse after drug withdrawal**
   - Commercial ELISA available based on recombinant antigen
2. **Antibodies to asialoglycoprotein receptor (anti-ASGPR)**
   - Transmembrane glycoprotein on hepatocyte surface
   - Present in 88% of autoimmune hepatitis regardless of type
   - Associated with higher frequency of relapse after corticosteroid withdrawal
   - **Correlated with inflammatory activity within liver tissue and useful in defining end points of therapy**
   - Commercial assay in development
3. **Antibodies to actin (anti-actin)**
   - Directed against polymerized F-actin
   - Present in 74% with type 1 autoimmune hepatitis and 86% with SMA
   - Associated with early age of onset, HLA B8 and *DRB1*03*, and death from liver failure or need for liver transplantation (19% versus 0%) compared with patients with ANA
   - **Possible defining characteristic of subgroup with poor outcome, but prognostic value assay dependent**
   - Commercial ELISA available, but best assay for diagnosis and prognosis not standardized
4. **Antibodies to liver cytosol type 1 (anti-LC1)**
   - Directed against foraminotransferase cyclodeaminase
   - Mainly in patients up to 20 years old (rare in patients older than 40 years)
   - Commonly associated with anti-LKM1 (32%)
   - Serum levels fluctuating with disease activity and response to treatment
   - Associated with frequent concurrent immune diseases, rapid progression to cirrhosis, and severe inflammation
   - Possibly useful as markers of severity and/or residual liver inflammation in type 2 autoimmune hepatitis
   - No commercial assay available
5. **Other antibodies investigated as prognostic markers**
   - *Anti-chromatin* in 39%; more common in men than women; more common during active than inactive disease; more frequent in patients who relapse

- *Antibodies to double-stranded (ds) DNA* present in 34% to 64% of ANA-positive patients by ELISA and in 23% by IIF; ELISA defining subgroup of ANA-positive patients who deteriorate during corticosteroid therapy more commonly than seronegative patients
- *Antibodies against cyclic citrullinated peptides* in 11%; associated with a higher frequency of rheumatoid arthritis, greater occurrence of histologic cirrhosis at presentation, and death from hepatic failure

Treatment

INDICATIONS (Table 5.5)

1. **Treatment is indicated in all patients with active liver inflammation.** The degree of hepatic dysfunction as assessed by increased international normalized ratio (INR), hypoalbuminemia, or hyperbilirubinemia does not compel therapy in the absence of inflammatory activity.
2. Disease severity, as assessed by laboratory tests of liver inflammation (serum AST/ALT and γ-globulin levels) and histologic patterns of liver injury (interface hepatitis, bridging necrosis, multilobular necrosis, active cirrhosis), influences the urgency of treatment.
3. Asymptomatic mild disease can have clinically unsuspected aggressive intervals and rapid response to treatment.
4. **Untreated asymptomatic patients with mild disease have poorer 10-year survival than do treated patients with severe disease (67% versus 98%) and warrant therapy.**

TREATMENT REGIMENS (Table 5.6)

1. **Prednisone alone or a lower dose of prednisone plus azathioprine is effective in all forms of autoimmune hepatitis; the combination regimen is preferred because of a lower risk of corticosteroid-related side effects (10% versus 44%) (Fig. 5.5).**
2. The combination regimen with azathioprine requires determinations of leukocyte and platelet counts at regular intervals (every 1 to 3 months) throughout the treatment period to monitor for bone marrow toxicity.

TABLE 5.5 ■ **Treatment indications**

Urgent	Nonurgent	Not indicated
Incapacitating symptoms or acute severe (fulminant) onset	Mild or no symptoms	No symptoms
AST/ALT ≥10-fold ULN	AST/ALT <10-fold ULN and γ-globulin <2-fold ULN	Portal hepatitis
AST/ALT >5-fold ULN and γ-globulin ≥2-fold ULN	Interface hepatitis	Inactive cirrhosis
Bridging necrosis	Active cirrhosis	Decompensated inactive cirrhosis with intractable ascites, hepatic encephalopathy, and/or variceal bleeding
Multilobular necrosis		

ALT, serum alanine aminotransferase level; AST, serum aspartate aminotransferase level; ULN, upper limit of the normal range.

TABLE 5.6 ■ Standard treatment regimens

Regimens	Drugs		Relative contraindications
Prednisone and azathioprine	Prednisone (daily dose): 30 mg × 1 wk 20 mg × 1 wk 15 mg × 2 wk 10 mg maintenance until end point	Azathioprine (daily dose): 50 mg maintenance until end point	Severe cytopenia Thiopurine methyltransferase deficiency Pregnancy Active neoplasm
Prednisone only	60 mg × 1 wk 40 mg × 1 wk 30 mg × 2 wk 20 mg maintenance	None	Obesity Osteopenia Emotional instability Brittle diabetes mellitus Labile hypertension Postmenopausal state Acne

3. Follow-up assessments should occur every 6 months during treatment, or sooner if symptoms of liver failure or drug intolerance are noted.
4. **No findings at presentation preclude a satisfactory response to treatment**; ascites and encephalopathy identify patients with a poor prognosis but do not contraindicate therapy.
5. Patients with multilobular necrosis on histologic examination who fail to resolve at least one laboratory parameter or improve pretreatment hyperbilirubinemia during a 2-week treatment period have high immediate mortality; they should be evaluated for liver transplantation if features of decompensation are present.
6. Patients who improve by the foregoing parameters have an excellent immediate survival; their drug treatment should be continued until the end point is reached (see later).
7. **In Europe, prednisolone in an equivalent dose is preferred over prednisone.**

DRUG ACTIONS

1. Prednisolone is the active metabolite of prednisone and is responsible for the beneficial and toxic effects.
   ■ Conversion of prednisone to prednisolone is reduced in cirrhosis, but not sufficiently to affect treatment response and to warrant administration of prednisolone.
   ■ Prednisolone complexes with the glucocorticoid receptor in cytosol, and the complex translocates to the nucleus.
   ■ The prednisolone–glucocorticoid receptor complex interacts with the 5'-untranslated promoter region of glucocorticoid response genes and inhibits cytokine gene expression that affects type 1 and type 2 cytokine pathways.
   ■ Blanket immunosuppression is achieved, but the short biologic half-life justifies daily administration.
   ■ Side effects are associated with the level of unbound prednisolone and are increased by hypoalbuminemia (decreased binding sites) and hyperbilirubinemia (competitive inhibition of binding).
2. 6-Thioguanines are the active metabolites of azathioprine and complement the actions of prednisolone.
   ■ Azathioprine is converted to 6-mercaptopurine, which is converted to 6-thioguanines by hypoxanthine guanine phosphoribosyl transferase.

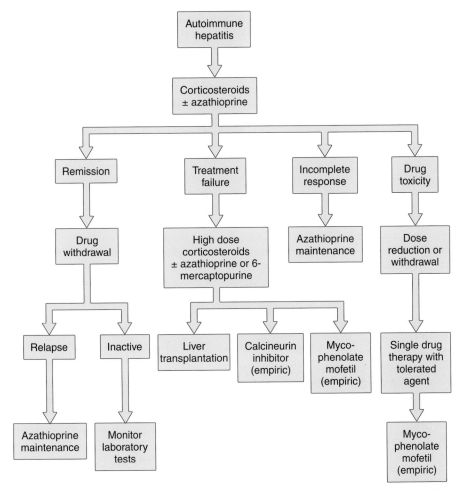

Fig. 5.5 Treatment algorithm for autoimmune hepatitis. The diagnosis of autoimmune hepatitis justifies treatment with prednisone alone or a lower dose in combination with azathioprine (corticosteroids with or without azathioprine). Treatment is continued until remission, treatment failure, incomplete response, or drug toxicity. Depending on treatment response, additional treatment may be necessary, including the empiric use of nonstandard salvage therapies for treatment failure or drug toxicity (calcineurin inhibitors or mycophenolate mofetil). Mycophenolate mofetil has been effective for patients with azathioprine intolerance. Liver transplantation is the most effective salvage therapy and should not be deferred in decompensated patients.

- 6-Thioguanines interfere with purine nucleotide synthesis and impair proliferation of activated T and B lymphocytes.
- 6-Thioguanines selectively inhibit inflammatory gene expression in activated T lymphocytes and induce T-cell apoptosis.
- Thiopurine methyltransferase mediates elimination of 6-mercaptopurine and affects the therapeutic efficacy and toxicity of 6-thioguanines.
- Genes encoding thiopurine methyltransferase are highly polymorphic, and *TPMT*3A* or *TPMT*3B* encodes lower enzyme activities than do other polymorphisms.

- A homozygous deficiency of thiopurine methyltransferase is present in 0.3% of the normal population; a heterozygous (intermediate) deficiency is present in 11% of the normal population.
- Deficiency in enzyme activity retards the inactivation of azathioprine, favors production of 6-thioguanines, increases the potency of a given dose, and/or enhances toxicity.
- No correlation exists between genotypic and phenotypic determinations of thiopurine methyltransferase activity and the frequency of side effects in autoimmune hepatitis treated with azathioprine (50 to 150 mg daily).

DRUG-RELATED SIDE EFFECTS

1. Corticosteroid-induced complications include cosmetic (facial rounding, dorsal hump formation, striae, weight gain, acne, alopecia, facial hirsutism), metabolic (diabetes, obesity, hyperlipidemia, hypertension), skeletal (osteopenia, vertebral compression, avascular necrosis), psychiatric (emotional instability, psychosis), and somatic (cataract formation, pancreatitis, opportunistic infection, malignant disease) changes.
2. Corticosteroid-induced cosmetic changes are most common (80% after 2 years of therapy).
3. Severe corticosteroid-induced side effects are infrequent and usually require at least 18 months of treatment with prednisone (20 mg daily).
4. Severe corticosteroid-induced side effects warrant premature discontinuation of treatment in 13% (mainly because of intolerable obesity, cosmetic changes, or osteoporosis).
5. Postmenopausal women are at risk for vertebral compression, especially during retreatment after relapse.
6. Regular weight-bearing exercise, calcium (1 to 1.5 g/day), and vitamin D_3 (400 U/week) comprise an appropriate adjuvant program for preservation of bone density in all adult patients; alendronate (70 mg once each week) is indicated for progressive osteopenia.
7. Azathioprine-induced complications include cholestatic hepatotoxicity, nausea, emesis, rash, opportunistic infection, pancreatitis, and severe myelosuppression in up to 10% treated with 50 mg daily; side effects are frequently reversible with dose reduction or termination of therapy.
8. Cytopenia is most common side effect of azathioprine; the most dire consequence is bone marrow failure; the frequency of cytopenia is 46%; severe hematologic abnormalities warrant drug withdrawal in 6%.
9. Azathioprine is a category D drug for pregnancy; it is a nonessential drug for disease control during pregnancy.
10. Oncogenicity is a theoretical complication of azathioprine therapy; the risk of extrahepatic malignancy is 1.4-fold that of age- and sex-matched normal populations; no predominant malignant cell type is reported.
11. Complications of treatment (weight gain, cushingoid appearance, fluid retention, cytopenia, worsening liver tests) may be difficult to distinguish from complications of liver disease (cytopenia is most commonly associated with cirrhosis).
12. **Thiopurine methyltransferase activity should be determined in patients with pretreatment cytopenia or cytopenia developing during azathioprine treatment.**

TREATMENT END POINTS (Table 5.7)

1. Standard therapy is continued until remission, treatment failure, incomplete response, or drug toxicity (see Fig. 5.5).
2. Histologic resolution lags behind clinical and laboratory resolution by 3 to 6 months; therapy must be extended to accommodate this lag.

TABLE 5.7 ■ **Standard treatment end points**

Feature	Remission	Treatment failure	Incomplete response	Drug toxicity
Definition	Ideal end point: no symptoms, normal liver tests, normal liver tissue Satisfactory end point: no symptoms, AST/ALT ≤2-fold ULN, other tests normal, no interface hepatitis	Increase AST/ALT and/or bilirubin >67% and/or worse histologic activity	Improvement but insufficient to satisfy remission criteria after 3 yr	Intolerable side effects, vertebral compression or progressive cytopenia
Occurrence	77% within 2 yr (age-related)	9%	13%	13%
Action	Gradual drug withdrawal over 6 wk	Prednisone 60 mg daily or prednisone 30 mg and azathioprine 150 mg daily	Long-term treatment (low-dose prednisone or indefinite azathioprine)	Dose reduction or elimination of offending agent Continued therapy with tolerated agent
Outcome	Relapse in 50% within 6 mo or sustained remission	Gradual dose reduction to maintenance levels Clinical and laboratory improvement in 70% Histologic improvement in 20% Indefinite therapy	Indefinite therapy	Indefinite therapy with single tolerated drug or low-dose offending agent

ALT, serum alanine aminotransferase level; AST, serum aspartate aminotransferase level; ULN, upper limit of the normal range.

3. **Liver biopsy examination is necessary before drug withdrawal establish remission**; significant residual inflammatory activity occurs in 55% of patients with normal laboratory study results.
4. The degree of histologic improvement during therapy influences relapse frequency:
   ■ Reversion to normal liver architecture is associated with a 20% frequency of relapse.
   ■ Improvement to portal hepatitis is associated with a 50% frequency of relapse.
   ■ Progression to cirrhosis during therapy or persistence of interface hepatitis is associated with a 100% frequency of relapse.
   ■ Residual portal plasma cells are associated with an increased frequency of relapse (31% versus 7%); the positive predictive value for relapse of 92% is counterbalanced by a sensitivity for relapse of 31%.
5. **The ideal treatment end point is defined by complete resolution of symptoms, normalization of all liver injury test results (serum AST/ALT, bilirubin, and γ-globulin levels), and reversion of hepatic architecture to normal.** This ideal result is possible in only 40%; it does not preclude relapse after drug withdrawal, and it can result in serious side effects if it is relentlessly pursued.
6. **A satisfactory treatment end point is defined by improvement in the serum AST/ALT level to less than twice ULN, normalization of the serum bilirubin and γ-globulin concentrations, and disappearance of interface hepatitis from the liver tissue.** A satisfactory end point achievable in most patients; it is associated with reduction or prevention of hepatic fibrosis, improved long-term survival, and sustainable long-term remission without medication in some cases.

TABLE 5.8 ■ **Withdrawal schedule after remission**

Weeks after remission	Combination regimen		Single-drug regimen
	Prednisone (mg/day)	Azathioprine (mg/day)	Prednisone (mg/day)
1	7.5	50	15
2	7.5	50	10
3	5	50	5
4	5	25	5
5	2.5	25	2.5
6	2.5	25	2.5
Thereafter	None	None	None

7. Corticosteroid withdrawal after an ideal or satisfactory end point is gradual over a 6-week period after the treatment end point (Table 5.8). Laboratory tests (serum AST/ALT, bilirubin, and γ-globulin levels) should be performed every 3 weeks during treatment withdrawal and every 3 weeks thereafter for 3 months. Tests should then be performed every 6 months for 1 year after remission and then at annual intervals if remission is sustained.

TREATMENT RESULTS

1. **Remission (see Fig. 5.5)**
   - 77% achieving ideal or satisfactory end point within 24 months
   - Average duration of treatment to an ideal or satisfactory response: 22 months
   - Rapidity of response affected by age (94% of patients aged 60 years or more achieving an ideal or satisfactory end point within 24 months, whereas only 64% of adult patients aged less than 40 years responding within this interval)
   - Sustained remission after initial treatment in 21% with long-term follow-up
2. **Relapse after drug withdrawal (see Fig. 5.5)**
   - Occurring in 50% within 6 months and in 70% to 86% within 3 years
   - Defined by recrudescence of symptoms, with an increase in serum AST/ALT level at least threefold ULN or reappearance of interface hepatitis
   - Most common manifestation a serum AST/ALT level at least threefold ULN (liver biopsy not needed)
   - Reinstitution of original treatment inducing another remission, but relapse commonly recurring after termination of therapy, with possible disease progression
   - Repeated treatment and relapse associated with increasing cumulative frequency of treatment-related side effects (70% or more), progression to cirrhosis (38%), and death from liver failure or requirement for liver transplantation (20%)
   - **Long-term maintenance therapy with azathioprine (2 mg/kg daily) justified after the first relapse**
   - Indefinite low-dose prednisone (up to 10 mg daily; median dose, 7.5 mg daily) warranted if patient has azathioprine intolerance (Table 5.9)
   - Sustained inactive disease possible after relapse and withdrawal of maintenance therapy; withdrawal only if stable inactive disease for at least 1 year on treatment

TABLE 5.9 ■ **Long-term treatment regimens after multiple relapses**

Features	Low-dose prednisone	Azathioprine only
Indication	Clinical and laboratory remission after previous relapse and repeat standard therapy	Clinical and laboratory remission after previous relapse and repeat standard therapy
Schedule	Reduce prednisone dose by 2.5 mg/mo until lowest level to prevent symptoms and maintain AST <3-fold ULN (no interface hepatitis) Gradual azathioprine withdrawal	Increase azathioprine to 2 mg/kg daily Gradual prednisone withdrawal
Outcome	Improved steroid-related side effects, 85% New side effects, 0% Liver-related mortality, 9%	Weight loss, 43% Hypertension improved, 13% Liver-related mortality, 1%
Limitations	Possible long-term steroid-related complication	Corticosteroid withdrawal arthralgias, 53% Lethargy, 10% Malignancy, 7% Myelosuppression, 6% Uncertain teratogenicity

AST, serum aspartate aminotransferase level; ULN, upper limit of the normal.

3. **Treatment failure (see Fig. 5.5)**
   - Occurring in 9% during initial treatment
   - Connoting deterioration despite adherence with therapy
   - Warranting treatment with high-dose prednisone alone (60 mg daily) or prednisone (30 mg daily) in conjunction with azathioprine (150 mg daily)
   - High-dose regimen inducing clinical and biochemical improvement in 70% within 2 years
   - Histologic resolution in only 20%
   - Indefinite therapy frequently necessary, with risk of side effects and liver failure
   - Liver transplantation justified at the first sign of decompensation (usually ascites)
   - Reconfirmation of original diagnosis necessary by excluding viral infection, variant syndrome of PSC or PBC, nonalcoholic (corticosteroid-related) fatty liver disease, and drug-induced liver disease

4. **Incomplete response (see Fig. 5.5)**
   - Occurring in 13% during initial treatment
   - Connoting improvement insufficient to satisfy remission criteria after 3 years
   - Warranting empirical trial with low-dose prednisone (up to 10 mg daily) or long-term azathioprine (2 mg/kg daily) to maintain serum AST/ALT level less than threefold ULN and no interface hepatitis

5. **Survival**
   - 10-year life expectancies for treated patients with and without cirrhosis at presentation of 89% and 90%, respectively; overall 10-year survival of 93%
   - **Survival of treated patients comparable to that of an age- and sex-matched normal cohort from the same geographic region (94% over 10 years)**
   - Treatment response unaltered by histologic cirrhosis

6. **Hepatocellular carcinoma**
   - Occurring in 0.5% of patients screened for viral infection and followed long term
   - 10-year probability of developing hepatocellular carcinoma of 2.9%

- Developing only in patients with cirrhosis for at least 10 years
- **Risk factors in white North American patients: male gender, portal hypertension with ascites, varices, or thrombocytopenia, immunosuppressive treatment for at least 3 years, and cirrhosis of at least 10 years' duration**
- Ultrasonography at 6-month intervals recommended for individuals with risk factors

LIVER TRANSPLANTATION (see Fig. 5.5)

1. Transplantation is effective in decompensated patients in whom corticosteroid therapy has failed.
2. Autoantibodies and hypergammaglobulinemia disappear by 2 years after transplantation.
3. Five-year patient survival and graft survival range from 83% to 92%; actuarial 10-year survival is 75%.
4. **Disease recurs in 12% to 46%, usually 1 to 8 years after transplantation (median, 2 years) and mainly in recipients who are inadequately immunosuppressed.**
5. Frequency of recurrence increases from 12% at 1 year to 36% after 5 years; progression to cirrhosis and graft failure is possible; asymptomatic histologic recurrence may precede clinical recurrence by 1 to 5 years.
6. Recurrence responds to adjustments in immunosuppressive regimen or reintroduction of corticosteroids; graft survival and patient survival after recurrence range from 78% to 89%; refractory recurrence may require another calcineurin inhibitor, rapamycin, or retransplantation.
7. HLA *DRB1*03* or *DRB1*04* is more common in recipients with recurrence than in recipients without recurrence (100% versus 40%).
8. The frequency of acute (81% versus 47%), steroid-resistant (38% versus 13%), and chronic (11% versus 2%) graft rejection is higher in autoimmune hepatitis than in alcoholic liver disease.
9. Gradual corticosteroid withdrawal is possible in 68%, and complications of hypercholesterolemia, hypertension, and diabetes are decreased; corticosteroid withdrawal is commonly deferred until after the first year.
10. **De novo autoimmune hepatitis occurs in 3% to 5% of adult and pediatric recipients who undergo transplantation for non-autoimmune disease.**
11. Recurrent and de novo autoimmune hepatitis must be considered in all cases of graft dysfunction.

PROMISING ALTERNATIVE DRUGS (Table 5.10)

1. **Cyclosporine (see Fig. 5.5)**
   a. This calcineurin inhibitor reduces transcription of IL-2, impairs signal transduction from engaged T-cell antigen receptor, and dampens lymphocyte proliferation.
   b. Empirical use as salvage therapy (5 to 6 mg/kg daily) in patients refractory to or intolerant of corticosteroids is effective within 1 year (small numbers).
   c. Relapse is usual after drug withdrawal, and cyclosporine treatment may be indefinite.
   d. Long-term consequences, including renal insufficiency, hypertension, and malignancy, are unknown; the target population, dosing schedule, and monitoring strategy are undefined.
   e. Representative clinical experiences:
      - Pediatric: Serum ALT levels returned to normal in 80% after 6 months and in 100% after 1 year; growth dynamics improved; and no side effects occurred when used as first-line therapy for 6 months followed by conventional corticosteroid treatment.

TABLE 5.10 ■ **Promising immunosuppressive drugs**

Drug	Dose	Actions and uses
Cyclosporine	5–6 mg/kg daily	Calcineurin inhibitor that reduces transcription of IL-2, impairs signal transduction from engaged T-cell antigen receptor, and dampens lymphocyte proliferation Empiric use as salvage therapy and as front-line therapy in treatment trials with children and adults
Tacrolimus	3 mg twice daily	Calcineurin inhibitor that prevents dephosphorylation of transcription factors for cytokine production and limits expression of IL-2 receptors Inhibits proliferation of activated T lymphocytes Small open-label trial achieved biochemical improvement at modest risk
Mycophenolate mofetil	1 g twice daily	Inhibits inosine monophosphate dehydrogenase and depletes guanine nucleotides necessary for DNA synthesis and lymphocyte proliferation Effective salvage therapy in small open-label trial Substitute for azathioprine if thiopurine methyltransferase deficiency
6-Mercaptopurine	1.5 mg/kg daily	Bypasses conversion step from azathioprine Converted directly to 6-thioguanines by enzyme-dependent pathway Anecdotal use in treatment failure and azathioprine intolerance
Budesonide	3 mg three times daily	Second-generation corticosteroid with high first-pass hepatic clearance Low systemic availability and metabolites lack glucocorticoid activity Results of randomized clinical trial have been published, and budesonide with azathioprine is superior to prednisone with azathioprine Ineffective as prednisone-sparing agent for treatment-dependent patients

IL, interleukin.

■ Adult: Mean serum AST and ALT levels decreased, and the histologic activity index improved in the absence of side effects in 19 children and adults treated for 26 weeks as front-line or salvage therapy.
   f. This agent is not incorporated into the conventional treatment algorithm as first-line or salvage therapy.
2. **Tacrolimus (see Fig. 5.5)**
   ■ This calcineurin inhibitor prevents dephosphorylation of transcription factors for cytokine production and limits expression of IL-2 receptors, thereby impairing proliferation of activated T lymphocytes.
   ■ An open-label trial (3 mg twice daily for 3 months) reduced serum AST and ALT levels by 70% and 80%, respectively, in 21 patients with only modest changes in leukocyte and platelet counts and renal function.
   ■ This empirical salvage option is expensive and potentially toxic.
3. **Mycophenolate mofetil (see Fig. 5.5)**
   ■ This ester prodrug of mycophenolic acid acts as purine antagonist.
   ■ It impairs conversion of inosine monophosphate to xanthosine monophosphate by inhibiting inosine monophosphate dehydrogenase.
   ■ It depletes guanine nucleotides necessary for DNA synthesis and lymphocyte proliferation, decreases expression of IL-2 receptors, inhibits immunoglobulin production, and impairs function of adhesion molecules.

- Ten small experiences in patients intolerant of or refractory to conventional treatment showed improvement in 39% to 84% of patients and frequent ability to reduce the dose of or discontinue corticosteroids; drug intolerance or ineffectiveness was noted in 34% to 78%.
- Overall experience in four reports indicated that improvements of varying degrees can be achieved in 45% of treated patients.
- This agent is effective mainly in children with autoimmune hepatitis and normal bile ducts and in adults with intolerance to azathioprine; it is ineffective in PSC, autoimmune sclerosing cholangitis, and adults refractory to azathioprine treatment.
- The target population, optimal dosing schedule, safety profile, cost analysis, and monitoring regimen are unclear.

4. **6-Mercaptopurine (see Fig. 5.5)**
   - This agent bypasses the conversion step from azathioprine and is converted directly to 6-thioguanines.
   - 6-Thioguanine nucleotides interfere with DNA and RNA synthesis as purine antagonists.
   - Competing enzymatic pathways convert to inactive metabolites of 6-thiouric acid by xanthine oxidase or 6-methyl mercaptopurine by thiopurine methyltransferase.
   - Therapeutic efficacy and toxicity are affected by deficiency in thiopurine methyltransferase activity or drugs that inhibit xanthine oxidase (allopurinol).
   - It may be effective in patients unresponsive to azathioprine in combination with prednisone, for uncertain reasons.
   - Empirical use in treatment failure is at 25 mg/day, followed by a slow increase to 1.5 mg/kg/day.

5. **Budesonide**
   - This second-generation corticosteroid has high (90%) first-pass hepatic clearance, low systemic availability, and metabolites devoid of glucocorticoid activity.
   - It improved ALT and immunoglobulin levels in a small trial (6 to 8 mg daily for 6 to 10 weeks, and then at an individualized dose for up to 9 months), with low frequency of side effects.
   - Results of a randomized controlled trial in 203 treatment-naïve patients indicated more frequent normalization of ALT levels and lower frequency of corticosteroid-related side effects in patients treated with budesonide (3 mg three times daily) and azathioprine (1 to 2 mg/kg) for 6 months than in patients treated with a conventional corticosteroid regimen.
   - It is ineffective as salvage therapy for corticosteroid-dependent patients because disease worsened or drug intolerance developed, prednisone withdrawal symptoms were common, and extrahepatic immune manifestations were variably controlled.
   - It may be used as first-line therapy for mild disease or in patients at risk for corticosteroid-related complications, especially osteoporosis.
   - Side effects may relate to previous treatment with prednisone (altered pharmacokinetics) or cirrhosis and portosystemic shunting (impaired drug clearance).

6. **Other immunosuppressive agents**
   - Cyclophosphamide (1 to 1.5 mg/kg daily), methotrexate (7.5 mg per week), rapamycin, rituximab, intravenous immunoglobulin, deflazacort, ursodeoxycholic acid, 6-thioguanines, and various steroid pulse schedules have been used in isolated instances as salvage therapies.
   - The benefit-to-risk ratio is uncertain; rigorous clinical trials are necessary.

POTENTIAL SITE-SPECIFIC INVESTIGATIONAL THERAPIES

Numerous investigational therapies in various stages of development are summarized in Table 5.11.

TABLE 5.11 ■ **Site-specific investigational interventions**

Site-specific intervention	Putative actions	Precedents
Competing peptides	Blocks antigen-binding groove of class II MHC DR molecule and limits CD4 T-helper cell activation	Rheumatoid arthritis
Soluble cytotoxic T-lymphocyte antigen-4	Competes with CD28 of the CD4 T-helper cell for B7 ligands of antigen-presenting cell Blocks the second signal of immunocyte activation	Bone marrow recipients
T-cell vaccination	Eliminates disease-specific, liver-infiltrating, cytotoxic T-cell clone responsible for liver injury	Animal model
Oral tolerance	Suppresses type 1 cytokine response by selectively recruiting CD4 T cells that favor type 1 cytokine response (low-dose antigen) Induces CD4 T-cell anergy or apoptosis (high-dose antigen)	Multiple sclerosis, rheumatoid arthritis, diabetes, autoimmune thyroiditis
Cytokine manipulations	Modulates cytokine milieu by monoclonal antibodies or recombinant cytokines to counteract the type 1 cytokine response favoring cellular cytotoxicity	Inflammatory bowel disease, chronic hepatitis C
Human bone marrow mesenchymal stem cell infusion	Engrafts failed liver, differentiates into functioning hepatocytes, reduces oxidative stress, accelerates repopulation of native liver with normal hepatocytes	Immunodeficient mice with liver failure
T-regulatory (CD4+CD25+) cell adoptive transfer	Blunts actions and proliferation of autoreactive T cells through direct contact or modification of cytokines	Documented human deficiencies Cell culture source
Small inhibitory ribonucleic acids (siRNAs)	Synthesized to match sequences in target genes, promote cleavage of the gene product, and silence gene expression	Murine models of viral and fulminant hepatitis

MHC, major histocompatibilty complex.

FURTHER READING

Czaja AJ. Autoantibodies in autoimmune liver disease. *Adv Clin Chem* 2005; 40:127–164.

Czaja AJ. Autoimmune hepatitis. Part A: pathogenesis. *Expert Rev Gastroenterol Hepatol* 2007; 1:113–128.

Czaja AJ. Autoimmune hepatitis. Part B: diagnosis. *Expert Rev Gastroenterol Hepatol* 2007; 1:129–143.

Czaja AJ. Current and future treatments of autoimmune hepatitis. *Expert Rev Gastroenterol Hepatol* 2009; 3:269–291.

Czaja AJ. Emerging opportunities for site-specific molecular and cellular interventions in autoimmune hepatitis. *Dig Dis Sci* 2010; 55:2712–2726.

Czaja AJ. Features and consequences of untreated autoimmune hepatitis. *Liver Int* 2009; 29:816–823.

Czaja AJ. Genetic factors associated with the occurrence, clinical phenotype and outcome of autoimmune hepatitis. *Clin Gastroenterol Hepatol* 2008; 6:379–388.

Czaja AJ. Performance parameters of the diagnostic scoring systems for autoimmune hepatitis. *Hepatology* 2008; 48:1540–1548.

Czaja AJ. Rapidity of treatment response and outcome in type 1 autoimmune hepatitis. *J Hepatol* 2009; 51:161–167.

Czaja AJ. Safety issues in the management of autoimmune hepatitis. *Expert Opin Drug Saf* 2008; 7:319–333.

Czaja AJ. Special clinical challenges in autoimmune hepatitis: the elderly, males, pregnancy, mild disease, fulminant onset, and nonwhite patients. *Semin Liver Dis* 2009; 29:315–330.

Hennes EM, Zeniya M, Czaja AJ, et al. Simplified diagnostic criteria for autoimmune hepatitis. *Hepatology* 2008; 48:169–176.

Manns MP, Czaja AJ, Gorham JD, et al. Practice guidelines of the American Association for the Study of Liver Diseases: diagnosis and management of autoimmune hepatitis. *Hepatology* 2010; 51:2193–2213.

Montano-Loza A, Carpenter HA, Czaja AJ. Consequences of treatment withdrawal in type 1 autoimmune hepatitis. *Liver Int* 2007; 27:507–515.

Montano-Loza A, Carpenter HA, Czaja AJ. Improving the end point of corticosteroid therapy in type 1 autoimmune hepatitis to reduce the frequency of relapse. *Am J Gastroenterol* 2007; 102:1005–1012.

CHAPTER 6

Alcoholic liver disease

Janice H. Jou, MD ■ Anna Mae Diehl, MD

KEY POINTS

1   Alcoholic liver disease is one of the most prevalent forms of liver disease in the United States; worldwide, numerous epidemiologic studies have documented the correlation between per capita alcohol consumption and deaths from cirrhosis.

2   The risk of hepatotoxicity increases if a threshold level of alcohol consumption is exceeded, but even consistently high consumption infrequently causes cirrhosis. Variables affecting the development of cirrhosis include genetic polymorphisms of alcohol-metabolizing enzymes, gender differences, nutritional status, concomitant viral hepatitis, exposure to drugs or toxins, and immunologic factors.

3   Alcoholic liver disease encompasses a spectrum of histologic abnormalities: steatosis (fatty liver), steatohepatitis (alcoholic hepatitis), and cirrhosis (when fibrogenesis predominates). Steatosis and steatohepatitis are not necessarily progressive, and they may also develop in livers that are already cirrhotic.

4   Treatment of alcoholic liver disease includes discontinuation of alcohol consumption, treatment of extrahepatic complications of alcoholism (electrolyte abnormalities, withdrawal syndromes, cardiac dysfunction, poor nutrition, pancreatitis, gastropathy, infection), treatment of severe alcoholic hepatitis, and management of the sequelae of cirrhosis (ascites, portal hypertensive bleeding, and encephalopathy). Liver transplantation should be considered in the abstinent patient with decompensated cirrhosis.

Epidemiology

1. Alcohol is used by three fourths of Americans; alcohol abuse and dependence are common: approximately 10% of Americans who drink experience alcohol-related problems.

2. Alcoholic liver disease is one of the most serious medical consequences of long-term alcohol abuse and is the most common cause of cirrhosis in the Western world. In 2003, approximately 44% of deaths from cirrhosis in the United States were the result of alcoholic liver disease.

3. Alcohol abuse and dependence rates are higher for men (11%) than for women (4%) and are higher for nonblack than for black persons (nonblack men, 11%; nonblack women, 4%; black men, 8%; black women, 3%). Despite these differences, progression to cirrhosis occurs at a higher rate in the black population than in the nonblack population.

DIAGNOSIS OF ALCOHOL DEPENDENCE AND ABUSE

1. **Alcohol dependence** (three items required):
    ■ Alcoholic beverages often taken in larger amounts or over a longer period than intended
    ■ Persistent desire for alcohol or one or more unsuccessful attempts to cut down or control use
    ■ A great deal of time spent in obtaining alcohol, drinking it, or recovering from its effects
    ■ Recurrent use at times when alcohol use is physically hazardous (e.g., driving while intoxicated) or frequent intoxication or withdrawal symptoms despite major obligations at work, school, or home
    ■ Social, occupational, or recreational activities discontinued or reduced because of alcohol use
    ■ Continued alcohol use despite knowledge of having persistent or recurrent social, psychological, or physical problems that are caused or exacerbated by alcohol use
    ■ Marked tolerance: need for markedly increased amounts of alcohol (at least a 50% increase) to achieve intoxication or desired effect or a markedly diminished effect with continued use of the same amount
    ■ Characteristic withdrawal symptoms
    ■ Alcohol taken to relieve or avoid withdrawal symptoms
2. **Alcohol abuse** (one item required):
    ■ Continued use despite knowledge of having a persistent or recurrent social, occupational, psychological, or physical problem that is caused or exacerbated by the use of the substance
    ■ Recurrent use in situations in which its use is physically hazardous

SCREENING FOR ALCOHOL PROBLEMS

CAGE questionnaire:
a. Have you ever felt you ought to **cut down** on your drinking?
b. Have people **annoyed** you by criticizing your drinking?
c. Have you ever felt bad or **guilty** about your drinking?
d. Have you ever had a drink first thing in the morning (**eye opener**) to steady your nerves or get rid of a hangover?
   Two or more positive responses make up a positive test result.

Risk Factors for Alcoholic Liver Disease

1. In all societies studied, a positive correlation exists between average per capita consumption of alcohol and the frequency of cirrhosis.
2. The amount ingested and the duration of intake correlate with the incidence of alcohol-related liver disease.
3. Once a **threshold** level of consumption is exceeded (estimated to be **60 to 80 g/day for men** and **20 g/day for women**), the risk of hepatotoxicity increases dramatically.
4. Consistently high intake of alcohol uncommonly induces cirrhosis; less than 20% of men consuming more than two six-packs of beer per day for 10 years become cirrhotic.
5. Several advisory committees have recommended that alcohol consumption be limited no more than two drinks per day for healthy men and no more than one drink per day for healthy nonpregnant women.

SPECIFIC RISK FACTORS

1. **Gender:** Women experience more toxicity per dose than men, but this cannot be explained solely by differences in body composition or alcohol distribution. Gastric mucosal alcohol dehydrogenase activity is lower in women than in men; this may permit greater hepatic metabolism of ingested alcohol in women.
2. **Genetic variability in alcohol-metabolizing enzymes:** Polymorphisms of the **alcohol dehydrogenase** and **aldehyde dehydrogenase** enzymes seem to protect certain persons from ethanol toxicity. For example, Asians frequently inherit a "slow" aldehyde dehydrogenase isoenzyme, thereby increasing serum levels of acetaldehyde; this causes flushing, nausea, and dysphoria (disulfiram-like reaction) and may explain why habitual alcohol use and alcoholic liver disease are rare in Asians.
3. **Nutrition:** Ethanol interferes with intestinal absorption and storage of nutrients and reduces appetite for nonalcoholic sources of calories; this may result in deficiencies of protein, vitamins, and minerals.
4. **Presence of infections with hepatotropic viruses and other chronic liver diseases:** Acute and chronic hepatitis B or C accelerate the progression of alcoholic liver disease. Fatty liver disease related to obesity and/or insulin resistance (i.e., nonalcoholic fatty liver disease) can also coexist with alcoholic liver disease, and the two may combine to cause more serious liver damage than would occur if either disease was present alone.
5. **Concurrent exposure to drugs or toxins:** Long-term consumption of alcohol induces the activity of microsomal enzymes and thus potentiates the metabolism of drugs, solvents, and xenobiotics. For example, therapeutic doses of acetaminophen can cause severe hepatic damage in alcoholic individuals; similarly, tolbutamide, isoniazid, and industrial solvents accelerate alcoholic liver disease.
6. **Immunologic derangements:** Alcoholic liver disease is modulated by alterations in the cellular immune system; these include increased reactivity of T and B cells and increased expression of major histocompatibility complex (MHC) class I and class II DR antigens. Increased levels of the immune modulatory cytokines tumor necrosis factor (TNF), interleukin-1, and interleukin-6 are also seen. Alterations of the humoral immune system include increased levels of circulating immunoglobulins, the presence of autoantibodies (against nuclear, smooth muscle, liver cell membrane, liver-specific proteins, and alcoholic hyaline antigens), and the development of antibodies against neoantigens, proteins altered by reaction to acetaldehyde, malondialdehyde, and various radicals.
7. **Continued alcohol ingestion:** Patients who have developed some form of alcoholic liver injury and who persistently consume alcohol have a high risk of progression to cirrhosis. Abstinence, conversely, almost guarantees clinical improvement and, in many cases, regression of histologic injury.

Clinical Features

HISTORY

1. A history of habitual alcohol consumption is useful in suggesting alcohol as the cause of liver disease.
2. The type of alcoholic beverage consumed does not influence the likelihood of developing hepatotoxicity. The amount of ethanol (in grams) consumed in spirits, wine, or beer can be

estimated by multiplying the volume of the beverage in milliliters by the percentage of that beverage that is pure ethanol (spirits = 40%, wine = 12%, beer = 5%) times the specific gravity (0.8) of ethanol.

3. The CAGE questionnaire is sensitive for detecting alcohol abuse.

4. Accelerated disease progression is likely when alcohol abuse is accompanied by one or more of the following: viral hepatitis, acetaminophen intake, obesity, exposure to solvents, a family history of alcoholic liver disease, hemochromatosis, Wilson disease, or alpha-1 antitrypsin deficiency.

SYMPTOMS AND SIGNS OF ALCOHOLIC LIVER DISEASE

1. The clinical features of alcoholic liver disease are variable, ranging from a complete absence of symptoms to the florid features of advanced liver failure and portal hypertension. Because portal hypertension may occur in alcoholic hepatitis in the absence of established cirrhosis, alcoholic hepatitis can be difficult to distinguish from alcoholic cirrhosis without liver biopsy.

2. Patients can have one or more of the following: fever, weakness, anorexia, nausea and vomiting, malaise, confusion, sleep–wake cycle alterations, hepatomegaly, splenomegaly, cachexia, jaundice, spider telangiectasias, Dupuytren's contractures, gynecomastia, testicular atrophy, parotid/lacrimal gland enlargement, asterixis, Muercke's lines, white nails, and decreased libido; none of these features is specific or pathognomonic for alcoholic liver disease.

3. **Other sequelae of excess alcohol may be present, including alcoholic cardiomyopathy, pancreatitis and pancreatic insufficiency, and neurotoxicity.**

LABORATORY ABNORMALITIES (Table 6.1)

TABLE 6.1 ■ **Laboratory abnormalities in alcoholic liver disease**

Parameter	Result
AST/ALT ratio	>2 and both generally <300 U/L
Alkaline phosphatase	Increased to very high
Bilirubin	Normal to very high
Prothrombin time	Normal to very high
Albumin	Normal to decreased
Ammonia	Normal to high
Hematocrit	Typically mild macrocytic anemia; may be normal
White blood cell count	Leukemoid reactions can be associated with steatohepatitis
Platelets	Normal to decreased
Triglycerides	Typically increased, especially in active drinkers
Potassium, phosphate, magnesium	Often deficient in active drinkers
Glucose	Hyperglycemia common

ALT, alanine aminotransferase; AST, aspartate aminotransferase.

Diagnosis

1. The diagnosis of alcoholic liver disease is typically established clinically in patients with evidence of liver disease and history of significant alcohol use. Given the dearth of pathognomonic symptoms and signs of alcoholic liver disease, the elimination of other potential causes of liver injury is mandatory.
2. Imaging is not helpful in implicating alcohol as the cause of liver disease, although imaging for surveillance of hepatocellular carcinoma in the setting of alcoholic cirrhosis is recommended.
3. Liver biopsy is not necessary for the diagnosis of alcoholic liver disease, but it may be helpful in staging of fibrosis and in ascertaining whether other chronic liver diseases are contributing.
4. The histologic spectrum of alcoholic liver disease is summarized in the following section. These entities are not always discrete or necessarily progressive. In fact, all forms of alcohol-induced liver damage, including advanced fibrosis and cirrhosis, tend to regress gradually when alcohol use is discontinued.

Histology and Spectrum of Disease

FATTY LIVER (STEATOSIS)

This disorder is a consequence of alcohol oxidation. Fatty liver results when the intracellular redox potential and redox-sensitive nutrient metabolism are disturbed. An excessive accumulation of reducing equivalents favors metabolic pathways that lead to the accumulation of intracellular lipid. The excess lipid is stored in large droplets within individual hepatocytes. With abstinence, the normal redox potential is restored, the lipid is mobilized, and fatty liver resolves completely. Although reports have noted fatal outcomes and progression to cirrhosis, fatty liver is generally considered a benign, reversible condition (Fig. 6.1).

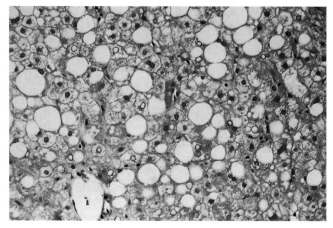

Fig. 6.1 Histopathology of fatty liver (steatosis) in alcoholic liver disease (H&E).

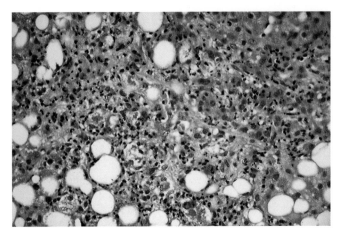

Fig. 6.2 Histopathology of alcoholic hepatitis. This histologic section shows macrovesicular steatosis, Mallory-Denk bodies, neutrophilic inflammation, and fibrosis (H&E).

ALCOHOLIC HEPATITIS

1. This disease is characterized by steatosis, hepatocellular necrosis, and acute inflammation. The steatosis is most pronounced in zone 3 of the hepatic acinus. Characteristic eosinophilic fibrillar material (Mallory's hyaline, or Mallory-Denk bodies) may be seen in swollen (ballooned) hepatocytes. These condensations of cytoskeletal intermediary filaments result from the formation of acetaldehyde-tubulin adducts. Although characteristic of alcoholic hepatitis, they are not specific and are also seen in other forms of hepatitis. Focally intense lobular infiltration of polymorphonuclear leukocytes distinguishes alcoholic hepatitis from other types of liver disease. In most other types of hepatitis, the inflammatory infiltrate is composed of mononuclear cells predominately localized around the portal triads.
2. Until relatively recently, alcoholic hepatitis was believed to be the prerequisite for alcoholic cirrhosis. However, it is now known that acetaldehyde may initiate fibrogenesis in the absence of demonstrable necroinflammation. Nonetheless, the severity of the clinical syndrome that occurs in some patients with alcoholic steatonecrosis and the potential of this lesion to progress to cirrhosis have made it the target of many therapeutic trials (Fig. 6.2).

CIRRHOSIS

1. Cirrhosis is considered the end stage of alcoholic liver disease. However, most patients with alcoholic fatty liver never progress to cirrhosis despite continued and prolonged consumption of alcohol. In others, fibrogenic damage ensues (Fig. 6.3). In some of these individuals, features of all three histologic "stages" coexist.
2. Alcoholic liver damage is typically associated with the deposition of collagen around the terminal hepatic vein (i.e., perivenular fibrosis) and along the sinusoids. This results in a "chicken wire" pattern of scarring that is rarely seen in other types of cirrhosis.
3. Long-term consumption of alcohol also impairs the regenerative response that is normally triggered by liver cell death. This results in small nodules of regenerating parenchyma. For this reason, **micronodular cirrhosis** is seen in actively drinking patients.
4. Abstinence releases the liver from the antiproliferative actions of alcohol and is associated with the development of **macronodular cirrhosis.**

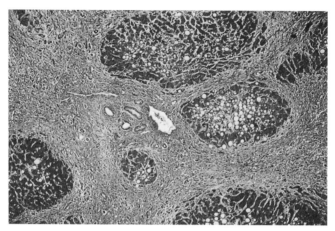

Fig. 6.3 Histopathology of alcoholic cirrhosis (H&E).

Indices of Liver Dysfunction for Alcoholic Hepatitis

Formulae for estimating the short-term prognosis of patients with alcoholic hepatitis:

1. **Composite Clinical Laboratory Index (CCLI):** Orrego et al, in 1978, defined a group of parameters that correlate with mortality in hospitalized patients with alcoholic hepatitis. Calculation of the CCLI permits a linear estimate of acute mortality (Table 6.2).

2. **Maddrey's discriminant function (DF):** Maddrey et al, in 1978, simplified the assessment of outcome of alcoholic liver disease by developing a DF:

$$DF = 4.6 \times (\text{the difference between the patient's and control prothrombin time}) + \text{serum bilirubin}$$

   ■ **Patients with a DF greater than 32 have a 50% mortality rate during their current hospitalization.** This index offers the advantage of few variables and easy computation (and therefore easy recall), but it is relatively imprecise.

3. **Model for End-stage Liver Disease (MELD):** The composite score uses a mathematical formula incorporating the patient's bilirubin, international normalized ratio, and creatinine. A MELD score greater than 18 portends a worse prognosis in alcoholic hepatitis.

4. **Early change in bilirubin level and Lille score:** A decrease in total bilirubin level at 7 days indicates improving liver function and predicts increased 6-month survival (82.8% versus 5.8%). If total bilirubin does not decrease at 7 days, the eventual response to steroids is low, and steroids can likely be discontinued. The Lille score is a composite score combining pretreatment parameters with response of bilirubin after 7 days of corticosteroids. A score greater than 0.45 indicates a lack of response to steroids and poor 6-month survival.

Treatment

GENERAL MEASURES

1. **Discontinuation of alcohol use and resumption of a nutritious diet remain the cornerstones of therapy for alcoholic patients even after cirrhosis has developed.**

TABLE 6.2 ■ **Composite clinical laboratory index for alcoholic hepatitis**

Parameter	Score
Hepatomegaly	1
Splenomegaly	1
Ascites	
1+	1
2+	2
3+	3
Encephalopathy	
Grade 1	1
Grade 2	2
Grade 3	3
Clinical bleeding	1
Spider telangiectasias	1
Palmar erythema	1
Collateral circulation	1
Peripheral edema	1
Anorexia	1
Weakness	1
AST >200 U/L	1
ALT (U/L)	
>100	1
>200	2
Alkaline phosphatase >80 IU/L	1
Albumin <2.59 g/dL	1
Prothrombin time (sec prolonged)	
<3	1
3–5	2
>5	3
Bilirubin (mg/dL)	
1.2–2	1
2–5	2
>5	3

Initial CCLI ≥13 correlates with severe liver disease and/or cirrhosis.
The following normalization rate (NR) is used to assess effectiveness of therapy and/or follow disease progression:
NR = (Change in CCLI/days to reach lowest score) ×100
Example: Day   1   4   12   20   28
*   Score   12   10   8.0   6.0   6.0*
NR = (12 – 6.0)/20 × 100 = 30
(The higher the NR, the faster the recovery.)

ALT, alanine aminotransferase; AST, aspartate aminotransferase; CCLI, Composite Clinical Laboratory Index.

2. Vigorous efforts to enroll patients in a detoxification program are justified.
3. Hospitalization benefits those patients with significant extrahepatic complications of alcoholism, notably electrolyte abnormalities, cardiac dysfunction, pancreatitis, hemorrhagic gastropathy, major alcohol withdrawal syndromes, and infection.
4. The risk of hepatocellular carcinoma is increased in any patient with cirrhosis but is especially high in alcoholic patients. Although it is recommended that serial ultrasound examinations with or without measurement of serum alpha fetoprotein levels may be helpful in detecting hepatocellular carcinoma at an early stage, little evidence indicates that such surveillance measures improve survival in patients with alcoholic liver disease. Chronic infection with hepatitis B or C virus also has a significant role in predisposition to liver cancer. The effect of antiviral therapy on the evolution of hepatocellular carcinoma in alcoholic patients with chronic viral infection is unknown.

SPECIFIC THERAPY FOR ALCOHOLIC HEPATITIS

1. **Corticosteroids:** Two prospectively randomized, placebo-controlled trials demonstrated that patients with clinically severe alcoholic hepatitis benefit from treatment with corticosteroids once serious infection and gastrointestinal bleeding have been controlled. A Cochrane systematic review found that mortality was decreased with the use of steroids with a DF greater than 32 or hepatic encephalopathy:
   - **A 4-week (28 day) course of prednisolone 40 mg daily more than halved the 1-month mortality rate of patients with Maddrey's DF greater than 32 or hepatic encephalopathy.**
   - These results were obtained in carefully selected patients who did not have clinically significant diabetes, pancreatitis, cancer, or viral hepatitis. The efficacy of corticosteroids in patients with these comorbid conditions and alcoholic hepatitis has not been established.
2. **Pentoxifylline (PTX):** This nonselective phosphodiesterase inhibitor is approved (at a dose of 400 mg orally three times daily) by the Food and Drug Administration for use as a rheologic agent. Its use for acute alcoholic hepatitis was initially suggested by the University of Southern California Liver Unit in 1991. Findings were reconfirmed in a randomized double-blind placebo-controlled trial from the same unit; 101 patients with a DF greater than 32 were enrolled (49 in the PTX arm versus 52 controls):
   - **PTX significantly reduced 4-week mortality to 24.5% from 46.1% (in the placebo group); it also reduced the frequency of hepatorenal syndrome from 34.6% (in placebo) to 8.2%.**
   - The mechanisms through which PTX exerted its effects are unclear but are thought to be mediated at least in part by modification of cytokine synthesis and/or effect (e.g., TNF).
   - These findings are significant and highly promising because the study was well designed, with good follow-up after discharge. Although further studies are needed, PTX should be included in the list of therapies (with corticosteroids) for the management of acute alcoholic hepatitis.
3. **Diet:** Ethanol interferes with intestinal absorption and storage of nutrients and reduces appetite for nonalcoholic sources of calories; this may result in deficiencies of protein, vitamins, and minerals. Such malnutrition correlates with mortality in patients with alcoholic liver disease.
   - Trials of supplemental amino acid therapy have yielded conflicting results.
   - Parenteral amino acids have been reported to improve nutritional status, serum bilirubin levels, and aminopyrine breath test results but not to increase the rates of short-term or long-term survival.

4. **Other supplements:** Patients who are actively drinking are generally severely depleted of magnesium, potassium, and phosphate. This deficiency can precipitate multiorgan system dysfunction. Therefore, these elements should be repleted promptly.
5. **Thiamine:** This must be administered to prevent Wernicke's encephalopathy.
6. **Other treatments:** Therapies are aimed at neutralizing the proinflammatory cytokine, TNF alpha (anti-TNF alpha antibodies), reducing oxidative stress (propylthiouracil and cyanidanol), improving hepatic regeneration (anabolic steroids), and preventing fibrosis (d-penicillamine and colchicine). None reproducibly improves short-term survival, and at least one (treatment with anti-TNF antibodies) actually worsened mortality. Hence, these agents are not recommended for general clinical use.

SPECIFIC THERAPY FOR DECOMPENSATED ALCOHOLIC CIRRHOSIS

1. **Drug therapy:** Few long-term treatment trials of patients with alcoholic liver disease have been conducted, and these were confounded by noncompliance and large dropout rates.
   - A Cochrane systematic review concluded that, contrary to earlier reports, **colchicine** had significant deleterious effects on outcome in patients with fibrosis or cirrhosis from alcohol ingestion, viral hepatitis, or a cryptogenic condition. Patients taking colchicine had a higher incidence of adverse events.
   - A Canadian prospective randomized controlled trial evaluated **propylthiouracil** and demonstrated improved long-term survival.
   - Studies of drug therapy included small numbers of patients and may have been too small to detect uncommon adverse reactions. At present, these drugs are not recommended treatments for chronic alcoholic liver disease.
2. **Antioxidant therapy:** Several antioxidants have been tried in the setting of chronic alcoholic liver disease, with or without cirrhosis, with varying, incompletely satisfying effects. Substantial benefit has not been proven with the following agents:
   - **S-Adenosylmethionine (SAM-e)**
   - **Vitamin E**
   - **Silymarin** (milk thistle–derived antioxidant)
   - **Polyenylphosphatidylcholine (PPC)**
3. **Liver transplantation:**
   - Transplantation clearly improves survival in patients with decompensated alcoholic cirrhosis when compared with medically treated controls.
   - Patients with a history of alcohol dependence or alcohol abuse and end-stage liver disease should be considered for liver transplantation (see Chapter 31).
   - Abstinent patients (for longer than 6 months) who are evaluated by a multidisciplinary committee and are determined to be at low risk for recidivism and noncompliance are good candidates for liver transplantation.
   - A signed contract stipulating abstinence is occasionally helpful in maintaining commitment.
   - Screening programs now in place have reduced recidivism rates to less than 10% after liver transplantation.
   - Emerging evidence suggests that an accelerated form of alcoholic liver disease may develop in patients who resume alcohol abuse after transplantation.

FURTHER READING

Akriviadis E, Bolta R, Briggs W, et al. Pentoxifylline improves short-term survival in severe acute alcoholic hepatitis: a double-blind, placebo-controlled trial. *Gastroenterology* 2000; 119:1637–1648.

Carithers RL, Herlong HF, Diehl AM, et al. Methylprednisolone therapy in patients with severe alcoholic hepatitis: a randomized multicenter trial. *Ann Intern Med* 1989; 110:685–690.

Israel Y, Orrego H, Niemela O. Immune responses to alcohol metabolites: pathogenic and diagnostic implications. *Semin Liver Dis* 1988; 8:81–90.

Jain A, DiMartini A, Kashyap R, et al. Long-term follow-up after liver transplantation for alcoholic liver disease under tacrolimus. *Transplantation* 2000; 70:1335–1342.

Leiber CS. Biochemical factors in alcoholic liver disease. *Semin Liver Dis* 1993; 13:136–153.

Louvet A, Naveau S, Abdelnour M, et al. The Lille model: a new tool for therapeutic strategy in patients with severe alcoholic hepatitis with steroids. *Hepatology* 2007; 45:1348–1354.

Lucey MR, Merion RM, Henley KD, et al. Selection for and outcome of liver transplantation in alcoholic liver disease. *Gastroenterology* 1992; 102:1736–1741.

Lumeng L, Crabb DW. Genetic aspects and risk factors in alcoholism and alcoholic liver disease. *Gastroenterology* 1994; 107:572–578.

Maddrey W, Boitnott J, Bedine M, et al. Corticosteroid therapy in alcoholic hepatitis. *Gastroenterology* 1978; 75:193–199.

Mezey E. Interaction between alcohol and nutrition in the pathogenesis of alcoholic liver disease. *Semin Liver Dis* 1991; 11:340–348.

Orrego H, Kalant H, Israel Y, et al. Effect of short-term therapy with propylthiouracil in patients with alcoholic liver disease. *Gastroenterology* 1978; 75:105–115.

O'Shea RS, Dasarathy S, McCullough AJ, et al. AASLD practice guidelines: alcoholic liver disease. *Hepatology* 2010; 51:307–328.

Pares A, Planas R, Torres M, et al. Effects of silymarin in alcoholic patients with cirrhosis of the liver: results of a controlled, double-blind, randomized and multicenter trial. *J Hepatol* 1998; 28:615–621.

Pereira SP, Howard LM, Muiesan P, et al. Quality of life after liver transplantation for alcoholic liver disease. *Liver Transpl* 2000; 6:762–768.

Rambaldi A, Saconato HH, Christensen E, et al. Systematic review: glucocorticosteroids for alcoholic hepatitis. A Cochrane Hepato-Biliary Group systematic review with meta-analyses and trial sequential analyses of randomized clinical trials. *Aliment Pharmacol Ther* 2008; 27:1167–1178.

CHAPTER 7

Fatty liver and nonalcoholic steatohepatitis

Brent A. Neuschwander-Tetri, MD

KEY POINTS

1   Hepatic steatosis, or the accumulation of triglyceride droplets in hepatocytes, is found in one third to one half of all adults in the United States and can be a cause of elevated serum aminotransferase levels (typically less than 250 U/L).

2   Steatosis without significant inflammation or fibrosis on biopsy is a benign hepatic condition, although it is a sign of insulin resistance and risk for development of cardiovascular disease and diabetes mellitus.

3   Steatosis associated with necroinflammatory changes identified on a liver biopsy specimen, called nonalcoholic steatohepatitis (NASH) when alcohol consumption is minimal or none, can cause progressive hepatic fibrosis, cirrhosis, and liver failure.

4   Nonalcoholic fatty liver disease (NAFLD) is the umbrella term that includes both steatosis without inflammation and NASH.

5   A liver biopsy is warranted to diagnose NASH or other causes of occult liver disease when elevated aminotransferase levels are unexplained, especially in the patient with obesity or type 2 diabetes mellitus.

6   Hepatic steatosis is reliably identified by imaging techniques when the degree of fatty infiltration is substantial. Ultrasonography reveals increased liver echogenicity, whereas noncontrast computed tomography (CT) imaging reveals decreased liver density compared with the spleen.

7   Focal steatosis is a variant typically detected incidentally during sonographic or CT imaging of the abdomen. The appearance is usually characteristic, although biopsy confirmation is occasionally required to exclude malignancy when the imaging appearance is atypical.

8   Nontriglyceride lipotoxicity caused by metabolites of free fatty acids likely causes the liver injury recognized as NASH; steatosis may be an adaptive mechanism of temporarily storing fatty acids as triglyceride to prevent lipotoxic injury.

Overview

TERMINOLOGY

1.   *Nonalcoholic fatty liver disease* is a term used to describe excessive liver triglyceride accumulation when alcohol consumption is minimal (less than two to four drinks daily).

2.   No uniformly accepted term exists for NAFLD that is not NASH; terms such as *benign steatosis*, *simple steatosis*, and *nonalcoholic fatty liver* (NAFL) are commonly used.

3. NASH is diagnosed when a liver biopsy specimen shows steatosis and characteristic necroinflammatory changes in a patient who has fewer than two to four drinks daily; the presence of fibrosis is not required, but characteristic perisinusoidal fibrosis supports a diagnosis of steatohepatitis.
4. NASH is *not* a diagnosis of exclusion; it can often be found in the presence of other liver diseases such as chronic hepatitis C.

Pathogenesis

NASH is thought to be a disease of lipotoxic injury to hepatocytes caused by nontriglyceride metabolites of free fatty acids. Triglyceride in the lipid droplets may actually be a protective response to store fatty acids in an inert form. The specific metabolites of free fatty acids that cause lipotoxic injury have not been fully identified. Possibilities include ceramides, diacylglycerols, lysophosphatidyl choline species, and phosphatidic acid species.

The causes of hepatic lipotoxicity are attributable to one or more of the following abnormalities in the trafficking of fatty acids in the body:

INCREASED PERIPHERAL MOBILIZATION OF FATTY ACIDS

1. Adipose tissue releases free fatty acids in response to cyclic adenosine monophosphate (cAMP)–mediated signaling from glucagon, epinephrine, and adrenocorticotropic hormone; released fatty acids are transported to the liver bound to albumin in the circulation.
2. Insulin is a major inhibitory signal that normally prevents adipose tissue lipolysis after meals; adipocyte insulin resistance allows inappropriate postprandial lipolysis in adipose tissue with release of free fatty acids into the circulation.
3. Prolonged starvation is associated with appropriate release of fat from peripheral stores that can overwhelm the liver's ability to handle it, thus leading to steatosis and NASH.

INCREASED HEPATIC SYNTHESIS OF FATTY ACIDS

The liver disposes excess carbohydrates, especially fructose, by converting carbohydrate to fatty acids through de novo lipogenesis; excess carbohydrates from dietary sources (e.g., sugar-sweetened beverages) or provided parenterally (e.g., total parenteral nutrition) predispose to hepatic lipotoxicity.

IMPAIRED HEPATIC CATABOLISM OF FATTY ACIDS

1. Impaired mitochondrial beta-oxidation of fatty acids is a major factor in alcoholic steatosis and has also been shown to contribute to the development of NASH.
2. Factors that cause microvesicular steatosis may do so through impaired mitochondrial function (e.g., valproic acid, alcohol, and acute fatty liver of pregnancy).
3. Other oxidative pathways (cytochrome P-450, peroxisomal) facilitate disposal of fatty acids.

IMPAIRED SYNTHESIS OF TRIGLYCERIDE AND ITS SECRETION AS VERY-LOW-DENSITY LIPOPROTEINS FROM THE LIVER

1. Fatty acids delivered to the liver but not metabolized are reesterified to form triglycerides.
2. Fatty acid esterification to triglyceride ensures that the level of fatty acids within hepatocytes remains low, thus averting cellular injury from fatty acid metabolites.

3. Monounsaturated fatty acids (MUFAs) are needed to make triglyceride; impaired MUFA synthesis in the liver may predispose to lipotoxicity.
4. Once triglyceride is formed, various components are needed to form and secrete intact VLDL.
5. Any deficiency or metabolic aberration that interferes with any one of these steps can cause accumulation of hepatic triglyceride and hepatic steatosis.
6. Autophagy may be an important pathway of handling accumulated triglyceride to release free fatty acids by lysosomal lipases in hepatocytes.

Clinical Features

SYMPTOMS

1. Patients with benign steatosis or nonalcoholic steatohepatitis (NASH) are usually asymptomatic, whereas patients with alcoholic hepatitis are nearly always symptomatic.
2. Right upper quadrant pain or fullness of varying severity occurs in approximately one third of patients with nonalcoholic fatty liver disease (NAFLD); liver capsule distention probably underlies the pain.
3. Patients occasionally present with right upper quadrant pain as a chief complaint; hepatic steatosis may be diagnosed as the cause only after imaging studies exclude other potential intrahepatic or biliary causes.

PHYSICAL FINDINGS

1. Hepatomegaly is common but can be difficult to detect on physical examination of the obese patient.
2. Signs of chronic liver disease such as spider telangiectasias, muscle wasting, jaundice, and ascites point to the presence of cirrhosis.
3. Acanthosis nigricans, identified as increased pigmentation around the neck and on the elbows, knuckles, or other joints, is associated with insulin resistance.

Risk Factors

1. **Insulin resistance** (Tables 7.1 and 7.2)
    - Most patients with NAFLD have underlying insulin resistance (Fig. 7.1).
    - NAFLD may be the first indication that a child or adult has insulin resistance.
    - Most risk factors for NAFLD are associated with insulin resistance.
    - Severe insulin resistance is a risk factor for NASH.

TABLE 7.1 ■ **Body habitus and frequency of hepatic steatosis**

Body habitus	Hepatic steatosis (%)
Normal	21
>10% over ideal body weight	75
Morbidly obese	90–95

2. **Obesity**
   - An increased ratio of abdominal fat to hip fat predicts NAFLD.
   - NASH is found in 8% to 20% of obese individuals with NAFLD.
   - NAFLD occurs in 90% to 95% of severely obese children and adults.
3. **Type 2 diabetes mellitus**
   - NAFLD is unusual in type 1 diabetes mellitus unless glycemic control is poor or the patient is also obese and insulin resistant.
   - Type 2 diabetes mellitus is a risk factor for NASH in patients with NAFLD.
4. **Lipid abnormalities**
   - Fasting hypertriglyceridemia partially reflects increased trafficking of fat through the liver and increased hepatic secretion of very-low-density lipoprotein (VLDL) and thus is commonly found in NAFLD; this condition does not directly cause NAFLD.
   - The role of hypercholesterolemia in the causation of NAFLD is uncertain; the goal of treating hypercholesterolemia is reduction of cardiovascular risks.
5. **Gender**
   - Female gender is *not* a risk factor for NAFLD.
   - Steatosis is equally prevalent among male and female patients on computed tomography (CT) and at autopsy.
   - A greater prevalence of NASH in women has not been confirmed by clinical studies.
6. **Medications**
   - Tamoxifen can cause NASH; the decision to stop tamoxifen should be individualized depending on the severity of liver disease and the risk of recurrent breast cancer.
   - Corticosteroids have been implicated as contributing to NAFLD, but supporting data are weak.
7. **Lifestyle**
   - Sedentary behavior is associated with insulin resistance and NAFLD.

TABLE 7.2 ■ **Causes of nonalcoholic steatohepatitis**

Nutritional abnormalities
  Obesity
  Total parenteral nutrition
  Choline deficiency
  Rapid weight loss
  Kwashiorkor

Drugs
  Tamoxifen
  Corticosteroids
  Chloroquine

Metabolic diseases
  Insulin resistance
  Abetalipoproteinemia
  Hypobetalipoproteinemia
  Wilson disease
  Weber-Christian disease

Surgical alterations of gastrointestinal anatomy
  Jejunoileal bypass
  Jejunocolic bypass
  Extensive small bowel loss
  Gastroplasty

Occupational exposure
  Hydrocarbons

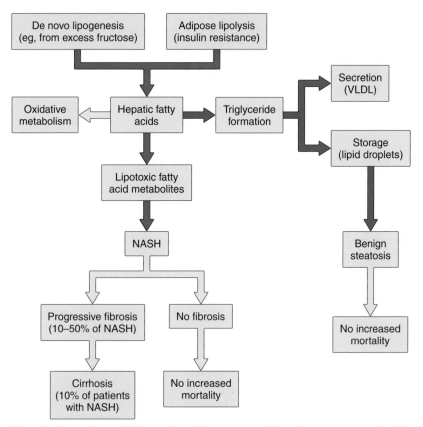

Fig. 7.1 Algorithm for the nontriglyceride lipotoxicity hypothesis of the pathogenesis of nonalcoholic steatohepatitis (NASH) showing the outcomes associated with lipotoxic liver injury. Accumulation of triglyceride as fat droplets, once thought to be a necessary step, is now considered to be a parallel but not pathogenic process and may actually be protective by drawing fatty acids away from the formation of lipotoxic intermediates. Dietary carbohydrate and inappropriate peripheral lipolysis are the major factors predisposing to an increased burden of fatty acids handled by the liver. Adipose insulin resistance is the major cause of inappropriate adipocyte lipolysis. Fatty acids are also disposed of through oxidative pathways (mitochondria, peroxisomes, cytochrome P-450), and this generates reactive oxygen species (ROS), but the role of ROS in causing hepatocellular injury in NASH remains uncertain. Pathways predisposing to NASH are shown in *red,* and pathways preventing NASH are shown in *green.* VDLD, very-low-density lipoprotein

- Excessive consumption of high-fructose corn syrup, such as in soft drinks, is associated with insulin resistance and NAFLD.
- Animal data suggest that dietary trans-fats may contribute to NASH.

Diagnosis

HISTORY

1. A patient suspected of having NASH should be interviewed regarding the following (see Table 7.2):
   - Alcohol consumption

TABLE 7.3 ■ **Steatohepatitis and serum aminotransferase patterns**

Alcoholic hepatitis	AST > ALT, typically >2:1 ratio
Nonalcoholic steatohepatitis	ALT > AST, sometimes >2:1 ratio

ALT, alanine aminotransferase; AST, aspartate aminotransferase.

- Exercise habits and barriers to regular exercise
- Sugar-sweetened beverage consumption
- Frequency of eating fast food
- History of gestational diabetes mellitus
- Family history of diabetes mellitus
2. The nature and frequency of right upper quadrant abdominal pain should be specifically queried.

LABORATORY FEATURES

1. No blood tests point unequivocally to steatosis or NASH.
2. Elevated aminotransferase (aspartate aminotransferase [AST], alanine aminotransferase [ALT]) levels are commonly the only biochemical indicators of steatosis and NASH.
3. Aminotransferase levels can be normal in both steatosis and NASH, as has been demonstrated in liver biopsy specimens of obese persons undergoing bariatric surgery.
4. The AST/ALT ratio can be helpful in distinguishing alcoholic hepatitis from NAFLD or NASH (Table 7.3); an AST/ALT ratio greater than 2 suggests alcoholic hepatitis, whereas patients with NASH typically have ALT levels that exceed AST levels in the absence of cirrhosis; AST is typically greater than ALT in NASH with cirrhosis.
5. Serum aminotransferase levels and other liver biochemical tests are not helpful in identifying the presence of liver fibrosis or cirrhosis; aminotransferase levels often normalize as NASH progresses to cirrhosis.
6. Serum alkaline phosphatase may be elevated up to twice the upper limit of normal.
7. Viral, autoimmune, and metabolic causes of liver disease must be evaluated as potential contributors to elevated aminotransferase levels.

IMAGING

Imaging studies cannot distinguish benign steatosis from NASH, although NASH is usually diffuse, whereas steatosis can be either focal or diffuse. Focal or diffuse steatosis is often an incidental imaging finding.

1. **Ultrasonography**
   - The liver is echogenic or "bright."
   - Ultrasonography detects steatosis only when fat accumulation is substantial.
   - Cirrhosis can also cause an echogenic appearance of the liver, but the texture is typically coarser.
2. **Computed tomography**
   - A liver with steatosis is low in density compared with the spleen on noncontrast images.
3. **Magnetic resonance imaging**
   - This imaging technique is the most sensitive noninvasive measure of liver fat.

- Phase shifting can be useful for identifying focal fat based on its loss of intensity on T1-weighted images.

4. **Focal fat**
   - This is found in up to one third of patients with CT evidence of hepatic steatosis.
   - It can be peripheral (especially in the diabetic patient receiving insulin by peritoneal dialysis), central, or periportal.
   - It is typically aspherical or geometric in shape.
   - It does not exert a mass effect on adjacent structures.
   - Fine-needle biopsy occasionally is needed to establish the diagnosis.

5. **Focal sparing**
   - This is defined as regions of normal liver in an otherwise steatotic liver.
   - It appears relatively hypoechoic by sonography (compared with surrounding bright liver).
   - It appears relatively hyperdense by CT.
   - The shape is typically geometric.
   - The location is commonly in the caudate lobe or adjacent to the gallbladder.
   - It can be caused by an aberrant gastric vein draining directly into the liver that spares an area of insulin-rich portal blood.

6. **Problems identifying other lesions in the steatotic liver**
   - Hemangiomas, which are usually characteristically hyperechoic by ultrasonography, can appear relatively hypoechoic in a steatotic liver.
   - Identifying dilatation of intrahepatic bile ducts can be difficult because of loss of contrast between the usually hyperechoic bile duct wall and the liver parenchyma.

LIVER BIOPSY

1. Liver biopsy is often needed to evaluate unexplained elevation of aminotransferase levels. Unless a therapeutic trial of discontinuance of specific medications, aggressive lifestyle modification, or avoidance of occupational exposures is planned, liver biopsy should not be delayed for arbitrary waiting periods.

2. Liver biopsy is usually not indicated when imaging suggests steatosis and aminotransferase levels are normal.

3. **Histologic findings in nonalcoholic steatohepatitis**
   - **Steatosis:** Fat droplets (triglyceride) within hepatocytes can be large, displacing cellular contents to the periphery.
   - **Inflammation:** Mixed neutrophilic and mononuclear cell infiltrates are present within the lobule; portal chronic inflammation can occur, especially in children and after treatment; ballooning enlargement of hepatocytes with rarefaction of cytoplasmic contents is a marker of hepatocyte injury.
   - **Mallory-Denk bodies**: These eosinophilic cytoplasmic aggregates of keratins are typically smaller than those seen in alcoholic hepatitis and are usually found in ballooned hepatocytes.
   - **Glycogen nuclei**: These clear intranuclear vacuoles fill the nucleus.
   - **Fibrosis:** This is similar to alcoholic liver disease, with perivenular deposition around the central vein and a "chicken wire" pattern of sinusoidal fibrosis; it occurs in approximately one third of patients with NASH and signifies a risk for progression to end-stage liver disease; it is staged as 1 (perisinusoidal **or** periportal only), 2 (perisinusoidal **and** periportal), 3 (bridging), or 4 (cirrhosis).

Prognosis (Fig. 7.1)

STEATOSIS

Steatosis alone is a benign condition, although it may be associated with clinically significant right upper quadrant abdominal pain.

NONALCOHOLIC STEATOHEPATITIS

- The risk of developing fibrosis and cirrhosis is 10% to 50% in patients with NASH.
- The risk of developing cirrhosis when fibrosis is absent on initial biopsy is low.
- Hepatocellular carcinoma is increasingly recognized in patients with advanced NASH with fibrosis or cirrhosis.

Treatment

WEIGHT LOSS AND EXERCISE

1. For the overweight or obese person with hepatic steatosis or NASH, gradual and sustained weight loss results in resolution of steatosis and normalization of aminotransferase levels.
2. Weight loss achieved with protein malnutrition does not improve hepatic steatosis.
3. Weight loss achieved with bariatric surgery improves NASH, but patients must adhere to postoperative dietary guidance to avoid nutritional deficiencies.
4. Improved glycemic control in type 2 diabetes mellitus without weight loss is not helpful.
5. Regular exercise improves insulin sensitivity and improves NAFLD.

MEDICATIONS

No medications are approved for the treatment of NASH. The following drugs have been examined in clinical trials:

- Thiazolidinediones appear to be beneficial for some patients, probably by improving adipocyte insulin sensitivity and preventing inappropriate lipolysis; side effects of thiazolidinediones include weight gain, exacerbation of heart failure, and possibly osteoporosis.
- Vitamin E may be helpful in some patients.
- Other agents under evaluation include metformin, high-dose ursodiol, omega-3 fatty acids, pentoxifylline, exenatide, and silymarin.
- Statin use is not contraindicated in patients with NASH.

FURTHER READING

Belfort R, Harrison SA, Brown K, et al. A placebo-controlled trial of pioglitazone in subjects with nonalcoholic steatohepatitis. *N Engl J Med* 2006; 355:2297–2307.

Brunt EM. Pathology of fatty liver disease. *Mod Pathol* 2007; 20(Suppl 1):S40–S48.

Cohen DE, Anania FA, Chalasani N, et al. An assessment of statin safety by hepatologists. *Am J Cardiol* 2006; 97:77C–81C.

Cusi K. Role of insulin resistance and lipotoxicity in non-alcoholic steatohepatitis. *Clin Liver Dis* 2009; 13:545–563.

Gastaldelli A, Harrison SA, Belfort-Aguilar R, et al. Importance of changes in adipose tissue insulin resistance to histological response during thiazolidinedione treatment of patients with nonalcoholic steatohepatitis. *Hepatology* 2009; 50:1087–1093.

Harrison SA, Day CP. Benefits of lifestyle modification in NAFLD. *Gut* 2007; 56:1760–1769.

Jou J, Choi SS, Diehl AM. Mechanisms of disease progression in nonalcoholic fatty liver disease. *Semin Liver
Dis* 2008; 28:370–379.

Kashi MR, Torres DM, Harrison SA. Current and emerging therapies in nonalcoholic fatty liver disease.
Semin Liver Dis 2008; 28:396–406.

Neuschwander-Tetri BA. Lifestyle modification as the primary treatment of NASH. *Clin Liver Dis* 2009;
13:649–665.

Neuschwander-Tetri BA. Hepatic lipotoxicity and the pathogenesis of NASH. *Hepatology* 2010; 52:774–788.

Neuschwander-Tetri BA, Unalp A, Creer MH, et al. Influence of local reference populations on upper limits
of normal for serum alanine aminotransferase levels. *Arch Intern Med* 2008; 168:663–666.

Nolan CJ, Larter CZ. Lipotoxicity: why do saturated fatty acids cause and monounsaturates protect against
it? *J Gastroenterol Hepatol* 2009; 24:703–706.

Ratziu V, Giral P, Jacqueminet S, et al. Rosiglitazone for nonalcoholic steatohepatitis: one-year results of
the randomized placebo-controlled Fatty Liver Improvement with Rosiglitazone Therapy (FLIRT) trial.
Gastroenterology 2008; 135:100–110.

Socha P, Horvath A, Vajro P, et al. Pharmacological interventions for nonalcoholic fatty liver disease in adults
and in children: a systematic review. *J Pediatr Gastroenterol Nutr* 2009; 48:587–596.

CHAPTER 8

Drug-induced and toxic liver disease

Thomas D. Schiano, MD ■ Martin Black, MD

KEY POINTS

1 Drug-induced liver injury (DILI) accounts for 7% of reported drug adverse effects, 2% of hospitalizations for jaundice, 1% of cases of acute liver failure (ALF), and most cases of hepatitis in patients older than 50 years of age. Ten percent of those with jaundice will die.

2 The spectrum of DILI ranges from subclinical liver disease with mildly elevated liver chemistry test results to subacute liver failure and ALF requiring liver transplantation. DILI can mimic almost every type of acute and chronic liver disease.

3 Many different medications and toxins have been implicated in causing ALF, and the prognosis is poor without liver transplantation.

4 Over-the-counter preparations and herbal medications may have significant hepatotoxicity, and their use should be determined in cases of unexplained acute or chronic liver disease.

5 Early suspicion of DILI is essential because morbidity is greatly increased if the medication is continued after symptoms develop or liver chemistry test abnormalities appear.

6 The main treatment for drug hepatotoxicity is withdrawal of the offending agent. Patients should be counseled regarding signs of DILI, especially with use of agents with well-recognized hepatotoxic potential.

Overview

1. **Drug-induced liver injury (DILI) is one of the most common causes of elevated liver chemistry values.**
2. Patients with DILI and jaundice at initial presentation experience worse outcomes.
3. The Drug-Induced Liver Injury Network (DILIN) was created by the National Institutes of Health in 2003. Initial DILIN findings showed that 73% of cases resulted from taking a single prescription medication, 9% were attributable to herbal or dietary supplements, and 18% resulted from taking multiple agents.
4. Among patients with DILI caused by a single prescription drug, **the major offending agents were antimicrobials (46%), central nervous system agents (15%), immunomodulating agents (5%), analgesics (5%), and lipid-lowering agents (3%).**
5. In Asia, most cases of DILI result from taking complementary and alternative medications (CAM).
6. The **incidence of DILI is greater in older individuals,** probably related to altered pharmacokinetic factors.
7. Polypharmacy may contribute to an increased risk of adverse drug reactions through alterations of cytochrome P-450.

8. Although most DILI cases in children are mild, pediatric patients have the potential to progress to ALF.
9. Children with viral infection have an unusual sensitivity to aspirin (Reye's syndrome); however, the most common agents causing DILI in children are antiepileptic drugs, such as valproate, and psychotropic agents.
10. Patients with chronic liver disease have an increased incidence of DILI and a worse outcome.
11. DILI is the single most common adverse drug reaction leading to discontinuation during development of new medications, failure of new drugs to obtain regulatory approval, and withdrawal of existing drugs from the market.

Clinical Presentation

1. DILI may occur as an unexpected idiosyncratic reaction to a medication's therapeutic dose or as an expected consequence of the agent's intrinsic toxicity.
2. Hepatotoxicity may be the only manifestation of the adverse drug effect, or it may be accompanied by injury to other organ systems or by systemic manifestations.
3. Acute liver injury may develop within days of ingestion of a known hepatotoxin or after several weeks of taking a drug that provokes an immunoallergic reaction. Liver tests may have a necroinflammatory, cholestatic, or a mixed pattern with features of both parenchymal and cholestatic injury.
   - Aminotransferases (aspartate aminotransferase [AST] and alanine aminotransferase [ALT]) and lactate dehydrogenase may be elevated 10 to 100 times the upper limit of normal (ULN) in acute hepatocellular injury, whereas alkaline phosphatase levels are usually less than 3 times the ULN.
   - Cholestatic drug injury resembles obstructive jaundice in its clinical manifestations and biochemical parameters. Serum alkaline phosphatase, gamma glutamyltranspeptidase, and direct bilirubin are variably elevated with or without aminotransferase elevation (usually no higher than five to eight times ULN).
   - Subclinical hepatic injury reflected only by minor liver enzyme elevation (e.g., AST and ALT in the range of 100 to 250 U/L) is a common phenomenon and may not worsen and may even subside despite continued administration of a medication.
   - Table 8.1 shows the histopathologic conditions associated with particular hepatotoxic agents.

Characterization of Drug-Induced Liver Injury

INTRINSIC HEPATOTOXICITY

This is almost always **dose dependent and reproducible in laboratory animals.** Examples of agents include acetaminophen, carbon tetrachloride, and alcohol.

IDIOSYNCRATIC HEPATOTOXICITY

1. This **occurs unpredictably in a small number of recipients** of a medication and accounts for most cases of DILI. Some dose dependency exists, and toxicity is not reliably reproduced in laboratory animals. Examples of agents include isoniazid (INH), sulfonamides, valproate, and phenytoin.
2. Liver injury may manifest after **latent periods of varying duration.**

TABLE 8.1 ■ **Clinicopathologic patterns of drug-induced liver injury***

Disorder	Hepatotoxic agents
Acute	
Hepatitis-like syndromes (acute necroinflammation)	Dapsone, disulfiram, isoniazid, carbamazepine NSAIDs, allopurinol, bupropion, lisinopril, losartan, paroxetine, phenytoin, sulfonamides, statins, trazodone, pyrazinamide, HAART, valproic acid
Fulminant hepatic failure	Acetaminophen, fialuridine (FIAU), halothane, isoniazid, sustained-release niacin, nitrofurantoin, propylthiouracil, valproic acid, flutamide
Cholestasis	Ampicillin, chlorpromazine, prochlorperazine, cimetidine, ranitidine, estrogens, cytarabine, trimethoprim–sulfamethoxazole, thiabendazole, tolbutamide, anabolic steroids, erythromycins
Mixed necroinflammatory and cholestatic	Carbimazole, chlorpropamide, dicloxacillin, methimazole, azathioprine, naproxen, phenylbutazone, sulindac, phenytoin, thioridazine, captopril, cyproheptadine, enalapril, fosinopril, irbesartan, terbinafine, phenobarbital
Granulomatous hepatitis	Allopurinol, dapsone, diazepam, diltiazem, hydralazine, penicillin, phenylbutazone, phenytoin, quinidine, procainamide, clopidogrel, sulfonamides
Macrovesicular steatosis	Alcohol, corticosteroids, L-asparaginase, methotrexate, nifedipine, tamoxifen
Microvesicular steatosis	Alcohol, amiodarone, aspirin, zidovudine, didanosine, piroxicam, tetracyclines, tolmetin, valproic acid
Budd–Chiari syndrome	Estrogens
Ischemic necrosis	Cocaine, sustained-release niacin, methylenedioxyamphetamine
Chronic	
Chronic active hepatitis	Alpha-methyldopa, nitrofurantoin, oxyphenisatin
Fibrosis/cirrhosis	Alcohol, alpha-methyldopa, isoniazid, methotrexate
Peliosis hepatis	Anabolic/androgenic steroids, azathioprine, hydroxyurea, oral contraceptives, tamoxifen
Phospholipidosis	Amiodarone, perhexiline, diltiazem, nifedipine
Primary biliary cirrhosis	Chlorpromazine, haloperidol, prochlorperazine
Sclerosing cholangitis	Floxuridine (FUDR) by hepatic artery infusion
Steatohepatitis	Amiodarone, diethylstilbestrol, tamoxifen, irinotecan
Sinusoidal obstruction syndrome	Azathioprine, busulfan, cyclophosphamide, daunorubicin, oxaliplatin, pyrrolizidine alkaloids, 6-thioguanine
Autoimmune hepatitis	Minocycline, statins
Hepatoportal sclerosis	Didanosine
Nodular regenerative hyperplasia	Didanosine, azathioprine, 6-thioguanine, 6-mercaptopurine
Vanishing bile duct syndrome	Azithromycin, amoxicillin-clavulanic acid, anabolic steroids, allopurinol
Oncogenic	
Cholangiocarcinoma	Thorotrast
Focal nodular hyperplasia	Estrogens, oral contraceptives
Hepatic adenoma	Estrogens, oral contraceptives

Continued

TABLE 8.1 ■ Clinicopathologic patterns of drug-induced liver injury*—cont'd

Disorder	Hepatotoxic agents
Hepatocellular carcinoma	Alcohol, anabolic/androgenic steroids
Hepatoblastoma	Estrogens
Angiosarcoma	Arsenic, vinyl chloride, Thorotrast
Inflammatory pseudotumor	Anabolic steroids

*This list is not meant to be comprehensive.
HAART, highly active antiretroviral therapy; NSAIDs, nonsteroidal anti-inflammatory drugs.

3. Susceptibility results from an interplay among factors such as the toxic potential of the drug, environmental and host genetic risk factors that determine drug disposition, and metabolism and tissue susceptibility to toxicity.
4. Immunologically mediated injury can be accompanied by a mononucleosis-like illness and extrahepatic hallmarks of generalized hypersensitivity such as fever, rash, and eosinophilia; these features usually develop after a sensitization period of several weeks.
5. Symptoms recur if the agent is used again.

MITOCHONDRIAL HEPATOTOXICITY

This decreases fatty acid oxidation and/or energy production and leads to cell death. Examples of agents include diclofenac, amiodarone, tacrine, troglitazone, and topoisomerases.

Pathophysiology

1. The liver is exposed to high concentrations of ingested drugs, particularly those with a high first-pass metabolism.
2. Hepatic uptake of drugs may occur by specific transport mechanisms; most drugs are lipophilic and diffuse across the hepatocellular sinusoids.
3. Many of the mechanisms in the pathophysiology of DILI at the molecular level are shown in Table 8.2.
4. Normally, the liver metabolizes drugs to more polar forms, thus facilitating their excretion in aqueous fluids. Sometimes these metabolites may be toxic (e.g., in acetaminophen overdose), but they are generally converted to less toxic compounds by detoxification enzymes.
5. Individual susceptibility to drug hepatotoxicity is influenced by multiple variables that affect the biotransformation of drugs, and usually more than one of these is involved in any one patient (Table 8.3).

Biotransformation

This is a process by which therapeutic agents are rendered more hydrophilic, thus facilitating their excretion from the body. Biotransformation takes place in several steps, classified as phase 1, phase 2, and phase 3 reactions.

TABLE 8.2 ■ **Mechanisms of drug-induced liver injury occurring at the molecular level**

Peroxidation of lipids

Denaturation of protein

Adenosine triphosphate depletion

Mitochondrial dysfunction

Free radical generation

Electrophilic radical generation and hapten formation

Biotransformation through cytochrome P-450

Binding of active metabolites to nuclear or cytoplasmic molecules

Binding or blockage of transfer RNA

Binding or blockage of bile transporters

Attachment to membrane receptors

Disruption of calcium homeostasis

Disruption of the hepatocellular cytoskeleton

TABLE 8.3 ■ **Factors influencing an individual's susceptibility to drug-induced liver injury**

Age

Long-term alcohol use

Drug–drug interactions

Duration of use and total dose of drug

Enzyme induction

Enzyme polymorphism

Ethnic and racial factors

Gender

Human leukocyte antigen (HLA) type

Nutritional status

Pregnancy

Renal function

Systemic disease

Underlying liver disease

PHASE 1 REACTIONS

1. These are **mediated by cytochrome P-450,** are primarily oxidative, and yield active intermediate metabolites that may be responsible for liver injury. The cytochrome P-450 family of isoenzymes found primarily within the endoplasmic reticulum results in aliphatic and aromatic hydroxylation, dealkylation, or dehydrogenation. Products of these reactions may sometimes undergo further metabolism through phase 2 reactions.

2. Many medications may alter cytochrome P-450 activity and thus promote drug toxicity. Cytochrome P-450 enzymes catalyze the rate-limiting steps in the elimination of many drugs.

PHASE 2 REACTIONS

1. These are **mainly conjugative,** converting the active metabolite to nontoxic, more hydrophilic products by linkage with glutathione, sulfate, or glucuronide. This is the only step required for the hepatic metabolism of some compounds; however, most drugs first undergo cytochrome P-450 metabolism.
2. **Phase 1 reactions may thus be regarded as "toxification" and phase 2 as "detoxification."** Drug injury may result from toxification (increased active metabolites) or inadequate detoxification.

PHASE 3 REACTIONS

These **involve excretion and transport.** Substances formed from drug detoxification become substrates for the export pump of the multidrug resistance protein family that mediates adenosine triphosphate–dependent secretion across the canalicular membrane into bile.

Diagnosis of Drug-induced Liver Injury

1. A detailed drug history, including dosage, duration of therapy, and other concomitantly administered drugs, is essential.
2. Other causes of liver disease must be excluded by careful assessment of clinical, radiologic, histologic, biochemical, and serologic findings.
3. The possibility of drug injury superimposed on preexisting liver disease must be considered.
4. Elevation of serum lactate dehydrogenase levels is more indicative of toxic liver injury than of viral-related disease, although this finding is nonspecific.
5. Nonspecific histologic lesions suggestive of drug injury include granulomas (Fig. 8.1), eosinophils within an inflammatory infiltrate (Fig. 8.2), a sharp zone of demarcation between necrosis and unaffected parenchyma, and a disproportionately severe degree of damage in relation to the patient's condition and the extent of liver chemistry test abnormalities.

Hepatotoxicity of Specific Medications

More than 1000 drugs have been implicated in causing acute or chronic liver injury, ranging from subclinical elevation of liver chemistry tests to ALF. The following is a summary of some of the more frequently used medications having hepatotoxic potential and those with the best-characterized mechanisms of injury.

ACETAMINOPHEN (PARACETAMOL, TYLENOL)

1. This is typically well tolerated without side effects. Overdose is the most common cause of DILI leading to ALF.
2. The amount ingested as a single dose required for hepatic injury is quite variable. **A toxic dose may be 10 to 20 g, whereas in alcoholic patients it can be as low as 5 to 10 g.**
3. Acetaminophen is present in many over-the-counter (e.g., Nyquil) and prescription (e.g., Vicodin) preparations.
4. The greatest risks for hepatotoxicity are influenced by the dose of acetaminophen ingested and the interval between drug ingestion and administration of the antidote.

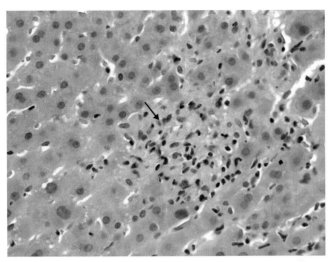

Fig. 8.1 Histopathology of granulomatous hepatitis. A noncaseating epithelioid granuloma found in a lobule (H & E). *(Courtesy of M. I. Fiel, MD.)*

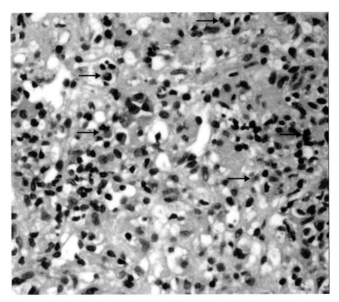

Fig. 8.2 High-power photomicrograph of a mixed inflammatory infiltrate with a prominent eosinophilic component in a patient with drug-induced liver injury (H & E). *(Courtesy of M. I. Fiel, MD.)*

5. Alcoholism is a significant risk factor for toxicity, and appreciable liver injury sometimes occurs with therapeutic use or unwitting overdose ("therapeutic misadventure"). Malnutrition or fasting may play a role in acetaminophen hepatotoxicity by reducing glutathione stores.
6. The use of concurrent medications that induce cytochrome P-450 may heighten the risk and severity of liver injury associated with acetaminophen overdose.

Clinical Phases after Massive Ingestion

1. Acute **gastrointestinal symptoms occur 30 minutes to 24 hours after ingestion.**
2. Cessation of gastrointestinal symptoms is followed by a period of well-being for approximately 48 hours. Right-sided abdominal pain, oliguria, elevated liver chemistry test results, and prolonged prothrombin time then occur.
3. **Hepatic necrosis occurs 3 to 5 days after ingestion.** Aminotransferase levels may peak at greater than 20,000 U/L. Renal failure from proximal and distal renal tubular damage occurs in up to 20% of patients, and ALF develops in up to 30%.
4. Recovery phase occurs 5 to 10 days after ingestion without residual histologic damage.

Prognosis

1. Risk of liver injury can be assessed based on the serum acetaminophen level obtained more than 4 hours after ingestion (Fig. 8.3).
2. Criteria for predicting death or the need for liver transplantation:
   - pH lower than 7.3 irrespective of stage of encephalopathy or
   - Prothrombin time international normalized ratio (INR) greater than 6.5 and serum creatinine higher than 3.4 mg/dL in patients with stage 3 or 4 encephalopathy
   - Factor V level of 10% or less (may be a sensitive predictor of adverse outcome)

Mechanism of Hepatotoxicity

Acetaminophen is metabolized by conjugation to glucuronide and sulfate. A relatively small amount is metabolized by cytochrome P-450 to form oxidative metabolites, which are further conjugated before elimination. When large quantities are ingested, the glucuronide and sulfate conjugation pathways become saturated, and more metabolism by cytochrome P-450 occurs. Increased formation of one of the oxidative metabolites, N-acetyl-p-benzoquinoneimine (NAPQI), leads to depletion of intracellular glutathione (which normally inactivates the potent electrophile) and allows it to bind covalently to certain cell macromolecules and thus disrupts mitochondrial function (Fig. 8.4). Depletion of glutathione before ingestion, by starvation or alcohol ingestion, may further potentiate NAPQI toxicity.

Treatment

1. Goals are to reduce further absorption of ingested acetaminophen and to replete hepatic glutathione by use of N-acetylcysteine (NAC).
2. **Recommended use of NAC is 70 mg/kg orally and then every 4 hours for an additional 17 doses.**
3. Intravenously, NAC is given by a loading dose of 150 mg/kg in 5% dextrose over 15 minutes and a maintenance dose of 50 mg/kg over 4 hours followed by 100 mg/kg over 16 hours.
4. NAC is safe and beneficial when given up to 24 hours after overdose or even later for patients with already established severe DILI.
5. Activated charcoal and gastric lavage can be used to prevent absorption of acetaminophen, but they are effective only when used within 1 hour of ingestion for charcoal and within 4 hours for gastric lavage.
6. If a serum acetaminophen concentration cannot be obtained, patients should be treated if they ingested a toxic dose greater than 150 mg/kg or greater than 12 g.
7. Patients should receive a full course of NAC if they have an unknown history regarding the acetaminophen dose or a nonacute overdose (longer than 4 hours earlier), which precludes use of the nomogram for treatment decisions.

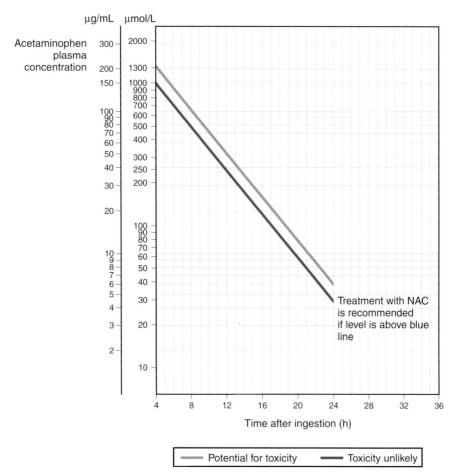

Fig. 8.3 Acetaminophen toxicity nomogram. The Rumack-Matthew nomogram was created to predict whether patients would develop hepatotoxicity after acetaminophen overdose and is intended as a guide for early management of a single acute overdose. Acetaminophen levels should be measured at least 4 hours after ingestion. Hepatotoxicity is predicted when the plasma acetaminophen concentration lies above the probable hepatotoxicity line, a semilogarithmic plot joining the acetaminophen concentration of 200 mg/L at 4 hours with the concentration of 50 mg/L at 12 hours. *(From Rumack BH, Mathew, H. Acetaminophen poisoning and toxicity. Pediatrics 1975; 55:871–876.)* NAC, N-acetylcysteine.

NONSTEROIDAL ANTI-INFLAMMATORY DRUGS

1. Despite the extremely low incidence of hepatotoxicity induced by nonsteroidal anti-inflammatory drugs (NSAIDs), widespread use of these agents makes them an important class of potentially hepatotoxic drug.
2. The prevalence of isolated **minor increases in liver chemistry test results is 1% to 15%,** and these changes are often considered a class effect of these agents. Nearly all NSAIDs have been implicated in causing liver injury, ranging from mild to severe.
3. Most NSAIDs produce injury in an unpredictable fashion by an idiosyncratic mechanism. The risk of clinically significant acute liver injury is low, injury is almost always reversible, and fatal reactions are rare.

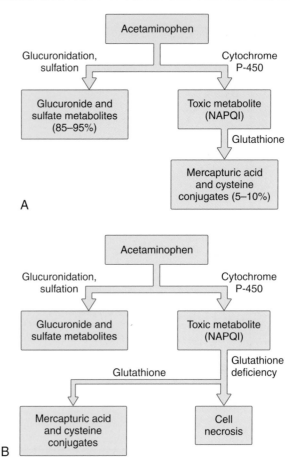

Fig. 8.4 Acetaminophen metabolism for therapeutic (nontoxic) amounts (**A**) and toxic (overdose) amounts (**B**). NAPQI, *N*-acetyl-*p*-benzoquinoneimine

ASPIRIN

1. Liver chemistry abnormalities are almost always mild, asymptomatic, and reversible.
2. In 30% of cases, aminotransferase levels are less than 100 U/L, and in 45% they are between 300 and 500 U/L. Liver histology shows focal necrosis and mild nonspecific inflammation.
3. Liver injury is dose dependent, related to serum salicylate levels, and caused by intrinsic toxicity of the salicylate moiety. Ninety percent of patients with toxic cases have a serum level greater that 15 mg/dL, which is easily achieved with the large doses of aspirin used in the treatment of some rheumatologic disorders.

ANTIMICROBIAL AGENTS

INH, macrolide antibiotics, penicillin and its derivatives, and sulfonamides are the most frequent agents responsible for antimicrobial-related hepatotoxicity. Hepatic injury may be necroinflammatory (INH), cholestatic (macrolides, clavulanic acid), or a combination of the two (sulfonamides).

Antibiotics

1. Hepatotoxicity is usually self-limited and idiosyncratic.
2. Penicillin hepatotoxicity is more frequently necroinflammatory than cholestatic. Carbenicillin and oxacillin are frequent offenders, and oxacillin is known to cause cholestatic hepatitis. First-generation cephalosporins rarely have hepatotoxic potential; ceftriaxone has been implicated in the formation of biliary sludge.
3. **Amoxicillin-clavulanic acid (Augmentin) is the most frequently reported antibiotic associated with DILI,** which can occur within 2 weeks of starting the drug. Delayed onset of symptoms can be seen up to 8 weeks following cessation of therapy. The type of hepatic injury observed varies according to the time from onset of therapy, in which hepatocellular injury predominates at 1 week, cholestatic injury at 2 to 3 weeks, and mixed liver injury after 3 weeks. The probability of persistent liver damage and death or need for liver transplantation is approximately 10%. Progressive vanishing bile duct syndrome following discontinuation of therapy has also been seen.
4. The estolate, ethylsuccinate, propionate, and stearate esters of erythromycin have all been implicated in the development of cholestatic jaundice. Serum alkaline phosphatase levels may rise to high levels, with modest elevations in aminotransferase levels. These abnormalities slowly resolve after cessation of the drug.
5. Sulfonamides (including sulfasalazine) most frequently cause necroinflammatory injury, but they may also provoke cholestatic, mixed, or granulomatous hepatitis. Trimethoprim-sulfamethoxazole (Bactrim, Septra) causes predominantly cholestatic injury that may be severe and last for many months. The clinical presentation may involve multiple organ systems, including concurrent renal failure.
6. Fluoroquinolones have been reported to cause DILI but less frequently than other groups of antibiotics.

Antituberculous Agents

1. Isoniazid
   - The **incidence of jaundice is approximately 1%.** Jaundice is rare in patients younger than age 20 years, and the incidence is greater than 2% in patients more than 50 years old. Alcoholic patients and patients with underlying liver disease or malnutrition, pregnant or immediately postpartum women, and persons taking other potentially hepatotoxic medications or having viral hepatitis are at greatest risk.
   - **Up to a threefold elevation in aminotransferase levels may be seen in 10% to 20% of patients** during the first 2 months of therapy. One half of cases of symptomatic INH hepatotoxicity occur within the first 2 months.
   - Continuing INH after clinical liver injury occurs may result in ALF with a high mortality. **Treatment should be interrupted in patients with ALT three times the ULN or higher in the presence of symptoms or five times the ULN if asymptomatic.**
   - The mechanism of hepatotoxicity is by cytochrome P-450 transformation of the parent compound into a toxic acetyl radical.
2. Rifampin
   - Injury is mainly hepatocellular but may have a mixed pattern.
   - This drug has rare hepatotoxic potential when taken alone. However, when taken with INH, hepatotoxicity is greater than with either drug alone. This combination may result in clinical hepatitis in 5% to 8% of patients.
   - Toxicity with concurrent INH use results from cytochrome P-450 induction by rifampin and results in greater conversion of INH to toxic metabolites.
3. Streptomycin and ethambutol have very rare hepatotoxic potential, whereas pyrazinamide has been incriminated in liver injury.

Antiviral Agents

1. Fialuridine (FIAU): In 1993, this investigational agent for the treatment of chronic hepatitis B induced severe toxic reactions characterized by ALF, lactic acidosis, pancreatitis, myopathy, and neuropathy related to widespread mitochondrial injury in 15 patients.
2. Interferon: This may provoke elevation of hepatic enzymes in patients with chronic hepatitis B or C or in patients with concurrent autoimmune hepatitis. Pegylated interferon has been noted to induce de novo autoimmune hepatitis and an accelerated form of chronic ductopenic rejection after liver transplantation.
3. Antiretroviral therapy (ART) in human immunodeficiency (HIV) infection:
   - The overall incidence of hepatotoxicity in patients with HIV infection who are receiving ART is 3% to 18%.
   - All three classes of ART, nucleotide reverse transcriptase inhibitors (NRTIs), non-nucleoside reverse transcriptase inhibitors (NNRTIs), and protease inhibitors (PIs), have been associated with DILI (Fig. 8.5 and Table 8.4).
   - In patients receiving ART, liver tests should be monitored closely, especially during the first 4 to 6 weeks, for evidence of hypersensitivity reactions. Liver biopsy demonstrating microvesicular steatosis may support NRTI-associated mitochondrial injury. A threshold aminotransferase elevation of 5 to 10 times the ULN should prompt discontinuation.

HORMONAL AGENTS

1. Oral contraceptives cause frequent, reversible liver chemistry test abnormalities; some patients may develop overt cholestatic jaundice. The molecular basis of injury may be an alteration of the basolateral membrane of the hepatocyte with a resultant decrease in bile flow. Other conditions associated with use of oral contraceptive include the following:
   - Cholestasis of pregnancy

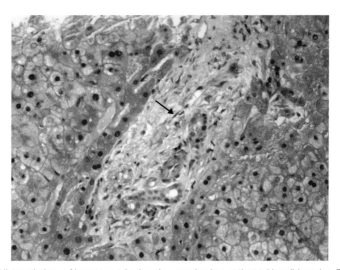

Fig. 8.5 Histopathology of hepatoportal sclerosis occurring in a patient taking didanosine. Two portal tracts show fibro-obliteration of the portal vein radicles (phlebosclerosis) (trichrome stain ×100). *(Courtesy of M. I. Fiel, MD.)*

- Hepatic adenoma (risk increases with duration of use and is higher in women more than 35 years old)
- Budd–Chiari syndrome (may be related to the thrombogenic effect of the estrogenic component)
- Focal nodular hyperplasia (relationship not firmly established)
2. Anabolic and androgenic steroids:
   - Peliosis hepatis
   - Cholestatic jaundice
   - Hepatic adenoma (possible association)
   - Hepatocellular carcinoma
3. Flutamide: This oral anti-androgen used in the treatment of metastatic prostate cancer is associated with an idiosyncratically mediated modest elevation of aminotransferases and rarely, massive hepatocellular necrosis.

HALOTHANE

1. Although the incidence of hepatotoxicity is low, fear of this complication dramatically limited its use, and today this drug is rarely used.

TABLE 8.4 ■ **Hepatotoxicity of antiretroviral anti agents used to treat human immunodeficiency virus infection and specific precautions**

Antiretroviral class	Precautions with regard to hepatotoxicity
Protease inhibitors (PIs) Ritonavir (Norvir) Lopinavir/Ritonavir (Kaletra) Amprenavir (Agenerase) Saquinavir (Fortovase) Indinavir (Crixivan) Fosamprenavir (Lexiva) Nelfinavir (Viracept) Atazanavir (Reyataz) Tipranavir (Aptivus) Darunavir (Prezista)	Hepatotoxicity with high-dose ritonavir (600 mg twice daily) Less hepatotoxicity with low-dose ritonavir (<200 mg twice daily) used in PI boosting regimens Avoid the combination of amprenavir with ritonavir (competing CYP 450 3A4 metabolism) Indirect hyperbilirubinemia with indinavir and atazanavir; avoid the combination of indinavir with atazanavir Severe hepatotoxicity with tipranavir reported; caution advised with use of tipranavir in patients with underlying liver disease
Nucleoside reverse transcriptase inhibitors (NRTIs) Zalcitabine (ddC) Didanosine (ddI) Stavudine (d4T) Lamivudine (3TC) Zidovudine (AZT) Abacavir (Ziagen) Tenofovir (Viread) Abacavir/lamivudine/zidovudine (Trizivir) - Abacavir/lamivudine (Epzicom)	Lactic acidosis (especially with ddC, ddI, d4T) ddI associated with noncirrhotic portal hypertension Avoid ddI-d4T combination Increased risk of lactic acidosis with ribavirin in conjunction with ddI or d4T Avoid ribavirin-ddI combination in advanced fibrosis because of the risk of hepatic decompensation
Non-nucleoside reverse transcriptase inhibitors (NNRTIs) Nevirapine (Viramune) Efavirenz (Sustiva) Delavirdine (Rescriptor)	Increased risk of hepatotoxicity with nevirapine in patients with HBV/HCV infection or in women with a CD4+ count >350/mm^3 or men with a CD4+ count >400/mm3

HBV, hepatitis B virus; HBC, hepatitis C virus.
From Chang CY, Schiano TD. Drug hepatotoxicity. *Aliment Pharmacol Ther* 2007; 25:1135–1151.

2. Hepatotoxicity was extremely uncommon after a first exposure (1 per 10,000 cases), typically occurring within 2 weeks of surgery. Repeated exposures over a short period of time increased the risk of hepatotoxicity.

3. The mechanism of liver injury appeared to involve formation of a toxic metabolite (probably generated by cytochrome P-450 metabolism). Liver damage occurred directly from or as a result of the capacity of halothane metabolites to function as neoantigens able to elicit typical hypersensitivity manifestations (e.g., fever, eosinophilia).

Other halogenated anesthetics such as enflurane and isoflurane have infrequently been reported to cause liver injury similar to that of halothane.

NEUROLOGIC AND ANTIPSYCHOTIC AGENTS

In general, phenothiazines, other neuroleptics (e.g., haloperidol), and less frequently benzodiazepines and barbiturates (e.g., phenobarbital) can cause cholestatic liver injury probably secondary to delayed hypersensitivity. Hepatocellular injury can be produced by tricyclic antidepressants (e.g., amitriptyline), as well as by anticonvulsants such as carbamazepine, phenytoin, and valproic acid.

1. **Chlorpromazine** (Thorazine)
   - The incidence of drug-induced jaundice may be as high as 1% to 5%, and asymptomatic liver chemistry test abnormalities have been reported in up to 25% of patients.
   - Onset of jaundice typically occurs within 1 to 4 weeks of initiation of treatment. Recovery usually occurs within 2 to 8 weeks with discontinuation of the drug, although symptoms resembling those of primary biliary cirrhosis can persist.
   - Bilirubin levels may be as high as 5 to 15 mg/dL, and alkaline phosphatase may be up to 10 times the ULN, with moderate elevations of aminotransferase levels.
   - Pronounced hypercholesterolemia is common. Histologically, centrilobular cholestasis is seen with periportal inflammation, usually including eosinophils.

2. **Carbamazepine** (Tegretol): This is structurally similar to tricyclic antidepressants. It is reported to produce mild to moderate liver chemistry test elevations in up to 20% of patients within the first 6 to 8 weeks of therapy.

3. **Phenytoin** (Dilantin)
   - Asymptomatic aminotransferase elevations are common, with clinically significant liver injury in 0.1% of patients.
   - Most patients with clinical hepatotoxicity have hypersensitivity-type symptoms, including eosinophilia, fever, leukocytosis, lymphadenopathy, and rash (pseudolymphoma). Cholestatic liver injury and ALF have also been reported.

4. **Valproic acid** (Depakene)
   - This is a common cause of asymptomatic aminotransferase elevations, which are usually mild, reversible, and dose dependent.
   - Fatal valproate hepatotoxicity is not dose dependent, occurs in young patients who are often receiving other anticonvulsants, and appears to be idiosyncratic. Liver biopsy shows microvesicular steatosis accompanied by centrilobular necrosis.

CARDIOVASCULAR AGENTS AND GLYCEMIC AGENTS

1. **Amiodarone**
   - **Up to fivefold aminotransferase elevations are seen in 40% of patients receiving long-term therapy.** Hepatomegaly is typical, but jaundice is generally absent. A relationship

appears to exist among the dose of amiodarone, the plasma level of the drug, and the development of abnormal liver tests. The drug should be discontinued when aminotransferase levels are twice normal, and a liver biopsy should be considered.

- Acute and even fatal hepatotoxicity, probably immunoallergic, may occur.
- Chronic injury usually has an insidious onset; aminotransferase levels are usually mildly elevated. Liver test abnormalities resolve slowly over several weeks to months after the drug is withdrawn.
- Liver histology shows changes mimicking those of alcoholic hepatitis with steatosis, Mallory's bodies, focal necrosis, and centrizonal fibrosis. Phospholipidosis (recognition requires electron microscopic examination) typically results from entrapment of the drug within lysosomes.

2. **Alpha-methyldopa** (Aldomet)
   - This can cause a spectrum of liver disease ranging from transient aminotransferase elevations to chronic hepatitis and even ALF. The frequency of symptomatic liver injury is 1% of cases; 80% of these patients develop acute hepatocellular injury, 5% have cholestatic injury, and the remainder have chronic hepatitis.
   - Chronic hepatitis can be histologically indistinguishable from autoimmune hepatitis.

3. **Angiotensin-converting enzyme (ACE) inhibitors**
   - Captopril, enalapril, fosinopril, and lisinopril have each been implicated in causing hepatic injury. Hepatotoxicity occurs infrequently, usually in the setting of medical comorbidities and polypharmacy.

4. **Other cardiac medications**
   - Verapamil and nifedipine can cause abnormal liver tests, whereas diltiazem, quinidine, and procainamide can cause granulomatous hepatitis.

GLYCEMIC AGENTS

1. **Thiazolidinediones**
   - Troglitazone was removed from the market in 2000 because of numerous reports of DILI, sometimes fatal.
   - Pathogenesis appears to be mitochondrial injury and impaired bile salt transporter.
   - Cases of hepatotoxicity with both pioglitazone and rosiglitazone have been reported.

2. **Metformin:** Impaired hepatic function is a risk factor for the development of lactic acidosis in patients receiving metformin.

LIPID-LOWERING AGENTS

1. **Statins**
   - Their use was once thought to be precluded in patients with liver disease, but **statins have now been found to be generally safe.**
   - Mildly elevated aminotransferase levels occur in patients taking statins, but clinically significant elevation occurs infrequently. These changes are generally dose related, occur with the first 12 weeks of therapy, and improve spontaneously in many cases.
   - DILI typically manifests with elevated aminotransferase levels, although mixed or cholestatic injury patterns have been reported, as well as cases of autoimmune hepatitis.
   - Chronic liver disease, fatty liver, and compensated cirrhosis are not contraindications to statin therapy. However, their use should be avoided in patients with decompensated cirrhosis. These drugs are not contraindicated after liver transplantation.

2. **Niacin**
   - This is widely available over the counter and is one of the least expensive antilipidemic agents.
   - Hepatotoxicity is infrequent, occurring at doses that exceed 3 g/day. Its spectrum can range from asymptomatic aminotransferase elevation that resolves within a month of cessation of use to ALF.
   - Sustained-release formulations are more convenient than regular niacin, and their use has been advocated to improve compliance. However, over the years severe hepatotoxicity, including ALF, associated with the use of sustained-release niacin has been reported.

IMMUNOSUPPRESSIVE MEDICATIONS USED FOR TREATMENT OF INFLAMMATORY BOWEL DISEASE

1. **Methotrexate**
   - Hepatotoxicity, including hepatic steatosis, fibrosis, and cirrhosis, has been recognized for several decades in patients treated for psoriasis.
   - Cumulative dose appears to be the greatest risk factor for the development of cirrhosis. A total dose of 1.5 g is associated with significant liver disease.
   - In contrast to psoriasis (for which a correlation between liver test abnormalities and histopathology is lacking), elevated aminotransferase levels are not uncommon in patients with rheumatoid arthritis and inflammatory bowel disease (IBD) who are receiving methotrexate. In rheumatoid arthritis, preexisting liver chemistry abnormalities, concurrent alcohol consumption, and intrinsic liver disease are risk factors for significant DILI and the need for a drug holiday. In IBD, methotrexate-induced liver test abnormalities typically resolve during therapy and only rarely necessitate discontinuation of the agent.
   - Routine surveillance liver biopsy is not recommended in patients with rheumatoid arthritis or IBD who are receiving methotrexate.
   - Cyclosporine is an infrequent cause of DILI, usually manifested by cholestasis and prominent hyperbilirubinemia.
2. **Thiopurines (azathioprine/6-mercaptopurine/6-thioguanine)**
   - These drugs have been associated with a wide range of hepatotoxic reactions including nodular regenerative hyperplasia, veno-occlusive disease, and, most commonly, cholestasis and asymptomatic elevation of aminotransferase levels.
   - Hepatotoxicity seems to correspond to high thioguanine methyltransferase (TPMT) activity. High TPMT enzyme activity preferentially shunts thioguanine metabolism toward an increase in the production of the metabolite 6-methylmercaptopurine ribonucleotide (6-MMP); this can be detected on a commercially available assay.
   - Concurrent use of allopurinol affects thioguanine metabolism.
3. **Biologic therapy**
   - As a class, tumor necrosis factor (TNF) antagonists are known to cause elevated aminotransferase levels and need to be used cautiously in patients with liver disease.
   - Agents such as etanercept (Enbrel), adalimumab (Humira), and infliximab (Remicade) have also been associated with triggering autoimmune hepatitis, and numerous cases of ALF have been reported.
   - **Screening patients for chronic hepatitis B before starting biologic therapy or any chemotherapeutic regimen is mandatory, to prevent reactivation of hepatitis B by using an oral antiviral agent.**

CHEMOTHERAPEUTIC AGENTS

1. Alkylating agents are uncommonly associated with DILI. Cyclophosphamide and ifosfamide do require dose reduction in the setting of liver dysfunction. Cyclophosphamide is infrequently hepatotoxic; alkylating agents such as melphalan, chlorambucil, nitrogen mustards, and busulfan do not depend on hepatic metabolism.
2. Antitumor antibiotics such as doxorubicin and daunorubicin can cause hepatocellular injury and steatosis, so dose reductions are recommended in patients with liver disease.
3. Antimetabolites such as thiopurines, cytarabine, and 5-fluorouracil depend on hepatic metabolism, and thus dose reductions are often necessary in patients with liver dysfunction.

COMPLEMENTARY AND ALTERNATIVE MEDICINES

1. This approach is used much more frequently as remedies for various medical conditions, especially in the treatment of liver disease. Because herbal products are not marketed as drugs, they are not subjected to rigorous safety and efficacy testing.
2. **Use of herbal medicine should be a part of any history in a patient with liver disease.**
3. Initial clinical symptoms often can be nonspecific, and constitutional symptoms can occur much earlier than jaundice.
4. Many products may have a good safety record, and liver injury occurs when recommended toxic dose thresholds are exceeded.
5. Treatment consists of withdrawal of the offending agent. Continued use of the agent after hepatotoxicity has occurred may result in cirrhosis or ALF.
6. Although the histopathology of herbal and complementary and alternative agents may mimic any acute or chronic liver disease (Table 8.5), these agents should be strongly considered obscure causes of liver injury. Uncommon histologic patterns of liver injury that should arouse the suspicion of toxicity related to herbal remedies or complementary and alternative medicine are zonal necrosis, necrosis with associated steatosis or bile duct injury, and vascular injury.
7. These agents may cause liver injury directly or through their interaction with cytochrome P-450.

OCCUPATIONAL HEPATOTOXINS

1. Occupational hepatotoxins are now infrequently encountered because of increased awareness by physicians, workers, and regulatory agencies such as the Occupational Safety and Hazard Administration (OSHA) and the National Institute for Occupational Safety and Hazard (NIOSH).
2. A list of known hepatotoxic chemicals is shown in Table 8.6, and many occupations involve exposure to these potentially hepatotoxic chemicals.
3. Many cases of occupational hepatotoxicity may go unrecognized because they are not suspected, not properly investigated, or simply are not reported.
4. A single severe exposure often leads to an acute clinical presentation, whereas prolonged exposure of a lesser degree may lead to subacute or chronic liver disease.
5. Occupational hepatotoxicity can clinically and histologically mimic almost any known liver disease.

ENVIRONMENTAL HEPATOTOXINS

1. **Mushroom poisoning**
   - Western Europe, where amateur wild mushroom gathering is a popular pastime, has the highest incidence. In the United States, most poisonings occur in the Pacific Northwest, although *Amanita* species have been identified in oak woodlands throughout the country.

TABLE 8.5 ■ **Histopathologic patterns of hepatotoxicity related to environmental, botanical, and complementary and alternative medicines**

Histopathologic pattern	Agent
Autoimmune hepatitis	Ma-huang
Chronic hepatitis, with or without fibrosis	Germander
	Greater celandine
	Jin Bu Huan
Cirrhosis	Chaparral
	Germander
	Greater celandine
	Jin Bu Huan
Cholestatic hepatitis	Black cohosh
	Chaparral
	Greater celandine
	Jin Bu Huan
	Kava
Acute liver failure	*Atractylis gummifera*
	Black cohosh
	Callilepis laureola (impila)
	Chaparral
	Chinese herbal medicine
	Cocaine
	Germander
	Green tea extract
	Hydroxycut
	Kava
	Lipokinetix
	Pennyroyal
	Sustained-release niacin
	Teucrium polium
Hepatocellular carcinoma	Aflatoxin
Massive hepatic necrosis	Cocaine
	Germander
	Greater celandine
	Kava
	Pennyroyal
Microvesicular steatosis	Margosa oil
Vascular lesions: sinusoidal obstruction syndrome	Pyrrolizidine alkaloids
Zonal necrosis	*Atractylis gummifera*
	Callilepis laureola
	Cocaine
	Germander
	Jin Bu Huan
	Pennyroyal oil
	Teucrium polium

Amanita phalloides accounts for more than 90% of fatalities. Consumption of a single mushroom can lead to ALF and death.

■ *Amanita phalloides* exerts its hepatotoxicity through two distinct toxins, phalloidin and amatoxin. Neither is destroyed by cooking or gastric acidity. These toxins result in cell necrosis, most commonly involving the liver and kidneys.

TABLE 8.6 ■ **Some hepatotoxic chemicals and their uses**

Chemical	Uses
Arsenic and inorganic salts	As pesticides and alloys; in production of dyes, ceramics, drugs, fireworks, paint, petroleum, ink and semiconductors
Beryllium	In alloys, cathode ray tubes, ceramics, electrical equipment, gas mantles, missiles, nuclear reactors, and refractory materials
Carbon tetrachloride	As degreasers, fat processors, fire extinguishers, fumigants, production of solvents; in fluorocarbons, inks, insecticides, lacquer, propellants, refrigerants, rubber and wax
Dioxane	As solvents, degreasers, cement components; in production of adhesives, deodorants, detergents, emulsions, fats, glue, lacquer, oil, paint, polish, shoe cream, varnish remover, waxes; in histology laboratories
Phosphorus (yellow)	In munitions, pyrotechnics, explosives, smoke bombs, fertilizers, rodenticides, bronze alloys, semiconductors, and luminescent coatings
Picric acid (2,4,6-trinitrophenol)	As a copper etcher, and a forensic and biology laboratory chemical; in batteries, colored glass, disinfectants, drugs, dyes, explosives, matches, photography chemicals, and tanneries
Polychlorinated biphenyls	In cable insulation, dyes, electric equipment, herbicides, lacquers, paper treatment, plasticizers, resins, rubber textiles, flame proofing, transformers, and wood preservation
2,3,7,8-Tetrachloro-dibenzo-p-dioxin	Contaminant of commercial preparations of 2,4,5-trichlorophenoxyacetic acid, polychlorinated biphenyls, and other chlorinated compounds
Tetrachloroethane	As a dry-cleaning agent, fumigant, solvent, degreaser; in production of gaskets, lacquers, paints, phosphorus, resins, varnish, wax
Tetrachloroethylene	As a solvent, degreaser, chemical intermediate, fumigant; in production of cellulose esters, gums, rubber, soap, vacuum tubes, wax, wool
Thorotrast	Previously used radiologic contrast agent
2,4,5-Trinitrotoluene	As an explosive
Vinyl chloride	As a chemical intermediate and solvent; in production of polyvinyl chloride and resins

From Schiano TD, Hunt K. Occupational and environmental hepatotoxicity. In: Boyer TD, Wright TL, Manns MP, eds. *Zakim and Boyer's Hepatology: A Textbook of Liver Disease,* 5th edn. Toronto, Saunders; 2006:561–577.

- A latent asymptomatic period ranges from 6 to 24 hours, followed by a gastrointestinal phase lasting 12 to 24 hours, heralded by severe crampy abdominal pain, nausea, vomiting, and watery diarrhea. A second latent phase lasts 12 to 24 hours, in which clinical symptoms improve but liver dysfunction is first noted. Finally, rapid progression to ALF from massive hepatocellular necrosis occurs (Fig. 8.6).
- Induction of emesis and administration of charcoal with gastric lavage may reduce the toxin load, but most patients present several hours after ingestion.
- High-dose penicillin G in combination with silymarin (an extract of the milk thistle *Silybum marianum*) has been used in some patients with resultant improvement of hepatic dysfunction. However, liver transplantation is almost always necessary, so early evaluation and referral to a transplant center are crucial.

2. **Pyrrolizidine alkaloids**
   - More than 300 have been identified; *Senecio*, heliotropine, *Crotalaria*, and *Symphytum* (comfrey species) are well-known hepatotoxins.

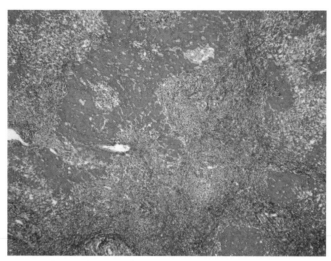

Fig. 8.6 Histopathology of massive hepatic necrosis. A representative photomicrograph from a liver explant from a patient who ingested an *Amanita* species mushroom and who required liver transplantation. Note the confluent necrosis and absence of viable hepatocytes (trichrome stain). *(Courtesy of M. I. Fiel, MD.)*

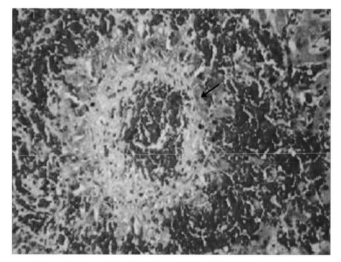

Fig. 8.7 Histopathology of sinusoidal obstructive syndrome. High-power magnification of a terminal venule with obliteration of the lumen by fibrous tissue (trichrome stain ×400). *(Courtesy of M. I. Fiel, MD.)*

- Large outbreaks have been reported with contamination of wheat; many alkaloids are used as supplements or in traditional herbal medicines.
- These agents may cause acute liver injury and sinusoidal obstruction syndrome (Fig. 8.7) or ongoing chronic liver injury and cirrhosis. Pulmonary hypertension may also ensue.

3. **Cocaine**
   - This can cause profound elevation of serum aminotransferase levels. It may mimic acetaminophen overdose and results in ALF. Cocaine exerts its hepatotoxicity by the creation of toxic free radicals through cytochrome P-450, so use of NAC may be helpful.
   - Intoxication should be considered along with ischemic hepatitis, acetaminophen overdose, and mushroom poisoning in the differential diagnosis of acute hepatitis with extremely elevated serum aminotransferase levels that rise into the several thousand range.
4. **Aflatoxin:** This is produced by the fungus *Aspergillus flavus*, which is a contaminant of nuts, corn, wheat, barley, rice, cottonseed, and soy beans. Epidemiologic studies point to an association between the quantity ingested (from contaminated food) and the incidence of hepatocellular carcinoma. It may act synergistically as a cocarcinogen with hepatitis B virus. Its carcinogenicity is mediated by a unique mutation in codon 249 of the p53 oncogene.

FURTHER READING

Bell LN, Chalasani N. Epidemiology of idiosyncratic drug-induced liver injury. *Semin Liver Dis* 2009; 29:337–347.

Chalasani N, Fontana RJ, Bonkovsky HL, et al. Causes, clinical features, and outcomes from a prospective study of drug-induced liver injury in the United States. *Gastroenterology* 2008; 135:1924–1934, 1934.e1–e4.

Chang CY, Schiano TD. Drug hepatotoxicity. *Aliment Pharmacol Ther* 2007; 25:1135–1151.

Chun LJ, Tong MJ, Busuttil RW, Hiatt JR. Acetaminophen hepatotoxicity and acute liver failure. *J Clin Gastroenterol* 2009; 43:342–349.

Cooper SC, Aldridge RC, Shah T, et al. Outcomes of liver transplantation for paracetamol (acetaminophen)-induced hepatic failure. *Liver Transpl* 2009; 15:1351–1357.

Daly AK, Day CP. Genetic association studies in drug-induced liver injury. *Semin Liver Dis* 2009; 29:400–411.

Gupta NK, Lewis JH. The use of potentially hepatotoxic drugs in patients with liver disease. *Aliment Pharmacol Ther* 2008; 28:1021–1041.

Kleiner DE. The pathology of drug-induced liver injury. *Semin Liver Dis* 2009; 29:364–372.

Perrone C. Antiviral hepatitis and antiretroviral drug interactions. *J Hepatol* 2006; 1(Suppl):S119–S125.

Pugh AJ, Barve AJ, Falkner K, et al. Drug-induced hepatotoxicity or drug-induced liver injury. *Clin Liver Dis* 2009; 13:277–294.

Reuben A. Hy's law. *Hepatology* 2004; 39:521–528.

Russo MW, Galanko JA, Shrestha R, et al. Liver transplantation for acute liver failure from drug induced liver injury in the United States. *Liver Transpl* 2004; 10:1018–1023.

Russo MW, Scobey M, Bonkovsky HL. Drug-induced liver injury associated with statins. *Semin Liver Dis* 2009; 29:412–422.

Saukkonen JJ, Cohn DL, Jasmer RM, et al. An official ATS statement: hepatotoxicity of antituberculosis therapy. *Am J Respir Crit Care Med* 2006; 174:935–952.

Seeff LB. Herbal hepatotoxicity. *Clin Liver Dis* 2007; 11:577–596.

CHAPTER 9

Cirrhosis and portal hypertension: an overview

Catherine Petruff Cheney, MD, AGAF ■ Eric Mathew Goldberg, MD ■ Sanjiv Chopra, MBBS, MACP

KEY POINTS

1 The major causes of cirrhosis include chronic hepatitis B, chronic hepatitis C, alcohol, hemochromatosis, and nonalcoholic steatohepatitis (NASH).

2 An etiologic classification of cirrhosis is more clinically relevant than a morphologic one (micronodular, macronodular, mixed), because the cause can be determined in most cases, and important management issues such as family counseling, vaccination, and specific therapy are best addressed once the cause has been determined.

3 Important and potentially life-threatening complications of cirrhosis include ascites, spontaneous bacterial peritonitis, variceal hemorrhage, hepatic encephalopathy, hepatorenal syndrome, hepatopulmonary syndrome, and hepatocellular carcinoma.

4 The Child–Turcotte–Pugh classification is useful in assessing prognosis and estimating the potential risk of variceal bleeding and operative mortality.

5 The Model for End-stage Liver Disease (MELD), a more recently developed prognostic assessment based on international normalized ratio (INR), serum creatinine level, and serum bilirubin level, is currently used to determine the appropriateness and timing of liver transplantation.

Cirrhosis

DEFINITION

1. The word *cirrhosis* is derived from the Greek word *kirrhos*, meaning orange or tawny, and *osis*, meaning condition.
2. **World Health Organization definition of cirrhosis is a diffuse process characterized by fibrosis and the conversion of normal liver architecture into structurally abnormal nodules that lack normal lobular organization.**
3. Structural changes in the liver may cause impairment of hepatic function manifested as
   ■ jaundice
   ■ portal hypertension and varices
   ■ ascites
   ■ hepatorenal syndrome
   ■ spontaneous bacterial peritonitis
   ■ hepatic encephalopathy
   ■ progressive hepatic failure

4. This definition distinguishes cirrhosis from other types of liver disease that have either nodule formation or fibrosis, but not both. These hepatic disorders may be characterized by portal hypertension in the absence of cirrhosis. **Nodular regenerative hyperplasia**, for example, is characterized by diffuse nodularity without fibrosis, whereas chronic **schistosomiasis** is characterized by Symmers' pipestem fibrosis with no nodularity.

CLASSIFICATION

1. Morphologic classification is less useful because of considerable overlap.
   - Micronodular cirrhosis, with uniform nodules less than 3 mm in diameter: causes include alcohol, hemochromatosis, biliary obstruction, hepatic venous outflow obstruction, jejuno-ileal bypass, and Indian childhood cirrhosis.
   - Macronodular cirrhosis, with nodular variation greater than 3 mm in diameter: causes include chronic hepatitic C, chronic hepatitis B, alpha-1 antitrypsin deficiency, and primary biliary cirrhosis,
   - Mixed cirrhosis, a combination of micronodular and macronodular cirrhosis: micronodular cirrhosis frequently evolves into macronodular cirrhosis.
2. Etiologic classification is preferred.
   - This method of classification is the most useful clinically; by combining clinical, biochemical, genetic, histologic, and epidemiologic data, the likely etiologic agent can be ascertained.
   - **The two most common causes of cirrhosis are excessive alcohol use and viral hepatitis**. Table 9.1 lists the etiologic classification and tests used to determine the cause.
   - Most cases of cryptogenic cirrhosis may be "burned out" nonalcoholic steatohepatitis (NASH). It is now established that NASH may occur in patients with cryptogenic cirrhosis who undergo liver transplantation, a finding suggesting that NASH is a disease recurrence.

PATHOLOGY

Liver biopsy is performed in selected patients with chronic liver disease when the clinical, biochemical, and radiologic data are not definitive for cirrhosis.

1. Gross examination: the liver surface is irregular, with multiple yellowish nodules; depending on the severity of the cirrhosis, the liver may be enlarged because of multiple regenerating nodules or, in the final stages, small and shrunken.
2. Pathologic criteria for diagnosis of cirrhosis
   - Nodularity (regenerating nodules)
   - Fibrosis (deposition of connective tissue creates pseudolobules)
   - Fragmentation of the sample
   - Abnormal hepatic architecture
   - Hepatocellular abnormalities
   - Pleomorphism
   - Dysplasia
   - Regenerative hyperplasia
3. Information obtained from histologic examination
   - Establishment of the presence of cirrhosis
   - Determination of the cause of cirrhosis in some cases
   - Assessment of grade of histologic activity
4. Specific histologic methods for determining the cause of cirrhosis
   - Immunohistochemistry (e.g., hepatitis B virus)
   - Polymerase chain reaction (PCR) techniques (e.g., hepatitis C virus)

TABLE 9.1 ■ **Etiology and diagnostic workup of the common causes of cirrhosis**

Etiology	Diagnostic evaluation
Infection	
Hepatitis B	HBsAg, anti-HBs, anti-HBc, HBV DNA
Hepatitis C	Anti-HCV, HCV RNA
Hepatitis D	Anti-HDV
Toxins	
Alcohol	History, AST/ALT ratio, liver biopsy
Cholestasis	
Primary biliary cirrhosis	AMA, IgM, liver biopsy
Secondary biliary cirrhosis	MRCP, ERCP, liver biopsy
Primary sclerosing cholangitis	MRCP, ERCP, liver biopsy
Autoimmune	
Autoimmune hepatitis	ANA, IgG level smooth muscle antibodies, liver-kidney microsomal antibodies, liver biopsy
Vascular	
Cardiac cirrhosis	Echocardiogram, liver biopsy
Budd–Chiari syndrome	CT, US, MRI/MRA,
Sinusoidal obstruction syndrome	History of offending drug use, liver biopsy
Metabolic	
Hemochromatosis	Iron studies, *HFE* gene mutation, liver biopsy
Wilson disease	Serum and urinary copper, ceruloplasmin, slit lamp eye examination, liver biopsy
Alpha-1 antitrypsin deficiency	Alpha-1 antitrypsin level, protease inhibitor type, liver biopsy
NASH	Liver biopsy
Cryptogenic	Exclude NASH, drugs

ALT, alanine aminotransferase; AMA, antimitochondrial antibodies; ANA, antinuclear antibodies; anti-HBc, antibody to hepatitis B core antigen; anti-HBs, antibody to hepatitis B surface antigen; anti-HCV, antibody to hepatitis C virus; anti-HDV, antibody to hepatitis D virus; AST, aspartate aminotransferase; CT, computed tomography; ERCP, endoscopic retrograde cholangiopancreatography; HBsAg, hepatitis B surface antigen; IgG, immunoglobulin G; IgM, immunoglobulin M; MRA, magnetic resonance angiography; MRCP, magnetic resonance cholangiopancreatography; MRI, magnetic resonance imaging; NASH, nonalcoholic steatohepatitis; US, ultrasonography.

- Quantitative copper measurement (Wilson disease)
- Periodic acid–Schiff (PAS)–positive, diastase-resistant globules (alpha-1 antitrypsin deficiency)
- Quantitative iron measurement (hemochromatosis)

CLINICAL FEATURES

The manifestations of cirrhosis are protean. Patients with cirrhosis may come to clinical attention in numerous ways:

1. Stigmata of chronic liver disease on physical examination (e.g., palmar erythema, spider telangiectasias)

2. Abnormal serum chemistry test results and hematologic indices (e.g., serum aminotransferases, bilirubin, alkaline phosphatase, albumin, prothrombin time, and platelet count)
3. Radiographic abnormalities (e.g., small, shrunken, nodular liver on ultrasound or computed tomographic [CT] examination)
4. Complications of decompensated liver disease (e.g., ascites, variceal hemorrhage)
5. Cirrhotic appearance of the liver at the time of laparotomy or laparoscopy
6. Autopsy

A patient with cirrhosis may present with none, some, or all of the following findings:
1. **General features**
   - Fatigue
   - Anorexia
   - Malaise
   - Weight loss
   - Muscle wasting
   - Fever
2. **Gastrointestinal**
   a. Parotid enlargement
   b. Diarrhea
   c. Cholelithiasis
   d. Gastrointestinal bleeding
      - Esophageal/gastric/duodenal/rectal/stomal varices
      - Portal hypertensive gastropathy/enteropathy/colopathy
3. **Hematologic**
   a. Anemia
      - Folate deficiency
      - Spur cell anemia (hemolytic anemia seen in severe alcoholic liver disease)
      - Splenomegaly with resulting pancytopenia
   b. Thrombocytopenia
   c. Leukopenia
   d. Impaired coagulation
   e. Disseminated intravascular coagulation
   f. Hemosiderosis
4. **Pulmonary**
   a. Decreased oxygen saturation
   b. Altered ventilation–perfusion relationships
   c. Portopulmonary hypertension
   d. Hyperventilation
   e. Reduced pulmonary diffusion capacity
   f. Hepatic hydrothorax
      - Accumulation of fluid within the pleural space in association with cirrhosis and in the absence of primary pulmonary or cardiac disease
      - Usually right-sided (70%)
      - Typically associated with clinically apparent ascites, but can be found in patients without ascites
   g. Hepatopulmonary syndrome
      - Triad of liver disease, an increased alveolar–arterial gradient while breathing room air, and evidence for intrapulmonary vascular dilatations
      - Wide reported range of prevalence in cirrhotic patients from approximately 5% to 50%

- Characterized by dyspnea, platypnea, orthodeoxia, digital clubbing, and severe hypoxemia (PO_2 less than 80 mm Hg, and often less than 60 mm Hg)
- Intrapulmonary shunting demonstrated by contrast-enhanced ("bubble") echocardiography or technetium-99m macroaggregated albumin scanning; pulmonary arteriography rarely required
- Associated with significantly increased risk of mortality without liver transplantation; risk increases with the degree of hypoxemia (Chapter 31)
- The Model for End-stage Liver Disease (MELD) exception points may be given to patients with significant hypoxemia (PO_2 less than 60 mm Hg)
- Complete resolution typical after liver transplantation; time course of improvement variable and often delayed up to 1 year

5. **Cardiac:** hyperdynamic circulation
6. **Renal**
   - Secondary hyperaldosteronism leading to sodium and water retention
   - Renal tubular acidosis (more frequent in alcoholic cirrhosis, Wilson disease, and primary biliary cirrhosis)
   - Hepatorenal syndrome
7. **Endocrinologic**
   a. Hypogonadism
      - Male patients: loss of libido, testicular atrophy, impotence, decreased amounts of testosterone
      - Female patients: infertility, dysmenorrhea, loss of secondary sexual characteristics
   b. Feminization (acquisition of estrogen-induced characteristics)
      - Spider telangiectasias
      - Palmar erythema
      - Gynecomastia
      - Changes in body hair patterns
   c. Diabetes
8. **Neurologic**
   a. Hepatic encephalopathy
      - Variants include spastic paraplegia and acquired non-wilsonian hepatocerebral degeneration
   b. Peripheral neuropathy
   c. Asterixis
9. **Musculoskeletal**
   - Reduction in lean muscle mass
   - Hypertrophic osteoarthropathy: synovitis, clubbing, and periostitis
   - Hepatic osteodystrophy
   - Muscle cramps
   - Umbilical herniation
10. **Dermatologic**
    a. Spider telangiectases
    b. Palmar erythema
    c. Nail changes
       - Azure lunules (Wilson disease)
       - Muercke's nails: paired horizontal white bands separated by normal color
       - Terry's nails: white appearance to the proximal two thirds of the nail plate
    d. Pruritus
    e. Dupuytren's contractures

f. Clubbing
g. Jaundice
h. Paper money skin
i. Caput medusae
j. Easy bruising

COMPLICATIONS

- Ascites (see Chapter 11)
- Spontaneous bacterial peritonitis (see Chapter 11)
- Variceal hemorrhage (see Chapter 10)
- Hepatic encephalopathy (see Chapter 13)
- Hepatocellular carcinoma (see Chapter 27)
- Hepatorenal syndrome (see Chapter 12)

DIAGNOSIS

1. **Physical examination**
   a. Stigmata of chronic liver disease and/or cirrhosis
      - Spider telangiectasias
      - Palmar erythema
      - Dupuytren's contractures
      - Gynecomastia
      - Testicular atrophy
   b. Features of portal hypertension
      - Ascites
      - Splenomegaly
      - Caput medusae
      - Evidence of hyperdynamic circulation (e.g., resting tachycardia)
      - Cruveilhier–Baumgarten murmur: venous hum best auscultated in the epigastrium
   c. Features of hepatic encephalopathy
      - Confusion
      - Asterixis
      - Fetor hepaticus
   d. Other
      - Jaundice
      - Bilateral parotid enlargement
      - Scant chest and axillary hair
2. **Laboratory evaluation** (see also Chapter 1)
   a. Tests of hepatocellular injury
      - Aminotransferases (aspartate aminotransferase [AST] and alanine aminotransferase [ALT]): most forms of chronic hepatitis other than alcohol have an AST/ALT ratio of less than 1; however, as chronic hepatitis progresses to cirrhosis, the ratio of AST/ALT may reverse.
   b. Tests of cholestasis
      - Alkaline phosphatase
      - Serum bilirubin (conjugated and unconjugated)
      - Gamma glutamyltranspeptidase (GGTP)
      - 5′-Nucleotidase

    c. Tests of synthetic function
- Serum albumin
- Prothrombin time

    d. Special tests to aid in diagnosis
- Viral hepatitis serology (see Chapters 3 and 4)
- PCR techniques for detecting viral RNA or DNA
- Serum iron, total iron binding capacity (TIBC), ferritin, genetic testing for the *HFE* gene mutation (hemochromatosis)
- Ceruloplasmin, serum and urinary copper (Wilson disease)
- Alpha-1 antitrypsin level and protease inhibitor type
- Serum immunoglobulins (autoimmune hepatitis)
- Autoantibodies: antinuclear antibodies (ANA), antimitochondrial antibodies (AMA), anti–liver kidney microsomal antibodies (LKM), anti–smooth muscle antibodies (SMA) (autoimmune hepatitis, primary biliary cirrhosis)

    e. Screening test for hepatocellular carcinoma: serum alpha fetoprotein

3. **Imaging studies** (see also Chapter 1)

    a. Abdominal ultrasonography
- Noninvasive, relatively inexpensive
- Can easily detect ascites, biliary dilatation
- Screening test for primary hepatocellular carcinoma
- Duplex Doppler ultrasonography can further assess hepatic and portal vein patency

    b. CT
- Noninvasive, more expensive than ultrasound
- Findings in cirrhosis are nonspecific
- May be helpful in the diagnosis of hemochromatosis; increased density of the liver is suggestive

    c. Magnetic resonance imaging (MRI)
- Noninvasive, but expensive
- Excellent for further evaluation of suspicious liver lesions; can help differentiate focal fat from a possible hepatic malignancy
- Can easily assess hepatic vasculature without the need for nephrotoxic contrast agents; more reliable than Doppler ultrasound
- May suggest iron overload states (black hypointense liver)
- Magnetic resonance cholangiography (MRC) a noninvasive method to image the biliary tree

    d. Radionuclide studies
- Colloid liver spleen scan using technetium-99m sulfur colloid may aid in detection of cirrhosis; increased uptake of colloid in the bone marrow and spleen, with decreased uptake in the liver
- Seldom performed; supplanted by CT and MRI

    e. Esophagogastroduodenoscopy (EGD) to screen for gastroesophageal varices

4. **Liver biopsy** (see also Chapter 1)

    a. The gold standard for the diagnosis of cirrhosis

    b. Usually performed percutaneously; occasionally obtained through the transjugular approach or at laparoscopy

    c. Relatively low-risk procedure

    d. Complications: bleeding, infection, pneumothorax, pain, hypotension

TREATMENT

1. Specific treatments are available in certain instances:
   - Phlebotomy for hemochromatosis
   - D-Penicillamine for Wilson disease
   - Avoidance of alcohol for alcohol-induced cirrhosis
   - Combination of peginterferon alfa and ribavirin for chronic hepatitis C
   - Lamivudine, adefovir, entecavir, telbivudine or tenofovir for chronic hepatitis B (interferon usually avoided in cirrhosis caused by chronic hepatitis B)
   - Corticosteroids for autoimmune hepatitis
   - Ursodeoxycholic acid for primary biliary cirrhosis
2. In most cases, management focuses on the treatment of complications that arise in the setting of cirrhosis (e.g., variceal hemorrhage, hepatic encephalopathy, ascites, and spontaneous bacterial peritonitis).
3. Surveillence for hepatocellular carcinoma with serial ultrasound examinations and serum alpha fetoprotein measurements at frequent intervals (e.g., every 6 months) is generally recommended in patients with cirrhosis.
4. Vaccination of cirrhotic patients against hepatitis A and B is recommended if patients lack serologic evidence of immunity.
5. Cirrhotic patients should be advised to avoid alcohol and other hepatotoxins.
6. **In end-stage cirrhosis, liver transplantation can be a lifesaving procedure if the patient is an appropriate candidate (see Chapter 31).**

PROGNOSIS

1. This depends on the development of cirrhotic-related complications.
2. A classification scheme proposed to assess survival, **Child's classification**, has undergone various modifications; the system currently used by many hepatologists is the **Child–Turcotte–Pugh (CTP) scoring system** (Table 9.2).

TABLE 9.2 ■ **Modified Child–Turcotte–Pugh scoring system for cirrhosis**

Parameter	Numerical score		
	1	2	3
Ascites	None	Slight	Moderate/severe
Encephalopathy	None	Slight/moderate	Moderate/severe
Bilirubin (mg/dL)	<2.0	2–3	>3.0
Albumin (mg/L)	>3.5	2.8–3.5	<2.8
Prothrombin time (sec increased)	1–3	4–6	>6.0

Total numerical score	Child Pugh class
5–6	A
7–9	B
10–15	C

3. Patients with compensated cirrhosis may have a relatively long life expectancy if they do not exhibit evidence of decompensation; estimated 10-year survival in compensated patients is 47%, but estimated 5-year survival is only 16% when decompensation occurs.
4. In patients with cirrhosis and varices who have not yet had their first variceal hemorrhage, the risk of bleeding from varices can be predicted based on a scoring system that incorporates the CTP classification, the size of varices, and certain endoscopic stigmata such as red wale markings and cherry-red spots on varices (see Chapter 10).
5. In cirrhotic patients, the risk of general anesthesia and operative mortality also correlates with the CTP classification (see Chapter 30).
6. **MELD** is a prognostic assessment based on serum bilirubin, serum creatinine, and international normalized ratio (INR); it is currently used to determine optimal timing for liver transplantation (see Chapter 31).

EVALUATION

See Fig. 9.1.

Portal Hypertension

Definition: an increase in portal venous pressure
- Normal portal pressure: 5 to 10 mm Hg
- Portal hypertension: greater than 12 mm Hg
- Normal portal blood flow: 1 to 1.5 L/minute
- Increased resistance to portal blood flow leading to formation of portosystemic collateral vessels that divert portal blood flow to the systemic circulation, thus effectively bypassing the liver

CLASSIFICATION (Table 9.3)

1. Portal hypertension has causes other than cirrhosis.
2. The major classification scheme employed is based on the location of the block to portal flow: **prehepatic, intrahepatic, and posthepatic**; intrahepatic causes are further separated into **presinusoidal, sinusoidal, and postsinusoidal** (Fig. 9.2); this method of classification has some overlap.

CLINICAL CONSEQUENCES

1. Varices: gastroesophageal, anorectal, retroperitoneal, stomal, other
2. Portal hypertensive gastropathy, enteropathy, and colopathy
3. Caput medusae
4. Ascites and hepatic hydrothorax
5. Congestive splenomegaly
6. Hepatic encephalopathy

MEASUREMENT OF PORTAL PRESSURE

1. In most cases, the diagnosis of portal hypertension can be based on physical findings; however, in some instances actual measurement of the portal pressure is required.

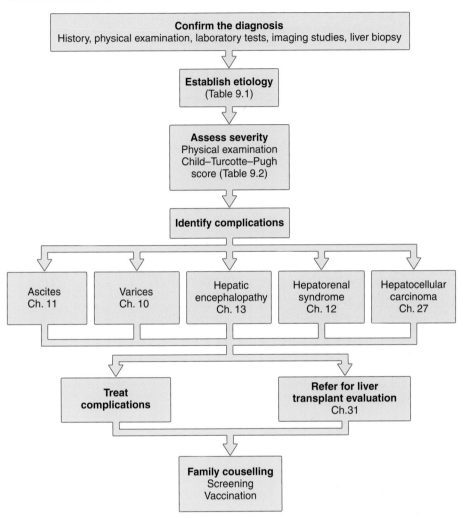

Fig. 9.1   Evaluation of the patient with cirrhosis.

2. Patency of the portal vein should be assessed before measurement of portal pressure; this may be accomplished by duplex Doppler ultrasound or magnetic resonance angiography (MRA).
3. Direct measurement of portal pressure is invasive, expensive, complicated, and accurate.
   ■ Operative portal vein measurement: requires laparotomy and is affected by many variables including anesthesia
   ■ Percutaneous transhepatic measurement
   ■ Transjugular measurement
4. Indirect measurement of portal pressure is the preferred method and is less invasive, safer, and less complicated.
   a. Hepatic vein catheterization

TABLE 9.3 ■ Causes of portal hypertension

1. Prehepatic
   Portal vein thrombosis
   Cavernous transformation of the portal vein
   Splenic vein thrombosis
   Splanchnic arteriovenous fistula
   Idiopathic tropical splenomegaly
2. Intrahepatic (some overlap exists)
   a. Presinusoidal: affects portal venule
      Schistosomiasis (most common cause of portal hypertension worldwide)
      Congenital hepatic fibrosis
      Sarcoidosis
      Chronic viral hepatitis
      Primary biliary cirrhosis (early)
      Myeloproliferative diseases
      Nodular regenerative hyperplasia
      Hepatoportal sclerosis (idiopathic portal hypertension)
      Malignant disease
      Wilson disease
      Hemochromatosis
      Polycystic liver disease
      Amyloidosis
      Toxic agents: copper, arsenic, vinyl chloride, 6-mercaptopurine
   b. Sinusoidal: affects sinusoids
      All causes of cirrhosis (see Table 9.1)
      Acute alcoholic hepatitis
      Severe viral hepatitis
      Acute fatty liver of pregnancy
      Vitamin A intoxication
      Systemic mastocytosis
      Peliosis hepatis
      Cytotoxic drugs
   c. Postsinusoidal: affects central vein
      Sinusoidal obstruction syndrome
      Alcoholic central hyaline sclerosis
3. Posthepatic
   a. Hepatic vein thrombosis
      Budd–Chiari syndrome
      Vascular invasion by tumor
   b. Inferior vena caval obstruction
      Inferior vena cava web
      Vascular invasion by tumor
   c. Cardiac disease
      Constrictive pericarditis
      Severe tricuspid regurgitation

- Involves cannulation of the hepatic vein, balloon occlusion of the hepatic vein, and measurement of the wedged hepatic vein pressure (WHVP)
- **Portal venous pressure gradient**: defined as the **difference between the portal pressure and that in the inferior vena cava**
- WHVP actually a measure of sinusoidal pressure, not portal pressure
- Portal pressure possibly underestimated in cases of presinusoidal portal hypertension
- Can measure hepatic blood flow

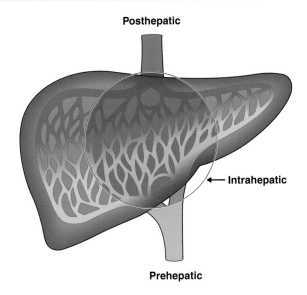

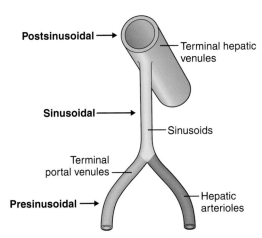

Fig. 9.2   Sites of block in portal hypertension.

b. Intrasplenic measurement
- Involves percutaneous puncture of the spleen
- Not routinely performed

TREATMENT OF COMPLICATIONS

See Chapters 10 to 13 and 31.

EVALUATION

See Fig. 9.3.

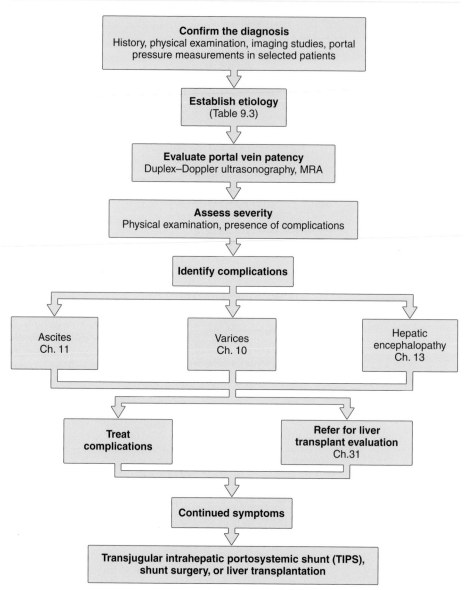

Fig. 9.3 Evaluation of the patient with portal hypertension. MRA, magnetic resonance angiography.

FURTHER READING

Albers I, Hartman H, Bircher J. Creutzfeldt. Superiority of the Child–Pugh classification to quantitative liver function tests for assessing prognosis of liver cirrhosis. *Scand J Gastroenterol* 1989; 24:269–276.

Anthony PP, Ishak KG, Nayak NC, et al. The morphology of cirrhosis: recommendations on definition, nomenclature, and classification by a working group sponsored by the World Health Organization. *J Clin Pathol* 1978; 31:395–414.

Bosch J, Navasa M, Garcia-Pagan JC, et al. Portal hypertension. *Med Clin North Am* 1989; 73:931–952.

Christensen E, Schicting P, Fauerholdt L, et al. Prognostic value of Child–Turcotte criteria in medically treated cirrhosis. *Hepatology* 1984; 4:430–435.

D'Amico G, Pagliaro L, Bosch J. The treatment of portal hypertension: a meta-analytic review. *Hepatology* 1995; 22:332–351.

Gines P, Quintero E, Arroyo V, et al. Compensated cirrhosis: natural history and prognostic factors. *Hepatology* 1987; 7:122–128.

Goldberg E, Chopra S. Diagnostic approach to the patient with cirrhosis. *UpToDate* 2009. Available at http://www.uptodate.com/patients/content/topic.do?topicKey=~UERfCNtHA22Nug.

Kamath PS, Wiesner RH, Malinchoc M, et al. A model to predict survival in patients with end-stage liver disease. *Hepatology* 2001; 33:464–470.

Londono MC, Cardenas A, Guevera M, et al. MELD score and serum sodium in the prediction of survival in patients with cirrhosis awaiting liver transplantation. *Gut* 2007; 56:1283–1290.

Marmur J, Bergquist A, Stal P. Liver transplantation of patients with cryptogenic cirrhosis: clinical characteristics and outcome. *Scand J Gastroenterol* 2010; 45:60–69.

Poonawala A, Nair SP, Thuluvath PJ. Prevalence of obesity and diabetes in patients with cryptogenic cirrhosis: a case control study. *Hepatology* 2000; 32:689–692.

Wiesner R, Edwards E, Freeman R. Model for end-stage liver disease and allocation of liver donors. *Gastroenterology* 2003; 124:91–96.

CHAPTER 10

Portal hypertension and gastrointestinal bleeding

Norman D. Grace, MD ■ Elena M. Stoffel, MD ■ James Puleo, MD

KEY POINTS

1 Patients with cirrhosis who develop large esophageal varices as a consequence of portal hypertension have a 25% to 35% risk of a variceal hemorrhage and a 15% to 20% mortality rate associated with each bleeding episode. Mortality depends on the clinical status of the patient and the severity of the bleeding episode.

2 Nonselective beta-adrenergic blockers are effective and are a first-line therapy for the primary prevention of variceal hemorrhage in patients with cirrhosis and portal hypertension. Endoscopic variceal ligation is an excellent alternative, especially for patients with varices who have contraindications to or cannot tolerate beta blockers.

3 Endoscopic therapy (variceal band ligation) and pharmacologic therapy (somatostatin/octreotide/ vapreotide, terlipressin) are effective in controlling acute bleeding episodes. The combination of endoscopic and pharmacologic therapy offers an advantage over the use of either therapy alone.

4 Endoscopic variceal band ligation is the endoscopic treatment of choice for the prevention of recurrent variceal bleeding.

5 Pharmacologic maintenance therapy with nonselective beta-adrenergic blockers is effective for the prevention of recurrent variceal bleeding in selected patients, defined by a hemodynamic response to therapy. Serial measurement of portal pressure is helpful in assessing the effectiveness and making changes in therapy when indicated.

6 The combination of endoscopic and pharmacologic treatment is the preferred option for prevention of recurrent variceal bleeding.

7 For patients in whom medical therapy fails to prevent recurrent variceal hemorrhage, options include transjugular intrahepatic portosystemic shunt (TIPS), surgical portosystemic shunt, and liver transplantation. Selection of the appropriate rescue procedure is dictated by the clinical status of the patient, the availability of expertise for performance of the procedure, and, in the case of liver transplantation, appropriateness of the candidate and availability of a donor organ.

Portal Hypertension: Overview

PATHOPHYSIOLOGY

1. Portal hypertension is defined as an increase in the portal venous pressure gradient (PVPG) and is a function of portal venous blood flow and hepatic and portocollateral resistance.

2. In patients with cirrhosis, portal hypertension is initiated by an increase in hepatic and portocollateral resistance. This resistance is modulated by an increase in levels of intrahepatic

endothelin, a potent vasoconstrictor, and a decrease in levels of intrahepatic nitric oxide, a vasodilator.

3. Hepatic resistance may be modified by changes in perivenular and presinusoidal myofibroblasts as well as the smooth muscle component of portocollateral vessels.

4. Portal hypertension is exacerbated by the development of systemic vasodilatation, which leads to plasma volume expansion, an increase in cardiac output, and hyperdynamic circulation. Systemic vasodilatation is a result of an increase in systemic levels of nitric oxide and, to a lesser extent, increased circulatory levels of glucagon, prostaglandins, tumor necrosis factor (TNF) alpha, and other cytokines and alterations in the autonomic nervous system. Angiogenic factors modulate the development of collateral vessels secondary to increased portal vein pressure.

5. **Any increase in portal blood flow and/or hepatic or portocollateral resistance will increase portal pressure. Conversely, any decrease in portal blood flow and/or hepatic resistance will decrease portal pressure. This forms the basis for the pharmacologic treatment of portal hypertension.**

PHARMACOTHERAPY

1. Two classes of drugs—vasoconstrictors and vasodilators—are used for treatment of portal hypertension.

2. **Vasoconstrictors** (vasopressin, somatostatin, nonselective beta blockers) produce a decrease in splanchnic blood flow that leads to a reduction in portal venous blood flow and portal pressure.

3. **Vasodilators** (nitroglycerin, long-acting nitrates, angiotensin inhibitors [losartan, irbesartan]), prazosin) alter resistance by inducing changes in the intrahepatic perivenular and perisinusoidal myofibroblasts as well as the smooth muscle component of portocollateral vessels.

4. Combined use of vasoconstrictors and vasodilators offers the potential benefit of additive reductions in portal pressure, but their use may be limited by the side effects of treatment (i.e., systemic hypotension).

EPIDEMIOLOGY OF ESOPHAGOGASTRIC VARICEAL HEMORRHAGE

1. Some 50% of patients with alcoholic cirrhosis will develop esophageal varices within 2 years of diagnosis, and 70% to 80% will do so within 10 years. In patients with cirrhosis secondary to hepatitis C, the risk of varices is somewhat less; 30% will develop esophageal varices within 6 years of the initial diagnosis of cirrhosis.

2. Some 25% to 35% of patients with cirrhosis and large esophageal varices will experience an episode of variceal bleeding; most bleeding episodes occur within the first year after the diagnosis of varices.

3. In patients with cirrhosis who survive the initial episode of esophagogastric variceal hemorrhage (EVH) with conservative medical management, the risk of recurrent EVH is 65% to 70%; most episodes of recurrent bleeding occur within 6 months of the index hemorrhage.

4. EVH accounts for approximately one third of deaths in patients with cirrhosis and portal hypertension; the mortality rate for each episode of EVH is 15% to 20%, depending on the clinical status of the patient.

5. Treatment to prevent recurrent EVH should be initiated immediately following control of the acute EVH.

RISK FACTORS FOR FIRST VARICEAL HEMORRHAGE

- Large esophageal varices
- The presence of endoscopic red color signs (red weals, cherry-red spots, hematocystic spots); these are essentially small varices on the surface of large varices
- Hepatic decompensation as evaluated by the Child–Turcotte–Pugh classification or the Model for End-stage Liver Disease (MELD) score (ascites is a particular risk factor)
- Active alcohol consumption in patients with alcoholic liver disease

PREDICTIVE VALUE OF PORTAL HEMODYNAMIC MEASUREMENTS

1. Measurement of the hepatic venous pressure gradient (HVPG) is an easy and reproducible method for estimating PVPG. HVPG is the difference between the wedged or occluded hepatic venous pressure and the free hepatic venous pressure. HVPG has a high correlation with PVPG in patients with cirrhosis when hepatic resistance is sinusoidal or postsinusoidal, as in patients with alcoholic cirrhosis. HVPG tends to underestimate PVPG when the defect is presinusoidal, as in primary biliary cirrhosis.
2. **An HVPG of 10 mm Hg or greater is necessary for esophageal varices to form and bleed.**
3. According to Laplace's law, variceal wall tension (T) is a function of the transmural pressure (TP) times the radius (r) of the varix divided by the variceal wall thickness (w):

$$T = (TP_1 - TP_2) \times r / w$$

This calculation combines measurements of variceal size and pressure and has the highest predictive value for determining the risk of EVH.
4. The risk of recurrent EVH correlates with the level of HVPG: **the higher the HVPG, the greater the risk of recurrent EVH.**
5. HVPG is also prognostic for survival: **the higher the HVPG, the worse the survival.** HVPG also predicts the development of hepatic decompensation and the development of hepatocellular carcinoma.
6. Serial measurements of HVPG are predictive of the risk of recurrent EVH. **Patients who have a decrease in HVPG to a level less than 12 mm Hg either spontaneously or in response to pharmacologic therapy are not at risk for recurrent EVH and other complications of portal hypertension. Patients in whom HVPG decreases by 20% or more over the first few months after the index hemorrhage, usually in response to pharmacologic therapy, have a marked decrease in the risk of recurrent EVH, whereas patients who have less than a 20% decrease in HVPG while receiving pharmacologic therapy maintain a high risk of recurrent EVH.**

Prevention of Initial Variceal Hemorrhage

PHARMACOLOGIC

1. **For patients with large esophageal varices and no prior history of variceal hemorrhage, nonselective beta-adrenergic blockers have been shown to decrease the risk of initial variceal bleeding by approximately 40% and are the treatment of choice for the primary prevention of variceal hemorrhage.**

2. Nonselective beta blockers (propranolol, nadolol, timolol) should be offered to compliant patients who have no contraindications to the use of beta blockers, such as severe chronic obstructive lung disease or congestive heart failure.
3. For patients unable to tolerate beta blocker therapy, no drugs given as monotherapy have shown benefit.
4. In routine practice, the dose of the nonselective beta blocker should be achieved by a stepwise increase in dosage, adjusted to patient tolerance. **If portal hemodynamic studies are readily available, serial measurements of HVPG in response to beta blocker therapy may be of value in determining the therapeutic dose and potential clinical benefit of beta blockers.**
5. Therapy with nonselective beta blockers should be continued indefinitely. A follow-up study of individuals with nonbleeding esophageal varices who discontinued propranolol after 2 to 3 years revealed that their risk of variceal hemorrhage increased to that of untreated individuals, with increased mortality compared with an untreated population.

ENDOSCOPIC

1. **Endoscopic variceal band ligation (EVL)** may prevent an initial episode of variceal hemorrhage with success rates comparable with those achieved with propranolol.
2. Studies to date show no advantage to a combination of endoscopic and pharmacologic treatment with EVL and nonselective beta blockers for prevention of an initial variceal hemorrhage.

SURGICAL

1. Although portosystemic shunt surgery markedly decreases the risk of variceal hemorrhage, randomized controlled trials clearly demonstrated an increased frequency of hepatic encephalopathy and liver failure and a decrease in overall survival associated with such surgical procedures. Therefore, prophylactic shunt surgery is not indicated for the prevention of variceal hemorrhage. Similarly, transjugular intrahepatic portosystemic shunt (TIPS) is not indicated for the prevention of an initial variceal hemorrhage.
2. Decisions about candidacy for liver transplantation should be dictated by the overall clinical status of the patient. The presence of varices by itself is not an indication for liver transplantation.

Treatment of Acute Variceal Hemorrhage

INITIAL

1. Resuscitation of the patient is critical in the management of the patient with cirrhosis and suspected variceal hemorrhage and should include the following measures:
   - Establish adequate venous access for blood and fluid replacement.
   - Insert a nasogastric or Ewald tube to assess the severity of bleeding and to lavage gastric contents before endoscopy.
   - Treat clotting factor deficiencies with fresh frozen plasma if indicated.
   - Administer blood transfusions to establish hemodynamic stability. Caution should be taken not to overtransfuse the patient. In general, patients should be kept slightly undertransfused, usually with a hematocrit value of approximately 24, to avoid increasing portal pressure and exacerbating variceal bleeding.

- Establish airway protection in patients with massive bleeding or evidence of hepatic encephalopathy.
- Initiate antibiotic treatment to reduce the risk of infection (see Chapter 11). Before treatment, blood cultures, diagnostic paracentesis if ascites is present, and other studies as indicated should be performed.
- Initiate pharmacologic therapy with vasoactive drugs (e.g., octreotide or terlipressin) as soon as possible and before endoscopy.

2. **Endoscopy is the only reliable means for establishing the source of bleeding and should be performed as soon as the patient is adequately resuscitated.** The diagnosis of esophagogastric variceal bleeding is determined either by direct visualization of bleeding or, more often, by endoscopic stigmata in patients with varices and no other visible source of bleeding.

ENDOSCOPIC

1. EVL is the endoscopic treatment of choice in the treatment of acute esophageal variceal hemorrhage. EVL has been shown to have success rates of 80% to 90% in initial control of variceal hemorrhage and has few local complications, primarily mucosal ulceration.
2. The use of pharmacologic therapy in conjunction with endoscopic therapy improves the efficacy of endoscopic treatment in controlling acute bleeding.

PHARMACOLOGIC

1. The use of vasoactive drugs for the treatment of acute bleeding related to portal hypertension offers several advantages:
    - Treatment can be started in the emergency room or even en route to the hospital, when variceal bleeding is suspected.
    - Unlike endoscopic therapy in which the effects of treatment are local, vasoactive agents lower portal pressure.
    - The use of vasoactive agents before endoscopy may offer the endoscopist a clearer view of the varices because bleeding is less active.
    - Vasoactive agents can be useful for the treatment of sources of portal hypertensive bleeding other than esophageal varices, such as gastric varices more than 2 cm below the gastroesophageal junction or portal hypertensive gastropathy.
2. Pharmacologic agents include vasopressin, nitroglycerin, somatostatin, octreotide, vapreotide, and terlipressin (Table 10.1). Although in common usage throughout the world, none of these agents is approved by the Food and Drug Administration for this indication.
    - The combination of **vasopressin and nitroglycerin** has been shown to control variceal bleeding in a higher percentage of patients than vasopressin alone. More importantly, the addition of nitroglycerin ameliorates many of the systemic side effects of vasopressin and thus renders vasopressin more tolerable.
    - **Somatostatin**, given intravenously by bolus followed by continuous infusion, has been effective in controlling variceal bleeding in 60% to 80% of patients and has practically no serious side effects associated with its use.
    - Because somatostatin is not generally available in the United States, **octreotide**, its synthetic analogue with a longer half-life, is widely used instead in this country. A meta-analysis concluded that octreotide was superior to vasopressin/terlipressin in controlling acute variceal bleeding. Vapreotide and lanreotide are somatostatin analogues that are currently under investigation.

TABLE 10.1 ■ Pharmacologic treatment of acute variceal bleeding

Drug	Route	Administration	Dose
Terlipressin	IV	Initial bolus	2 mg/4 hr
		Subsequent bolus	1–2 mg/4 hr
Somatostatin	IV	Initial bolus	250–500 µg
		Continuous infusion	250–500 µg/hr
Octreotide	IV	Initial bolus	25–50 µg
		Continuous infusion	25–50 µg/hr

Treatment should be continued for 5 days

IV, intravenous.

- **Terlipressin**, a synthetic analogue of vasopressin, has a longer half-life than vasopressin and therefore can be given by intravenous bolus infusion. Randomized controlled trials have shown this drug to be more effective than vasopressin, with far fewer side effects. It is used widely in Europe, and approval by the Food and Drug Administration is pending.

The combination of endoscopic and pharmacologic therapy (octreotide) offers clinical advantages over the use of either therapy alone, with less rebleeding in the acute period (first 5 days) and lower transfusion requirements. However, combination therapy has not been shown to improve survival.

TIPS

In high-risk patients (Child's class C or Child's class B with active bleeding at endoscopy), the placement of TIPS using a coated stent within 24 hours of admission may result in less morbidity and improved survival compared to standard medical therapy.

BALLOON TAMPONADE

1. Endoscopic therapy has replaced balloon tamponade as initial therapy for variceal bleeding. However, balloon tamponade may still be of value as a temporizing treatment for failures of pharmacologic and endoscopic therapy, before more definitive treatment for the control of acute variceal bleeding is undertaken.
2. Success with balloon tamponade can often be achieved with inflation of just the gastric balloon, thereby avoiding the additional complications associated with use of the esophageal balloon.
3. Complication rates with the use of balloon tamponade relate to the experience of the team using the balloon. Specific precautions are required to minimize the risk of aspiration and asphyxiation. The balloon should not be kept inflated for more than 24 hours because of the risk of esophageal necrosis.

TREATMENT FOR FAILURES OF MEDICAL THERAPY

1. **A National Institutes of Health consensus conference supported the use of TIPS** for the rescue of the 10% to 20% of patients in whom medical therapy fails to control acute variceal hemorrhage.

2. In experienced hands, TIPS can be successful in 90% to 95% of patients, with relatively low immediate mortality compared with the use of surgical shunts.
3. Rebleeding and hepatic encephalopathy are long-term complications of TIPS, but are less of a risk with the advent of coated stents.
4. In a few selected centers, the early (within 12 hours of diagnosis) use of portosystemic shunt surgery has been advocated, with excellent results reported. However, this approach has not gained widespread acceptance.

Prevention of Recurrent Variceal Hemorrhage

Because of the high recurrence rate of variceal bleeding after control of initial bleeding, it is not surprising that medical therapy for the control of acute variceal bleeding has not been associated with improved survival. Treatment to prevent recurrent variceal bleeding has a greater potential to influence long-term survival.

1. The risk for recurrent variceal bleeding is highest in the first few weeks, and the risk of rebleeding remains significantly elevated during the first 6 months after the index hemorrhage.
2. **It is crucial that therapy to prevent recurrent bleeding be initiated as soon as the acute bleeding episode is adequately controlled.**

ENDOSCOPIC

1. **EVL** has replaced sclerotherapy as the endoscopic therapy of choice for the prevention of recurrent variceal bleeding. When compared with sclerotherapy, EVL is associated with lower rates of recurrent bleeding, mortality, and complications and requires fewer sessions for variceal obliteration.
2. The combination of EVL and sclerotherapy offers no advantage over EVL alone.
3. Patients who have had a variceal bleeding episode should undergo EVL at regular intervals (every other week) until the varices are obliterated, followed by regular surveillance with repeat endoscopic treatment if varices recur. The combination of endoscopic and pharmacologic therapy may decrease the risk of recurrent varices.

PHARMACOLOGIC (Table 10.2)

1. **Nonselective beta-adrenergic blockers (propranolol, nadolol)** have been shown to reduce the risk of recurrent variceal bleeding and to reduce mortality associated with bleeding.

2. Beta blocker therapy is indicated for patients
    - With good hepatic function (Child's classes A and B)
    - Deemed to be compliant with taking medication
    - With no contraindications to use of beta blockers (e.g., congestive heart failure, severe chronic lung disease)

3. The therapeutic dose of beta blockers is adjusted to the highest tolerated dose.
4. In centers where hepatic hemodynamic measurements are readily available, serial measurements (baseline and at 1 to 3 months) of the HVPG are predictive of the efficacy of treatment. Recurrent variceal bleeding is significantly reduced when
    - HVPG decreases to less than 12 mm Hg.
    - At least a 20% decrease in HVPG from baseline is noted.
5. If therapy with beta blockers does not achieve one of these end points, the addition of a second drug (e.g., a long-acting nitrate) may be considered in an attempt to reduce HVPG

TABLE 10.2 ■ **Pharmacologic treatment for prevention of variceal bleeding**

Drug	Initial dose	Therapeutic dose (range/day)
Propranolol	40 mg b.i.d.	40–400 mg
Nadolol	40 mg q.d.	40–160 mg
Timolol	10 mg q.d.	5 mg q.d.–40 mg
Isosorbide 5-mononitrate	20 mg b.i.d.	20 mg t.i.d.–20 mg q.i.d.

b.i.d., twice daily; q.d., once daily; q.i.d., four times daily; t.i.d., three times daily.

further. Carvedilol, a nonselective beta blocker with intrinsic anti–alpha-1-adrenergic activity, has been shown to decrease portal pressure to a greater extent than selective beta blockers and is reasonably well tolerated. Studies are needed to determine the clinical role of this agent.

COMBINED ENDOSCOPIC AND PHARMACOLOGIC

Combination endoscopic and pharmacologic treatment is the preferred option for the prevention of recurrent variceal bleeding. Several randomized controlled trials have shown endoscopic therapy plus nonselective beta blockers to be more effective than either or drug treatment or EVL alone for the prevention of rebleeding.

TREATMENT FOR FAILURES OF MEDICAL THERAPY

1. TIPS is effective at reducing portal pressure and is currently the preferred treatment for patients in whom initial medical therapy fails, especially for those patients who are poor operative risks.
2. For low-risk patients (Child's class A), portosystemic shunt surgery remains an alternative. In patients with nonalcoholic cirrhosis, a distal splenorenal shunt is preferable to a portosystemic shunt because of the lower frequency of hepatic encephalopathy associated with the selective shunt.
3. Liver transplantation should always be considered for patients with end-stage liver disease. Selection of candidates is dictated by the patient's clinical status, the cause of cirrhosis, abstinence from alcohol in patients with alcoholic cirrhosis, and the availability of a donor organ.
4. For patients who are candidates for liver transplantation, a TIPS procedure can be used as a bridge to transplantation.

Management of Nonesophageal Variceal Sources of Bleeding Related to Portal Hypertension

GASTRIC VARICES

1. Gastric varices that extend more than 5 cm below the gastroesophageal junction or are isolated to the fundus are at high risk for bleeding.
2. Endoscopic treatment for gastric varices is less effective than for esophageal varices. Use of cyanoacrylate glue has been effective in the management of bleeding gastric varices and is the treatment of choice. Complications of therapy have included bacteremia and glue embolization. The efficacy of other therapies, such as clips, snares, and thrombin, is under investigation.

3. Pharmacologic therapy should be considered for initial treatment of acute bleeding and prevention of recurrent bleeding.
4. Patients in whom pharmacologic therapy fails should be considered for TIPS or liver transplantation for appropriate candidates.

PORTAL HYPERTENSIVE GASTROPATHY

1. Portal hypertensive gastropathy is a common complication of cirrhosis and portal hypertension, but significant gastrointestinal bleeding from this source is relatively uncommon.
2. Endoscopically, portal hypertensive gastropathy ranges from a mild form characterized by a diffuse mosaic mucosal pattern to more severe forms characterized by brown spots, cherry-red spots, granular mucosa, and diffuse mucosal hemorrhages.
3. Prior treatment of esophageal varices with endoscopic therapy has been associated with an increase in the severity of portal hypertensive gastropathy.
4. Pharmacologic therapy is the only medical option for treating acute bleeding or preventing recurrent bleeding from portal hypertensive gastropathy. Endoscopic therapy has no role.
5. For the uncommon failures of medical therapy, TIPS and liver transplantation are the options for rescue.

FURTHER READING

Abraczinskas DR, Ookubo R, Grace ND, et al. Propranolol for the prevention of first esophageal variceal hemorrhage: a lifetime commitment? *Hepatology* 2001; 34:1096–1102.

Abraldes JG, Vellanueva C, Banares R, et al. Hepatic venous pressure gradient and prognosis in patients with acute variceal bleeding treated with pharmacologic and endoscopic therapy. *J Hepatol* 2008; 48:229–236.

Bureau C, Peron JM, Alric L, et al. "A la carte" treatment of portal hypertension: adapting medical therapy to hemodynamic response for the prevention of bleeding. *Hepatology* 2002; 36:1361–1366.

D'Amico G, Pagliaro L, Bosch J. Pharmacological treatment of portal hypertension: an evidence-based approach. *Semin Liver Dis* 1999; 19:475–505.

de Franchis R. Evolving consensus in portal hypertension: report of the Baveno IV consensus workshop on methodology of diagnosis and therapy in portal hypertension. *J Hepatol* 2005; 43:167–176.

Garcia-Tsao G, Bosch J. Management of varices and variceal hemorrhage in cirrhosis. *N Engl J Med* 2010; 362:823–832.

Garcia-Pagan JC, Caca K, Bureau C, et al. Early use of TIPS in patients with cirrhosis and variceal bleeding. *N Engl J Med* 2010; 362:2370–2379.

Garcia-Tsao G, Sanyal J, Grace ND, et al. Prevention and management of gastroesophageal varices and variceal hemorrhage in cirrhosis. *Hepatology* 2007; 46:922–938.

Gonzalez R, Zamora J, Gomez-Camarera J, et al. Combination endoscopic and drug therapy to prevent variceal rebleeding in cirrhosis. *Ann Intern Med* 2008; 149:109–122.

Grace ND, Groszmann RJ, Garcia-Tsao G, et al. Portal hypertension and variceal bleeding: report of a single topic symposium. *Hepatology* 1998; 28:868–880.

Groszmann RJ, Garcia-Tsao G, Bosch J, et al. Beta-blockers to prevent gastroesophageal varices cirrhosis. *N Engl J Med* 2005; 353:2254–2261.

Lo GH, Lai KH, Cheng JS, et al. Endoscopic variceal ligation plus nadolol and sucralfate compared with ligation alone for the prevention of variceal rebleeding: a prospective, randomized trial. *Hepatology* 2000; 32:461–465.

Lui HF, Stanley AJ, Forrest EH, et al. Primary prophylaxis of variceal hemorrhage: a randomized controlled trial comparing band ligation, propranolol, and isosorbide mononitrate. *Gastroenterology* 2002; 123:735–744.

Monescillo A, Martinez-Lagares E, Ruiz-del Arbol L, et al. Influence of portal hypertension and its early decompensation by TIPS placement in the outcome of variceal bleeding. *Hepatology* 2009; 40:793–801.

Sanyal AJ, Fontana RJ, DiBisceglie AM, et al. The prevalence and risk factors associated with esophageal varices in subjects with hepatitis C and advanced fibrosis. *Gastrointest Endosc* 2006; 64:855–864.

Tan PC, Hou MC, Lin HC, et al. A randomized trial of endoscopic treatment of acute gastric variceal hemorrhage: *N*-butyl-2-cyanoacrylate injection versus band ligation. *Hepatology* 2006; 43:690–697.

CHAPTER 11

Ascites and spontaneous bacterial peritonitis

Ke-Qin Hu, MD ■ Armine Avanesyan, MD ■ Bruce A. Runyon, MD

KEY POINTS

1 In the United States, 85% of cases of ascites occur in the setting of cirrhosis with portal hypertension; the development of ascites is associated with a 50% 2-year survival.

2 Evaluation of the patient with ascites begins with a thorough history and physical examination focused on identifying clinical clues to the underlying disease process.

3 Abdominal paracentesis with ascitic fluid analysis is a safe and cost-effective strategy in the differential diagnosis of ascites. Routine ascitic fluid tests include cell count, culture in blood culture bottles, albumin, and total protein, with additional testing depending on the clinical setting.

4 Treatment of patients with cirrhosis and ascites involves a stepwise approach including dietary sodium restriction and dual diuretic therapy. Second-line therapies include intermittent large-volume paracentesis (LVP), transjugular intrahepatic portosystemic shunt (TIPS), and liver transplantation.

5 Spontaneous bacterial peritonitis (SBP) is the prototype ascitic fluid infection and usually develops in the setting of preexisting ascites in patients with cirrhosis. The morbidity and mortality of ascitic fluid infection and the efficacy of early treatment warrant a high index of suspicion, early diagnosis by paracentesis with appropriate ascitic fluid analysis, and prompt non-nephrotoxic antibiotic treatment.

6 Selective intestinal decontamination with norfloxacin or trimethoprim–sulfamethoxazole has been demonstrated to prevent SBP in high-risk subgroups (i.e., prior SBP, active gastrointestinal hemorrhage, and low-protein ascitic fluid).

Overview of Ascites

DEFINITION

Ascites is defined as pathologic accumulation of fluid within the peritoneal cavity.

EPIDEMIOLOGY AND NATURAL HISTORY

1. **In the United States, 85% of cases of ascites occur in the setting of cirrhosis.** Table 11.1 lists common causes of ascites.
2. Ascites is the most common clinical manifestation of hepatic decompensation.

TABLE 11.1 ■ **Causes of ascites in the United States**

Cause	Percentage (%)
Cirrhosis	85
Miscellaneous portal hypertension-related	8
Cardiac ascites	3
Peritoneal carcinomatosis	2
Miscellaneous non–portal hypertension-related	2

3. Approximately 50% of patients with cirrhosis will develop ascites within 10 years.
4. Once ascites occurs, the 2-year survival rate is 50%.
5. Ascites becomes unresponsive to diuretic therapy in 10% of patients with cirrhosis.
6. Once ascites becomes refractory, the 1-year survival rate is 25%.

PATHOGENESIS IN THE SETTING OF CIRRHOSIS

1. Portal hypertension leads to excess formation of fluid within the congested hepatic sinusoids; the fluid overwhelms intrahepatic lymphatics and weeps across the liver.
2. The **overflow theory** proposes that a stimulus arising from the liver results in a primary increase in plasma volume through increased renal sodium retention.
3. The **underfill theory** proposes that when ascites formation begins, the intravascular fluid compartment contracts, with an increase in the plasma oncotic pressure and a decrease in portal venous pressure; this results in a secondary increase in renal sodium retention in an attempt to compensate.
4. The **peripheral arterial vasodilatation theory** is a modification of the underfill theory and proposes that peripheral arterial vasodilatation results in an increase in vascular capacitance and a decrease in *effective* plasma volume, which results in the secondary increase in renal sodium retention.

Evaluation of the Patient with Ascites

HISTORY

1. History often reveals clues to alcoholic liver diseases or chronic viral hepatitis.
2. A thorough history is necessary to rule out a cause other than liver disease, such as heart failure, tuberculosis, or nephrotic syndrome (Table 11.2).
3. History related to ascites
   ■ The most common symptom of ascites is an increase in abdominal girth accompanied by weight gain, frequently with lower extremity edema.
   ■ Acute onset of uncontrollable ascites can be associated with the Budd–Chiari syndrome.
   ■ Ascites associated with fever and/or abdominal pain may indicate ascitic fluid infection or malignancy.
   ■ A history of heart failure raises the possibility of cardiac ascites; alcoholic cardiomyopathy can mimic alcoholic cirrhosis superficially.

TABLE 11.2 ■ **Clinical clues to causes of ascites other than cirrhosis**

Cause	Clinical clues
Cardiac ascites	Setting and examination findings suggestive of heart failure
Malignant ascites	Setting of known malignancy and absence of stigmata of liver disease; often abdominal pain and profound weight loss
Tuberculous ascites	Persistent abdominal pain and fever; often extraperitoneal tuberculosis
Nephrotic syndrome	Anasarca and substantial proteinuria in a diabetic patient
Pancreatic ascites	Follows episode of severe acute pancreatitis or occurs in the setting of chronic pancreatitis

PHYSICAL EXAMINATION

1. Physical signs suggestive of cirrhosis and portal hypertension (e.g., spider telangiectases, palmar erythema, abdominal wall collateral vessels, splenomegaly, or asterixis)
2. Physical findings in ascites
   ■ Presence of a full, bulging abdomen
   ■ Shifting dullness evident when peritoneal fluid is greater than 1500 mL
   ■ Abdominal wall hernias common in patients with ascites

ABDOMINAL ULTRASONOGRAPHY

1. Detection of as little as 100 mL of ascitic fluid
2. Confirmation or refutation of the presence of portal hypertension (e.g., spleen greater than 12 cm maximum dimension and enlarged portal vein)
3. Valuable in differentiating obesity from ascites and detecting ovarian or mesenteric masses

GRADE AND TYPE OF ASCITES

1. Grading ascites
   ■ Grade 1: detectable only by careful physical examination
   ■ Grade 2: easily detected but relatively small amount
   ■ Grade 3: obvious but not tense
   ■ Grade 4: tense
2. Refractory ascites
   a. Ascites that cannot be mobilized or early recurrence of ascites (i.e., after therapeutic paracentesis) that cannot be satisfactorily prevented by medical therapy
   b. Two types of refractory ascites
      ■ **Diuretic resistant**: lack of response to dietary sodium restriction and intensive diuretic treatment
      ■ **Diuretic intractable**: development of diuretic-induced complications that preclude the use of effective diuretic doses

3. Bloody ascites
   - Red blood cell count higher than 10,000/mm^3 in ascitic fluid
   - Most commonly associated with slightly traumatic paracentesis
4. Chylous ascites
   - Ascitic fluid milky, with triglyceride content greater than 200 mg/dL

Ascitic Fluid Analysis

DIAGNOSTIC PARACENTESIS

- Paracentesis is safe despite the coagulopathy that is usually present.
- Diagnostic paracentesis is the final confirmation of the presence of ascites.
- Careful ascitic fluid analysis is essential for the differential diagnosis of ascites.

1. Indications
   - New-onset ascites
   - Routine on hospital admission or readmission of patients with ascites
   - Symptoms or signs suggestive of ascitic fluid infection (i.e., fever, abdominal pain, elevated white blood cell count, encephalopathy, and renal impairment)
2. Technically, diagnostic paracentesis involves passing a steel 22-gauge needle, by a Z-tract technique, below the level of percussed dullness, either in the left lower quadrant (two finger-breadths cephalic and two fingerbreadths medial to the anterior superior iliac spine) or in the midline between the symphysis pubis and umbilicus.
3. Complications include fluid leak at the site (if a Z-tract is not used), abdominal wall hema-toma, and inadvertent bowel perforation.
4. Routine prophylactic use of fresh frozen plasma or platelets before paracentesis is not recom-mended because bleeding is very uncommon. Coagulopathy may preclude paracentesis only when clinically evident primary hyperfibrinolysis or disseminated intravascular coagulation (DIC) is present.

ASCITIC FLUID TESTS

Ascitic fluid tests commonly ordered are shown in Table 11.3.
1. Ascitic fluid cell count is the most important test.

- Fluid with 250 or more polymorphonuclear neutrophils (PMNs)/mm^3 (and a predomi-nance of PMNs) is presumed infected.

TABLE 11.3 ■ **Ascitic fluid tests**

Routine	Optional	Unusual	Unhelpful
Cell count	Gram stain	Tuberculosis smear/culture	pH and lactate
Culture	Glucose	Cytology	Cholesterol
Albumin	Lactate dehydrogenase	Triglyceride	Alpha fetoprotein
Total protein	Amylase	Bilirubin	Fibronectin

- Any inflammatory cause of ascites can lead to neutrocytic ascites (250 or more PMNs/mm³).
- For bloody ascites, 1 PMN is subtracted from the cell count for every 250 red blood cells, to correct for PMNs that enter the fluid with the blood.

2. Culture results are optimized by immediate inoculation of aerobic and anaerobic blood culture bottles with 10 mL of ascitic fluid at the bedside (sensitivity is approximately 90%).

3. Ascitic fluid albumin measurement is necessary to calculate the **serum–ascites albumin gradient (SAAG).**

   - A SAAG of 1.1 g/dL or more is 97% accurate in detecting portal hypertension; this value narrows the differential diagnosis (Table 11.4).

4. Ascitic fluid total protein measurement assists in determining the cause of ascites (Table 11.5) and the risk of ascitic fluid infection (values lower than 1.0 g/dL indicate a high risk).

EVALUATION OF THE UNDERLYING LIVER DISEASE

1. Determining the underlying origin of cirrhosis is an essential part of clinical evaluation for ascites that may result in effective treatment of the cause of ascites.
2. The underlying liver disease should be staged by Child–Turcotte–Pugh and Model for End-stage Liver Disease (MELD) scores.

Treatment of Ascites in Patients with Cirrhosis

GENERAL PRINCIPLES

1. One should establish the diagnosis of the underlying liver disease, determine prognosis, and optimize treatment; liver transplantation should be considered in appropriate candidates.

TABLE 11.4 ■ **Differential diagnosis of ascites based on the serum–ascites albumin gradient**

High gradient (≥1.1 g/dL)	Low gradient (<1.1 g/dL)
Cirrhosis	Peritoneal carcinomatosis
Alcoholic hepatitis	Tuberculous peritonitis
Cardiac ascites	Pancreatic ascites
Massive liver metastases	Biliary ascites
Fulminant hepatic failure	Nephrotic syndrome
Budd–Chiari syndrome	Connective tissue diseases
Portal vein thrombosis	Intestinal obstruction/infarction
Sinusoidal obstruction syndrome	Postoperative lymphatic leak
Acute fatty liver of pregnancy	
Myxedema	
"Mixed" ascites	

TABLE 11.5 ■ **Ascitic fluid clues regarding the cause of ascites**

Cause of ascites	Ascitic fluid clues
Cirrhotic ascites	SAAG ≥1.1 g/dL AFTP <2.5 g/dL (usually)
Cardiac ascites	SAAG ≥1.1 g/dL AFTP ≥2.5 g/dL
Peritoneal carcinomatosis	SAAG <1.1 g/dL AFTP ≥2.5 g/dL Cytology generally yields malignant cells
Tuberculous ascites	SAAG <1.1 g/dL (without cirrhosis) AFTP >2.5 g/dL (without cirrhosis) WBC >500/mm^3, lymphocyte predominance
Chylous ascites	SAAG <1.1 g/dL AFTP ≥2.5 g/dL Triglycerides in ascites > serum (usually >200 mg/dL)
Nephrotic syndrome	SAAG <1.1 g/dL AFTP <2.5 g/dL
Pancreatic ascites	SAAG <1.1 g/dL AFTP ≥2.5 g/dL Amylase in ascites > amylase in serum (often >1000 U/L)

AFTP, ascitic fluid total protein; SAAG, serum–ascites albumin gradient; WBC, white blood cell count.

2. Possible **precipitating factors** of the ascites should be identified:
   - Dietary indiscretion
   - Gastrointestinal bleeding with volume and blood resuscitation
   - Hepatocellular carcinoma with or without portal vein thrombosis
   - Use of nonsteroidal anti-inflammatory drugs (NSAIDs)
   - Iatrogenic (i.e., saline administration)
   - Noncompliance with diuretics

3. Understanding sodium balance is the key to successful treatment.
   - Sodium balance occurs when sodium intake = sodium loss.
   - Sodium intake = dietary intake + all medically related sodium administration.
   - Sodium loss = insensible (~5 mmol/day) + fecal (~5 mmol/day) + urinary sodium excretion.

4. **Sodium restriction is the mainstay of treatment of ascites.**
   - Sodium should be restricted in all patients with cirrhosis and significant ascites.
   - Sodium intake of 2 g/day (88 mmol/day) is a realistic goal.
   - A low-salt diet alone will eliminate ascites in only approximately 10% of patients.

5. **Diuretic therapy**
   a. This is **required in approximately 90% of patients** with ascites, especially those with
      - Moderate to tense ascites
      - A positive sodium balance while on a sodium-restricted diet
   b. The preferred regimen is a combination of two diuretics acting on different sites of the nephron; serial monitoring (Table 11.6) is needed to determine optimal doses.

6. By suppressing the renin-angiotensin-aldosterone system, midodrine may improve arterial blood volume and natriuresis; further studies are needed to determine its therapeutic role.

7. Assessment of urinary excretion is used to monitor treatment response (see Table 11.6).

TABLE 11.6 ■ **Factors used to assess treatment response and complications in patients with ascites**

Physical examination	24-hr urine	Blood chemistry
Weight	Volume	Sodium
Ascitic fluid volume	Sodium excretion	Potassium
Peripheral edema		Creatinine
Encephalopathy		

- A 24-hour urine collection should be obtained for quantitation of sodium, potassium, and creatinine. The goal is sodium excretion greater than 78 mmol/day (88 mmol/day when approximately 10 mmol/day of nonurinary losses is added to 78 mmol/day of urinary losses).
- Completeness of collection is assessed by creatinine excretion of more than 10 mg/kg per day in women and more than 15 mg/kg per day in men. If the specimen is incomplete, a urinary ratio of sodium to potassium greater than 1 usually correlates with a 24-hour sodium excretion of more than 78 mmol.
- A negative sodium balance with a weight loss of 0.5 kg per day is a reasonable goal; however, patients with peripheral edema can tolerate greater rates of sodium excretion and more rapid weight loss.
- Urinary sodium excretion greater than 78 mmol/day in a patient in whom treatment is failing indicates dietary noncompliance as the cause.
- Diuretics should be increased after 3 days if the patient has had no increase in urinary sodium excretion or decrease in body weight.

8. Complications limiting diuretic management of ascites include (see Table 11.6)
   - Azotemia (most common limiting factor)
   - Electrolyte abnormalities (severe potassium and sodium abnormalities)
   - Intravascular hypovolemia
   - Hepatic encephalopathy

STEPWISE DIURETIC APPROACH

Treatment based on sodium restriction and diuretics is the mainstay of the therapy for cirrhotic patients with ascites; approximately 90% of patients respond to this therapy.

1. **Spironolactone** (a potassium-sparing diuretic that acts at the aldosterone-sensitive sodium channels in the distal nephron and collecting ducts) is the **diuretic of choice** for single-agent therapy of ascites.
   - It is a less potent natriuretic than furosemide; hypokalemia is less likely to develop.
   - The prolonged half-life of spironolactone (up to 5 to 7 days) allows once-daily dosing.
   - The maximum daily dose is 400 mg.
2. Combination diuretic regimens

The combination of spironolactone and furosemide is the most effective regimen for managing cirrhotic ascites in terms of shortest hospitalization times and maintenance of normokalemia.

- **Starting doses are spironolactone 100 mg and furosemide 40 mg once daily**. This ratio of potassium-sparing/wasting diuretics leads to the fewest potassium abnormalities.

- Doses of both drugs should be increased while maintaining the same ratio (e.g., spironolactone 200 mg and furosemide 80 mg daily).
- Maximum doses are spironolactone 400 mg and furosemide 160 mg once daily.

REFRACTORY ASCITES

Large-volume paracentesis (LVP) is usually used at least temporarily in patients with refractory ascites. Concomitant administration of intravenous albumin may decrease the frequency of post-paracentesis circulatory dysfunction in selected patients. Transjugular intrahepatic portosystemic shunt (TIPS) should be relegated to patients who require frequent LVP and have a favorable post-TIPS outcome as predicted by the MELD score. Liver transplantation should be considered in all appropriate candidates.

1. LVP
    - This is defined as removal of 5 L or more of fluid by therapeutic paracentesis.
    - LVP should not need to be performed more often than every 2 weeks even in patients with no urinary sodium excretion.
    - LVP is associated with more rapid resolution of tense ascites than diuretic therapy.
    - Intravenous volume expanders are unnecessary for paracenteses of less than 5 L of fluid.
    - Volume expanders (usually 6 to 8 g of 25% albumin infusion/L of fluid removed) are used for paracenteses of more than 5 L of fluid, although this approach remains controversial.
2. TIPS (see also Chapter 10)
    a. TIPS significantly and promptly reduces the portacaval pressure gradient.
    b. It is effective in approximately 90% of patients with refractory ascites; improvement is noted within 1 to 3 months.
    c. Most patients need continued diuretic treatment after TIPS.
    d. Compared with LVP, TIPS is associated with:
        - Better long-term control of refractory ascites
        - Improved transplant-free survival
        - Higher frequency of hepatic encephalopathy (40%)
3. Peritoneovenous shunting (PVS): Because of poor long-term patency, excessive complications, and no survival advantage, PVS is now a nearly abandoned procedure.
4. Liver transplantation
    - Liver transplantation is the only lifesaving therapy for patients with refractory ascites, whose 1-year survival rate is 25% without this treatment.
    - Better outcomes occur when patients undergo transplantation without hepatorenal syndrome.

Spontaneous Bacterial Peritonitis and other Ascitic Fluid Infections

OVERVIEW

1. Patients with cirrhosis and ascites have a 10% annual risk of ascitic fluid infection.
2. The five variants of ascitic fluid infection may have different prognostic significance and require different management strategies (Table 11.7). Spontaneous bacterial peritonitis (SBP) is the most common type of ascitic fluid infection.
3. A high index of suspicion is necessary to ensure early detection and initiation of antibiotics; paracentesis must be performed to diagnose ascitic fluid infection.

TABLE 11.7 ■ **Classification of ascitic fluid infection**

Category	Ascitic fluid analysis
Spontaneous bacterial peritonitis (SBP)	PMNs ≥250/mm^3, single organism
Culture-negative neutrocytic ascites (CNNA)	PMNs ≥250/mm^3, negative culture
Monomicrobial non-neutrocytic bacterascites (MNB)	PMNs <250/mm^3, single organism
Polymicrobial bacterascites	PMNs <250/mm^3, multiple organisms
Secondary bacterial peritonitis	PMNs ≥250/mm^3, multiple organisms

PMN, polymorphonuclear neutrophils.

4. Early initiation of appropriate broad-spectrum non-nephrotoxic antibiotics has significantly decreased the mortality rate (currently 5%) of ascitic fluid infection.
5. The MELD score may be independently associated with an increased risk of SBP; for every one-point increase in MELD score, the risk of SBP increased by 11% in one study.
6. Proton pump inhibitors have been reported to be associated with an increased risk of SBP in patients with cirrhosis and ascites.

PATHOGENESIS

1. Bacterial seeding of ascitic fluid is the common denominator of ascitic fluid infections; the two most likely routes are as follows:
   a. Translocation of bacteria through the intestinal wall
      ■ This accounts for more than 70% of ascitic fluid infections.
      ■ It is promoted by abnormal gut flora, mucosal edema, and altered gut permeability.
   b. Hematogenous seeding of the ascitic fluid
      ■ One half of SBP episodes are accompanied by bacteremia involving the same organism isolated from the ascitic fluid.
      ■ The causative organism can sometimes be cultured from urine or sputum.
2. Colonization of ascitic fluid ("bacterascites")
   ■ This has two different outcomes: clearance by intraperitoneal phagocytic cells or progressive bacterial growth with peritonitis (i.e., SBP).
   ■ Bacterascites normally resolves as a result of opsonization of the bacteria and subsequent clearance by intraperitoneal phagocytic cells.
3. Bacterial flora of SBP
   ■ *Escherichia coli*, pneumococci, and *Klebsiella* caused 80% of SBP cases in the past; in this era of selective intestinal decontamination, gram-positive organisms cause more than 50% of bacterial infections.
   ■ Anaerobes cause only 1% of cases of SBP.
4. Risks for ascitic fluid infection:
   ■ A prior episode of SBP: most important risk factor; two thirds of patients will develop a recurrence of infection within the following year
   ■ Gastrointestinal bleeding (specifically variceal hemorrhage)
   ■ Ascitic fluid total protein lower than 1.0 g/dL

CLINICAL FEATURES AND DIAGNOSIS

1. Ascitic fluid infections develop primarily in patients with preexisting ascites in the setting of cirrhosis.
2. Approximately 87% of patients with SBP have symptoms or signs of infection, including fever (69%), abdominal pain (59%), and mental status change (54%).
3. Occurrence of any symptoms and/or signs of infection in a patient with ascites should prompt diagnostic paracentesis.
4. Lactoferrin is a product of activated PMNs that acts as a surrogate marker for PMNs and may provide a simple and rapid test for diagnosing SBP, if it becomes commercially available.
5. Dipsticks that measure leukocyte esterase can detect an elevated PMN count in 90 to 180 seconds at the bedside and permit immediate initiation of antibiotics; most of the studies performed to date have used a dipstick designed for urine, but an ascitic fluid–specific dipstick is showing excellent sensitivity and specificity.

CLASSIFICATION (See Table 11.7)

1. **SBP** has a positive ascitic fluid culture (almost always a single organism) and a PMN count in ascites of at least 250 cells/mm^3 in the absence of an intra-abdominal surgical source of infection.
2. **Culture-negative neutrocytic ascites (CNNA)** has a negative ascitic fluid culture, an ascitic fluid neutrophil count of at least 250 cells/mm^3, and no apparent intra-abdominal source of infection.
   a. It occurs most commonly in the setting of suboptimal culture technique.
   b. With a sensitive culture technique, it most commonly represents resolution of transient bacterial colonization of the ascitic fluid because of the fluid's inherent antibacterial properties.
   c. Bacterial growth may continue, leading to SBP and positive fluid culture.
   d. **CNNA and SBP have comparable mortality rates; therefore, similar management is warranted.**
   e. Recent antibiotic exposure (even one dose) may suppress bacterial growth in the culture.
   f. Causes of neutrocytic ascites other than SBP should be considered:
      - Peritoneal carcinomatosis
      - Pancreatitis
      - Tuberculous peritonitis
      - Peritonitis related to connective tissue disease
      - Hemorrhage into ascitic fluid
3. **Monomicrobial non-neutrocytic bacterascites (MNB)** is a variant of SBP with a positive ascitic fluid culture (single organism) associated with a normal ascitic fluid PMN count (i.e., lower than 250 cells/mm^3).
   - Patients with MNB generally have less severe liver disease than do those with SBP.
   - The outcome of bacterascites is determined by the presence or absence of associated clinical symptoms or signs; asymptomatic bacterascites typically resolves spontaneously without antibiotic treatment; **symptomatic bacterascites should be managed in the same manner as SBP.**
   - When an ascitic fluid culture unexpectedly yields an organism, paracentesis should be repeated promptly to evaluate for the development of a neutrocytic response, which mandates antibiotic treatment.

4. **Polymicrobial bacterascites** indicates **inadvertent perforation of the bowel** by the paracentesis needle, with an ascitic fluid culture demonstrating multiple organisms in the setting of a normal neutrophil count (i.e., lower than 250 cells/mm^3).
   - Inadvertent bowel perforation by paracentesis occurs rarely, typically in the setting of an extremely difficult paracentesis, and may be obvious when air or stool is aspirated during the tap.
   - Most inadvertent bowel perforations resolve spontaneously without development of secondary peritonitis; however, paracentesis should be repeated to evaluate for a neutrocytic response and the need for antibiotics.
   - Management of patients with a neutrocytic ascitic fluid response is with empirical broad-spectrum antibiotics to cover gram-negative enteric, gram-positive, and anaerobic organisms.
5. **Secondary bacterial peritonitis** is differentiated from SBP by the presence of a **known or suspected surgically treatable intra-abdominal source of infection** (e.g., perforated viscus or intra-abdominal abscess). The ascitic fluid PMN count is at least 250 cells/mm^3, and the culture grows multiple gut organisms.
   a. Other ascitic fluid findings indicate secondary bacterial peritonitis:
      - Total protein greater than 1.0 g/dL
      - Glucose lower than 50 mg/dL
      - Lactate dehydrogenase greater than the upper limit of normal for serum
   b. Secondary peritonitis should also be suspected if repeat paracentesis performed after 48 hours of appropriate antibiotic treatment reveals an ascitic fluid PMN count higher than the baseline value.
   c. Management includes empirical broad-spectrum antibiotics to cover gram-negative enteric, gram-positive, and anaerobic bacteria; evaluation to localize the perforation is indicated.
   d. Prompt surgical intervention is mandatory; medical therapy alone is insufficient.

TREATMENT

1. Empiric treatment is indicated before culture results become available when the ascitic fluid PMN count is 250 cells/mm^3 or higher.
   - The most common causative organisms in the past included *E. coli* (43%), *Streptococcus* species (23%), and *Klebsiella pneumoniae* (11%).
   - Anaerobic organisms rarely lead to ascitic fluid infections except in secondary peritonitis.
   - The flora responsible for ascitic fluid infections continues to change, presumably as a result of antibiotic pressures.

   - Aminoglycosides carry an unacceptable risk of nephrotoxicity and are considered contraindicated in cirrhotic patients with ascites.

   - Fungi do not cause spontaneous bacterial peritonitis except in patients with acquired immunodeficiency syndrome (AIDS); fungi are usually cultured from ascitic fluid in cases of secondary peritonitis.
2. **Third-generation cephalosporins are the recommended treatment.**

   - **Cefotaxime**, a non-nephrotoxic broad-spectrum third-generation cephalosporin, provides coverage for more than 94% of the flora responsible for SBP and is the **antibiotic of choice** for empirical treatment.
   - The recommended dose is 2 g intravenously every 8 hours over 5 days.

   - Ascitic fluid cultures rapidly become sterile after even one dose of cefotaxime.

- The antibiotic spectrum may be narrowed once culture results become available and the sensitivities of the causative organism are known.
- Alternative antibiotic regimens include amoxicillin-clavulanic acid (in Europe) and fluoroquinolones.

3. A follow-up paracentesis is indicated whenever
   - Secondary (surgical) bacterial peritonitis is suspected
   - The typical clinical response to cefotaxime (i.e., fall in serum white cell count, defervescence, etc.) does not occur

4. Secondary bacterial peritonitis or SBP caused by an organism resistant to cefotaxime can lead to persistently positive ascitic fluid cultures and ascitic fluid PMN counts higher than pretreatment values.

5. Survival rates in patients with SBP have improved.

6. Introvenous volume expanders in patients with SBP have shown benefit.
   - SBP is associated with marked increases of cytokines, including tumor necrosis factor alpha and interleukin-6, and production of nitric oxide, a potent vasodilator.
   - These changes are associated with clinical deteriorations in blood pressure, renal function, coagulation, and hepatic function.
   - Intravenous volume expanders (e.g., albumin) increase central volume and maintain renal perfusion.
   - One study reported that administration of intravenous albumin 1.5 g/kg at the time SBP is diagnosed and 1.0 g/kg on day 3 of antibiotic treatment decreased the risk of renal insufficiency and SBP-related mortality; it is reasonable to administer albumin in this setting while awaiting additional studies.

Prophylaxis of Ascitic Fluid Infection

INDICATIONS

1. Patients at high risk for development of SBP include those with (1) a previous episode of SBP, (2) gastrointestinal hemorrhage, and (3) ascitic fluid total protein less than 1.0 g/dL during hospitalization.

2. Selective intestinal decontamination to prevent SBP has been suggested in these situations (Table 11.8).

ANTIBIOTIC REGIMENS

1. **Norfloxacin**, a poorly absorbed fluoroquinolone, has been used to achieve selective intestinal decontamination in cirrhotic patients; norfloxacin has several characteristics that make it suitable for prophylaxis:
   - Poor absorption when taken orally
   - Effectiveness against enteric gram-negative organisms
   - Sparing of gram-positive and anaerobic organisms to maintain their protective role in the normal gut flora

2. Norfloxacin reduces the incidence of SBP, delays progression to hepatorenal syndrome, and improves overall survival (see Table 11.8).

TABLE 11.8 ■ **Indications for prophylaxis of ascitic fluid infection**

Indication	Duration of prophylaxis
Recovery from an episode of SBP	Indefinitely, or until ascites disappears
Gastrointestinal bleeding in a patient with cirrhosis	7 days
Ascitic fluid total protein <1.0 g/dL	During hospitalization (controversial)

Ascitic fluid protein <1.5 g/dL plus one of the following parameters:
  Child–Turcotte–Pugh score ≥9 and bilirubin >3 mg/dL
  Creatinine ≥1.2 mg/dL
  Blood urea nitrogen ≥25 mg/dL
  Serum sodium ≤130 mEq/L,
	Continue until decompensated liver disease improves or liver transplantation performed

SBP, spontaneous bacterial peritonitis.

3. In patients who have survived an episode of SBP:
   ■ Recurrence can be as high as 68% at 1 year without antibiotic prophylaxis.
   ■ Norfloxacin, 400 mg orally daily, has been shown to decrease the probability of recurrent SBP to 20% at 1 year.
   ■ Norfloxacin prophylaxis is cost effective in reducing recurrent SBP.
   ■ However, norfloxacin treatment does not alter the overall mortality in these patients.
4. In patients with cirrhosis and gastrointestinal hemorrhage:
   ■ The incidence of SBP can be as high as 45% to 66% at 1 year without antibiotic prophylaxis.
   ■ Antibiotic prophylaxis started immediately and continued for 7 days decreases the incidence of SBP to 10% to 20%.
   ■ Antibiotic prophylaxis may improve survival in these patients.
   ■ Intravenous ceftriaxone has been shown to be more effective than oral norfloxacin for SBP prophylaxis in patients with advanced cirrhosis and gastrointestinal hemorrhage.
5. In hospitalized patients with ascitic fluid total protein less than 1.0 g/dL:
   ■ The overall probability of new-onset SBP is 20% in 1 year.
   ■ Prophylaxis with norfloxacin 400 mg orally daily decreases in-hospital incidence of SBP from 22% to 0% without an effect on in-hospital mortality.
6. Trimethoprim–sulfamethoxazole, one double-strength tablet orally daily, has also been reported to be effective in preventing SBP.

CONCERNS

1. Routine long-term use of prophylactic norfloxacin leads to the rapid development of quinolone-resistant organisms in the fecal flora.
2. Long-term norfloxacin prophylaxis is associated with
   ■ Quinolone-resistant gram-negative bacilli in 50% of SBP cultures
   ■ A high incidence of urinary tract infection by quinolone-resistant gram-negative bacilli

FURTHER READING

Bajaj JS, Zadvornova Y, Heuman DM, et al. Association of proton pump inhibitor therapy with spontaneous bacterial peritonitis in cirrhotic patients with ascites. *Am J Gastroenterol* 2009; 104:1130–1134.

Fernandez J, Arbol LR, Gomez C, et al. Norfloxacin vs ceftriaxone in the prophylaxis of infections in patients with advanced cirrhosis and hemorrhage. *Gastroenterology* 2006; 131:1049–1056.

Fernandez J, Navasa M, Planas R, et al. Primary prophylaxis of spontaneous bacterial peritonitis delays hepatorenal syndrome and improves survival in cirrhosis. *Gastroenterology* 2007; 133:818–824.

Garcia-Tsao G. Current management of the complications of cirrhosis and portal hypertension: variceal hemorrhage, ascites, and spontaneous bacterial peritonitis. *Gastroenterology* 2001; 120:726–748.

Guarner C, Sola R, Soriano G, et al. Risk of first community-acquired spontaneous bacterial peritonitis in cirrhotics with low ascitic fluid protein levels. *Gastroenterology* 1999; 117:424–419.

Guarner C, Garcia-Tsao G, Navasa M, et al. Diagnosis, treatment and prophylaxis of spontaneous bacterial peritonitis: a consensus document. *J Hepatol* 2000; 32:142–153.

Malinchoc M, Kamath PS, Gorden FD, et al. A model to predict poor survival in patients undergoing transjugular intrahepatic portosystemic shunts. *Hepatology* 2000; 31:864–871.

Moore KP, Wong F, Gines P, et al. The management of ascites in cirrhosis: report on the consensus conference of the International Ascites Club. *Hepatology* 2003; 38:258–266.

Obstein KL, Campbell MS, Reddy KR, et al. Association between model for end-stage liver disease and spontaneous bacterial peritonitis. *Am J Gastroenterol* 2007; 102:2732–2736.

Parsi MA, Saadeh SN, Zein NN, et al. Ascites fluid lactoferrin for diagnosis of spontaneous bacterial peritonitis. *Gastroenterology* 2008; 135:803–807.

Rössle M, Ochs A, Gülberg V, et al. A comparison of paracentesis and transjugular intrahepatic portosystemic shunting in patients with ascites. *N Engl J Med* 2000; 342:1701–1707.

Runyon BA. Management of adult patients with ascites due to cirrhosis: an update. AASLD Practice Guideline. *Hepatology* 2009; 49:2087–2107.

Runyon BA. Ascites and spontaneous bacterial peritonitis. In: Feldman M, Friedman LS, Sleisenger MH, eds. *Sleisenger and Fordtran's Gastrointestinal and Liver Disease: Pathophysiology, Diagnosis, Management*, 7th edn. Philadelphia: Saunders; 2002:1517.

Soriano G, Castellote J, Alvarez C, et al. Secondary bacterial peritonitis in cirrhosis: a retrospective study of clinical analytical characteristics, diagnosis and management. *J Hepatol* 2010; 52:39–44.

Sort P, Navasa M, Arroyo V, et al. Effect of intravenous albumin on renal impairment and mortality in patients with cirrhosis and spontaneous bacterial peritonitis. *N Engl J Med* 1999; 341:403–409.

CHAPTER 12

Hepatorenal syndrome

Mónica Guevara, MD, PhD ■ Juan Rodés, MD, FRCP

KEY POINTS

1. Hepatorenal syndrome (HRS) is a severe complication of patients with cirrhosis and ascites.
2. The annual incidence of HRS in patients with ascites is approximately 8%.
3. The diagnosis of HRS is associated with a poor prognosis and very short survival.
4. Liver transplantation is the treatment of choice for HRS.

Overview

1. The term *hepatorenal syndrome* (HRS) was initially applied to many different disorders involving the liver and the kidney.
2. During the 1960s and the 1970s, nephrologists in the United States popularized the term to define renal failure in cirrhosis.
3. In 1996, the International Ascites Club delineated the first diagnostic criteria to define HRS.
4. In 2007, these criteria were revisited and changed (Table 12.1).

Definition

1. Renal failure, estimated by a level of serum creatinine greater than 1.5 mg/dL, occurring in a patient with advanced liver disease and portal hypertension
2. HRS characterized by
   - A marked decrease in glomerular filtration rate (GFR) and renal plasma flow (RPF) in the absence of other identifiable causes of renal failure
   - Marked abnormalities in systemic hemodynamics
   - Activation of endogenous vasoactive systems

Pathogenesis

1. The pathogenesis of HRS is not completely understood.
2. Several mechanisms have been implicated (Fig. 12.1):
   - Disturbance in systemic hemodynamics
   - Increased activity of vasoconstrictor systems
   - Reduced or insufficiently increased activity of vasodilator factors

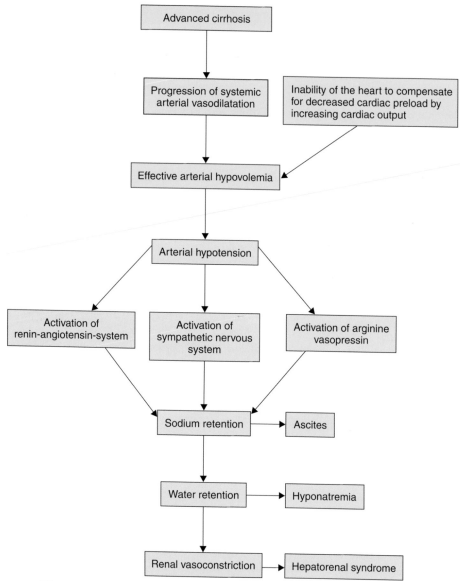

Fig. 12.1 Pathogenesis of hepatorenal syndrome according to the vasodilatation theory.

3. **Systemic hemodynamics**
   - Hemodynamic alteration results from severe arterial vasodilation located mainly in the splanchnic territory.
   - The hemodynamic profile is characterized by hypervolemia, low arterial pressure, and low systemic vascular resistance.
   - In the setting of increased activity of vasoconstrictor systems, marked renal vasoconstriction develops.

- Vasoconstriction occurs not only in renal circulation but also in brachial, femoral, and cerebral blood flow, probably as a compensatory mechanism to counteract splanchnic vasodilation.
- HRS has been traditionally assumed to develop in the setting of progression of the hyperdynamic circulation with high cardiac output; however, in few studies assessing cardiovascular function in patients with HRS or refractory ascites, cardiac output was found to be significantly reduced compared with patients without HRS.

4. **Vasoconstrictor systems**
   a. Renin-angiotensin-aldosterone system (RAAS) and sympathetic nervous system (SNS)
      - RAAS and SNS activity are increased in most cirrhotic patients with ascites.
      - These systems are particularly activated in patients with HRS.
      - The activity of both systems, RAAS and SNS, correlates inversely with renal blood flow.
      - Experimental studies have demonstrated the compensatory nature of the increased vasoconstrictor activity.
      - Pharmacologic blockage of the effectors of these systems induces reduction in systemic vascular resistance and arterial hypotension, findings suggesting that their increased activation is crucial to maintain systemic hemodynamics.
   b. Antidiuretic hormone arginine vasopressin [AVP]
      - This hormone contributes to water retention and dilutional hyponatremia.
   c. Endothelin (ET)
      - This endothelial-derived peptide is also increased in cirrhosis.
      - The most important effect of ET is renal vasoconstriction, which can decrease RBF and GFR.
      - Among patients with cirrhosis, those with HRS show the highest levels of ET.
      - The role of ET in the pathogenesis of HRS remains to be clarified.
   d. Others: adenosine, leukotrienes, and isoprostanes

5. **Vasodilatory factors**
   a. Renal prostaglandins (PGs)
      - PGs are the most important intrarenal vasodilators.
      - PGs contribute to maintain renal perfusion in cirrhotic patients.
      - Inhibition of synthesis of PGs induces a profound derangement of RPF and GFR.
      - Cirrhotic patients with HRS have reduced production of renal PGs.
      - Renal vasoconstriction results from the imbalance between renal vasoconstrictors and vasodilators.
   b. Nitric oxide (NO)
      - NO is locally synthesized within the kidney.
      - Under normal conditions, NO plays a role in the regulation of glomerular microcirculation, sodium excretion, and renin release.
      - Inhibition of NO does not induce renal vasoconstriction as a result of the compensatory increase of renal PGs.
      - Inhibition of both NO and PGs induces renal vasoconstriction in patients with cirrhosis and ascites.
      - NO interacts with PGs to maintain renal perfusion in cirrhotic patients with ascites.
   c. Natriuretic peptides
      - These vasodilators are involved in the maintenance of renal perfusion.
      - Atrial natriuretic peptide (ANP) is the major natriuretic hormone.
      - ANP is elevated in decompensated cirrhosis, and patients with HRS have the highest levels.
      - Increased ANP may act as a homeostatic mechanism to counteract the effect of vasoconstrictor systems.

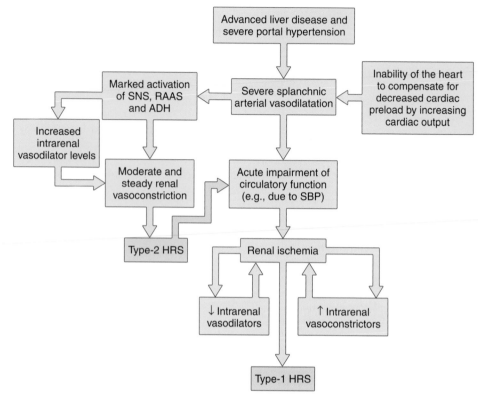

Fig. 12.2 Pathogenesis of type 1 and type 2 hepatorenal syndrome. ADH, antidiuretic hormone; RAAS, renin-angiotensin-aldosterone system; SBP, spontaneous bacterial peritonitis; SNS, sympathic nervous system

Pathogenesis

VASODILATATION THEORY

1. This is the most widely accepted theory of the pathogenesis of HRS (Fig. 12.2).
2. Portal hypertension, the initial event in the pathogenesis of HRS, induces arterial vasodilation by mechanisms not completely understood.
3. Arterial vasodilatation is located mainly in the splanchnic circulation.
4. Vasodilation induces decreased effective arterial blood volume and increased activity of vasoconstrictor systems.
5. Activation of the vasoconstrictor system further increases to compensate for circulatory dysfunction.
6. HRS is the extreme manifestation of circulatory dysfunction and may be the result of
   - marked activation of vasoconstrictor systems
   - decreased activity of vasodilatory factors
   - increased production of intrarenal vasoconstrictors

Facts that Sustain Support for the Vasodilatation Theory

1. Administration of vasoconstrictor drug analogues of AVP, which induce vasoconstriction mainly in the dilated splanchnic arterial circulation, is associated with:

TABLE 12.1 ■ **Diagnostic criteria for hepatorenal syndrome**

1. Cirrhosis with ascites
2. Serum creatinine level greater than 133 µmol/L (1.5 mg/dL)
3. Lack of improvement in serum creatinine level (i.e., lack of a decrease to a level of ≤ 133 µmol/L) after ≥2 days following diuretic withdrawal and volume expansion with albumin; recommended dose of albumin: 1 g/kg of body weight per day up to a maximum of 100 g/day
4. Absence of shock
5. Lack of current or recent treatment with nephrotoxic drugs
6. Absence of parenchymal kidney disease as indicated by proteinuria >500 mg/day, microhematuria (>50 red blood cells/high-power field), and/or abnormal renal ultrasonography

  ■ Normalization of the activity of vasoconstrictor systems
  ■ Improvement in systemic hemodynamics
  ■ Improvement in renal function and reversal of HRS
2. Transjugular intrahepatic portosystemic shunt (TIPS) placement, which reduces the portal venous pressure gradient, induces an improvement in renal function in patients with HRS.

Diagnosis

1. The diagnosis of HRS is based on the demonstration of a marked reduction in GFR and the exclusion of other types of renal failure.
2. In 2007, the International Ascites Club modified the diagnostic criteria used to define HRS. These are the current criteria used to define HRS (Table 12.1).

Other Causes of Acute Kidney Injury in Cirrhosis

ACUTE TUBULAR NECROSIS

1. This is characterized by an abrupt impairment in renal function.
2. Cirrhotic patients frequently experience clinical situations that predispose to the development of acute tubular necrosis (ATN), such as hypovolemic or septic shock, major surgical procedures, or exposure to nephrotoxic drugs.
3. Although no specific markers for ATN have been described, the presence of the following criteria may be useful for diagnosis:
   ■ High urine sodium concentration
   ■ Urine/serum osmolality ratio lower than 1
   ■ Abnormal urine sediment, with epithelial cells and casts

GLOMERULAR DISEASE

1. Despite the high incidence of glomerular abnormalities on histologic examination of kidney in patients with cirrhosis, signs or symptoms of glomerular dysfunction seldom develop.
2. The presence of glomerular abnormalities seems to be independent of the origin of cirrhosis.

3. Patients with more severe glomerular abnormalities develop mainly proteinuria and/or hematuria.

DRUG-INDUCED KIDNEY INJURY

1. Aminoglycosides and nonsteroidal anti-inflammatory drugs are the most common drugs inducing renal failure in cirrhotic patients.
2. Drug-induced renal failure has a clinical profile similar to that of ATN.

PRERENAL AZOTEMIA

1. Intravascular volume depletion can lead to prerenal azotemia.
2. Causes of intravascular volume depletion include vomiting, diarrhea, and diuretic overuse.
3. It is difficult to differentiate prerenal azotemia from HRS based on urinary sodium or urinary volume; thus these parameters were removed from the diagnostic criteria of HRS.
4. Improvement in renal function after albumin expansion (see earlier) allows the differentiation of prerenal azotemia from HRS.
5. A negative response to albumin expansion is a major diagnostic criterion of HRS.

Clinical Features

HRS is classified as type 1 or type 2 according to both the intensity and the manner of progression of renal failure. These types exhibit different prognosis and survival, and each type should be treated differently.

TYPE 1

1. This is characterized by a severe and rapidly progressive renal failure defined as doubling of serum creatinine, reaching a level greater than 2.5 mg/dL in less than 2 weeks.
2. Patients usually have severe liver failure (jaundice, encephalopathy, and coagulopathy).
3. It may occur following a precipitating factor (severe bacterial infection, gastrointestinal hemorrhage, or therapeutic paracentesis without plasma expansion).
4. It is the complication with the poorest prognosis in cirrhosis.
5. Median survival time is only 2 weeks.

TYPE 2

1. Moderate and stable renal failure occurs.
2. It is associated with relatively preserved liver failure.
3. The main clinical consequence is refractory ascites.
4. Median survival is approximately 6 months.

Treatment

1. Liver transplantation is the treatment of choice in patients with HRS.
2. Patients with HRS who undergo transplantation have more complications, spend more days in the intensive care unit, and have a higher in-hospital mortality rate than patients without

HRS who undergo liver transplantation. However, patients with HRS who are treated with vasopressin analogues and albumin before liver transplantation have a post-transplant outcome similar to that of transplant recipients with normal renal function.

3. Patients with type 1 HRS have an expected survival of less than 2 weeks; this poor prognosis makes the applicability of liver transplantation very unlikely unless survival could be increased by other measures, that is, treatment with vasoconstrictors and albumin.

4. Patients with type 2 HRS usually have a sufficiently prolonged survival to allow liver transplantation.

5. The Model for End-stage Liver Disease (MELD) score has been implemented to assign organ allocation in patients on the waiting list for liver transplantation. This score takes into account serum bilirubin level, international normalized ratio (INR) and serum creatinine level. Before the era of MELD, liver transplantation in patients with HRS was difficult. These patients have a short survival, and to reach liver transplantation, they must have a high priority on the waiting list. Because patients currently undergo liver transplantation according to their MELD score, patients with HRS who are candidates for transplantation now may have the procedure because they can be prioritized on the waiting list, thus increasing the probability of liver transplantation.

TYPE 1 (Fig. 12.3)

1. **Terlipressin:**
   - Type 1 HRS is reversible following treatment with terlipressin, a vasoconstrictor analogue of antidiuretic hormone, and intravenous albumin.
   - Vasoconstriction of splanchnic circulation is the presumed mechanism of action of terlipressin.
   - A delay of several days occurs between the improvement in circulatory function and the increase in GFR.
   - Concurrent systemic vasoconstriction may potentially cause ischemic side effects.
   - Reversal of HRS improves survival, and a significant number of patients may undergo liver transplantation.

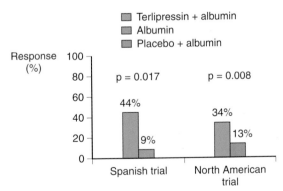

Fig. 12.3 Response to treatment with terlipressin and albumin in patients with hepatorenal syndrome in two randomized clinical trials. *(From Martín-Llahí M, Pepín MN, Guevara M, et al. Terlipressin and albumin vs albumin in patients with cirrhosis and hepatorenal syndrome: a randomized study.* Gastroenterology *2008; 134:1352–1359; and Sanyal AJ, Boyer T, Garcia-Tsao G, et al. A randomized, prospective, double-blind, placebo-controlled trial of terlipressin for type 1 hepatorenal syndrome.* Gastroenterology *2008; 134:1360–1368.)*

- Recurrence of HRS after treatment with terlipressin is not frequent, and readministration of the same treatment should be considered.
- Approximately 40% of patients with HRS respond to treatment with terlipressin and albumin, and thus new therapeutic strategies are needed for the large number of patients without response to treatment (Fig. 12.3).
- A study showed that serum bilirubin lower than 10 mg/dL and an early increase in arterial pressure predict a response to treatment with terlipressin and albumin in type 1 HRS.

2. **Catecholamines** (midodrine and norepinephrine) are also effective for the treatment of HRS; more studies are needed to confirm the efficacy of these agents before they can be recommended.

3. **TIPS** improves renal function in patients with HRS.
   - It is recommended for patients who cannot receive vasoconstrictor drugs and have no contraindications to TIPS.

4. **Hemodialysis** is not effective in the treatment of HRS; it should be used only if patients have specific clinical indications (hypervolemia, tubular acidosis, hyperkalemia).

5. **Extracorporeal albumin dialysis,** a system that uses an albumin-containing dialysate that is recirculated and perfused through a charcoal and anion-exchanger column, has been shown to improve renal function in patients with type 1 HRS. However, one study showed that molecular adsorbent recirculating system (MARS) treatment is not associated with an increase in GFR.

TYPE 2

1. No studies are specifically designed to evaluate the effect of vasoconstrictor treatment on renal function in patients with type 2 HRS.

2. Management is mainly focused on the treatment of refractory ascites usually found in these patients.

3. Only two pilot studies specifically assessed TIPS in type 2 HRS.
   - In one study, a marked reduction of serum creatinine was observed in eight out of nine patients treated by TIPS. This finding was associated with a significant improvement in the control of ascites. Four of these patients died, two within the first month and two 12 and 14 months after TIPS; the remaining five patients had longer survival.
   - The second study included 14 patients with type 1 HRS and 17 with type 2 HRS treated by TIPS. A significant improvement in serum creatinine and creatinine clearance was observed in the whole group of 31 patients, as well as an improvement in the control of ascites in 24 cases. Six patients developed TIPS dysfunction, and 11 developed hepatic encephalopathy during follow-up. The 1-year probability of survival in the 17 patients with type 2 HRS treated by TIPS was 70%; TIPS is therefore effective in reversing type 2 HRS, although more data on complication rate and survival are needed.

Prevention

In four specific situations, HRS may be successfully prevented (Table 12.2).

1. Therapeutic paracentesis: the administration of plasma volume expanders, specifically albumin, after total paracentesis (greater than 5 L) in patients with cirrhosis and ascites decreases the incidence of renal failure and hyponatremia.

2. Spontaneous bacterial peritonitis (SBP): the administration of albumin (1.5 g/kg intravenously at the diagnosis of infection and 1 g/kg intravenously 48 hours later) together with

TABLE 12.2 ■ **Effective interventions for preventing hepatorenal syndrome**

Condition	Intervention	Effect
Therapeutic paracentesis	Albumin (8 g/L of ascites removed)	Reduces the risk of HRS and hyponatremia
Spontaneous bacterial peritonitis	Albumin (1.5 g/kg IV at diagnosis of the infection and 1 g/kg after 2 days)	Reduces the risk of HRS and Improves survival
Primary prophylaxis of spontaneous bacterial peritonitis.	Long-term oral norfloxacin (400 mg/day)	Reduces the risk of type 1 HRS
Severe acute alcohol hepatitis	Pentoxifylline (400 mg t.i.d. p.o.)	Reduces the risk of HRS and Improves survival

HRS, hepatorenal syndrome; IV, intravenously; p.o., orally; t.i.d., three times daily.

intravenous cefotaxime 1 gm twice daily for 5-7 days in patients with cirrhosis and SBP markedly reduces the incidence of impairment in circulatory function and the occurrence of type 1 HRS.

3. Primary prophylaxis of SBP using long-term oral norfloxacin in patients with low protein ascites (less than 1.5 mg/dL) and serum bilirubin greater than 4 mg/dL associated with a Child–Pugh score higher than 9, or serum creatinine greater than 1.2 mg/dL, was associated with a significant decrease in 1-year probability of development of SBP (7% versus 61%) and type 1 HRS (28% versus 41%) and a significant increase in the 3-month and 1-year probability of survival (94% versus 62% and 60% versus 48%, respectively).

4. The administration of pentoxifylline (400 mg orally three times a day) to patients with severe acute alcoholic hepatitis reduced the occurrence of HRS (8% in the pentoxifylline group versus 35% in the placebo group) and the hospital mortality (24% versus 46%, respectively).

FURTHER READING

Angeli P, Volpin R, Gerunda G, et al. Reversal of type 1 hepatorenal syndrome with the administration of midodrine and octreotide. *Hepatology* 1999; 29:1690–1697.

Duvoux C, Zanditenas D, Hezode C, et al. Noradrenalin for treatment of type 1 hepatorenal syndrome (HRS) (abstract). *J Hepatol* 2001; 34:103A.

Fernandez J, Navasa M, Planas R, et al. Primary prophylaxis of spontaneous bacterial peritonitis delays hepatorenal syndrome and improves survival in cirrhosis. *Gastroenterology* 2007; 133:818–824.

Gines P, Uriz J, Calahorra B, et al. for the International Study Group on Refractory Ascites in Cirrhosis. Transjugular intrahepatic portosystemic shunting versus paracentesis plus albumin for refractory ascites in cirrhosis. *Gastroenterology* 2002; 123:1839–1847.

Gonwa TA, Morris CA, Goldstein RM, et al. Long-term survival and renal function following liver transplantation in patients with and without hepatorenal syndrome: experience in 300 patients. *Transplantation* 1991; 91:428–430.

Guevara M, Ginés P, Bandi JC, et al. Transjugular intrahepatic portosystemic shunt in hepatorenal syndrome: effects on renal function and vasoactive systems. *Hepatology* 1998; 28:416–422.

Guevara M, Ginés P, Fernandez-Esparrach G, et al. Reversibility of hepatorenal syndrome by prolonged administration of ornipressin and plasma volume expansion. *Hepatology* 1998; 27:35–41.

Martín-Llahí M, Pepín MN, Guevara M, et al. Terlipressin and albumin vs albumin in patients with cirrhosis and hepatorenal syndrome: a randomized study. *Gastroenterology* 2008; 134:1352–1359.

Mitzner SR, Stange J, Klammt S, et al. Improvement of hepatorenal syndrome with extracorporeal albumin dialysis MARS: results of a prospective, randomized controlled clinical trial. *Liver Transpl* 2000; 6:277–286.

Nazar A, Pereira GH, Guevara M, et al. Predictors of response to therapy with terlipressin and albumin in patients with cirrhosis and type 1 hepatorenal syndrome. *Hepatology* 2010; 51:219–226.

Ruiz-del-Arbol L, Monescillo A, Arocena C, et al. Circulatory function and hepatorenal syndrome in cirrhosis. *Hepatology* 2005; 42:439–447.

Salerno F, Gerbes A, Ginés P, et al. Diagnosis, prevention and treatment of hepatorenal syndrome in cirrhosis. *Gut* 2007; 56:1310–1318.

Sanyal AJ, Boyer T, Garcia-Tsao G, et al. A randomized, prospective, double-blind, placebo-controlled trial of terlipressin for type 1 hepatorenal syndrome. *Gastroenterology* 2008; 134:1360–1368.

Sort P, Navasa M, Arroyo V, et al. Effect of plasma volume expansion on renal impairment and mortality in patients with cirrhosis and spontaneous bacterial peritonitis. *N Engl J Med* 1999; 341:403–409.

Wong F, Richardson R. Molecular adsorbent recirculating system is ineffective in the management of type 1 hepatorenal syndrome in cirrhosis with ascites (abstract). *Hepatology* 2009; 48(Suppl):1057A.

CHAPTER 13

Hepatic encephalopathy

Ravi K. Prakash, MD, MRCP (UK) ■ Kevin D. Mullen, MD, FRCPI

KEY POINTS

1 The key to the diagnosis of hepatic encephalopathy is recognition that significant liver disease is present.

2 The occurrence of any neuropsychiatric symptoms or signs in a patient with significant liver dysfunction should be considered hepatic encephalopathy until proven otherwise.

3 Patients with suspected overt hepatic encephalopathy are managed by a four-pronged strategy: general care of the unconscious patient, exclusion of other causes of encephalopathy, correction of precipitating factors, and initiation of empirical therapy.

4 Hepatic encephalopathy associated with acute liver failure (type A) is rare, and its clinical course and treatment are distinct from those in chronic liver disease.

5 Many hypotheses on the pathogenesis of hepatic encephalopathy exist; however, operationally the ammonia concept is perfectly suited to the clinician caring for patients with hepatic encephalopathy.

6 The diagnosis of hepatic encephalopathy is mainly clinical and is not based on blood ammonia levels.

Definition and Classification

1. **Overt hepatic encephalopathy (OHE):** a wide spectrum of neurologic and neuropsychiatric abnormalities in patients with significant liver dysfunction
2. **Covert/minimal hepatic encephalopathy (covert HE):** a disorder in which patients with cirrhosis have normal mental and neurologic status on clinical examination but exhibit reversible and quantifiable neuropsychologic and/or neuropsychiatric abnormalities

Table 13.1 depicts the Working Party classification of HE.

Pathophysiology

1. Failure of hepatic detoxification of neuroactive compounds arising from the gut; cross-circulation experiments in an animal model favor this theory.
2. **Specific hypotheses of HE**
   ■ **Ammonia:** This compound is mainly derived from nitrogenous products in the diet, bacterial metabolism of urea, and deamination of glutamine by the enzyme glutaminase. Ammonia enters the portal circulation from the gut and is converted to urea in the liver.

TABLE 13.1 ■ 1998 Hepatic Encephalopathy Working Party proposed classification of hepatic encephalopathy

Type	Description	Subcategory	Subdivision
A	Encephalopathy associated with acute liver failure	—	—
B	Encephalopathy with portosystemic bypass and no intrinsic hepatocellular disease	—	—
C	Encephalopathy associated with cirrhosis or portal hypertension/portosystemic shunts	Episodic	Precipitated Spontaneous Recurrent
		Resistant	Mild Severe Treatment dependent
		Covert	

In the presence of significant portosystemic shunting, with or without hepatocellular dysfunction, ammonia concentration rises in blood and crosses the blood–brain barrier. Exposure to increased brain ammonia results in structural alterations in astrocytes that cause swelling and brain edema. Over a long period of exposure to high ammonia levels, astrocytes develop structural changes known as Alzheimer type II astrocytes.

■ **Inflammation:** It is now clearly evident that inflammatory mediators and cytokines play an important role along with hyperammonia in the pathogenesis of HE; possible mechanisms include cytokine-mediated changes in blood–brain barrier permeability, microglial activation and the subsequent production of neurosteroids, and altered activity of peripheral benzodiazepine binding sites.

■ **Increased benzodiazepine-like compounds in the brain**

■ **Accumulation of manganese in the basal ganglia:** This is implicated in altered dopaminergic neurotransmission and extrapyramidal symptoms.

■ **Alterations in central nervous system (CNS) tryptophan metabolites** (e.g., serotonin): These changes may underlie some of the classic descriptions of altered sleep–wake cycles seen in early stages of encephalopathy.

Clinical Features

1. Acute liver failure–associated encephalopathy
2. Covert HE: patients with normal neurologic examination but abnormal neuropsychiatric test performance
3. Single or recurrent HE (two episodes of HE within 1 year)
4. Persistent HE
   ■ Low-grade HE (covert HE + grade I HE): mental status changes without disorientation
   ■ High-grade HE (stage II to IV): mental status changes with disorientation
5. Acquired hepatocerebral degeneration
6. Spastic paraparesis

The last two presentations are very rare and are exceptions to the rule that HE is usually reversible; they generally occur in the background of fluctuating HE and major long-standing portosystemic shunts.

Diagnosis

1. Consideration of the possibility of HE arises when significant liver dysfunction is known or suspected to be present. Clinical or laboratory evidence of liver failure and/or portal hypertension is usually obvious. However, in a minority of patients, evidence of significant liver dysfunction may be subtle, as in the following conditions:
   a. Well-compensated cirrhosis (e.g., chronic hepatitis C, remote alcohol abuse)
   b. Noncirrhotic portal hypertension:
      ■ Splanchnic vein thrombosis
      ■ Schistosomiasis
      ■ Noncirrhotic portal fibrosis
      ■ Idiopathic portal hypertension
   c. Congenital hepatic fibrosis
   d. Congenital intrahepatic and extrahepatic portosystemic shunts
2. **Historical points suggesting occult liver disease and/or portosystemic shunting**
   a. Past history of injection drug use
   b. Family history of cirrhosis (hemochromatosis)
   c. Residence in areas endemic for schistosomiasis
   d. Umbilical sepsis (splanchnic vein thrombosis)
   e. History of pancreatitis (splenic vein thrombosis)
   f. Past history of hepatitis (hepatitis B or C, alcoholic hepatitis)
   g. Past history of use of hepatotoxic drugs (e.g., methotrexate, nitrofurantoin)
3. **Physical signs suggesting underlying significant liver disease**
   a. **Upper extremity**
      ■ Clubbing, leukonychia
      ■ Dupuytren's contracture, palmar erythema
      ■ Spider telangiectasias, tattoos, injection marks, asterixis
      ■ Scratch marks, pigmentation, ecchymoses
      ■ Loss of muscle mass
   b. **Eyes and face**
      ■ Conjunctival icterus, cyanosis, parotid enlargement
      ■ Kayser–Fleischer rings
   c. **Chest**
      ■ Spider telangiectasias, loss of axillary hair, gynecomastia
   d. **Abdomen**
      ■ Splenomegaly (usually less than 5 cm below costal the margin)
      ■ Hepatomegaly
      ■ Caput medusae
      ■ Ascites
   e. **Testicular atrophy**
   f. **Loss of escutcheon**
   g. **Loss of hair on the shins**
   h. **Pedal edema**

4. **Laboratory test abnormalities**
   a. Hepatic synthetic dysfunction: increased prothrombin time, low serum albumin
   b. Elevated ammonia levels (not routinely recommended)
   c. Hypergammaglobulinemia
   d. Pancytopenia, leukopenia, thrombocytopenia
   e. Elevated cerebrospinal fluid glutamine levels
   f. Decreased plasma branched chain/aromatic amino acid ratio
   g. Hepatitis C antibody–positive status
   h. Hepatitis B surface antigen–positive status

The foregoing historical points, physical signs, and laboratory tests can individually or in combination indicate the presence of underlying liver dysfunction even when results of traditional tests of hepatic function, such as serum albumin and prothrombin times, are normal. Patients with well-preserved synthetic function of the liver do not commonly develop overt HE; a major precipitating factor is needed to induce an episode in such patients.

Covert Hepatic Encephalopathy

1. Covert HE is defined as **abnormal performance on psychometric testing** when a standard neurologic examination is completely normal.
2. It is present in more than 50% of patients with cirrhosis.
3. It has a significant negative impact on quality of life and is associated with poor driving skills, impaired navigational skills, and increased traffic violations and accidents.
4. It is shown to increase the risk of progression to overt HE.
5. The International Society for Hepatic Encephalopathy recommends the Psychometric Hepatic Encephalopathy Score (PHES) as the gold standard for diagnosis of covert HE; impairment of greater than 2 SD in two or more tests in this battery is necessary for diagnosis of covert HE.
   - NCT A (Number Connection Test A): measures concentration, mental tracking, and visuomotor speed.
   - NCT B (Number Connection Test B): measures concentration, mental tracking, and visuomotor speed.
   - DST (Digit Symbol Test): assesses psychomotor and visuomotor speed.
   - LTT (Line Tracing Test): measures both speed and accuracy and has visuomotor and visuo-spatial components.
   - SDT (Serial Dotting Test): assesses psychomotor speed. It has failed to gain popularity because of the lack of availability of testing material and normative data for comparison in United States; the RBANS (Repeatable Battery for Assessment of Neuropsychologic Status) was developed in United States and is considered an equivalent test.
6. **Drawbacks of paper and pencil tests**
   - Difficulty in interpretation and scoring
   - Too much reliance on fine motor skills
   - Poor test of memory
7. **The following computerized tests are being evaluated for diagnosis of covert HE to address the foregoing drawbacks:**
   - Inhibitory Control Test
   - Cognitive Drug Research Factor Score
   - Critical Flicker/Fusion Frequency (CFF) Test

Overt Hepatic Encephalopathy

1. The diagnosis is made when alterations in consciousness and a generalized movement disorder occur in a patient with known or suspected significant liver dysfunction.
2. The West Haven Criteria for Classification of Hepatic Encephalopathy is a tool for assessment of mental state in this population.
3. Recommended tests that allow better distinction among the different grades of HE are shown in Table 13.2.
4. **Associated motor disorders**
   - Slow, monotonous speech pattern
   - Loss of fine motor skills
   - Extrapyramidal-type movement disorders
   - Hyperreflexia, extensor plantar response (Babinski's sign), clonus
   - Asterixis
   - Hyperventilation
   - Seizures
   - Confusion, coma
   - Decerebrate/decorticate posturing

TABLE 13.2 ■ **West Haven criteria for classification of hepatic encephalopathy**

Grade	Description	Recommended Tests
0	No abnormality detected	
Covert HE	Normal mental status and neurologic examination Abnormal psychometric tests	>2 SD on 2 or more tests in PHES ICT: >5 lures CFF: cutoff frequency 39 Hz
I	Trivial lack of awareness Euphoria or anxiety Shortened attention span Impairment of addition or subtraction	Naming ≤7 animals in 120 sec Orientation in time and space
II	Lethargy or apathy Disorientation for time Obvious personality change Inappropriate behavior	Disorientation in time (≥3 items incorrect): Day of the week Day of the month The month The year Orientation to place
III	Somnolence to semistupor Responsiveness to stimuli Confusion Gross disorientation Bizarre behavior	Disorientation to place (≥2 items incorrect): State/country Region/county City Place Floor/ward Disorientation to time Reduction of Glasgow coma score (8–14)
IV	Coma, inability to test mental state	Unresponsiveness to pain stimuli (Glasgow coma score <8)

CFF, Critical Flicker/Fusion Frequency; HE, hepatic encephalopathy; ICT, Inhibitory Control Test; PHES, Psychometric Hepatic Encephalopathy Score; SD, Standard deviation.

5. Even though slow, monotonous speech and loss of fine motor skills are considered the hall-marks of OHE, none of the foregoing signs are specific. Virtually any neuropsychiatric abnor-mality in a patient with significant liver dysfunction can reflect HE.

Laboratory Tests

1. **Blood ammonia: measurement is not recommended routinely because it does not change the approach to diagnosis or treatment of patients with suspected HE.**
   a. Venous ammonia has the same correlation with the severity of HE as does arterial ammonia.
   b. Measures that should be employed while collecting blood for ammonia assay:
      ■ Blood must be collected from a stasis-free vein; fist clenching or application of tourni-quet can falsely elevate ammonia levels by release of ammonia from skeletal muscle.
      ■ Care must be taken to avoid turbulence or hemolysis.
      ■ Blood must be collected in "green-top glass vacutainer" that contains lithium or sodium heparin; heparin inhibits release of ammonia from red blood cells.
      ■ Blood must be stored in ice bath and immediately transported for assay within 20 min-utes of collection.
      ■ Enzymatic assay is most commonly used by laboratories to test ammonia over a broad range from as low as 12 μmol/L to as high as 1 mmol/L.
   c. The five most common sources of laboratory error:
      ■ Improper collection technique
      ■ Delay in transportation
      ■ Hemolysis or use of heparin lock during venipuncture
      ■ Smoking by patient or laboratory staff
      ■ Pollution of laboratory atmosphere or laboratory glassware with ammonium-containing detergents
2. **Electroencephalography (EEG)**
   a. EEG is rarely used clinically; it has some value in research settings.
   b. The main EEG criterion of HE is slowing of mean frequency.
   c. Reported sensitivity varies from 43% to 100%.
   d. Advances in automated EEG measurements need further validation:
      ■ ANNESS (artificial neural network expert system software)
      ■ Spatiotemporal decomposition, designated SEDACA (short epoch, dominant activity, cluster analysis)
   e. The foregoing advances have been studied, particularly as measures of covert HE; they are excellent research tools but are still undergoing validation.
3. **CFF Test**
   ■ This test is based on the hypothesis that retinal gliopathy (hepatic retinopathy) could serve as a marker of cerebral gliopathy in HE.
   ■ It correlates well with paper and pencil psychometric tests used to diagnose covert HE.
   ■ It enables discrimination of stage 0 HE from covert HE and OHE at a cutoff frequency of 39 Hz, with a sensitivity of 55% and a specificity of 100%.
   ■ It allows for quantification of HE and is not affected appreciably by training.
   ■ It is useful for monitoring fluctuations in the severity of HE in response to precipitating factors or therapeutic interventions.
4. **Magnetic resonance imaging (MRI)**
   a. This shows evidence of cortical atrophy, which is worse in alcoholic liver disease.

b. Hyperintensity of basal ganglia is seen on T1-weighted images.
   ■ Signal abnormalities are thought to be caused by manganese deposition in basal ganglia.
   ■ These abnormalities resolve following liver transplantation.
c. Proton MR spectroscopy detects a consistent increase in the glutamine/glutamate signal along with depletion of myoinositol in the brain that normalizes after liver transplantation.
d. Newer techniques to assess brain edema in HE:
   ■ Magnetization transfer ratio (MTR)
   ■ Fast fluid attenuated inversion recovery (FLAIR) T2-weighted image
   ■ Diffusion weight imaging (DWI)
e. The MTR and T2/FLAIR techniques provide an indirect measure of total cerebral water content.
f. These techniques are helpful in demonstrating that varying degrees of astrocyte swelling occur in chronic liver disease and may be partially responsible for HE; this swelling somewhat correlates with the severity of neuropsychiatric impairment.
g. Cerebral water content has been shown to reverse after liver transplantation and lactulose treatment.
h. T2/FLAIR imaging has shown higher signal intensity in the white matter in and around the corticospinal tract that reverses following liver transplantation.
i. DWI can differentiate between intracellular and extracellular edema; some studies have shown an increase in interstitial edema in the brain.

Treatment

1. **Response to treatment confirms the diagnosis of HE post hoc.**
2. **Four-pronged strategy for acute treatment**
   ■ General supportive care of the unconscious patient
   ■ Exclusion of other causes of encephalopathy and treatment of any present
   ■ Identification and treatment of correctable precipitating factors
   ■ Initiation of empirical treatment
3. **Exclusion of other causes of encephalopathy**
   a. Patients with significant liver dysfunction are susceptible to many causes of encephalopathy other than HE:
      ■ Sepsis
      ■ Hypoxia
      ■ Hypercapnia
      ■ Acidosis
      ■ Uremia
      ■ Sensitivity to central nervous system (CNS) drugs
      ■ Gross electrolyte changes
      ■ Postictal confusion
      ■ Delirium tremens
      ■ Wernicke–Korsakoff syndrome
      ■ Intracerebral hemorrhage
      ■ CNS sepsis
      ■ Pancreatic encephalopathy
      ■ Drug intoxication
      ■ Cerebral edema/intracranial hypertension (usually seen in acute liver failure)
      ■ Hypoglycemia (usually seen in acute liver failure)

    b. Many patients simultaneously have other causes of encephalopathy as well as HE, a situation contributing to difficulty in diagnosing HE.

4. Identification of precipitating factors

    a. Most patients with significant liver disease (except for type A HE) have an identifiable precipitating factor responsible for inducing the onset of an episode of HE. Some precipitating factors can be easily envisaged to enhance the production and/or absorption of gut compounds. Correcting these conditions is a key aspect of the treatment of HE.

    b. Other precipitating factors are less obvious but may act by reducing hepatic function. Sepsis and CNS-active drugs can independently cause encephalopathy or precipitate HE.

- Sepsis
- Gastrointestinal hemorrhage
- Constipation
- Dietary protein overload
- Dehydration
- CNS-active drugs
- Hypokalemia/alkalosis
- Poor compliance with lactulose therapy
- Postanesthesia status
- Postportal decompression procedure
- Bowel obstruction or ileus
- Uremia
- Superimposed hepatic injury
- Development of hepatocellular carcinoma

5. Empiric therapy

    a. Gut cleansing with enemas and gastric aspiration or lavage

    b. Low-protein or zero-protein diet

    c. Delivery of lactulose 15 mL orally or by nasogastric tube every 2 hours until loose bowel movements initiated and then titrated from 30 mL orally two to three times daily down to two to three bowel movements per day. Lower doses may suffice if the patient is not comatose; higher doses are not more efficacious, and overtreatment can cause dehydration and electrolyte abnormalities that can result in worsening of HE.

    d. Empiric therapy may be effective by correcting precipitating factors; however, because no way of predicting the response to correcting precipitating factors exists, all patients should receive full empiric therapy.

6. Treatment response

    a. In virtually all cases of OHE in chronic liver disease, it should be possible to reverse encephalopathy. Failure to reverse HE after 72 hours of treatment may indicate the following:

- Another cause of encephalopathy has been missed or treated inadequately.
- A precipitating factor has been missed or treated inadequately or remains uncorrected.
- Effective empirical therapy has not been instituted.
- Excessive lactulose therapy has induced dehydration.

    b. The most common reason for ineffective therapy is lack of delivery of lactulose into the small intestine or right colon. Only intestinal obstruction or ileus should prevent adequate delivery. Reluctance to use nasogastric tube delivery of lactulose in the comatose patient because of fear of precipitating variceal bleeding is unwarranted.

7. **Second-line therapy if needed**
   a. Rifaximin: 550 mg orally twice daily
   b. Metronidazole: 250 mg orally four times daily (recommend only short term)
   c. Neomycin: 500 mg orally four times daily (use higher doses with caution)
   d. Vancomycin: 250 mg orally four times daily
   e. Sodium benzoate (not approved for use in the United States)
   f. Flumazenil (may be effective but very short duration of action)
8. **Problems peculiar to type A HE**
   a. Type A accounts for small fraction of HE cases per year.
   b. Treatment follows the same principles as in chronic liver disease, except for the following:
      ■ Precipitating factors are often not obvious, and, even if these factors are present, correction is usually not effective.
      ■ Overall response to empiric therapy is poor.
      ■ If deep coma occurs, the prognosis is poor without liver transplantation.
      ■ Cerebral edema and intracranial hypertension are common and often lethal.
      ■ Other concurrent causes of encephalopathy are common (e.g., hypoglycemia, acidosis, sepsis)
      ■ Approximately 20% of patients have an agitated delirium or seizure phase.
9. **Long-term treatment**
   a. Lactulose
   b. Rifaximin
   c. Vegetable-based protein
   d. Diet enriched with branched-chain amino acids
   e. Bromocriptine
   f. Zinc repletion
   g. Sodium benzoate
   h. Ornithine aspartate
10. The foregoing therapies are usually used for maintenance treatment. Failure of one generally leads to trying the next listed treatment. A long-term low-protein diet is not ideal beacuse protein restriction to avoid HE does not allow maintenance of nitrogen balance.
11. **Options for intractable or recurrent HE**
    a. **Liver transplantation**
       ■ Treatment for intractable HE
       ■ Treatment for recurrent HE or HE responsive only to a low-protein diet
    b. **Modification of existing portosystemic shunts**
       ■ Surgical shunts or transjugular intrahepatic portosystemic shunts (TIPS) may be amenable to closure, possibly in combination with other measures to prevent recurrent variceal bleeding or reduction in shunt diameter.
       ■ The foregoing can be achieved in selected cases by radiologic and/or surgical intervention, which is usually attempted only if the patient is not a liver transplant candidate.
       ■ Acquired spontaneous portosystemic shunts are occasionally amenable to occlusion (by embolization) or reduction in flow (e.g., splenic artery embolization).
       ■ Congenital portosystemic shunts are amenable to closure in some cases.
    c. **Other options**
       ■ Colonic exclusion: virtually abandoned
       ■ Arterialization or portal venous stump: abandoned
       ■ Radiologic portal vein thrombolysis plus TIPS
       ■ TIPS in Budd–Chiari syndrome

FURTHER READING

Atluri DK, Asgeri M, Mullen KD. Reversibility of hepatic encephalopathy after liver transplantation. *Metab Brain Dis* 2010; 25:111–113.

Bajaj JS. The modern management of hepatic encephalopathy. *Aliment Pharmacol Ther* 2010; 31:537–547.

Bajaj JS, Hafeezullah M, Franco J, et al. Inhibitory control test for the diagnosis of minimal hepatic encephalopathy. *Gastroenterology* 2008; 135:1591–1600.

Bajaj JS, Hafeezullah M, Hoffmann RG, et al. Minimal hepatic encephalopathy: a vehicle for accidents and traffic violations. *Am J Gastroenterol* 2007; 102:1903–1909.

Bajaj JS, Saeian K, Schubert CM, et al. Minimal hepatic encephalopathy is associated with motor vehicle crashes: the reality beyond the driving test. *Hepatology* 2009; 50:1175–1183.

Bajaj JS, Schubert CM, Heuman DM, et al. Persistence of cognitive impairment after resolution of overt hepatic encephalopathy. *Gastroenterology* 2010; 138:2332–2340.

Bajaj JS, Wade JB, Sanyal AJ. Spectrum of neurocognitive impairment in cirrhosis: implications for the assessment of hepatic encephalopathy. *Hepatology* 2009; 50:2014–2021.

Bass NM, Mullen KD, Sanyal A, et al. Rifaximin treatment in hepatic encephalopathy. *N Engl J Med* 2010; 362:1071–1081.

Ferenci P, Lockwood A, Mullen KD, et al. Hepatic encephalopathy: definition, nomenclature, diagnosis and quantification: final report on the Working Party at the 11th World Congress of Gastroenterology, Vienna, 1998. *Hepatology* 2002; 35:716–721.

Haussinger D, Schliess F. Pathogenetic mechanisms of hepatic encephalopathy. *Gut* 2008; 57:1156–1165.

Mardini H, Saxby BK, Record CO. Computerized psychometric testing in minimal hepatic encephalopathy and modulation by nitrogen challenge and liver transplant. *Gastroenterology* 2008; 135:1582–1590.

Mullen KD, Amodio P, Morgan MY. Therapeutic studies in hepatic encephalopathy. *Metab Brain Dis* 2007; 22:407–423.

Prasad S, Dhiman RK, Duseja A, et al. Lactulose improves cognitive functions and health–related quality of life in patients with cirrhosis who have minimal hepatic encephalopathy. *Hepatology* 2007; 45:549–559.

Romero-Gomez M, Boza F, Garcia-Valdecasas MS, et al. Subclinical hepatic encephalopathy predicts the development of overt hepatic encephalopathy. *Am J Gastroenterol* 2001; 96:2718–2723.

Rovira A, Alonso J, Córdoba J. MR findings in hepatic encephalopathy. *AJNR Am J Neuroradiol* 2008; 29:1612–1621.

CHAPTER 14

Primary biliary cirrhosis

Gideon M. Hirschfield, MB, BChir, MRCP, PhD ■ E. Jenny Heathcote, MBBS, MD, FRCP, FRCP(C)

KEY POINTS

1 Primary biliary cirrhosis (PBC) is a chronic cholestatic liver disease that usually affects middle-aged women.

2 The cause of PBC likely reflects a combination of environmental and genetic factors.

3 The human leukocyte antigen (HLA) and interleukin-12 signaling axis are particularly relevant biologically in the origin of this autoimmune small duct cholangitis.

4 Most patients are asymptomatic at the time of diagnosis; symptom severity does not always correlate with disease severity.

5 The combination of persistently cholestatic liver chemistry studies, normal biliary imaging, and the presence of antimitochondrial antibody are usually sufficient to diagnose PBC. Liver biopsy is not recommended by consensus guidelines unless doubt exists over the diagnosis or antimitochondrial antibody is absent.

6 Treatment guidelines recommend that ursodeoxycholic acid, the only treatment for PBC approved by the Food and Drug Administration, be given to patients with PBC. The absence of a biochemical response to treatment is associated with a poorer outcome, but additional therapies for such patients are lacking. Randomized data failed to provide support for the use of methotrexate or colchicine, and fenofibrate use remains anecdotal. New agents (farnesoid X–receptor agonists) appear promising.

7 Liver transplantation is an effective treatment of PBC for patients meeting standard minimal listing criteria for transplantation; intractable pruritus is occasionally an indication in the absence of liver failure.

Epidemiology

1. Primary biliary cirrhosis (PBC) is a female-predominant (90% to 95%) disease seen in all ethnicities.

2. An estimated 1 in 1000 white women who are more than 40 years old have PBC. One robust UK estimate of annual incidence was 32.2 per million per year, with an estimated prevalence of 334.6 per million

3. The age of onset typically ranges from 30 to 70 years, and the diagnosis of PBC is increasingly made through routine screening. Diagnosis before menarche has not been reported.

Genetics

1. Genetic factors play a role in PBC, although the disorder is not the consequence of a single genetic mutation.
2. Approximately 1 in 20 patients has a family member affected with PBC. Patients and their family members are more likely to have other autoimmune diseases, particularly celiac disease and scleroderma.
3. Lack of complete concordance for PBC in identical twins adds to the evidence that environmental factors are also important; factors proposed include retroviral infection, xenobiotics, and molecular mimicry from infection. Smoking is an important risk factor for disease severity and progression.
4. An association with the class II human leukocyte antigen (HLA) locus is universally recognized but not understood mechanistically.
5. Genome-wide association testing and replication studies have identified the *IL12A*, *IL12RB2*, *IRF5*, and *17q21* loci as particularly relevant to PBC pathogenesis, thus implicating the Th1 and Th17 cell lineages, as well as demonstrating shared risk variants with other autoimmune diseases (e.g., celiac disease, systemic lupus erythematosus, asthma).
6. Suggestions that changes in X chromosome function and number affect disease susceptibility have not been supported by genome-wide studies; men with PBC have a clinical course identical to that of women.

Immunologic Abnormalities

Genetic studies of PBC support the concept that immunologic abberations underly this archetypal autoimmune disease. Immunologic changes identified in patients with PBC include the following:
1. **Antimitochondrial antibody (AMA)**
   a. Detected in 95% of patients with PBC
   b. Does not affect the course or treatment of PBC
   c. Can be seen in other liver diseases, including acute liver failure, drug injury and autoimmune hepatitis
   d. Not one antibody but a family of antibodies that react with different antigens within the mitochondria
      - Antimitochondrial antibody PDH-E2
        - The major autoantibody found in PBC
        - Directed principally against the dihydrolipoamide acyltransferase component (E2) of the ketoacid dehydrogenase complexes on the inner mitochondrial membrane
        - Pyruvate dehydrogenase the best known of these enzyme complexes
      - Anti-M4, anti-M8, and anti-M9
        - Other AMA described in PBC
        - Their existence not confirmed in a study that employed highly purified cloned human mitochondrial proteins as antigens
   e. Significance of AMA
      - The relationship between AMA and immunologic bile duct injury remains unclear.
      - Biochemical changes to the pyruvate dehydrogenase complex during biliary epithelial cell apoptosis appear important in explaining the relevance of AMA in PBC.
      - Pyruvate dehydrogenase and the other mitochondrial antigens are aberrantly expressed on the luminal surface of biliary epithelial cells from patients with PBC but not from control subjects or patients with primary sclerosing cholangitis.

- Pyruvate dehydrogenase E2 is expressed in bile duct epithelial cells before T-lymphocyte cytotoxicity occurs.
- Mitochondrial antigens are not tissue specific.
- No correlation exists between the presence or titer of AMA and the severity of the course of PBC; antibody titer can fall with treatment.
- High titers of AMA can be produced in experimental animals by immunization with pure human pyruvate dehydrogenase, but these animals do not develop liver disease; induction of autoimmune cholangitis following a chemical (2-octynoic acid) xenobiotic immunization has been reported.
- Genetic manipulation of mice (e.g., anion exchanger 2 knockout, NOD c3c4 congenic mice) leads to AMA production and autoimmune biliary disease with some features reminiscent of PBC.

2. **Other circulating autoantibodies**
   a. Antinuclear antibodies (ANA)
      - The pattern of immunofluorescence is highly specific to PBC, thus making the presence of multiple nuclear dot ANA (sp100) or the membrane rim ANA pattern (gp210) potentially diagnostic in AMA-negative patients.
   b. Anticentromere antibodies
   c. Studies suggest that gp210-positive patients tend to have a more aggressive disease course with liver failure, whereas anticentromere antibody–positive patients tend to have a portal hypertensive phenotype.

3. **Increased levels of serum immunoglobulins**
   - Increased level of serum immunoglobulin M (IgM) that is immunoreactive and highly cryoprecipitable
   - Possible false-positive results with assays to detect immune complexes

4. **Association with other autoimmune diseases**
   - Scleroderma
   - Sjögren's syndrome
   - Celiac disease
   - Thyroiditis or hypothyroidism
   - Rheumatoid arthritis or systemic lupus erythematosus (evidence for both less compelling)

5. **Abnormalities of cellular immunity**
   - Impaired T-cell regulation
   - Decreased numbers of circulating T lymphocytes
   - Reduced T-regulatory cells; increased Th17 cells in liver
   - Sequestration of T lymphocytes within hepatic portal triads

Pathogenesis

1. *Chronic nonsuppurative granulomatous cholangitis* is a better description of the disease than PBC, and at least two related processes appear to lead to hepatic damage (Fig. 14.1).
2. The first process is the chronic, often granulomatous, destruction of small bile ducts, presumably mediated by activated lymphocytes. It seems likely that the initial destructive bile duct lesion in PBC is caused by cytotoxic T lymphocytes. A component of autoimmune hepatitis cannot be excluded, and clinically a few patients (variably reported at 5% to 10%) have some evidence of this.

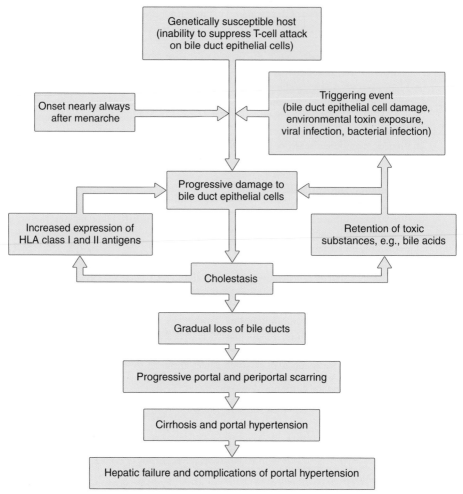

Fig. 14.1 Algorithm for the possible pathogenesis of primary biliary cirrhosis (PBC). The cause of PBC remains unknown, although genetic and immunologic factors appear to play a role. HLA, human leukocyte antigen.

- Bile duct cells in patients with PBC express increased amounts of class I HLA-A, HLA-B, and HLA-C and class II HLA-DR antigens, in contrast to normal bile duct cells.
- The bile duct lesion resembles disorders that are known to be mediated by cytotoxic T lymphocytes, such as graft-versus-host disease and rejection of allografts.
3. The second process includes chemical damage to hepatocytes in areas of liver where bile drainage is impeded by the destruction of the small bile ducts.
  - Retention of bile acids, bilirubin, copper, and other substances that are normally secreted or excreted into bile occurs.
  - The increased concentration of some of these substances, such as bile acids, may further damage liver cells.

■ The consequence of bile duct destruction eventually leads to portal inflammation and scarring and ultimately to cirrhosis and liver failure.

Pathology

GROSS FINDINGS

1. The liver is initially enlarged but smooth.
2. With progression of the disease, the liver enlarges further, becoming nodular and grossly cirrhotic with bile staining.
3. An increased prevalence of gallstones of approximately 40% is noted.
4. An increased prevalence of nodular regenerative hyperplasia is observed in the early stage of
   PBC; although varices and portal hypertension are most commonly associated with cirrhosis,
   presinusoidal portal hypertension can be seen as a result of this nodular regenerative hyperplasia in a few patients with PBC who do not have cirrhosis.
5. Enlarged lymph nodes resulting from benign reactive hyperplasia may be seen in the porta
   hepatis and around the aorta and inferior vena cava; this finding should not be mistaken for
   lymphoma.

HEPATIC HISTOLOGY

1. Four histologic stages of PBC are described, and all have conceptual utility.
2. Histologic staging is less relevant than biochemical response to treatment and liver function
   in clinical treatment, however, and is therefore not routinely evaluated in clinical practice.
   Additionally, noninvasive markers of fibrosis, particular transient elastography, have potential
   utility.
3. Considerations in interpreting liver biopsy staging:
   a. The liver may not be uniformly affected; thus, liver biopsy is subject to sampling
      variation.
   b. Several stages may be seen on one biopsy specimen; by convention, staging is based on the
      most advanced lesion seen on the biopsy specimen.
   c. Given that PBC is increasingly diagnosed at an earlier stage, it is less likely that character-
      istic pathologic observations can be made on needle biopsy specimens.
   d. Histologic stages are as follows:
      ■ Stage I
        – Injured bile ducts are usually surrounded by a dense infiltrate of mononuclear cells,
          most of which are lymphocytes (Fig. 14.2).
        – These florid, asymmetrical destructive lesions of interlobular bile ducts are irregu-
          larly scattered throughout the portal triads and are often seen only on large surgical
          biopsy specimens of the liver in which adequate representation of small bile ducts
          occurs.
        – Inflammation is confined to the portal triads.
      ■ Stage II
        – The lesion is more widespread but less specific.
        – Reduced numbers of normal bile ducts within portal triads and increased numbers
          of atypical, poorly formed bile ducts with irregularly shaped lumina may be evident
          (Fig. 14.3).
        – Diffuse portal fibrosis and mononuclear cell infiltrates are seen within triads.

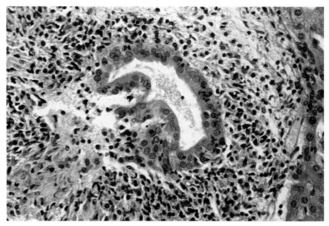

Fig. 14.2 Histopathology of stage I florid bile duct lesion. The epithelial cell lining of a small duct is infiltrated with lymphocytes (H&E).

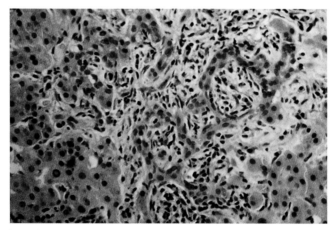

Fig. 14.3 Histopathology of stage II primary biliary cirrhosis. Atypical bile duct hyperplasia is seen. Tortuous bile ducts are visible, with an inflammatory cell infiltrate consisting of primarily lymphocytes and few neutrophils (H&E).

    – Inflammation may spill into the surrounding periportal areas.
    – **A diminished number of bile ducts in an otherwise unremarkable needle biopsy of the liver should alert one to the possibility of PBC.**
  ■ Stage III
    – This is similar to stage II, except fibrous septa extend beyond triads and form portal-to-portal bridges (Fig. 14.4).
  ■ Stage IV
    – This represents the end stage of the lesion, with frank cirrhosis and regenerative nodules (Fig. 14.5).
    – Findings may be indistinguishable from other types of cirrhosis. However, a paucity of normal bile ducts in areas of scarring suggests the possibility of PBC.

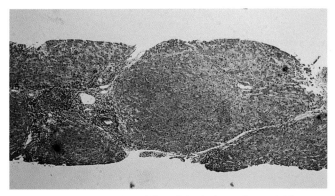

Fig. 14.4 Histopathology of stage III primary biliary cirrhosis. A portal-to-portal fibrous septum is shown on this low power view (Masson trichrome).

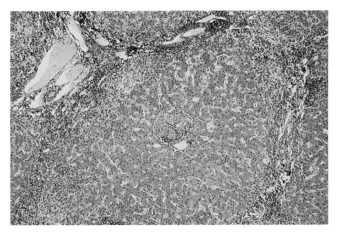

Fig. 14.5 Histopathology of stage IV primary biliary cirrhosis. A noncaseating granuloma is visible in the center of a nodule. Portal triads are linked by bands of connective tissue and inflammatory cells (Masson trichrome).

Clinical Features

SYMPTOMS

Up to about two thirds of patients are asymptomatic at the time of diagnosis.
Symptoms and signs of PBC partly reflect cholestasis.

1. **Fatigue**
   - Most common symptom, but variably reported depending on method of ascertainment
   - Not specific to PBC and seen in other hepatic and nonhepatic disease
   - Should consider nonhepatic disease such as depression, anemia, sleep apnea, hypothyroidism, and hypoadrenalism
2. **Pruritus**
   - Pathogenesis unknown; itching not solely from retention of the naturally occurring primary and secondary bile acids but likely caused by another substance normally secreted into bile

- Increased opioidergic tone related to chronic cholestasis suggested as a potential etiologic factor
- Characteristically worse at bedtime
- May initially occur during the third trimester of pregnancy and persist after delivery
- Paradoxically often improved as disease progresses
- Ursodeoxycholic acid (UDCA) not a treatment for pruritus and may exacerbate itching

3. **Osteoporosis**
   - Osteopenic bone disease occurs in at least 25% of patients with PBC; the pathogenesis is still unclear but seems to reflect low bone turnover, and severity of liver disease is important.
   - Osteomalacia is now very uncommon.
   - Clinical symptoms of osteoporosis are unusual, but when present they relate to spontaneous or low-impact fractures.

4. **Malabsorption**
   - This is now a very uncommon clinical manifestation, but previously it was recognized in patients with long-standing cholestasis.
   - Impaired secretion of bile causes diminished concentration of bile acids within the intestinal lumen; bile acid concentration may fall to less than the critical micellar concentration and be inadequate for complete digestion and absorption of neutral triglycerides in the diet.
   - Patients complain of nocturnal diarrhea, foul-smelling bulky stools, and/or weight loss despite a good appetite and increased caloric intake.
   - Malabsorption of the fat-soluble vitamins A, D, E and K and calcium may be present; night blindness is a particularly important symptom of vitamin A deficiency.
   - Pancreatic insufficiency may also contribute to malabsorption; this is most likely in patients with concomitant sicca syndrome.

5. **Sicca complex**
   - This combination of dry eyes, dry mouth, and vaginal dryness is a frequent complaint in patients with PBC.
   - Some patients have true primary Sjögren's syndrome, although most do not.

6. **Right-sided abdominal pain**
   - Nonspecific pain is described by up to one third of patients, without overt clinical or radiologic explanation.

PHYSICAL EXAMINATION

1. Findings may vary and depend on the stage of the disease; examination is usually normal in asymptomatic patients.
2. Hepatomegaly and splenomegaly are seen with progressive disease; a few patients may have splenomegaly early as a result of portal hypertension secondary to nodular regenerative hyperplasia.
3. Skin abnormalities
   a. Hyperpigmentation, if seen, may resemble tanning and is caused by melanin, not bilirubin, in early-stage PBC.
   b. Excoriations may be diffuse from scratching caused by intractable pruritus.
   c. Jaundice usually manifests later in the course of the disease.
   d. Xanthelasmas and xanthomata correlate with hypercholesterolemia; xanthelasmas are more common than xanthomata (Figs 14.6 and 14.7).
      - Less than 5% of patients will eventually develop xanthomata.
      - Xanthomata are found on the palms of the hands and soles of the feet, over extensor surfaces of the elbows and knees, in tendons of the ankles and wrists, and on buttocks.

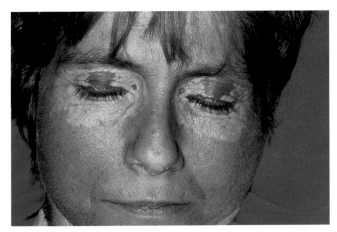

Fig. 14.6   Extensive bilateral xanthelasmas in a middle-aged woman.

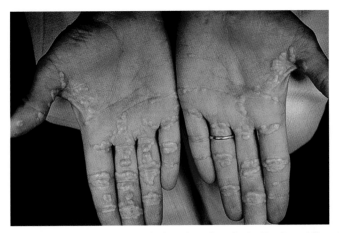

Fig. 14.7   Bilateral plantar xanthomatas in the palms of a patient with primary biliary cirrhosis.

4. Eyes: Kayser–Fleischer rings are rare and result from copper retention.
5. End-stage PBC: spider telangiectases, temporal and proximal limb muscle wasting, ascites, and edema usually occur with cirrhosis and portal hypertension.

NATURAL HISTORY AND PROGNOSIS

1. Median survival of symptomatic patients ranges from 7½ to 10 years in different studies and is 7 years for histologic stages III and IV.
2. Median survival of asymptomatic patients ranges from 10 to 16 years in various studies.
3. Most asymptomatic patients develop symptoms, usually within 2 to 4 years.
4. The presence or titer of AMA does not influence survival.
5. If patients achieve a biochemical response to treatment with UDCA (e.g., 1 year after treatment, bilirubin is less than the upper limit of normal [ULN] and aspartate aminotransferase

[AST] is less than twice the ULN and alkaline phosphatase [ALP] is less than three times the ULN), then 10-year survival is excellent, at 90%.

Diagnosis

LABORATORY TESTS

1. Liver biochemical tests
   - A cholestatic pattern (ALP/AST ratio usually less than 3 and AST or alanine aminotransferase [ALT] less than five times the ULN) is observed.
   - Biochemical tests alone are never diagnostic of PBC.
   - Elevation of serum ALP and gamma glutamyltranspeptidase elevations are the earliest abnormalities; the degree of elevation may relate to the severity of duct injury and the likelihood of treatment response.
   - Serum aminotransferases are often elevated in the course of the disease; persistent elevations on treatment may relate to poorer long-term outcomes.
   - Serum bilirubin is usually normal early in the course but becomes elevated if the disease progresses; it remains the strongest predictor of outcome.
2. **AMA is positive in 95% of patients.**
3. Other associated findings
   - Serum albumin and prothrombin concentrations are normal in the early stages and abnormal in the late stage.
   - Serum IgM is elevated.
   - Cholesterol is elevated in at least 50% of patients, presumed secondary to cholestasis, and without evidence that patients have higher cardiovascular mortality.
   - High-density lipoproteins are elevated.
   - Hepatic and urinary copper are elevated.
   - Hypothyroidism: elevated thyroid-stimulating hormone is the best way to screen for hypothyroidism.

LIVER BIOPSY

1. Biopsy is no longer routinely performed but can aid in confirming the diagnosis and providing an estimate of disease severity at presentation.
2. In patients without AMA (and where specific ANA testing is not available), or in those with potential alternative explanations for liver biochemical test findings, biopsy should be considered.

IMAGING TESTS

These tests are useful to rule out bile duct obstruction and to screen for gallstones if significant pain is present.

1. Ultrasound: noninvasive and usually adequate to rule out bile duct obstruction
2. Computed tomography: in patients in whom ultrasound examination is technically not feasible
3. Cholangiography: not needed except in AMA-negative patients in whom primary sclerosing cholangitis is a possible diagnosis; magnetic resonance cholangiography preferred in this setting

PRINCIPLES OF DIAGNOSIS

1. The diagnosis is based on history, physical findings, laboratory tests, and sometimes a liver biopsy.
2. The combination of cholestatic liver chemistries and a positive AMA test result gives a high positive predictive value for the histologic diagnosis of PBC. The diagnosis of PBC is now generally based on laboratory findings. Rising rates of obesity may, however, necessitate additional investigation; 0.5% of the healthy population is AMA positive, and up to 30% of healthy individuals may have fatty liver, which biochemically can be reflected by a rise in ALP.

DIFFERENTIAL DIAGNOSIS

1. Gallstones
2. Mechanical, extrahepatic bile duct obstruction such as tumors, cysts, and postsurgical strictures
3. Primary sclerosing cholangitis (if AMA negative)
4. Nonalcoholic or alcoholic fatty liver
5. Cholestatic viral hepatitis
6. Granulomatous hepatitis
7. Autoimmune hepatitis
8. Vanishing bile duct syndrome
9. Benign, recurrent intrahepatic cholestasis
10. Drug-induced cholestasis

Treatment

SYMPTOMS OF CHRONIC CHOLESTASIS

1. Pruritus (Table 14.1)
   a. Antihistamines
      - These are occasionally symptomatically helpful early in the course of PBC when itching is not severe and the sedative side effects are favorable.
   b. Cholestyramine
      - This nonabsorbed resin relieves pruritus in most patients.
      - Therapy should be directed at symptomatic relief, with a usual dose of 4 g twice daily, generally taken mixed with water or juice before and after breakfast.
      - Depending on the severity of cholestasis, it may take up to 14 days from the initiation of cholestyramine before the itching remits.
      - Other medications need to be taken 1 hour before or 2 to 4 hours after cholestyramine, to avoid inadvertent binding to cholestyramine.
   c. Colestipol hydrochloride (ammonium resin)
      - This is as effective as cholestyramine and may be used in patients who find cholestyramine unpalatable; some find colestipol equally unpalatable.
   d. Other antipruritogenic agents that may control itching in some patients (listed in order of suggested use):
      - Rifampin (150 to 300 mg twice daily)
      - Sertraline (50 to 100 mg once daily)
      - Naloxone (opioid antagonist): based on data suggesting itching may be mediated by opioidergic neurotransmission
      - Nalmefene (opioid antagonist)

TABLE 14.1 ■ **Drug treatment of pruritus**

Drug	Mechanism of action	Dose	Side effects
Cholestyramine	Bile acid resin	4–16 g orally/day	Unpalatability, constipation, can interfere with absorption of medications
Colestipol	Bile acid resin	5 g orally three times/day	Constipation, can interfere with absorption of medications
Rifampin	Competes with bile acids for hepatic uptake	300–600 mg orally/day	Idiosyncratic hepatotoxicity
Sertraline	SSRI	50–100 mg/day	Dry mouth
Naloxone	Opioid antagonist	0.2 µg/kg IV/min for 24 hr	Self-limited opioid withdrawal–like syndrome
Nalmefene	Opioid antagonist	60–120 mg orally/day	Self-limited opioid withdrawal–like syndrome
Naltrexone	Opioid antagonist	50 mg orally/day	Self-limited opioid withdrawal–like syndrome

IV, intravenously; SSRI, selective serotonin reuptake inhibitor.

- Naltrexone (opioid antagonist)
- Phototherapy with ultraviolet B light
- Large-volume plasmapheresis (almost always helpful but inconvenient and expensive)
- Molecular adsorbents recirculation system (MARS; effective where available)
- Liver transplantation
2. Malabsorption of fat-soluble vitamins
   a. Malabsorption frequency is roughly proportional to the severity and duration of cholestasis and is now rarely a clinical concern.
   b. Vitamins A, D, E, and K levels should be measured in jaundiced patients with PBC; patients with low levels should be treated.
   c. Treatment: vitamins should be administered orally as far apart from cholestyramine as possible, because cholestyramine may bind and inhibit their absorption.
      - Oral vitamin K: 5 mg/day
      - Vitamin A: 10,000 to 25,000 IU/day
      - 25-OH vitamin D: 20 µg three times weekly; check serum levels of 25-OH vitamin D after several weeks
      - Supplemental calcium
      - Vitamin E: 400 to 1000 IU/day
3. Steatorrhea
   - This is treated by a low-fat diet supplemented with medium-chain triglycerides (MCT) to maintain a reasonable caloric intake.
   - Most patients tolerate 60 mL of MCT oil per day.
   - Some patients with PBC and the sicca syndrome may have concomitant pancreatic insufficiency; this can be treated with pancreatic replacement therapy.
   - Patients may develop iron deficiency anemia, which reflects unrecognized gastrointestinal blood loss, usually from changes of portal hypertension in the stomach (gastropathy or gastric antral vascular ectasia). Colonoscopy to exclude a lower gastrointestinal cause is appropriate before arriving at this conclusion.

TABLE 14.2 ■ **Drug treatment of primary biliary cirrhosis**

Drug	Mechanism of action	Dose	Benefits	Side effects	Comments
Ursodeoxycholic acid	Choleretic	13–15 mg/kg/day orally	Improves liver bio-chemistry, slows histologic progression, and probably improves long-term survival	Diarrhea, weight gain, thinning of hair	Most widely used agent

4. Osteoporosis
   - Osteoporosis is a manifestation of PBC, but it also a frequent finding in healthy women of similar age.
   - Bone mineral density should be assessed with dual x-ray absorptiometry when the diagnosis of PBC is made.
   - A retrospective study showed beneficial effects of hormone replacement therapy in postmenopausal women with PBC.
   - A prospective, controlled pilot study showed that therapy with the bisphosphonate etidronate prevented corticosteroid-induced osteoporosis.
   - Liver transplantation is proven treatment and has resulted in increased bone mineral density, but improvement is rarely noted until 1 year after transplantation. Bone mineral density decreases for up to 6 months after transplantation because of immunosuppression with glucocorticoids and physical inactivity.

UNDERLYING DISEASE (Table 14.2)

1. UDCA
   - UDCA is the most widely used drug for PBC but is not curative, nor does it treat the disease per se. Consensus favors its use, but robust convincing data are lacking, reflecting a very slowly progressive disease for which the end points of death or transplantation are now relatively uncommon. The greatest overall benefit is likely in patients with early disease, although a survival benefit is demonstrable only in those with advanced disease.
   - UDCA is safe and well tolerated; mild weight gain (3 kg), bloating, and thinning of hair are noted. If a patient responds biochemically to treatment, no recognized treatment "fatigue" occurs. Stopping UDCA leads to a return in liver biochemical changes, usually back to baseline, in keeping with a mechanism of action that does not treat the underlying disease per se.
   - In four controlled trials, UDCA, at 13 to 15 mg/kg body weight/day orally, improved serum bilirubin, ALP, aminotransferase, and IgM levels.
   - Individual studies also favor an effect on improved survival, slower histologic progression, and reduced progression of portal hypertension.
   - When data were pooled in three important studies, UDCA clearly prolonged the time before liver transplantation was required compared with placebo, but the improvement was modest.
   - In a fourth, multicenter, study conducted in the United States, efficacy was limited to a subgroup of patients with stage I and II disease whose initial serum bilirubin level was less than 2 mg/dL.

- One meta-analysis of clinical trials did not show that mortality or liver transplantation, or pruritus, fatigue, quality of life, liver histology, or portal pressures, were significantly improved by UDCA, given at a dose of 8 to 15 mg/kg per day for 3 months to 5 years.
- Some studies, however, clearly showed that patients with a biochemical response to UDCA have normal life expectancy; the definition of response to therapy varies but generally includes the change in ALP value.
- Further support for UDCA comes from the falling rates of transplantation for PBC parallel to the widespread use of UDCA.
2. Colchicine: early data were encouraging, but a Cochrane review of all available studies failed to find any strong evidence to support the use of this agent.
3. Methotrexate: early data were encouraging, but a Cochrane review of all available studies failed to find any strong evidence to support the use of this drug.
4. New therapies
   - For patients without a biochemical response to therapy with UDCA, new drugs are needed.
   - Suggestions have included budesonide, fenofibrates, and rituximab; however, data are not available to support routine use of these drugs.
   - Farnesoid X–receptor agonists appeared promising in phase II studies, and genetic insights into disease may lead to targeted, disease-related therapy.

CIRRHOSIS SURVEILLANCE

1. Varices are usually associated with cirrhosis, but presinusoidal portal hypertension is recognized.
   - Optimal timing for determining when to screen by endoscopy is debated but uses disease severity (e.g., Mayo score), platelet count, and spleen size.
   - Patients with fatigue may find beta blockade troublesome, thus necessitating prophylactic banding of varices.
2. Hepatocellular carcinoma is reported in cirrhotic patients with PBC; screening guidelines include PBC and recommend surveillance at 6- to 12-month intervals by ultrasound if patients are cirrhotic.

LIVER TRANSPLANTATION

1. Patients with end-stage PBC are excellent candidates for liver transplantation; the Model for End-stage Liver Disease (MELD) score is generally an appropriate way to identify patients likely to benefit.

2. **End-stage PBC** is generally defined as cirrhosis complicated by the following:
   - Gastroesophageal variceal hemorrhage
   - Intractable ascites
   - Hepatic encephalopathy
   - Serum albumin less than 3.5 g/dL
   - Serum bilirubin greater than 4 mg/dL

3. One-year survival after liver transplantation in PBC patients is approximately 90%.
4. PBC may recur in the allograft, although recurrence is infrequent and rarely clinically of relevance. Cyclosporine may protect against recurrent disease as compared with tacrolimus.

FURTHER READING

Corpechot C, Abenavoli L, Rabahi N, et al. Biochemical response to ursodeoxycholic acid and long-term prognosis in primary biliary cirrhosis. *Hepatology* 2008; 48:871–877.

Gershwin ME, Mackay IR. The causes of primary biliary cirrhosis: convenient and inconvenient truths. *Hepatology* 2008; 47:737–745.

Gong Y, Huang ZB, Christensen E, Gluud C. Ursodeoxycholic acid for primary biliary cirrhosis. *Cochrane Database Syst Rev* 2008:(3):CD000551.

Hirschfield GM, Liu X, Xu C, et al. Primary biliary cirrhosis associated with HLA, IL12A, and IL12RB2 variants. *N Engl J Med* 2009; 360:2544–2555.

Huet PM, Vincent C, Deslaurier J, et al. Portal hypertension and primary biliary cirrhosis: effect of long-term ursodeoxycholic acid treatment. *Gastroenterology* 2008; 135:1552–1560.

Invernizzi P, Selmi C, Poli F, et al. Human leukocyte antigen polymorphisms in Italian primary biliary cirrhosis: a multicenter study of 664 patients and 1992 healthy controls. *Hepatology* 2008; 48:1906–1912.

Irie J, Wu Y, Wicker LS, et al. NOD.c3c4 congenic mice develop autoimmune biliary disease that serologically and pathogenetically models human primary biliary cirrhosis. *J Exp Med* 2006; 203:1209–1219.

Kuiper EM, Hansen BE, de Vries RA, et al. Improved prognosis of patients with primary biliary cirrhosis that have a biochemical response to ursodeoxycholic acid. *Gastroenterology* 2009; 136:1281–1287.

Lindor K. Ursodeoxycholic acid for the treatment of primary biliary cirrhosis. *N Engl J Med* 2007; 357:1524–1529.

Lindor KD, Gershwin ME, Poupon R, et al. Primary biliary cirrhosis. *Hepatology* 2009; 50:291–308.

Mayo MJ, Parkes J, Adams-Huet B, et al. Prediction of clinical outcomes in primary biliary cirrhosis by serum enhanced liver fibrosis assay. *Hepatology* 2008; 48:1549–1557.

Nakamura M, Kondo H, Mori T, et al. Anti-gp210 and anti-centromere antibodies are different risk factors for the progression of primary biliary cirrhosis. *Hepatology* 2007; 45:118–127.

Pares A, Caballeria L, Rodes J. Excellent long-term survival in patients with primary biliary cirrhosis and biochemical response to ursodeoxycholic acid. *Gastroenterology* 2006; 130:715–720.

Salas JT, Banales JM, Sarvide S, et al. Ae2a, b-deficient mice develop antimitochondrial antibodies and other features resembling primary biliary cirrhosis. *Gastroenterology* 2008; 134:1482–1493.

Shi J, Wu C, Lin Y, et al. Long-term effects of mid-dose ursodeoxycholic acid in primary biliary cirrhosis: a meta-analysis of randomized controlled trials. *Am J Gastroenterol* 2006; 101:1529–1538.

CHAPTER 15

Primary sclerosing cholangitis

Christopher L. Bowlus, MD

KEY POINTS

1 Primary sclerosing cholangitis (PSC) is a chronic cholestatic disease that is frequently found in association with inflammatory bowel disease, usually ulcerative colitis.

2 The diagnosis of PSC is based on clinical, biochemical, and, most importantly, cholangiographic findings in the absence of secondary causes of sclerosing cholangitis.

3 The etiology of PSC remains unknown, but both genetic and environmental factors are involved, and evidence points toward a defective inflammatory response to intestinal microbial antigens.

5 The progression of PSC is highly variable but typically leads to dominant biliary strictures, cirrhosis, choledocholithiasis, and cholangiocarcinoma (CCA). The risk of colon cancer is increased in patients with PSC and ulcerative colitis.

6 Medical, endoscopic, and surgical therapies have not had a major impact on survival or the prevention of complications of PSC.

7 Liver transplantation is associated with a 5-year survival rate of 85%. Although recurrence of PSC after liver transplantation has been described and appears to be increasing in frequency, the need for retransplantation is uncommon.

Overview

1. Primary sclerosing cholangitis (PSC) is a chronic cholestatic liver disease characterized by fibrosing inflammation of both the intrahepatic and extrahepatic biliary tree.

2. The histopathologic evolution of PSC results in damage to the bile ducts and ultimately leads to cholestasis, cirrhosis, liver failure, and premature death from liver failure unless liver transplantation is performed.

3. Long-term follow-up of patients with PSC has revealed a high frequency of colon and bile duct cancers, both of which are probably related to chronic inflammation.

4. Although multiple medical, endoscopic, and surgical therapies have been evaluated for the treatment of PSC, currently no therapy has demonstrated improvement in survival. Liver transplantation continues to be an important therapeutic intervention for the management of patients with end-stage PSC.

Terminology and Diagnostic Criteria

1. PSC is an idiopathic entity of biliary sclerosis distinguished from secondary sclerosing cholangitis resulting from identifiable causes (Table 15.1).

TABLE 15.1 ■ **Secondary causes of sclerosing cholangitis**

Cholangiocarcinoma

Choledocholithiasis and recurrent pyogenic cholangitis

Ischemia resulting from biliary surgery or trauma

Chemical injury of the bile ducts (e.g., intra-arterial chemotherapy)

Infectious agents

Congenital anomalies of the bile ducts

Cholangiopathy related to acquired immunodeficiency syndrome

Histiocytosis X

Diffuse intrahepatic malignancy

■ Diagnosis of PSC is based on a cholestatic biochemical profile, with cholangiography by magnetic resonance cholangiography (MRC), endoscopic retrograde cholangiography (ERC), or percutaneous transhepatic cholangiography demonstrating multifocal strictures and segmental dilatations in the absence of secondary causes of sclerosing cholangitis. MRC is sufficient for diagnosis in most cases, but ERC remains the gold standard.

■ Liver biopsy is not indicated in cases with typical cholangiographic findings (Fig. 15.1).

2. *Small duct* PSC refers to patients with histologic changes consistent with the classic form of PSC but without abnormal bile ducts on cholangiogram.

3. PSC/autoimmune hepatitis (AIH) overlap has features of both PSC and AIH and typically affects children and young adults. In some cases, AIH precedes the development of PSC.

4. Immunoglobulin G_4 (IgG_4)–related sclerosing cholangitis is a disease related to autoimmune pancreatitis and may be a separate entity from PSC.

Clinical Features

1. Demographic features
   a. The median age at diagnosis of PSC is approximately 35 to 40 years of age, but PSC can occur in children and older adults.
   b. Approximately two thirds of patients are male.
      ■ Among patients with PSC, 60% to 80% have inflammatory bowel disease (IBD), most commonly ulcerative colitis or Crohn's colitis, with features including extensive colitis, rectal sparing, backwash ileitis, or a quiescent course of disease.

2. Signs and symptoms: PSC at the time of presentation is highly variable, as outlined in Table 15.2.

3. Tables 15.3 and 15.4 show the frequencies of abnormal biochemical test results and autoantibodies, respectively, at the time of diagnosis.

4. Histologic features of PSC include periductal fibrosis, inflammation, and bile duct proliferation alternating with ductal obliteration and ductopenia.

5. Radiologic features most commonly seen in PSC include:
   ■ diffusely distributed multifocal annular strictures with intervening segments of normal or slightly ectatic ducts
   ■ short, bandlike strictures
   ■ diverticulum-like sacculations

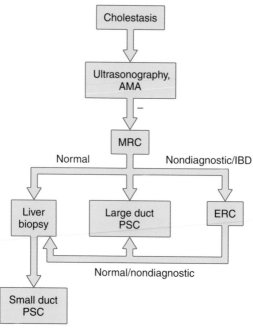

Fig. 15.1 Algorithm for the evaluation of patients with cholestatic liver biochemistry test results, nondiagnostic ultrasound, and negative antimitochondrial antibodies (AMA). If magnetic resonance cholangiography (MRC) is of good quality, the specificity is greater than 95%. Although the sensitivity of MRC is high (approximately 85%), if the quality is poor or if the index of suspicion is high, as in patients with inflammatory bowel disease, endoscopic retrograde cholangiography should be pursued. AMA, antimitochondrial antibodies; ERC, endoscopic retrograde cholangiography; MRC, magnetic resonance cholangiography; PSC, primary sclerosing cholangitis

TABLE 15.2 ■ **Symptoms and signs of primary sclerosing cholangitis at diagnosis**

		Frequency (%)
No symptoms		44
Symptom	Fatigue	75
	Weight loss	40
	Abdominal pain	37
	Pruritus	30–70
	Jaundice	30–65
	Fever	17–35
	Variceal bleeding	4–15
	Ascites	4–5
Sign	Hepatomegaly	34–62
	Jaundice	30–65
	Hyperpigmentation	25
	Splenomegaly	20–30
	Xanthomata	4

TABLE 15.3 ■ Liver biochemical test results in primary sclerosing cholangitis at diagnosis

Test	Abnormal results (%)
Serum alkaline phosphatase	91–99
Serum aminotransferases	95
Serum bilirubin	41–65
Hypergammaglobulinemia	30
Serum albumin	20
Prothrombin time	10

TABLE 15.4 ■ Autoantibodies in primary sclerosing cholangitis

Antibody	Frequency (%)
Perinuclear antineutrophil cytoplasmic antibodies (pANCA)	50–80
Antinuclear antibodies (ANA)	35
Antismooth muscle antibodies (ASMA)	15
Antiendothelial cell antibodies	13–20
Anticardiolipin antibodies	7–77
Thyroperoxidase	7–16
Thyroglobulin	4–66
Rheumatoid factor	4

Diseases Associated with Primary Sclerosing Cholangitis

1. Various diseases are associated with PSC (Table 15.5).
2. IBD is the most common and most important of these associations.
   ■ The diagnosis of IBD usually precedes the diagnosis of PSC; however, PSC may occur before the diagnosis of IBD or years after proctocolectomy. Furthermore, IBD can occur for the first time after liver transplantation for PSC.
   ■ No differences have been found in the course or severity of PSC in patients with or without IBD.
   ■ Patients with PSC and ulcerative colitis who undergo proctocolectomy and who have an ileal pouch–anal anastomosis have an increased risk of pouchitis compared with those patients who have ulcerative colitis alone.
   ■ The risk of colorectal cancer is increased in patients with PSC and ulcerative colitis compared with patients with ulcerative colitis alone (Fig. 15.2). Surveillance colonoscopy is recommended once the diagnosis of PSC and IBD is made.
   ■ Treatment with ursodeoxycholic acid (UDCA) may decrease the risk of colorectal cancer in patients with PSC and ulcerative colitis.

TABLE 15.5 ■ Diseases associated with primary sclerosing cholangitis

Disease	Prevalence (%)
Inflammatory bowel disease	~80
Type 1 diabetes mellitus	10
Thyroid disorders	8
Psoriasis	4
Rheumatoid arthritis	3
Celiac disease	2
Systemic lupus erythematosus	2
Sarcoidosis	1
Any autoimmune disease	24
Autoimmune hemolytic anemia	< 1*
Systemic sclerosis/retroperitoneal fibrosis	< 1*
Immune thrombocytopenic purpura	< 1*

*Limited to case reports.

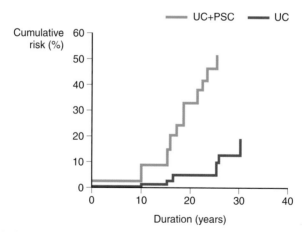

Fig. 15.2 Risk of colorectal cancer in patients with UC and PSC, compared with UC alone. *(From Jayaram H, Satsangi J, Chapman RW. Increased colorectal neoplasm in chronic ulcerative colitis complicated by primary sclerosing cholangitis: fact or fiction? Gut 2001; 48:430–434.) PSC, primary sclerosing cholangitis; UC, ulcerative colitis*

Epidemiology

1. The prevalence and incidence of PSC vary geographically and appear to correlate with the prevalence of IBD.
    ■ The incidence (0.9 to 1.3 per 100,000/year) and prevalence (8.5 to 14.2 per 100,000) of PSC have been reported to be similar in Oslo, Norway, in Wales, and in Olmsted County, Minnesota.

- The prevalence of PSC appears to be lower in southern Europe, Asia, and Alaska.
- The incidence of PSC appears to be increasing, but this observation may reflect a secondary ascertainment bias resulting from the increased use of ERC and MRC.
2. The prevalence of PSC in IBD cohorts is 2.4% to 7.5%.
3. The frequency of IBD in patients with PSC varies by geography.
   - The highest rates are in northern Europe and North America (75% to 98%), whereas rates are lower in southern Europe and Asia (21% to 44%).
   - The frequency of IBD in PSC is decreasing.

Etiology and Pathogenesis

The cause of PSC is unknown, but genetic and acquired factors are likely involved in the etiology. Although PSC has often been classified as an autoimmune disease, several characteristics, such as an absence of a female predilection, the lack of a disease-specific autoantibody, and a poor response to corticosteroids and other immunosuppressive therapies, are not supportive of this hypothesis. In contrast, PSC may be more likely an inflammatory disease similar to IBD, in which innate immune responses to bacterial pathogens are aberrant.

1. Genetic factors (Table 15.6)
   a. The 100-fold increased risk of PSC in first-degree relatives suggests an important genetic component.
   b. Genome-wide association studies demonstrated that the human leukocyte antigen (HLA) region has the greatest effect on PSC risk.
      - Approximately 40% of patients with PSC carry the HLA-B8 DR3 haplotype, compared with 20% of the unaffected population.

TABLE 15.6 ■ Genes associated with primary sclerosing cholangitis risk and progression

Associated with increased risk		
Gene/Region	Function/Mechanism	Odds Ratio
HLA-B8 DR3	The gene involved not yet identified; multiple genes possibly interact in this region and affect immune responses	4.8
HLA-C1	Decreased inhibition of natural killer cells through binding of killer immunoglobulin receptors	3.1
GPC6	Unknown, but possibly involved in modulating inflammatory responses of cholangiocytes	0.7
TGR5	G protein–coupled bile acid receptor that inhibits cytokine release by activated macrophages	1.14
Associated with disease progression		
Gene/Region	Function/Mechanism	Relative Risk
SXR	Steroid and xenobiotic receptor that mediates protection against bile acid injury; alleles are linked to survival, not susceptibility	1.8
MDR3 (ABCB4)	Canalicular phospholipid floppase; defects may impair biliary excretion of phosphatidylcholine	1.6

HLA, human leukocyte antigen

- HLA-B8 but not HLA-DR3 is associated with PSC in African Americans listed for liver transplantation, a finding suggesting that the causative variant is closer to the HLA B gene.
- Several, but not all, genes predisposing to IBD also increase the risk of PSC.
- Genes involved in signaling by bile acids have been associated with PSC risk and disease progression (*TGR5* and *SXR,* respectively).

2. Immunologic mechanisms
   a. Aberrant lymphocyte homing
      - Lymphocytes in livers from patients with PSC express the chemokine receptor CCR9 and $\alpha_4\beta_7$ integrin, which are markers of intestinal lymphocytes.
      - CXCL21 and MAdCAM-1 are ligands for CCR9 and $\alpha_4\beta_7$ integrin and are aberrantly expressed in livers from patients with PSC.
      - These cells have a memory phenotype suggesting that they are generated in the gut in during inflammation and then recirculated to liver, where they are recruited by chemokine receptors and adhesion molecules that are aberrantly expressed in the liver. This may explain why PSC can develop after colectomy.
   b. Activation of innate immune responses to bacterial pathogen-associated molecular patterns (PAMPs) likely circulating from a leaky and inflamed intestinal epithelium
      - PAMPs activate macrophages, dendritic cells, and natural killer (NK) cells through pattern recognition receptors, including Toll-like receptors (TLRs) and CD14 leading to the secretion of cytokines, which, in turn, activate NK cells (interleukin-12 [IL-12]) and promote recruitment and activation of lymphocytes.
      - IgG directed against biliary epithelial cells (BECs) has been found in the sera of some patients with PSC and induces the expression of TLR4 and TLR9 on BEC secretion of granulocyte-macrophage colony-stimulating factor, IL-1β and IL-8, which, in turn, may lead to the recruitment of neutrophils, macrophages, and T cells.
      - Cholangiocytes can also secrete inflammatory cytokines by activation of TLRs.
   c. Toxic bile
      - The absence of phospholipids results not only in unopposed bile acid toxicity but also in cholesterol supersaturated bile, which could facilitate oxidation of BECs.
      - Whether this is a primary insult or a secondary factor leading to progression of disease is unclear.

Natural History

PSC is most often a slowly progressive disease with a median survival from time of diagnosis of 12 to 16 years. Of patients who are asymptomatic at the time of diagnosis, 75% progress clinically or histologically, and 30% develop liver failure within a 6-year follow-up. Several prognostic models have been developed to define independent variables associated with survival (Table 15.7). Patients with small duct PSC have a favorable prognosis compared with those with large duct disease (Fig. 15.3).

1. The end stages of PSC are frequently associated with typical complications of portal hypertension including ascites, spontaneous bacterial peritonitis, and hepatic encephalopathy. As in other biliary types of liver injury, esophageal varices tend to appear early, even before cirrhosis.
2. CCA was reported to occur in up to 30% of patients. More recent studies reported a 10-year cumulative incidence of 7% to 9%, with the highest incidence within the first year of diagnosis. Risk factors for CCA include elevated serum bilirubin, variceal bleeding, proctocolectomy, duration of ulcerative colitis, and genetic variants in the *NKG2*D gene.

TABLE 15.7 ■ **Independent variables associated with survival in primary sclerosing cholangitis prognostic models from various studies**

		Cohort		
Mayo Clinic (*N* = 174)	King's College (*N* = 126)	Multicenter (*N* = 426)	Swedish (*N* = 305)	Revised multicenter (*N* = 405)
Age	Age	Age	Age	Age
Bilirubin	Hepatomegaly	Bilirubin	Bilirubin	Bilirubin
Histologic stage	Histologic stage	Histologic stage	Histologic stage	AST
Hemoglobin	Splenomegaly	Splenomegaly		Variceal bleeding
Inflammatory bowel disease	Alkaline phosphatase			Albumin

AST, aspartate aminotransferase.

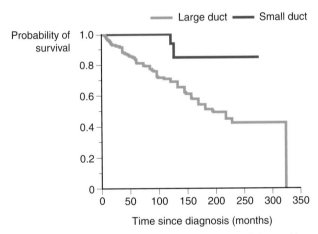

Fig. 15.3 Kaplan–Meier estimated survival curves for patients with small-duct and large-duct primary sclerosing cholangitis. *(From Bjornsson E, Boberg KM, Cullen S, et al. Patients with small duct primary sclerosing cholangitis have a favourable long-term prognosis. Gut 2002; 51:731–735.)*

Treatment

1. Medical therapy has been disappointing, and no controlled clinical trial has shown a benefit in survival.
   - UDCA has been the most extensively studied medication in large, long-term, randomized, placebo-controlled trials at doses of 13 to 15 mg/kg/day, 17 to 23 mg/kg/day, and 28 to 30 mg/kg/day. Biochemical improvement was common, but at the highest dose, UDCA treatment was associated with an increase in death and liver transplantation (Fig. 15.4).
   - Corticosteroids and other immunosuppressive medications have been studied but only in small trials and without significant effects. The exceptions are as follows: pediatric PSC/AIH overlap, in which immunosuppression resulted in reversal of biliary strictures on ERC; adult PSC/AIH overlap, in which corticosteroids may also be beneficial; and IgG$_4$-related cholangitis.

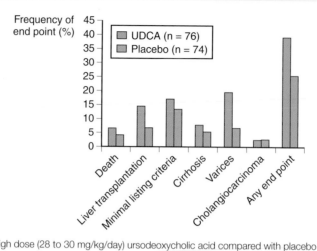

Fig. 15.4 High dose (28 to 30 mg/kg/day) ursodeoxycholic acid compared with placebo was associated with increased risk of reaching end points of death, liver transplantation, or minimal listing criteria (hazard ratio, 2.11; *P* = .038), as well as all primary end points (hazard ratio, 2.27; *P* = .008). *(From Lindor KD, Kowdley KV, Luketic VA, et al. High-dose ursodeoxycholic acid for the treatment of primary sclerosing cholangitis. Hepatology 2009; 50:808–814.)*

- Reports of beneficial effects of antibiotics in PSC included a randomized trial of metronidazole (with UDCA) in adults and a case series of open-label vancomycin in pediatric patients with PSC.
2. Although endoscopic therapy and radiologic therapy have been demonstrated to improve jaundice and to relieve bacterial cholangitis, the long-term benefit of such therapies in halting disease progression has not been demonstrated.
3. Biliary reconstructive surgical procedures have also been shown to relieve symptoms and have the advantage of excluding CCA. However, a long-term impact on prolonging disease progression has not been shown. Moreover, biliary reconstructive surgery has been associated with increased morbidity in patients who undergo liver transplantation and should be avoided if possible.
4. **Liver transplantation is currently the treatment of choice for patients with end-stage PSC.** Liver transplantation in patients with PSC is associated with patient survival rates of up to 90% at 1 year and 85% at 5 years (see Chapter 31).
    - Indications for liver transplantation are similar to those for other chronic liver diseases. Additional indications related to PSC include intractable pruritus, recurrent cholangitis, and early CCA.
    - Recurrence of PSC occurs in up to 20% to 25% of patients after 5 to 10 years. However, the diagnosis of recurrent PSC is difficult because of lack of standard diagnostic criteria and potential confounding factors that can mimic PSC including chronic rejection, cytomegalovirus infection, and hepatic artery thrombosis.

Complications and Their Treatment

1. Management of complications related to portal hypertension is similar to that of any other form of chronic liver disease.
2. Dominant strictures

- Approximately 30% to 40% of patients develop a *dominant stricture*, defined as a stenosis with a diameter of up to 1.5 mm in the common bile duct or of up to 1 mm in the hepatic duct.
- The most common site is the perihilar region and should raise the suspicion of CCA, although most dominant strictures are benign.
- Dominant strictures should be treated endoscopically or radiologically with balloon dilatation and stenting. In all cases, biliary histology and brush cytology should be obtained, to attempt to exclude CCA. Long-term stenting is rarely necessary.

3. Bacterial cholangitis frequently occurs in patients who have had a previous biliary surgical procedure and who have an obstructing dominant stricture.
   - Bacterial cholangitis should be treated with broad-spectrum intravenous antibiotics and drainage in the case of a dominant stricture.
   - For patients with frequent episodes of bacterial cholangitis unresponsive to dilatation of dominant strictures, prophylactic or on-demand therapy with ciprofloxacin, which achieves high biliary concentrations, is often effective.

4. CCA carries a poor prognosis and does not respond well to chemotherapy or radiation therapy. Most liver transplant programs consider CCA associated with PSC to be an absolute or relative contraindication to liver transplantation. Distinguishing a benign stricture from CCA can be difficult.
   - CA19-9 levels are often elevated in CCA but is also elevated in bacterial cholangitis. At a cutoff of 130 U/mL, the sensitivity and specificity are 79% and 98%, respectively.
   - Imaging studies rarely detect CCA but can be virtually diagnostic in patients with typical features of delayed venous enhancement.
   - Brush cytology has low sensitivity, ranging from 18% to 40%, but very high specificity. The presence of polysomy by fluorescence in situ hybridization may increase the sensitivity.
   - Positron emission tomography (PET) has no proven role in the diagnosis of CCA in PSC.
   - Evidence to recommend routine screening is insufficient, but annual imaging and CA19-9 measurement are often performed.

5. New-onset pruritus should initiate an evaluation for a dominant stricture or CCA. Identifying an effective agent in an individual patient often requires trials of several different medications.
   - Cholestyramine 4 g up to 16 g/day in divided doses (should be used as first-line therapy)
   - Rifampin 150 to 300 mg twice daily
   - Oral opiate antagonists (naltrexone 50 mg daily)
   - Sertraline 75 to 100 mg daily
   - Marinol
   - Antihistamines and phenobarbital not recommended

6. Gallbladder disease
   - Among patients with PSC, 25% will develop gallstones, usually black pigment stones. No association exists with disease stage or use of UDCA.
   - Patients with PSC are at increased risk of gallbladder carcinoma as well as CCA and should be screened annually with ultrasonography. Cholecystectomy should be considered in any patient with PSC who has a gallbladder polyp or mass.

7. Steatorrhea can be caused by a decrease in duodenal concentration of bile acids and thus a reduction in micellar formation or concurrent conditions such as chronic pancreatitis and celiac disease.

8. Fat-soluble vitamin deficiencies (A, D, E, and K) can be related to steatorrhea, but levels of fat-soluble vitamins A, D, and E should be measured even in the absence of steatorrhea and deficiencies treated with replacement therapy.

9. Peristomal varices are common in patients who have undergone a proctocolectomy for underlying IBD and who have an ileal stoma.

   ■ Bleeding from peristomal varices can be controlled by performing a surgical portosystemic shunt procedure or by placing a transjugular intrahepatic portosystemic shunt.

   ■ Complications of peristomal variceal bleeding can be prevented by performing an ileoanal anastomotic surgical procedure in patients with PSC who need a proctocolectomy.

10. Hepatic osteodystrophy should be screened for with bone density testing at diagnosis and every 2 to 3 years thereafter.

   ■ Osteopenia: treatment is with calcium, 1.0 to 1.5 g, and vitamin D, 1000 IU daily.

   ■ Osteoporosis: treatment is with calcium and vitamin D, and consideration must be given to administration of bisphosphonates.

Acknowledgment

Dr. Bowlus acknowledges Dr. Russell H. Wiesner, who authored this chapter in the second edition of the *Handbook of Liver Disease.*

FURTHER READING

Aron JH, Bowlus CL. The immunobiology of primary sclerosing cholangitis. *Semin Immunopathol* 2009; 31:383–397.

Baluyut AR, Sherman S, Lehman GA, et al. Impact of endoscopic therapy on the survival of patients with primary sclerosing cholangitis. *Gastrointest Endosc* 2001; 53:308–312.

Bergquist A, Said K, Broome U. Changes over a 20-year period in the clinical presentation of primary sclerosing cholangitis in Sweden. *Scand J Gastroenterol* 2007; 42:88–93.

Bjornsson E, Olsson R, Bergquist A, et al. The natural history of small-duct primary sclerosing cholangitis. *Gastroenterology* 2008; 134:975–980.

Chapman R, Fevery J, Kalloo A, et al. Diagnosis and management of primary sclerosing cholangitis. *Hepatology* 2010; 51:660–678.

Claessen MM, Vleggaar FP, Tytgat KM, et al. High lifetime risk of cancer in primary sclerosing cholangitis. *J Hepatol* 2009; 50:158–164.

European Association for the Study of the Liver. EASL Clinical Practice Guidelines: management of cholestatic liver diseases. *J Hepatol* 2009; 51:237–267.

Graziadei IW. Recurrence of primary sclerosing cholangitis after liver transplantation. *Liver Transpl* 2002; 8:575–581.

Karlsen TH, Franke A, Melum E, et al. Genome-wide association analysis in primary sclerosing cholangitis. *Gastroenterology* 2010; 138:1102–1111.

Kim WR, Therneau TM, Wiesner RH, et al. A revised natural history model for primary sclerosing cholangitis. *Mayo Clin Proc* 2000; 75:688–694.

Lindor KD, Kowdley KV, Luketic VA, et al. High-dose ursodeoxycholic acid for the treatment of primary sclerosing cholangitis. *Hepatology* 2009; 50:808–814.

Loftus EV Jr, Harewood GC, Loftus CG, et al. PSC-IBD: a unique form of inflammatory bowel disease associated with primary sclerosing cholangitis. *Gut* 2005; 54:91–96.

CHAPTER 16

Hemochromatosis

Jacob Alexander, MD ■ Kris V. Kowdley, MD, FACP

KEY POINTS

1 Hereditary hemochromatosis (HH) is an inherited disorder characterized by iron-mediated tissue injury secondary to impaired regulation of intestinal iron absorption.

2 HH is associated with mutations in genes encoding proteins, with the common feature of iron overload resulting from unregulated intestinal iron absorption.

3 Type 1 HH, or *HFE*-associated HH, is the most common form of HH and is inherited as an autosomal recessive trait.

4 Although the *HFE* gene mutation is highly prevalent in the white population, its penetrance is quite low; therefore, relatively few patients homozygous for the C282Y mutation in the *HFE* gene manifest the complete phenotype.

5 The features of iron overload are often unrecognized and diagnosed only in the setting of advanced disease, including diabetes mellitus, cirrhosis, and cardiomyopathy.

6 Patients in whom hemochromatosis is detected early and who are treated with iron depletion therapy (phlebotomy) have a normal life expectancy.

7 Suspected cases of HH should be evaluated with the following: biochemical markers of iron overload (serum transferrin iron saturation, and ferritin); *HFE* gene mutation analysis; and, in selected cases, liver biopsy (for staging or for diagnosis).

8 Patients with confirmed cases of HH should be treated with iron depletion therapy to maintain serum ferritin level in the range of 50 to 100 µg/L.

Epidemiology

1. In the white population, the C282Y mutation of the *HFE* gene, the genetic defect underlying the most common form of hereditary hemochromatosis (HH), is present in 1 in 200 to 1 in 250 in the homozygous form and in 1 in 8 to 1 in 12 in the heterozygous form.
2. The penetrance of the C282Y mutation is low (Table 16.1).
3. HH associated with other mutations is rare (Table 16.2).

Genetics

HH is associated with mutations in different genes involved in iron homeostasis (see Table 16.2).

TABLE 16.1 ■ Penetrance of the C282Y mutation

Penetrance	Definition	Frequency among C282Y homozygotes identified by population screening
Biochemical	Elevated serum transferrin-saturation and ferritin	50% of women 75% of men
Clinical	Hepatocellular carcinoma, hepatic fibrosis or cirrhosis, metacarpophalangeal arthritis, or elevated aminotransferase levels	Rare in women 28% of men

TABLE 16.2 ■ Mutations associated with hereditary hemochromatosis

Type of Hemochromatosis	Common name	Associated gene and gene product
Type 1	Classic hemochromatosis	HFE (HFE)
Type 2A	Juvenile hemochromatosis	HFE2 (haemojuvelin)
Type 2B	Juvenile hemochromatosis	HAMP (hepcidin)
Type 3	Tfr2-related hemochromatosis	Tfr2 (transferrin receptor-2)
Type 4	Ferroportin-related iron overload	SLC40A1 (ferroportin)

Classification

HFE HEMOCHROMATOSIS (TYPE 1)

1. The HFE gene is a major histocompatibility complex (MHC) class I–like gene and is located on the short arm of chromosome 6 telomeric to the A3 MHC class 1 histocompatibility locus.
   ■ Homozygous mutation of C282Y accounts for 90% to 95% of individuals with HH.
   ■ Homozygosity for H63D, another mutation of the HFE gene, is associated with less severe iron overload and rarely results in clinical HH.
   ■ C282Y/H63D compound heterozygosity accounts for 5% to 7% of HH.
2. HFE is primarily expressed in the crypt cells of the upper intestinal mucosa, where it interacts with the transferrin receptor and beta-2 microglobulin.
3. The exact roles of HFE in iron transport and pathogenesis of HH remain unclear.
4. C282Y homozygosity is associated with variable penetrance and clinical expression.
5. Factors known to influence iron absorption and accumulation may in part explain the clinical variability in phenotype:
   ■ Vitamin C (ascorbic acid) intake
   ■ Amount of iron in diet
   ■ Bioavailability of dietary iron
   ■ Type of dietary iron (heme iron absorption greater than nonheme)
6. The effect of modifying genes has also been postulated to contribute to the variable expression of disease.

NON-HFE HEMOCHROMATOSIS

1. HH associated with mutations in other genes (see Table 16.2) is rare.
2. Unlike the case of HFE HH, numerous different mutations are associated with each type of non-HFE HH.
3. **Type 2 HH** is associated with more severe iron overload and resultant tissue damage that develop earlier in life than in patients with HFE HH.
4. The manifestations of **type 3 HH** are similar to those of HFE HH.
5. **Type 4 HH** has distinct clinical and histologic manifestations:
   - Transferrin-iron saturation may be normal with elevated ferritin.
   - Iron is deposited predominantly in reticuloendothelial system (RES) cells in the liver.
   - Patients may tolerate phlebotomy poorly.
6. All forms of HH are inherited as autosomal recessive traits, except for type 4 HH, which is inherited as an autosomal dominant trait.

Pathophysiology

IRON ABSORPTION

1. **Only approximately 10% of dietary iron is absorbed** in physiologically normal persons, and this absorption is regulated in accordance with body iron stores.
2. Iron absorption is downregulated when serum transferrin saturation is high and following high dietary iron intake.
3. In HH, iron absorption is increased and is not downregulated as in normal individuals, and the result is in a positive iron balance.
4. Small bowel mucosal ferritin and ferritin mRNA levels are inappropriately decreased in HH; this pattern is normally associated with iron deficiency and is corrected by iron repletion.
5. Iron absorption involves uptake of iron from the intestinal lumen to the enterocytes, and then transfer from enterocytes to plasma, and both processes are increased in HH. *In vivo* kinetic studies indicated that increased transport of iron from the serosal side of the intestine into plasma drives the increased iron absorption.
6. The effect of the *HFE* mutation is thought to be mediated by lack of sufficient expression of hepcidin in the liver in response to iron stores at the level of the hepatocyte that leads to failure to inhibit iron absorption in the duodenum and resultant iron overload.

PARENCHYMAL IRON DEPOSITION IN TYPES 1 TO 3

1. **Iron is deposited in multiple organs** including liver, heart, pancreas, joints, skin, gonads, and other endocrine organs.
2. The major site of iron deposition in HH is the liver, consistent with its role as the major storage organ for iron.
3. Iron is deposited primarily in hepatocytes as ferritin and subsequently also as hemosiderin, with a decreasing gradient of iron absorption from periportal (zone 1) to pericentral (zone 3) hepatocytes.
4. Late in the disease, iron may be deposited in Kupffer cells and bile duct cells.
5. Saturation of serum transferrin precedes hepatic iron accumulation and is responsible initially for increased iron delivery to the tissues.

6. Later, non–transferrin-bound iron may play a role in iron delivery and toxicity.
7. There is also a possible defect of iron storage in reticuloendothelial cells.

EFFECT OF ALCOHOL INTAKE

1. Heavy alcohol intake is associated with higher serum iron markers, increased severity of clinical disease, and increased risk of cirrhosis and hepatocellular carcinoma (HCC) in C282Y homozygotes.
2. Liver fibrosis and cirrhosis occur at an earlier age and at lower levels of hepatic iron in these individuals.

LIVER DAMAGE

1. Progression of liver disease in HH is from fibrosis to cirrhosis to HCC.
2. Excess iron may mediate liver damage and/or promote liver fibrosis by several mechanisms:
   - Iron may catalyze the formation of free radicals that may damage cell organelles.
   - Iron may directly damage DNA and thus lead to mutations and carcinogenesis.
   - Iron may directly lead to hepatic fibrosis by increasing collagen synthesis.
3. Heavy alcohol intake may cause liver damage through accelerated tissue injury mediated by oxidative and nonoxidative mechanisms.
4. Liver disease in HH is characterized by progressive fibrosis, but without significant inflammation.
5. The presence of hepatitis (inflammatory changes) suggests coexistent viral infection or alcoholic liver disease.
6. Cirrhosis and HCC develop with long-standing iron overload; however, HCC without cirrhosis is very rare.
7. A correlation exists between elevated liver iron concentrations and fibrosis or cirrhosis.
8. Fibrosis or cirrhosis is observed in men who are more than 40 years of age and women more than 50 years of age, and earlier if pathogenetic cofactor (e.g., viral hepatitis or alcohol) is present.

Clinical Features

1. Before 1960, patients with HH were often diagnosed on presentation with classic features of "bronze diabetes mellitus," arthritis, liver disease, and heart failure.
2. With increased awareness of the disease, the diagnosis is now most commonly made in the asymptomatic phase through laboratory testing.
3. The diagnosis of asymptomatic HH is often made following discovery of elevated serum iron markers in the following clinical situations:
   - Elevated serum aminotransferase levels
   - Evaluation of serum iron markers
   - Family or population screening
4. When the diagnosis of HH is made after onset of symptoms, the most common symptoms at the time of diagnosis are as follows:
   - Weakness, lassitude, lethargy, or fatigue
   - Arthralgias or arthritis (women more commonly than men)
   - Nonspecific right upper quadrant pain
   - Loss of libido or potency (men)

5. Other manifestations include the following:
   - Increased skin pigmentation
   - Diabetes mellitus
   - Amenorrhea (women)
   - Liver involvement
   - Cardiac involvement
   - Infections

LIVER DISEASE

1. Increased hepatic iron concentration is present in patients with HFE HH and elevated serum ferritin.
2. The **severity of liver disease generally correlates with the severity of hepatic iron overload,** although coexisting liver diseases can add to the degree of liver injury.
3. Elevation of serum aminotransferase levels is generally mild, and levels frequently normalize once excess iron stores are removed.
4. If iron depletion is achieved and maintained before the development of hepatic fibrosis or cirrhosis, the risk of further liver complications is not increased.
5. Once cirrhosis has developed, patients remain at increased risk of HCC even after iron depletion.
6. Increased prevalence rates of chronic viral hepatitis B and C and heavy alcohol intake have been reported in patients with phenotypic HH.
7. Heavy alcohol use is associated with increased morbidity in patients with HH.

CARDIAC DISEASE

1. HH (especially type 2) can be associated with **cardiac dysfunction and arrhythmias.**
   - Cardiac dysfunction can manifest as restrictive cardiomyopathy or dilated cardiomyopathy.
   - Atrial and ventricular dysrhythmias can occur.
2. Cardiac involvement occurs relatively late in the course of HFE HH, and iron depletion before the development of dilated cardiomyopathy improves cardiac function. Thus, cardiac dysfunction is now seen less commonly because most patients are diagnosed and treated before cardiac involvement occurs.
3. Cardiomyopathy is a major cause of postoperative morbidity and mortality after liver transplantation.

DIABETES MELLITUS

1. Diabetes mellitus probably results from iron deposition in the pancreas.
2. It may be associated with increased plasma insulin levels, a finding suggesting peripheral insulin resistance (type 2) particularly with associated liver disease.

JOINT DISEASE

1. Joint disease is a **major cause of morbidity.**
2. It characteristically involves the second and third metacarpophalangeal joints; other metacarpophalangeal joints and wrist joints are also frequently involved; joints less commonly affected include shoulder, hip, knee, and ankle.

3. Pathologic features include joint space narrowing, chondrocalcinosis, subchondral cyst formation, and osteopenia.
4. It does not improve with iron depletion.

INFECTIONS

1. Patients with HH have **increased risk of bacterial, viral, and fungal infections.**
2. Increased risk of infections in HH is postulated to result from iron-mediated impairment of innate and acquired immune responses.
3. Unusual bacterial infections associated with HH:
   - *Vibrio vulnificus*
   - *Yersinia enterocolitica*
   - *Yersinia pseudotuberculosis*
   - *Listeria monocytogenes*

Natural History and Prognosis

1. Liver disease is slowly progressive but is usually mild (except with hepatitis or alcohol abuse) when the hepatic iron concentration is less than 200 μmol/g dry weight of liver.
2. Liver failure or HCC accounts for 60% of iron overload–related mortality.
3. Patients with HH and cirrhosis have a significantly increased risk of HCC (20- to 200-fold increased risk).
4. Cholangiocarcinoma may occasionally develop.
5. Concern exists about an increased risk of nonhepatobiliary cancers in HH, but the data are conflicting.
6. Some manifestations improve with iron depletion (malaise, fatigue, skin pigmentation, diabetes mellitus, abdominal pain), whereas others do not (arthropathy, hypogonadism, cirrhosis).
7. Patients without cirrhosis or diabetes mellitus have a normal life expectancy if they adhere to treatment.
8. Patients with cirrhosis or diabetes mellitus have a significantly decreased life expectancy, but the prognosis is improved with iron depletion therapy.
9. Patients with HH may need liver transplantation for end-stage liver disease or HCC.
10. Liver transplantation in patients with HH is associated with an increased risk of infections, especially fungal infections, and decreased survival.
11. HH is reportedly associated with even worse post-transplant outcomes than other causes of iron overload; however, outcomes of liver transplantation appear to have improved.

Diagnosis

CLINICAL SUSPICION AND LABORATORY TESTS

1. HH should be considered in these situations (Fig. 16.1):
   - Degenerative arthropathy
   - Unexplained hepatomegaly or liver disease
   - Unexplained hypogonadism
   - Elevated serum transferrin saturation or ferritin

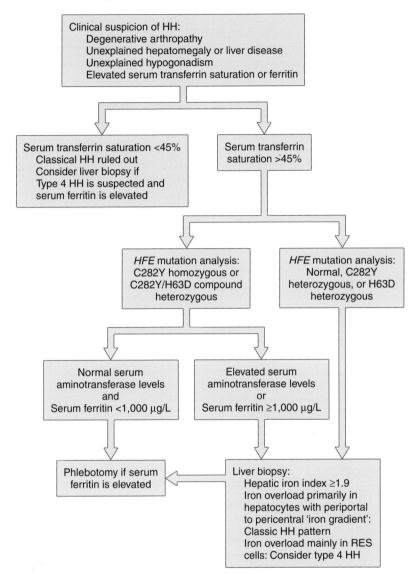

Fig. 16.1 Proposed algorithm for the diagnosis and treatment of hereditary hemochromatosis (HH). RES, reticuloendothelial system

2. Serum transferrin–iron saturation and ferritin are the first tests to be obtained when considering HH.
3. Serum transferrin–iron saturation is more sensitive and specific than ferritin for HH:
   ■ Elevated serum transferrin–iron saturation is the earliest manifestation of HH.
   ■ Serum ferritin is an acute phase reactant and can be elevated in inflammatory conditions and other chronic liver diseases (e.g., nonalcoholic steatohepatitis, chronic hepatitis C, alcoholic liver disease).

4. Circadian and postprandial variations of transferrin saturation can be a source of laboratory error, so the test is best done after overnight fasting.
5. A transferrin saturation of more than 45% warrants further evaluation for HH.
6. Isolated elevation of ferritin with normal transferrin–iron saturation may indicate type 4 HH.

GENOTYPING

1. *HFE* mutation analysis should be performed in all individuals with persistently elevated transferrin-iron saturation, especially if serum ferritin is also elevated.
2. The presence of C282Y homozygosity or C282Y/H63D compound heterozygosity confirms the diagnosis of HFE HH in the appropriate clinical setting.
3. Genetic tests for non-HFE HH are not currently available for clinical use.

LIVER BIOPSY

1. Liver biopsy may be required in two clinical situations:
   - For diagnosis when *HFE* genotyping is negative in a patient with suspected HH
   - For staging (presence or absence of cirrhosis) in a patient with confirmed HFE HH
2. Liver biopsy for diagnosis involves two studies (Table 16.3): the hepatic iron index and staining for hepatic iron.
3. Liver biopsy for staging is important because of the following:
   - Histopathologic study is the only reliable method for determining the presence or absence of cirrhosis in the absence of clinical signs.
   - The presence of cirrhosis is associated with an increased risk of mortality and HCC.
   - Knowledge of the presence or absence of cirrhosis may influence management (e.g., patients with cirrhosis need surveillance for HCC).
4. Staging with liver biopsy is required only in C282Y homozygotes with elevated serum aminotransferase levels or serum ferritin levels higher than 1000 μg/L because the likelihood of cirrhosis is low in the absence of these two findings.

OTHER TESTS

1. Hepatic magnetic resonance imaging can quantitatively estimate hepatic iron; it is devoid of the two principal disadvantages of liver biopsy: invasiveness, and sampling variability.

TABLE 16.3 ■ Assessment of hepatic iron overload by liver biopsy

Study	Comments
Hepatic iron index (hepatic iron concentration in μmol/g dry weight divided by the patient's age in years) measured in fresh or preserved tissue	Hepatic iron index ≥1.9 is frequently observed in patients with phenotypic HH, but in many C282Y homozygotes the index is <1.9.
Staining for hepatic iron (Perls' Prussian blue stain)	Staining for hepatic iron is important because sampling variability can yield a low hepatic iron index

HH, hereditary hemochromatosis.

2. Quantitative phlebotomy is useful for estimation of iron overload when liver biopsy is not required. Each phlebotomy usually removes 500 mL of blood (approximately 250 mg of iron); a need for removal of 4 g or more of iron before the onset of iron-limited erythropoiesis indicates the presence of significant iron overload.

Differential Diagnosis

1. Secondary iron overload can occur in the following situations:
   - Increased red blood cell turnover (e.g., disorders of ineffective erythropoiesis)
   - Repeated blood transfusions
   - Combination of the previous factors
2. Major causes of secondary iron overload can be classified as follows:
   a. Iron-loading anemias with or without transfusion
      - Thalassemia major
      - Sideroblastic anemia
      - Chronic hemolytic anemias
   b. Dietary iron overload (rare)
   c. Iron overload associated with chronic liver diseases
      - Alcoholic liver disease
      - Chronic hepatitis B and C
      - Nonalcoholic fatty liver disease
   d. Miscellaneous causes
      - Porphyria cutanea tarda
      - African iron overload
      - Neonatal hemochromatosis
      - Aceruloplasminemia
      - Atransferrinemia
3. The following features are helpful in differentiating secondary iron overload associated with chronic anemias from HH:
   - Liver biopsy in secondary iron overload shows iron overload primarily in Kupffer cells and reticuloendothelial cells, with a paucity of iron in hepatocytes. A periportal to pericentral "iron gradient" is also not observed in these conditions; however, a similar pattern may be observed in type 4 HH.
   - Quantitative phlebotomy demonstrates the onset of iron-limited erythropoiesis before removal of 4 g or more of iron.

Treatment

1. Iron depletion by serial phlebotomy is the cornerstone of therapy of HH.
2. Suggested protocol for serial phlebotomy:
   - Phlebotomy is performed, with removal of 500 mL of blood (approximately 250 mg of iron) weekly or biweekly until serum ferritin is 50 to 100 μg/L.
   - The hematocrit should be checked before each session, and serum ferritin should be assessed every 3 months (after every 10 to 12 phlebotomies).
   - If the hematocrit is less than 32%, phlebotomy should be postponed, and the frequency should be decreased to once in 2 weeks.
   - Once serum ferritin is lower than 50 μg/L, it should be checked every 3 to 4 months, and phlebotomy should be repeated as required to keep serum ferritin at 50 to 100 μg/L.

- The required frequency of maintenance phlebotomy depends on the rate of iron accumulation (generally required once in 2 to 4 months).
3. Precautions during phlebotomy:
   - Anemia should be prevented by monitoring hematocrit before each phlebotomy and ensuring adequate dietary protein, vitamin B_{12}, and folate intake.
   - High doses of ascorbic and citric acid, as well as a diet rich in iron, should be avoided. Moderate consumption of red meat is permissible.
   - Alcohol should be avoided while iron depletion therapy is in progress.
4. Because of increased susceptibility to *V. vulnificus* infection, patients should avoid eating uncooked seafood and exposing open wounds to warm coastal seawater. Susceptibility to *V. vulnificus* infection does not resolve with iron depletion therapy.
5. Iron chelators (deferoxamine, deferiprone, and deferasirox) are less effective, are more expensive, and are associated with adverse effects. Thus, these drugs are used only in patients with anemia or those who cannot tolerate phlebotomy.

Screening

FAMILY SCREENING

1. All first-degree relatives of patients with confirmed cases of HH should undergo screening.
2. *HFE* mutation analysis or fasting transferrin-iron saturation and ferritin is suggested for screening.
3. Relatives of patients with HFE HH who are negative for *HFE* mutations do not require any further testing.
4. Relatives who are positive for *HFE* mutations should be monitored with annual ferritin levels, and phlebotomy should be initiated when appropriate.

POPULATION SCREENING

1. Population screening for HH is controversial.
2. Genotypic screening (*HFE* mutation analysis) is not recommended, given the low penetrance of HH and concerns of psychological harm and genetic discrimination.
3. Phenotypic screening (transferrin-iron saturation) is suitable for population screening, but negative results in young adults should be interpreted with caution because those individuals may subsequently develop elevated transferrin-iron saturation.

FURTHER READING

Adams PC, Barton JC. Haemochromatosis. *Lancet* 2007; 370:1855–1860.

Allen KJ, Gurrin LC, Constantine CC, et al. Iron-overload-related disease in HFE hereditary hemochromatosis. *N Engl J Med* 2008; 358:221–230.

Fix OK, Kowdley KV. Hereditary hemochromatosis. *Minerva Med* 2008; 99:605–617.

Franchini M. Hereditary iron overload: update on pathophysiology, diagnosis, and treatment. *Am J Hematol* 2006; 81:202–209.

Olynyk JK, Trinder D, Ramm GA, et al. Hereditary hemochromatosis in the post-HFE era. *Hepatology* 2008; 48:991–1001.

Online Mendelian Inheritance in Man (OMIM). Johns Hopkins University, Baltimore. MIM No. 235200: 01/07/2010. Available at http://www.ncbi.nlm.nih.gov/omim/235200.

Pietrangelo A. Hemochromatosis: an endocrine liver disease. *Hepatology* 2007; 46:1291–1301.
Tavill AS. American Association for the Study of Liver Diseases, American College of Gastroenterology, American Gastroenterological Association. Diagnosis and management of hemochromatosis. *Hepatology* 2001; 33:1321–1328.
Weiss G. Genetic mechanisms and modifying factors in hereditary hemochromatosis. *Nat Rev Gastroenterol Hepatol* 2010; 7:50–58.

CHAPTER 17

Wilson disease and related disorders

John L. Gollan, MD, PhD, FRACP, FRCP, FACP ■ Alexander T. Hewlett, DO, MS

KEY POINTS

1. The Wilson disease (WD) gene is located on chromosome 13 and encodes a copper-transporting P-type adenosine triphosphatase (ATPase) protein, which is expressed primarily in the trans-Golgi network of the hepatocyte.

2. An impaired or deficient WD gene product is responsible for the lack of copper incorporation into ceruloplasmin and the defective biliary excretion of copper in WD.

3. Most patients with symptomatic WD present with hepatic or neuropsychiatric features; the principal hepatic manifestations include fulminant hepatic failure, chronic hepatitis, and cirrhosis.

4. In patients with a low serum ceruloplasmin level, the diagnosis of WD in the absence of Kayser–Fleischer rings requires determination of the hepatic copper concentration.

5. The use of DNA marker studies is limited largely to genetic screening of young family members or difficult diagnostic situations, with use of the index patient's DNA as a reference.

6. The drug of choice for treating WD remains D-penicillamine, but alternative drugs under selected circumstances include trientine, zinc, and tetrathiomolybdate. The use of combination therapy (e.g., trientine and zinc) appears promising.

7. Liver transplantation is indicated for patients with fulminant hepatitis or decompensated cirrhosis unresponsive to therapy.

Copper Metabolism (Figs 17.1 and 17.2)

1. Dietary copper (1 to 2 mg/day) is actively transported into the proximal small intestinal epithelial cells.
2. A fraction (25% to 60%) of copper is absorbed and transferred into the portal circulation, bound to serum albumin and amino acids. The remaining intraepithelial copper is bound to metallothioneins and is subsequently excreted as intestinal epithelial cells are sloughed. No significant enterohepatic circulation of copper occurs.
3. The Menkes gene *(ATP7A)* product likely plays an important role in copper absorption.
4. Only a small fraction of serum albumin–bound (nonceruloplasmin) copper is normally excreted by the kidney (less than 50 µg/24 hours); most is taken up by hepatocytes.
5. In the hepatocyte, copper is complexed with and detoxified by metallothioneins or glutathione and is used as a cofactor for specific cellular enzymes, incorporated into ceruloplasmin, or excreted into bile.

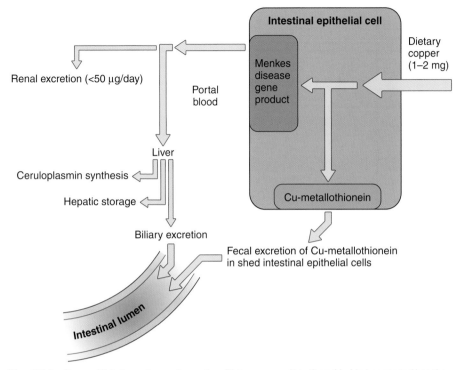

Fig. 17.1   Copper (Cu) absorption and excretion. Dietary copper (1 to 2 mg/day) is transported into the intestinal epithelial cell, with the Menkes gene product regulating absorption (25% to 60%). The remaining intraepithelial copper is bound to metallothionein and is subsequently excreted in stool as the intestinal epithelial cells are sloughed. A small amount of the absorbed copper is excreted in urine, but the majority is taken up by the hepatocyte, synthesized into ceruloplasmin, and stored in the liver or excreted in bile.

6. The site of copper incorporation into ceruloplasmin may be the Golgi apparatus. The WD gene *(ATP7B)* product, also known as the Wilson adenosine triphosphatase (ATPase), is presumed to be responsible for copper transport in this compartment and subsequent incorporation into ceruloplasmin.
7. The delivery of copper to specific intracellular locations is mediated by small cytosolic proteins termed *copper chaperones.*
8. As the copper content of the hepatocyte increases, the Wilson ATPase transfers from the trans-Golgi network to a vesicular compartment adjacent to the canalicular membrane.
9. Biliary excretion of copper occurs partly through a vesicular pathway. Another, perhaps less important, route of excretion is as copper-glutathione. A third potential excretory pathway is through a specific copper transporter in the plasma membrane.

Genetics

1. WD is an **autosomal recessive** disease with a gene frequency of 0.3% to 0.7%, thus accounting for a **heterozygote carrier rate of slightly greater than 1 in 100**. In 1985, the WD gene

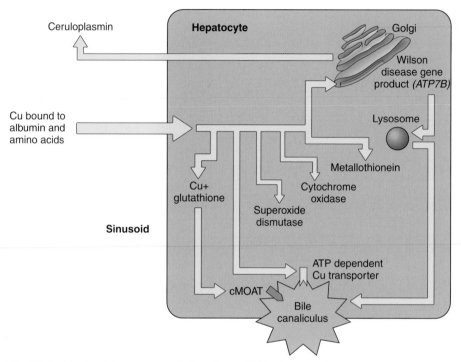

Fig. 17.2 Hepatocellular copper metabolism. Copper (Cu) is taken up by hepatocytes, where it interacts with glutathione and metallothionein. A portion of the intracellular copper is incorporated into metalloenzymes (e.g., superoxide dismutase, cytocrome cxidose), and some is transported into the trans-Golgi network by the WD gene protein (ATP7B), where it is incorporated into ceruloplasmin. It is postulated that copper is also routed from the trans-Golgi apparatus to a vesicular compartment in lysosomes for subsequent excretion in bile. Copper bound to glutathione is also excreted into the bile canaliculus through the organic anion transporter (cMOAT or MRP2) or by direct interaction with a postulated adenosine triphosphate (ATP)–dependent copper transporter.

was shown to be linked to the red cell enzyme, esterase D, an association that established the location on **chromosome 13.**

2. In 1993, three different groups of investigators isolated the WD gene by using positional cloning. The gene, designated *ATP7B,* spans an 80-kb region of the chromosome and encodes a 7.5-kb transcript that is expressed primarily in the liver, kidney, and placenta.

3. The gene product is a 1466-amino acid protein, a member of the cation-transporting P-type ATPase subfamily, and is highly homologous to the Menkes gene *(ATP7A)* product and the copper-transporting ATPase (cop A) found in copper-resistant strains of *Enterococcus hirae.*

4. More than **269 disease-causing mutations of the WD gene** have been identified to date. Most of the mutations are missense mutations. Comparatively few patients are homozygotes for the same mutation; however, **most are compound heterozygotes** (i.e., bearers of two different alleles).

   ■ Despite the clinical diversity of the disease, allelic heterogeneity at the *ATPB7* locus does not appear to account for the marked clinical variability observed in patients.

   ■ Although one normal allele is adequate to prevent clinical disease, heterozygotes for the WD gene may demonstrate subclinical abnormalities in copper metabolism.

Pathogenesis

1. Copper toxicity plays a primary role in the pathogenesis of this disorder. Affected organs invariably exhibit elevated copper levels.
2. Maintenance of normal copper homeostasis depends on the balance between gastrointestinal absorption and biliary excretion. Intestinal copper absorption in patients with WD does not differ from that of physiologically normal or cirrhotic subjects.
3. **Biliary excretion of copper is reduced in WD.** Studies indicate a possible defect in the entry of copper into lysosomes, but with normal delivery of lysosomal copper to bile. Investigators have suggested that copper transport into the trans-Golgi apparatus by the WD gene product is essential for its routing and excretion through the lysosomal pathway. This process, in turn, depends on the normal recycling of the WD protein between the trans-Golgi network and the vesicular compartment.
4. Deficiency of the plasma copper protein ceruloplasmin is unlikely to have a role in the pathogenesis of WD. The low serum ceruloplasmin level in patients with WD is believed to be the result of a lack of incorporation of copper into apoceruloplasmin, which has a shorter half-life than copper-bound ceruloplasmin.
5. Excess copper appears to exhibit toxicity by the generation of free radicals, which result in lipid peroxidation, depletion of antioxidants, and polymerization of Cu-thionein leading to necrosis and apoptosis. Morphologic abnormalities from oxidant damage have been identified, particularly in mitochondria (i.e., enlargement, dilatation of cristae, and crystalline deposits).
6. Pathologic copper deposition in the basal ganglia of the brain, particularly in the caudate nucleus and the putamen, results in the neurologic and psychiatric manifestations of the disease, whereas excessive deposition in Descemet's membrane of the cornea gives rise to Kayser–Fleischer rings.

Clinical Features

Patients with WD may be asymptomatic, although most present with hepatic or neurologic manifestations. **Clinical symptoms are rarely observed before age 5 years, and most untreated patients become symptomatic by the age of 40 years.** In a large series, the initial clinical manifestations were hepatic in 42%, neurologic in 34%, psychiatric in 10%, and hematologic in 12%. A few patients present with WD when they are more than 40 years old, and they normally present with neurologic symptoms that are commonly overlooked. Less commonly, patients present with renal, skeletal, cardiac, ophthalmologic, endocrinologic, or dermatologic symptoms.

HEPATIC

Hepatic manifestations tend to occur at a younger age (mean, 10 to 12 years) than neurologic manifestations. Three major patterns may occur: cirrhosis, chronic hepatitis, or fulminant hepatic failure:
1. Cirrhosis
   - This often occurs early in the course; symptoms may be minimal or absent, with nearly normal liver biochemical tests.
   - Later, the patient has an insidious, but relentless, progression to cirrhosis with liver failure.

- The association of WD with hepatocellular cancer was once considered rare, although several reports have appeared.
2. Chronic hepatitis
   - Young patients may present with features that are indistinguishable from viral or autoimmune chronic hepatitis.
   - Less than 5% of patients with chronic hepatitis who are less than 35 years old will have WD as the cause, and 5% to 30% of patients with WD present with features of chronic hepatitis.
   - **Modest elevation of serum aminotransferase levels in the presence of severe hepatocellular necrosis and inflammation is a distinctive feature of Wilsonian chronic hepatitis.**
   - The diagnosis may be difficult, because almost 50% of these patients have no evidence of Kayser–Fleischer rings and lack neurologic manifestations of the disease. Moreover, patients with severe hepatic inflammation may have normal serum ceruloplasmin levels.
   - The prognosis for treated patients is good even if they have developed cirrhosis.
3. Fulminant hepatic failure
   - Patients tend to be young, and the clinical picture may be indistinguishable from that of viral-induced massive hepatic necrosis.
   - Characteristic clinical features include intravascular hemolysis, splenomegaly, Kayser–Fleischer rings, and a fulminant course; patients rarely survive longer than days to weeks unless liver transplantation is performed.
   - **Serum aminotransferases are mildly to moderately elevated, with marked elevation of the serum bilirubin, a low serum alkaline phosphatase level, and evidence of Coombs-negative hemolytic anemia. Serum ceruloplasmin may be in the normal range; however, 24-hour urinary copper and free serum copper levels are usually elevated.**
   - Liver biopsy, if performed (in all likelihood through the transjugular route), will document an elevated hepatic copper content and usually the presence of cirrhosis.

NEUROLOGIC

1. This involvement tends to occur in the second to third decades of life.
2. **Kayser–Fleischer rings are almost invariably present on ophthalmologic (slit lamp) examination.**
3. Common early symptoms are dysarthria, clumsiness, tremor, drooling, gait disturbance, masklike facies, and deterioration of handwriting.
4. Rigidity with overt parkinsonian features, flexion contractures, grand mal seizures, and spasticity are seen less often and in the later stages of the disease.
5. Cognitive ability usually remains normal regardless of severe neurologic impairment.
6. Neurologic symptoms may improve markedly with treatment, although residual deficits are common despite adequate chelation therapy.
7. **Three subgroups** have been defined by clinical and magnetic resonance imaging (MRI) findings:
   - In a subgroup of patients with bradykinesia, rigidity, and cognitive impairment, MRI shows dilatation of the third ventricle.
   - A second group is characterized by ataxia, tremor, and reduced functional capacity; MRI reveals focal thalamic lesions.
   - A third subgroup exhibits dyskinesia, dysarthria, and an organic personality syndrome; MRI shows focal lesions in the putamen and globus pallidus.

PSYCHIATRIC

1. One third of all patients with WD may present with psychiatric symptoms; patients may be mistakenly diagnosed with a progressive psychiatric illness.
2. Psychiatric symptoms are present in virtually all neurologically affected patients, and the severity tends to parallel that of the neurologic abnormalities.
3. Early symptoms in teenagers may be limited to subtle behavioral changes and deterioration of academic and work performance.
4. Patients present later with personality changes, lability of mood, emotionalism, impulsive and antisocial behavior, depression, and increased sexual preoccupation.
5. Psychiatric symptoms usually resolve with chelation therapy.

OPHTHALMOLOGIC

1. Kayser–Fleischer rings
   - This golden brown or greenish discoloration in the limbic area is evident initially at the superior and inferior corneal poles and eventually becomes circumferential.
   - Electron-dense granules rich in copper and sulfur are deposited in Descemet's membrane.
   - Their presence or absence should be confirmed by an ophthalmologist with slit lamp examination.
   - They **occur in most symptomatic patients with WD and virtually always in those with neurologic manifestations; they are often absent in asymptomatic cases and in more than 40% of patients with hepatic disease**, particularly chronic hepatitis.
   - They are not pathognomonic of WD because they also are seen occasionally in patients with long-standing cholestasis from other causes.
   - The rings resolve in 80% of patients with chelation therapy over 3 to 5 years.
2. Sunflower cataracts
   - They are typically observed with Kayser–Fleischer rings, but less frequently.
   - Vision is unimpaired.
   - They resolve more rapidly than Kayser–Fleischer rings with treatment.

RENAL

1. Findings include proximal renal tubular acidosis or features of Fanconi's syndrome.
2. Distal renal tubular acidosis also may occur and is a likely factor accounting for the increased incidence of renal calculi in WD.
3. Hematuria, mostly microscopic, may be caused by nephrolithiasis or glomerular disease.
4. Proteinuria has been noted as a manifestation of WD, although nephrotic syndrome and Goodpasture's syndrome are more likely to be a side effect of D-penicillamine therapy (see later).
5. Chelation therapy usually results in marked improvement in renal function.

SKELETAL

1. More than half of patients with WD exhibit osteopenia caused by osteomalacia, osteoporosis, or both.
2. Symptomatic arthropathy occurs in 25% to 50% of patients; this degenerative joint disease resembles osteoarthritis and involves the spine and large joints.
3. Osteochondritis dissecans, chondromalacia patellae, and chondrocalcinosis have also been described.

MISCELLANEOUS

1. **Acute intravascular hemolysis** may be the presenting feature in up to 15% of patients; it is transient and self-limited but often associated with fulminant hepatic failure or chronic hepatitis.
2. **Cardiac involvement** was underestimated in the past; electrocardiographic abnormalities are present in one third of cases.
3. **Azure lunulae** (bluish discoloration of the lunules [bases] of finger nails) are unusual but characteristic findings.
4. The incidence of pigment and cholesterol gallstones is increased.
5. Delayed puberty, gynecomastia, and amenorrhea have been noted.

Diagnosis

WHEN TO SUSPECT

WD should be considered in persons between ages 3 and 40 years with
- Unexplained serum aminotransferase elevations, fulminant hepatic failure, chronic hepatitis with steatosis, cirrhosis, or poorly responsive autoimmune hepatitis
- Neurologic features of unexplained origin (abnormal behavior, incoordination, tremor, dyskinesia)
- A psychiatric disorder with signs of hepatic or neurologic disease, or refractoriness to therapy
- Kayser–Fleischer rings detected on routine eye examination
- Unexplained, acquired Coombs-negative hemolytic anemia
- A sibling or parent with the diagnosis of WD

DIAGNOSTIC TESTS

1. Ceruloplasmin
   a. Normal serum concentration is 20 to 40 mg/dL.
   b. Among patients with WD, 90% of all patients and 65% to 85% of patients presenting with hepatic manifestations have levels lower than the normal range.
   c. **The combination of a low serum ceruloplasmin level and Kayser–Fleischer rings is sufficient to establish a diagnosis of WD.**
   d. Normal levels are found in at least 15% of patients with WD and hepatic involvement, a finding reflecting an acute phase response to hepatic injury, and in patients with elevated serum estrogen levels secondary to pregnancy or exogenous administration
   e. A decreased level of ceruloplasmin is not pathognomonic of WD. The following non-Wilsonian causes also should be considered:
      - Diminished synthetic function as a consequence of severe liver disease
      - Nephrotic syndrome, protein-losing enteropathy, and intestinal malabsorption
      - 10% to 20% of asymptomatic heterozygote carriers of the WD gene (approximately 1 per 2000 in the general population)
      - Children up to age 2 years (physiologically low levels)
      - Hereditary aceruloplasminemia, which is unrelated to WD and associated with iron overload
2. Nonceruloplasmin serum copper
   - The mean free (nonceruloplasmin) serum copper concentration can be calculated by subtracting the amount of ceruloplasmin copper (0.047 µmol copper/mg of ceruloplasmin) from the total serum copper concentration.

■ Patients with WD have elevated concentrations of copper bound to serum albumin, amino acids, or transcuprein (nonceruloplasmin copper); however, total serum copper generally remains at less than 80 µg/dL.

■ **In untreated patients, non–ceruloplasmin-bound copper exceeds 25 µg/dL; in fulminant liver failure caused by WD, levels are markedly elevated.**

■ The test is useful for monitoring the adequacy of chelation therapy during maintenance treatment.

3. Urinary copper excretion

■ Normal urinary copper excretion is less than 40 µg/24 hours.

■ **Most patients with symptomatic WD have a urinary copper excretion greater than 100 µg/24 hours, and patients with fulminant hepatic failure often have levels that exceed 1000 µg/24 hours.**

■ Asymptomatic patients with WD may exhibit normal urinary copper excretion, and 16% to 23% of patients with WD who present with liver disease excrete less than 100 µg/24 hours. Thus, the predictive value of this test is limited.

■ Elevated levels may be seen in other hepatic disorders, such as primary biliary cirrhosis and chronic hepatitis, and in severe proteinuria from ceruloplasmin loss in urine.

■ The test is useful in confirming the diagnosis of WD and in monitoring compliance and response to chelation therapy.

■ D-Penicillamine, administered in a dose of 0.5 g before 24-hour urine collection, has been shown to increase urinary copper excretion, but it does not reliably distinguish WD from other liver diseases and has limited utility in adult populations.

4. Liver biopsy

a. Changes on light microscopy are nonspecific. Early features may include glycogen deposition in the nuclei of periportal hepatocytes and moderate fatty infiltration. The fatty changes increase progressively and in some cases may resemble steatosis induced by ethanol.

b. In more advanced cases, fibrosis or cirrhosis is present. In fulminant hepatitis and chronic hepatitis, submassive necrosis with Mallory's hyaline, also known as Mallory-Denk and cirrhosis is seen.

c. Histochemical staining of liver biopsy specimens for copper using rhodanine or rubeanic acid is of little value, unless results are positive, because during the initial stages of hepatocellular copper accumulation the metal is distributed diffusely in the cytosol and does not stain histochemically.

d. **A hepatic copper concentration greater than 250 µg/g dry liver (normal, 15 to 55 µg/g) accompanied by a low serum ceruloplasmin establishes the diagnosis of WD, with two caveats**:

■ The biopsy needle and the specimen container should be free of copper. A disposable needle made of steel or a Klatskin or Menghini needle, in each case washed in 0.1 M EDTA and rinsed with demineralized water, should be used.

■ The finding of a normal hepatic copper concentration excludes the diagnosis, but an elevated level alone may also be found in other liver diseases:

   – Cholestatic disorders (e.g., primary biliary cirrhosis, primary sclerosing cholangitis, intrahepatic cholestasis of childhood, and biliary atresia)

   – Non-Wilsonian hepatic copper toxicosis (e.g., Indian childhood cirrhosis, endemic Tyrollean infantile cirrhosis, and idiopathic copper toxicosis)

5. Incorporation of orally administered radiocopper into ceruloplasmin

■ Serum radioactivity (mainly as radiocopper-containing ceruloplasmin) is measured after oral administration of radiolabeled copper (^{64}Cu or ^{67}Cu) at 1, 2, 4, and 48 hours. Normally, one sees the prompt appearance of radiolabeled copper in serum, followed by the disappearance (as circulating copper is cleared by the liver for incorporation into newly synthesized ceruloplasmin), and then the progressive appearance of copper in circulating ceruloplasmin.

- In WD, the radioactivity does not reappear in serum as ceruloplasmin. Heterozygotes exhibit a slower and lower level of reappearance than do physiologically normal subjects.
- This test may be useful occasionally in diagnostic dilemmas, when liver biopsy is contraindicated, and in other hepatic disorders that exhibit an elevated hepatic copper concentration and/or Kayser–Fleischer rings; however, the test is difficult to perform because the isotope is not easily obtained.

6. Genetic diagnosis
   a. In family studies, haplotype analysis is available for the diagnosis in siblings of identified patients, with less than 1% to 2% error. Use of DNA marker studies (direct mutation analysis) in the diagnosis of WD, however, has several limitations:
      - The technique is relatively expensive, with limited laboratory availability.
      - WD is caused by many different disease-specific mutations.
      - **DNA marker studies can be performed only within families in which the diagnosis is already established in one family member, by using the index patient DNA as a reference.**
   b. Biochemical evaluation should still be performed when the diagnosis of WD is established by either haplotype analysis or by mutation analysis.
7. Scoring system: a scoring system was developed and validated by Ferenci et al to assist clinicians in determining when WD should be considered; the system uses a combination of symptoms, laboratory values, and finally mutational analysis.

DIAGNOSTIC APPROACH

See Fig. 17.3.

Treatment

DIET

1. A low-copper diet is rarely prescribed or necessary.
2. Tips to decrease dietary copper intake include the following:
   - Avoid foods with a high copper content (e.g., liver, chocolate, nuts, mushrooms, legumes, and shellfish).
   - Use deionized or distilled water if the drinking water copper content is greater than 0.2 ppm.
   - Avoid use of domestic water softeners and untested well water.

DRUGS

1. **British anti-Lewisite (BAL)**
   - This was the first effective copper chelating agent (3 mL of 10% BAL administered intramuscularly).
   - It was abandoned because it requires painful intramuscular injection.
   - The only rare situation in which BAL may be useful is in combination with D-penicillamine, when a patient demonstrates progressive neurologic deterioration while taking penicillamine (see use of tetrathiomolybdate).

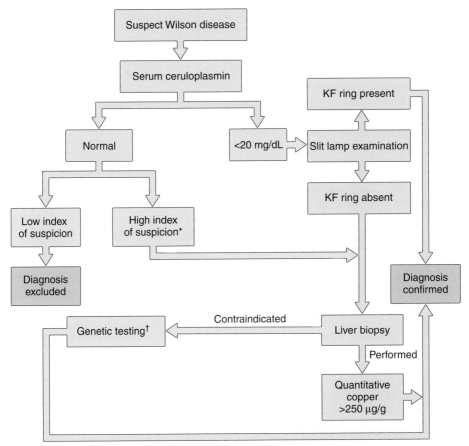

Fig. 17.3 Diagnostic algorithm for Wilson disease. In the past, radioactive copper testing was used, with lack of incorporation of orally administered radiocopper into ceruloplasmin supporting the diagnosis of wilson disease; this test is rarely used now. *Example: presence of Kayser–Fleischer (KF) ring, high urinary copper excretion, and neuropsychiatric symptoms with liver involvement. †Genetic testing is performed within families in which the diagnosis was already established in one family member by using the index patient's DNA as a reference.

2. **D-Penicillamine**
   - This amino acid derivative identified in the urine of patients taking penicillin remains the **first-line drug in WD.**
   - Mechanisms of action include copper chelation, detoxification, and possibly induction of cellular metallothionein synthesis, which enhances the proportion of nontoxic Cu-metallothionein.
   - The **initial dose is 1 to 2 g daily, with a standard maintenance dose of 1 g daily; it is best absorbed if taken on an empty stomach.**
   - Small doses of **pyridoxine** (25 mg/day) should be given daily, because of the weak antipyridoxine effect of D-penicillamine.
   - Approximately 20% of patients develop side effects within the first month of therapy. The most common side effect is a hypersensitivity reaction, consisting of fever, malaise, rash,

and occasionally lymphadenopathy; most patients can be desensitized for these symptoms by gradual reintroduction of the drug.

- Bone marrow suppression or significant (greater than 1 g/24 hours) or worsening proteinuria usually requires withdrawal of the drug.
- It may also cause significant worsening of neurologic features or precipitate autoimmune features such as myasthenia, polymyositis, or systemic lupus erythematosus. When such side effects occur, the drug should be discontinued and appropriate alternative therapy instituted.
- Dermatologic side effects include pemphigus, acanthosis nigricans, and elastosis perforans serpiginosa; the last of these, which also may occur with trientine, may respond to isotretinoin.

3. **Trientine**
   - This drug was introduced in 1969 as an alternative chelating agent to D-penicillamine.
   - Mechanisms of action include copper chelation and detoxification.
   - The daily dosage is similar to that of penicillamine: **1 to 2 g administered orally in three divided doses, taken on an empty stomach.**
   - Sideroblastic anemia is the only major side effect of this agent; other reported side effects include skin rash, gastrointestinal distress, and, rarely, rhabdomyolysis.
   - Most of the side effects of D-penicillamine, with the exception of elastosis perforans serpiginosa, subside when the patient is converted to trientine.
   - Because it is a less potent copper chelator than D-penicillamine and although it has a somewhat better safety profile, trientine should largely remain as **second-line therapy** until more comparative data are available

4. **Zinc**
   - The rationale for use of zinc is its ability to induce intestinal and hepatic metallothionein synthesis.
   - Zinc decreases copper absorption by increasing the formation of Cu-metallothionein in intestinal epithelial cells; copper is not absorbed in this form but is excreted as intestinal epithelial cells are shed, thus yielding a negative copper balance over time.
   - Zinc is relatively safe; side effects include gastrointestinal upset and headache.
   - The dose is **150 mg daily of zinc acetate, divided in two to three doses between meals.**
   - The **role of zinc in therapy is mainly in presymptomatic and neurologic patients, as a maintenance therapy in patients who have been previously decoppered and in combination therapy; also, zinc may be used as a temporary measure during pregnancy.**
   - Zinc monotherapy is not recommended as initial therapy for symptomatic patients, but good outcomes in those with predominately neurologic disease have been shown. However, outcomes are unsatisfactory in hepatic disease because of its poor decoppering effect.

5. **Ammonium tetrathiomolybdate**
   - This decreases intestinal copper absorption by forming complexes with intraluminal copper.
   - Following absorption, the drug forms nontoxic complexes with serum copper and prevents copper uptake by tissues.
   - Because its affinity for copper is higher than that of metallothionein, the drug can remove copper bound to metallothionein, thus potentially making it a more potent chelator than D-penicillamine and trientine.
   - The drug appears to be useful in removing redistributed copper during initial treatment with D-penicillamine or trientine when the patient has neurologic deterioration.
   - Tetrathiomolybdate, in combination with zinc, is currently undergoing comparison with the combination of trientine and zinc for effectiveness in patients with neurologic WD.
   - The potential side effects of bone marrow suppression and skeletal abnormalities (in animals) currently limit its usefulness and warrant further study before FDA approval and routine use can be recommended.

PREFERRED REGIMENS

1. Initial therapy
   - A baseline 24-hour urinary copper determination should be obtained.
   - Treatment is initiated with D-**penicillamine.**
   - The starting dose is 250 to 500 mg, gradually increasing to 1.0- to 1.5-g daily individual doses, which are usually required to achieve the desired level of copper excretion (rarely, a dose of 2.0 g is required).
   - Because of the potential for bone marrow suppression and nephrotic syndrome, a complete blood count and routine urinalysis should be performed every 2 weeks during the first 2 months of therapy.
   - Patients intolerant of D-penicillamine may be treated with trientine. Zinc or tetrathiomolybdate may be used when side effects caused by D-penicillamine are also known to be associated with trientine.
   - **Clinical signs of improvement may be delayed until at least 6 to 12 months of uninterrupted therapy.**
   - Patients with severe hepatic insufficiency unresponsive to pharmacotherapy should be considered for liver transplantation (see later).

2. Maintenance therapy
   - Once clinical symptoms and signs have stabilized, and urinary excretion of copper is less than 0.5 mg/24 hours or the nonceruloplasmin copper is reduced to less than 10 to 15 µg/dL, the dose of chelating agents should be reduced to the minimum essential dosage for maintenance.
   - **Typical daily maintenance doses for the current medications for adults are 750 to 1250 mg for penicillamine and trientine and 150 mg for zinc.**
   - A fall in the nonceruloplasmin copper to much less than 10 µg/dL may indicate severe copper depletion leading to reduced ferroxidase activity, which may result in hepatic iron accumulation; in this situation, the dose of chelating agent should be reduced.
   - Not uncommonly, one may note a lag in the recovery of the liver synthetic function and serum aminotransferase elevations for 3 to 6 months after the initiation of therapy.
   - Yearly slit lamp examination will document fading of Kayser–Fleischer rings, if the patient is adequately decoppered.
   - Alternative therapeutic agents, such as zinc and trientine, may be used, but experience with D-penicillamine is more extensive.
   - Treatment of asymptomatic patients with WD, diagnosed by screening of family members, may be started at age 3 years.
   - Lifelong therapy, without interruption, is essential in all patients with WD; cessation of therapy may result in rapid and irreversible hepatic and neurologic deterioration.

3. Pregnancy
   - **Therapy for patients with WD should be continued throughout pregnancy.**
   - D-penicillamine, trientine, and zinc all appear to be safe during pregnancy.
   - The **daily dose of D-penicillamine (or trientine) should not exceed 1.0 g during pregnancy,** and, if cesarean section is anticipated, the dose should be reduced to 0.5 g/day 6 weeks before delivery and until wound healing is complete.
   - Maintenance therapy with zinc does not require dose adjustment during pregnancy.

4. Patients with neurologic disease
   - Approximately 10% to 20% (up to 50% in one series) of patients presenting with neurologic disease have worsening of neurologic symptoms during initial treatment with D-penicillamine.
   - This phenomenon is most likely caused by the mobilization and redistribution of copper in the brain during initial treatment.

- Treatment with D-penicillamine should be continued in these patients, with gradual adjustment of the dose to increase urinary copper excretion.
- If neurologic manifestations continue to worsen, alternative approaches may include substituting tetrathiomolybdate for penicillamine; this medication is currently being evaluated as first-line therapy in patients with neurologic disease, but remains experimental.
- The differential diagnosis of neurologic deterioration during initial treatment with D-penicillamine also includes progression of the disease from subtherapeutic dosage or, rarely, a side effect of D-penicillamine, such as a lupus-like central nervous system vasculitis and cerebritis.

5. Combination therapy
   - Combination of medications with different and complementary modes of action, such as zinc with another oral chelating agent (e.g., trientine), is being tested as initial therapy for neurologic WD and is being compared with the combination of tetrathiomolybdate and zinc.
   - Anecdotal reports of combination therapy indicate encouraging results in symptomatic patients and in those with severe liver disease, thus obviating the need for liver transplantation in some patients.

LIVER TRANSPLANTATION

1. Liver transplantation results in complete reversal of the metabolic defect in copper metabolism, marked cupriuresis, and improvement in hepatic and neurologic manifestations.
2. In 55 patients with WD who underwent liver transplantation, the indications were fulminant hepatitis in 38%, hepatic insufficiency unresponsive to medical therapy in 58%, neurologic disease in 1 patient, and recurrent gastrointestinal bleeding in another.
3. In the absence of severe hepatic disease, liver transplantation for refractory neurologic manifestations should be considered experimental; however, several reports have noted improvement in these patients after liver transplantation.
4. In fulminant hepatic failure, the selection of patients is facilitated by determination of the prognostic index (Table 17.1); the outcome of liver transplantation in these selected patients is good, with 90% survival in one series.

FUTURE THERAPIES

1. Identification of the *ATP7*B gene and the mechanism of disease should make molecular-based therapies, including gene therapy, possible in the future.

TABLE 17.1 ■ **Prognostic index in Wilsonian fulminant hepatitis**

Score[*]	0	1	2	3	4
Bilirubin (mmol/L, NR 3–20)	<100	100–150	151–200	201–300	>300
AST (U/L, NL 7–40)	<100	100–150	151–200	201–300	>300
Prolongation of PT	<4	4–8	9–12	13–20	>30

AST, aspartate aminotransferase; NR, normal range; PT, prothrombin time.

[*]Patients with a prognostic index (total score) of 7 or greater should be considered for liver transplantation.

Adapted from Nazer H, Ede RJ, Mowat AP, Williams R. Wilson disease: clinical presentation and use of prognostic index. Gut 1986; 27:1377–1381.

2. Another potential therapy is hepatocyte cell transplantation; this has been applied in the animal model of WD, the LEC rat, in which complete metabolic correction was achieved.

Other Copper-Related Disorders

INDIAN CHILDHOOD CIRRHOSIS

1. This rapidly progressive cirrhosis manifests at 6 months to 5 years of age and is generally restricted to the Indian subcontinent.
2. Grossly increased hepatic, urinary, and serum copper concentrations are noted.
3. Environmental ingestion of excessive amounts of copper, resulting from the use of copper and brass vessels, is the likely cause of copper overload in this disorder, although a genetic predisposition appears to coexist in some patients.
4. This entity was one of the most common causes of chronic liver disease in India, but it is rarely seen now because of health education and avoidance of the use of brass vessels.

IDIOPATHIC COPPER TOXICOSIS

1. This is a rare disorder, with sporadic cases occurring worldwide.
2. Severe, progressive cirrhosis occurs in the absence of neurologic disease, with clinical onset usually by age 2 years.
3. Serum ceruloplasmin is normal; liver biopsy reveals cirrhosis with Mallory-Denk bodies and a hepatic copper concentration greater than 400 µg/g dry weight.
4. It may be caused by an unidentified genetic defect or excessive environmental copper exposure (e.g., contaminated spring water in endemic **Tyrollean infantile cirrhosis**).

MENKES DISEASE

1. This X-linked recessive disorder is characterized by impaired copper transport across the placenta, intestine, and blood–brain barrier that leads to a severe copper deficiency state (with deficient activity of essential cuproenzymes).
2. Symptoms usually appear before the age of 3 months.
3. It is characterized by growth retardation, hypothermia, skin and hair depigmentation, osteoporosis, tortuosity and dilatation of major arteries, varicosities of veins, and severe neurodegenerative disease.
4. It generally results in death by age 5 or 6 years.

FURTHER READING

Akil M, Brewer GJ. Psychiatric and behavioral abnormalities in Wilson's disease. *Adv Neurol* 1995; 65:171–178.

Durand F, Bernuau J, Giostra E, et al. Wilson's disease with severe hepatic insufficiency: beneficial effects of early administration of d-penicillamine. *Gut* 2001; 48:849–852.

Emre S, Atillasoy EO, Ozdemir S, et al. Orthotopic liver transplantation for Wilson's disease: a single center experience. *Transplantation* 2001; 72:1232–1236.

Ferenci P, Caca K, Loudianos G, et al. Diagnosis and phenotypic classification of Wilson disease. *Liver Int* 2003; 23:139–142.

Gollan JL, Gollan TJ. Wilson disease in 1998: genetic, diagnostic and therapeutic aspects. *J Hepatol* 1998; 28:28–36.

Huster D, Hoppert M, Lutsenko S, et al. Defective cellular localization of mutant ATPB7 in Wilson's disease patients and hepatoma cell lines. *Gastroenterology* 2003; 124:335–345.

Linn FH, Houwen RH, Hattum JV, et al. Long-term exclusive zinc monotherapy in symptomatic Wilson disease: experience of 17 patients. *Hepatology* 2009; 50:1442–1452.

Loudianos G, Gitlin JD. Wilson's disease. *Semin Liver Dis* 2000; 20:353–364.

O'Halloran TV, Culotta VC. Metallochaperones: an intra-cellular shuttle service for metal irons. *J Biol Chem* 2000; 275:25057–25060.

Roberts EA, Schilsky ML. A practice guideline on Wilson disease. *Hepatology* 2003; 37:1475–1492.

Roberts EA, Schilsky ML. Diagnosis and treatment of Wilson disease: an update. *Hepatology* 2008; 47:2089–2111.

Schilsky ML. Wilson disease: Current status and the future. *Biochemie* 2009; 91:1278–1281.

Steindl P, Ferenci P, Dienes HP, et al. Wilson's disease in patients presenting with liver disease: a diagnostic challenge. *Gastroenterology* 1997; 113:212–218.

Sternlieb I. Wilson's disease and pregnancy. *Hepatology* 2000; 31:531–532.

Zucker SD, Gollan JL. Wilson's disease and hepatic copper toxicosis. In: Zakim D, Boyer T, eds. *Hepatology: A Textbook of Liver Disease* 4th edn., Philadelphia: Saunders; 2003:1405–1439.

CHAPTER 18

Alpha-1 antitrypsin deficiency and other metabolic liver diseases

Christine E. Waasdorp Hurtado, MD ■ Ronald J. Sokol, MD ■ Hugo R. Rosen, MD, FACP

KEY POINTS

1 **Alpha-1 antitrypsin deficiency** (α-1 ATD) is the most common metabolic liver disease in childhood. The diagnosis should be considered in all adults and children with chronic hepatitis or cirrhosis of unknown origin. α-1 ATD is associated with chronic liver disease in 10% of affected adults and in 10% to 15% of affected children.

2 **Hereditary tyrosinemia** is characterized by progressive liver failure, renal tubular dysfunction, and hypophosphatemic rickets. Patients are at high risk for hepatocellular carcinoma if the disease is untreated. Treatment is available if the disease is identified early in life.

3 **Gaucher's disease** is the most common lysosomal storage disease. The clinical presentation and severity of liver involvement are variable.

4 **Cystic fibrosis** is the most common potentially fatal autosomal recessive disease in the white population. The prevalence of cirrhosis with portal hypertension is 10% to 20%.

5 **Porphyrias** are a heterogeneous group of genetic and acquired disorders of heme biosynthesis. The diagnosis should be considered in patients with abdominal pain and other gastrointestinal, renal, and neurologic complaints without an identified cause.

Overview

1. Acute and chronic liver diseases are increasingly identified as inherited, at least in part.
2. In most cases, a diagnosis can be made with a complete history, physical examination, and appropriate laboratory studies; some diagnoses require a liver biopsy.
3. Genetic and metabolic liver diseases account for approximately 10% of liver transplans in children.
4. Liver transplantation (LT) should be considered in children with metabolic liver disease associated with failure to thrive, target organ dysfunction (e.g., central nervous system or kidneys) caused by a toxic metabolic product, or progressive liver failure.
5. The presence of one genetic mutation for a specific liver disease can modify the severity of other diseases. The heterozygous state of alpha-1 antitrypsin deficiency (α-1 ATD) may increase the risk of progression in hepatitis B virus (HBV) and hepatitis C virus (HCV) infections, nonalcoholic fatty liver disease (NAFLD), cystic fibrosis (CF), and cryptogenic cirrhosis. Genetic polymorphisms are potential modifiers of hepatic cirrhosis.

Alpha-1 Antitrypsin Deficiency (α-1 ATD)

GENETICS

1. Alpha-1 antitrypsin (α-1 AT) is an inhibitor of neutrophil proteases and elastases.
2. α-1 AT is encoded by a gene on the long arm of chromosome 14 (14q31-32.2); α-1 ATD is an autosomal co-dominant disorder affecting 1 in 1800 live births.
3. PiMM (Pi = protease inhibitor), the normal variant, is the phenotype present in 95% of the population and is associated with normal serum levels of α-1 AT.
4. More than 100 allelic variants of α-1 AT are recognized. Not all variants are associated with clinical disease.
5. The Z α-1 AT protein is caused by a single nucleotide substitution (Glu to Lys). The variant is most common in persons of northern European descent.
6. **PiZZ and PiSZ phenotypes are associated with severe deficiency and liver disease,** whereas the PiMZ phenotype leads to an intermediate deficiency.
7. Low circulating levels of α-1 AT cause emphysema, whereas liver disease is caused by retention of the abnormally folded protein in the endoplasmic reticulum.

CLINICAL FEATURES

1. α-1 ATD predisposes children and adults to liver disease.
2. Liver involvement is often first identified in the newborn period as a result of persistent cholestatic jaundice. Affected infants tend to be small for gestational age. From 10% to 15% of persons with the PiZZ phenotype present with liver disease in the first years of life (Table 18.1).
   - Of those presenting with neonatal liver disease, 10% to 30% develop moderate to severe liver disease with coagulopathy, poor growth, and ascites in childhood.
   - In a prospective study from Sweden of children identified by newborn screening, 85% of PiZZ children demonstrated improvement in both clinical and laboratory signs of liver disease over an 18-year period. Only 5% to 10% of all PiZZ children developed significant liver disease (Fig. 18.1).
3. Serum aminotransferase, alkaline phosphatase, and gamma glutamyl transpeptidase (GGTP) levels may all be elevated.
4. Emphysema develops in 60% to 70% of adults with α-1 ATD over the age of 25 years, with the peak in the fourth and fifth decades.

TABLE 18.1 ■ **Findings in patients with alpha-1 antitrypsin deficiency (PiZZ or PiSZ phenotype)**

	Infancy (1–4 mo) (%)	At 18 yr of age (%)
Elevated serum alanine aminotransferase levels	48	10
Elevated serum gamma glutamyltranspeptidase levels	60	8
Clinical signs of liver disease	17	0

From Sveger T, Eriksson S. The liver in adolescents with alpha 1-antitrypsin deficiency. *Hepatology* 1995; 22:514–517.

PATHOGENESIS AND DIAGNOSIS

1. Liver disease is associated with retention of abnormally folded Z protein in the endoplasmic reticulum of hepatocytes. Liver disease occurs in the PiZZ and PiSZ phenotypes but rarely in persons with PiMZ. Liver disease does not occur with the other variants (e.g., PiSS).
2. Far fewer patients exhibit liver and lung disease associated with α-1 ATD than estimated by population human genetic estimations, a finding suggesting involvement of unidentified genetic and environmental factors and modifier genes in the development of tissue damage.
3. The pathogenesis of α-1 ATD–associated liver disease is not completely understood. The following theories have been proposed:
   - Accumulation of mutant protein in the endoplasmic reticulum may result in hepatotoxicity. This theory is supported by a transgenic mouse model and a study demonstrating delayed protein degradation of mutant α-1 AT Z protein in individuals with liver disease compared with those without liver disease.
   - Autophagy, a cellular mechanism for disposal of accumulated proteins, has been suggested to be defective in those with liver disease.
   - Other inherited traits for protein degradation and environmental factors (e.g., viral hepatitis) may increase accumulation of the defective protein and result in increased liver injury.
   - Liver disease is unlikely to be a consequence of a "proteolytic attack" mechanism, which is the likely mechanism responsible for lung injury.
4. The PiMZ state may predispose to more severe liver injury in various hepatic disorders (HBV and HCV infections, alcoholic liver disease, CF-associated liver disease, NAFLD).
5. The diagnosis is established by a serum α-1 AT level, phenotype (Pi typing), or genotype.
   - Serum levels of serum α-1 AT are generally decreased in affected patients; however, α-1 AT is an acute phase reactant and can be falsely elevated. Serum concentrations are rarely higher than 50 to 60 mg/dL in patients with the PiZZ phenotype.
   - Liver histology with diastase-resistant globules that are periodic acid–Schiff positive in the endoplasmic reticulum of periportal hepatocytes is classic for the disease, but these features should not be used for diagnosis because some patients with PiMZ also have these findings (see Fig. 18.1).

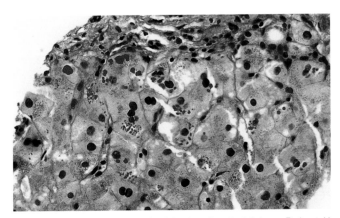

Fig. 18.1   Histopathology of liver involvement in alpha-1 antitrypsin deficiency. Periportal hepatocytes contain numerous eosinophilic diastase-resistant globules that are periodic acid–Schiff positive.

6. The diagnosis should be considered in all adults and children with chronic hepatitis or cirrhosis of unknown origin, children presenting with portal hypertension of unknown origin, and infants with neonatal cholestasis.

TREATMENT AND SCREENING

1. No specific therapies are available for α-1 ATD–associated liver disease at this time.
2. Infants with cholestasis may benefit from fat-soluble vitamin supplements (vitamins A, D, E, and K) and infant formula containing medium-chain triglyceride oil. In addition, treatment with ursodeoxycholic acid may increase bile flow and reduce liver injury associated with cholestasis, although no evidence indicates a direct long-term benefit in α-1 ATD.
3. **Avoidance of cigarette smoking,** including second-hand smoke, and of environmental pollution exposure is mandatory to slow the progression of lung disease. Replacement therapy with purified or recombinant α-1 AT by inhalation or infusion was successful in slowing the decline in forced expiratory volume in a nonrandomized trial, and this therapy is often used.
4. **LT** is the recommended treatment for α-1 ATD–associated end-stage liver disease and liver failure. The recipient assumes the donor Pi phenotype and is no longer at risk for emphysema. Long-term survival is excellent. LT should be pursued before lung decompensation precludes transplantation.
5. Somatic gene therapy, in which a normal α-1 ATD gene is transferred to an organ capable of synthesizing the mature protein that could be secreted into the circulation, is potentially useful for the treatment of lung disease. Gene therapy for treatment of liver disease requires delivery of peptides to the endoplasmic reticulum to prevent polymerization of mutant protein or manipulation of the degradation system in those at risk for liver disease. The technology is currently limited by poor transfer of gene products and unknown safety risks.
6. Small molecule pharmacologic chaperone therapy and manipulation of autophagy are currently being evaluated as possible future treatment strategies.
7. Screening is recommended for all relatives of patients with α-1 ATD to identify PiZZ or PiSZ family members and is mandatory for siblings of affected patients. Universal newborn screening has not been instituted.

Hereditary Tyrosinemia

GENETICS

1. This disease is caused by a deficiency in the fumarylacetoacetate hydrolase (FAH) gene, the terminal enzyme in phenylalanine and tyrosine degradation.
2. This autosomal recessive defect has an incidence of 1 in 100,000. The disorder is most prevalent in French Canadians in Quebec, Canada, where it has an incidence of 1 in 1800.
3. Many mutations of the FAH gene have been identified; no correlations exist between the genotype and the severity of disease. A founder mutation has been found in Quebec.

CLINICAL FEATURES

1. The disorder is characterized by **progressive liver failure, renal tubular dysfunction, and hypophosphatemic rickets.**

2. It may manifest as acute hepatic failure in infancy, neonatal cholestasis, rickets, or failure to thrive, or, later in childhood, as compensated or decompensated cirrhosis. The acute form usually manifests with poor growth, irritability, and vomiting. Death from liver failure by 1 to 2 years of age is not uncommon in untreated patients.
3. Patients have a characteristically prolonged prothrombin time despite mild elevations in aminotransferase and bilirubin levels. Serum alkaline phosphatase levels may be disproportionately elevated because of rickets caused by renal tubular involvement.
4. Neurologic crises develop and resemble acute intermittent porphyria, presumably from competitive inhibition of δ-aminolevulinic acid (ALA) dehydratase by succinylacetone.
5. Cardiomyopathy, particularly interventricular septal hypertrophy, is found in 30% of newly diagnosed patients. This complication resolves during treatment in most patients.
6. The incidence of hepatocellular carcinoma in untreated persons is high, even in the first 2 to 3 years of life.

PATHOGENESIS AND DIAGNOSIS

1. Tyrosine metabolites, including tyrosine and succinylacetone, proximal to the FAH blockage accumulate.
2. Succinylacetone and succinylacetate inhibit enzymes, including porphobilinogen synthase, and this process results in increased levels of ALA, which is responsible for acute neurologic crises.
3. The pathogenesis of liver injury caused by the accumulation of toxins is not understood.
4. Liver histology is characterized by macrovesicular steatosis, pseudoacinar formation of hepatocytes, hemosiderosis, and variable hepatocyte necrosis and apoptosis. Periportal fibrosis progresses to micronodular cirrhosis with regenerative nodules.
5. The diagnosis is established by the presence of elevated levels of succinylacetone in the urine or by genotyping. Other features include elevated plasma levels of tyrosine, methionine, and alpha fetoprotein, which are nonspecific findings. The diagnosis should be considered in patients with cirrhosis who have diminished hepatic synthetic function with mildly elevated aminotransferase levels. Renal tubular dysfunction results in glycosuria, proteinuria, amino aciduria, and hyperphosphaturia.

TREATMENT AND SCREENING

1. **Nutritional restrictions** are important, although they do not prevent or reduce the progression of liver disease. Phenylalanine, tyrosine, and methionine are restricted, with close monitoring of serum amino acids to ensure that levels remain in the normal range. Nutritional restrictions may benefit the kidneys.
   ▪ Vitamin D supplementation and phosphate supplementation prevent rickets.
2. **Pharmacologic treatment** is provided by Nitisone [NTBC; 2-(2-nitro-4-trifluoromethylbenzoyl)-1,3-cyclohexanedione]. NTBC inhibits 4-hydroxy phenyl-pyruvate dioxygenase, the second enzyme in tyrosine catabolic pathway proximal to the FAH block, and thus reduces production of the toxic products, such as succinylacetone. When NTBC treatment is started early in infancy, neurologic crises and liver failure are prevented and renal function is preserved. The effect on hepatocellular carcinoma remains unknown.
3. **LT** reverses the hepatic metabolic disease, prevents neurologic disease, and stabilizes renal involvement. LT is indicated if NTBC therapy fails, disease is advanced at diagnosis, or hepatocellular carcinoma has developed or is likely to develop.

Gaucher's Disease

GENETICS

1. This most common lysosomal storage disease is caused by a deficiency of the enzyme glucocerebrosidase. This deficiency results in accumulation of enzyme substrate (glucosylceramide) in the lysosomes of macrophages throughout the body (primarily the spleen, liver, bone marrow, and bone and, less often, the lungs, skin, conjunctiva, kidney, and heart).
2. It is an autosomal recessive defect affecting 1 in 40,000 in the United States.
3. The affected gene is located on long arm of chromosome 1(1q2.1). More than 300 mutations have been identified.

CLINICAL FEATURES

1. This is a continuum of disease with variation even among persons with the same genotype.
2. Three types of disease are recognized:
   - **Type I (non-neuropathic):** This type is most frequent, accounting for 95% of cases. The incidence in general population ranges from 1 in 20,000 to 1 in 200,000. The incidence in Ashkenazi Jews is 1 in 600. Patients present with hepatomegaly, splenomegaly (which may be profound), anemia, thrombocytopenia, osteopenia, and elevated serum aminotransferase levels. Progressive liver fibrosis and liver failure are rare.
   - **Type II and type III (neuropathic):** The incidence is less than 1 in 100,000. **Type II** causes progressive neurologic impairment at presentation and death by 2 years of age. **Type III** causes neurologic impairment varying from seizures to mild ataxia and dementia with associated hepatic dysfunction, but it is less severe than type II.
3. Liver involvement generally correlates with extrahepatic involvement. Storage cells are typically centrizonal. Patients may develop complications of portal hypertension.

DIAGNOSIS

1. Definitive diagnosis is made by an acid beta-glucosidase enzyme assay in leukocytes or fibroblasts or by genotyping.
2. Histopathologically, the disorder is characterized by lipid-laden histiocyte cells (Gaucher cells) in the spleen, hepatic sinusoids, bone marrow, and lymph nodes (Fig. 18.2).
3. The diagnosis should be considered in all adults and children with unexplained liver dysfunction, splenomegaly, hypersplenism, bleeding, and skeletal anomalies.
4. Prenatal diagnosis is possible with amniotic or chorionic villus sampling for genetic testing.

TREATMENT AND SCREENING

1. All patients (and siblings) with type III disease should be treated. Indications for treatment of type I disease include confirmation of the diagnosis (enzymatic or genetic) and at least two involved organ systems. Treatment is not effective for type II.
2. Enzyme replacement therapy: Imiglucerase is a recombinant acid beta-glucosidase.
3. Substrate reduction therapy: Oral treatment is indicated for patients in whom enzyme replacement therapy is not an option.
4. Bones should be monitored for disease with serial x-ray studies or magnetic resonance imaging (femur, spine, and symptomatic areas).

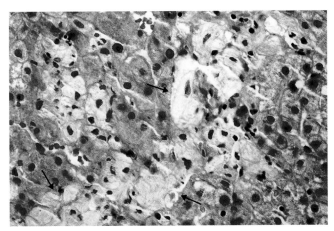

Fig. 18.2 Histopathology of liver involvement in Gaucher's disease. Lipid-laden histiocytic cells *(arrows)* are seen in the hepatic sinusoids (H&E).

5. LT is generally not required except in rare cases of liver failure.
6. Gene therapy is under investigation.

Glycogen Storage Disease (GSD)

GENETICS

Defects in enzymes involved in the degradation of glycogen to glucose result in excess glycogen accumulation.

1. **Type Ia** is caused by glucose-6-phosphatase deficiency (autosomal recessive). **Type Ib** is caused by abnormalities in endoplasmic reticulum translocase resulting in decreased glucose-6-phosphatase availability to substrate. **Type Ic** is caused by phosphate-pyrophosphate translocase deficiency. All type I defects result in decreased free glucose production. Excess glucose-6-phosphatase is shunted into pathways for synthesis of lactate, triglycerides, cholesterol, and uric acid, all of which are elevated in type I glycogen storage disease (GSD).
2. **Type III** is caused by genetic deficiency of the debrancher enzyme (amylo-1,6-glucosidase) with autosomal recessive inheritance. The gene is located on chromosome 1p21.
3. **Type IV** is caused by an autosomal recessive deficiency of the glycogen debrancher enzyme (amylo-1,4 1,6-transglucosidase) located on chromosome 3p12.
4. **Type VI** and **IX** involve defects in phosphorylase or phosphorylase kinase.

CLINICAL FEATURES

1. Children present with nonspecific gastrointestinal symptoms, short stature, hypoglycemia, and failure to thrive. Without intervention, progression to hepatomegaly (types I, VI, and IX), portal hypertension (type III and IV), or liver failure and death (type IV) between 2 and 4 years of age occurs.

2. Liver disease is seen in types I, III, IV, VI, and IX.
   - Type I: Deficiency of glucose-6-phosphatase leads to profound hypoglycemia during fasting. In addition, patients present with lactic acidemia, hyperuricemia, hypertriglyceridemia, hypercholesterolemia with accompanying massive hepatomegaly, short stature, and immaturity. Characteristic "doll's facies" is the result of excessive facial fat deposits. Enlarged kidneys are also seen.
   - Type Ib: This disorder is similar to type Ia, with the addition of neutrophil dysfunction or neutropenia. Hepatic adenomas may develop beyond the first decade in poorly treated patients.
   - Type III: This disorder has liver or muscle involvement. The presentation may be similar to, but milder than, type Ia, with hepatomegaly, hypoglycemia, hyperlipidemia, hyperuricemia, growth retardation, and similar laboratory test results. Hepatic fibrosis is more severe. Skeletal muscle weakness or cardiomyopathy may also be present.
   - Type IV (Andersen's disease): The disease is heterogeneous, with three presentations: (1) progressive liver failure and cirrhosis leading to early death, (2) chronic liver disease without progressive fibrosis, and (3) abnormal neuromuscular development. Most patients have cirrhosis and possible brain and cardiac involvement leading to death by 5 years of age.

PATHOGENESIS AND DIAGNOSIS

1. GSD is characterized by abnormal accumulation of glycogen in tissues, including liver, heart, skeletal, muscle, kidney, and brain.
2. The diagnosis is made by liver or muscle analysis for specific enzyme activity or by genetic testing.
3. The diagnosis is suggested by abnormal structure of glycogen observed by electron microscopy of liver or muscle tissue.

TREATMENT AND SCREENING

1. For patients with GSD types I and III who have hypoglycemia, frequent feedings of a high-starch, low–simple sugar diet or glucose polymers are used to maintain blood glucose levels. High-starch meals along with supplements of uncooked cornstarch are given throughout the day and at night.
2. Nocturnal nasogastric or gastrostomy tube drip feedings are also used to maintain normal serum glucose levels at night.
3. LT is the only effective treatment for patients with progressive liver failure and cirrhosis (types III and IV).
4. Patients with types VI and IX GSD usually do not require specific therapy.
5. Vector-mediated gene therapy holds promise in the future.

Cystic Fibrosis (CF)

GENETICS

1. This autosomal recessive disease affects 1 in 2000 to 1 in 3500 newborns, and it is the **most common potentially lethal inherited disease in the white population.**
2. Mutation occurs in the cystic fibrosis transmembrane conductance regulator (CFTR) gene, located on the long arm of chromosome 7. More than 1500 mutations have been identified, and $\Delta F508$ is the most common.
3. CFTR functions as a chloride channel and may regulate other cellular transport pathways.

CLINICAL FEATURES

1. The clinical presentation of CF varies greatly, with epithelial cells of different organs affected by the CFTR defect. Airways, sweat glands, pancreas, intestine, and liver are the most commonly affected tissues.

2. The pathognomonic lesion of CF-associated liver disease is focal biliary cirrhosis (present in up to 70% of adults with CF). The patchy distribution of cirrhotic transformation spares many areas of the hepatic tissue, thus preserving architecture and not causing significant symptoms. The focal nature explains the typically mild and insidious course of CF-associated liver disease.

3. Among patients with CF, 20% to 50% will develop clinical manifestations of liver disease. Neonatal cholestasis occurs in 3% to 5% of patients, and isolated hepatomegaly is found in 6% to 30%. Hepatic steatosis occurs in 23% to 67% of patients. Gallstones are found in 12% to 27% of patients. Portal hypertension and multilobular cirrhosis occur in 10% to 15% of patients with CF.

4. Median life expectancy in all patients with CF has increased to 40 years. With advances in medical management and duration of survival, the prevalence of recognized hepatobiliary involvement has increased.

PATHOGENESIS AND DIAGNOSIS

1. The pathophysiology of liver disease has not been fully elucidated. Proposed mechanisms include obstruction of intrahepatic bile ducts, altered bile acid metabolism, elevated cytokines, vitamin deficiencies, bacterial toxins, and hepatotoxic drugs.

2. The diagnosis is made either by the gold standard sweat chloride test or by CFTR genotype.

3. Liver biopsy has a limited role in CF because of the patchy nature of disease. Aminotransferase and alkaline phosphatase levels may be elevated at some time in most patients with CF, and these values have little correlation with progressive liver disease.

TREATMENT AND SCREENING

1. Ursodeoxycholic acid, administered at 15 mg/kg per day, has been shown to improve serum aspartate aminotransferase (AST), alanine aminotransferase (ALT), and GGTP levels, although long-term benefits are controversial.

2. Patients with severe steatosis and undernutrition may benefit from correction of pancreatic insufficiency with enzyme replacement.

3. Taurine supplementation has been suggested to be beneficial in patients with CF who are receiving long-term ursodeoxycholic acid treatment and who have severe pancreatic insufficiency and poor nutritional status.

4. Surgical options for patients with end-stage liver disease and portal hypertension include a transjugular portosystemic shunt, surgical portosystemic shunting, partial splenic embolization, splenectomy, and LT. Combined lung transplantation and LT may be performed.

5. Numerous novel therapies are under development, including a small molecule that induces ribosomes to produce functional CFTR during mRNA translation and recombinant growth factor. An animal study showed success with somatic gene transfer for correction of CFTR defects.

Porphyria

GENETICS

1. The porphyrias are a heterogeneous group of genetic and acquired disorders of the heme biosynthetic pathway (Table 18.2).
2. Three of the porphyrias are inherited in an autosomal recessive fashion, and five are inherited in an autosomal dominant fashion.

CLINICAL FEATURES

1. Porphyria consists of eight metabolic disorders classified according to the enzyme deficiency and tissue involvement (acute [neurovisceral], photocutaneous, and mixed forms). The presentation typically occurs during or after puberty; early childhood presentation has been reported.
2. **Acute porphyrias**: These are acute intermittent porphyria, variegate porphyria, hereditary coproporphyria, and ALA dehydratase porphyria.
   - They frequently begin in puberty and may diminish in the fifth decade.
   - Environmental agents and medications often precipitate attacks.

TABLE 18.2 ■ **The porphyrias**

Affected enzyme	Heme metabolic step	Resulting disease
	Glycine + succinyl CoA	
ALA synthase	↓	—
	ALA	
ALA dehydratase	↓	ALA dehydratase deficiency
	Porphobilinogen	
Porphobilinogen deaminase	↓	Acute intermittent porphyria
	Hydroxymethylbilane	
Uroporphyrinogen cosynthase	↓	Congenital erythropoietic porphyria
	Uroporphyrinogen III	
Uroporphyrinogen decarboxylase	↓	Porphyria cutanea tarda Hepatoerythropoietic porphyria
	Coprophyrinogen	
Coprophyrinogen oxidase	↓	Hereditary coproporphyria
	Protoporphyrinogen IX	
Protoporphyrinogen oxidase	↓	Variegate porphyria
	Protoporphyrin IX	
Ferrochelatase	↓	Erythropoietic protoporphyria
	Heme	

ALA, aminolevulinic acid; CoA, coenzyme.

From Bloomer JR. The porphyrias. In: Schiff ER, Sorrell MF, Maddrey WC, eds. *Schiff's Diseases of the Liver,* 9th edn. Philadelphia: Lippincott Williams & Wilkins; 2003:1231–1260.

- Symptoms include severe abdominal pain often associated with nausea, constipation, blood pressure derangements, hyponatremia, renal insufficiency, and neurologic complaints including peripheral neuropathy.
- Psychiatric symptoms may include depression, psychosis, and hysterical behaviors.
- Hepatic abnormalities range from mild elevations in AST and ALT levels during attacks to liver failure.

3. **Photocutaneous porphyrias**: These are erythropoietic protoporphyria, porphyria cutanea tarda (PCT), variegate porphyria, and hereditary coproporphyria.
   - Porphyrin accumulation leads to photosensitization and skin damage following sunlight exposure. The characteristic lesions include skin fragility, subepidermal bullae, hyperpigmentation, and hypertrichosis. Cutaneous porphyrias are not associated with neurologic or psychiatric complaints; however, liver involvement is seen.
   - Spontaneous PCT is associated with alcoholic liver disease, HCV infection, iron overload states, a mutated *HFE* allele (hereditary hemochromatosis), and Alagille's syndrome. PCT is associated with high rates of primary hepatocellular carcinoma.
4. **Mixed porphyrias** (combined acute and photocutaneous): Skin lesions occur in 50% of patients with variegate porphyria and in 30% of patients with hereditary coproporphyria.

PATHOGENESIS AND DIAGNOSIS

1. Metabolite accumulation leads to diverse clinical manifestations. Acute porphyria results from accumulation of one or both of the porphyrin precursors, ALA and porphobilinogen (PBG). In cutaneous porphyrias, the porphyrins accumulate.
2. The diagnosis can be challenging but is simplified by an improved understanding of the heme biosynthetic pathway, including metabolites.
3. Acute porphyrias are diagnosed by measurement of urinary ALA or PBG in a 24-hour urine collection. Levels 3 to 10 times the upper limit of normal (7 mg) are seen.
4. Erythrocyte porpholbilinogen deaminase levels are reduced in acute intermittent porphyria.
5. Urine uroporphyrin levels are elevated in congenital erythropoietic porphyria, PCT, and hepatoerythropoietic porphyria.
6. Elevated water-insoluble fecal protoporphyrin levels are used to diagnose variegate porphyria and erythropoietic protoporphyria.

TREATMENT AND SCREENING

1. Treatment is aimed at reduction of protoporphyrin levels in the liver:
2. Acute attacks:
   - Identify precipitants and avoid or remove them (Table 18.3).
   - Manage fluid and electrolytes and manage pain (avoid oxycodone).
   - Adequate caloric intake can lead to resolution of an attack resulting from glucose inhibition of ALA synthase activity.
   - Administer intravenous **hematin** for severe attacks. Hematin is a stable form of heme that inhibits ALA synthase and subsequent ALA and PBG accumulation.
   - Chenodeoxycholic acid increases protoporphyrin excretion into the bile.
   - LT has been used in severe cases, but the bone marrow continues to produce protoporphyrin, with resulting damage to the allograft. Therefore, bone marrow transplantation with or without LT has been suggested for patients with severe disease.
3. Photocutaneous porphyria:
   - Ultraviolet exposure should be avoided (use sunscreen and protective clothing).

TABLE 18.3 ■ **Precipitants of acute porphyria**

Environmental	Pharmacologic
Alcohol	Anticonvulsants: barbiturates, carbamazepine, phenytoin, valproate
Smoking	Antimicrobials: dapsone, doxycycline, metronidazole, rifampin, sulfonamides
Infection	Cardiovascular agents: amiodarone, nifedipine, verapamil
Stress	Diuretics: furosemide, spironolactone, thiazides
Menstruation	Drugs of abuse: cocaine, ecstasy, marijuana, and amphetamines
Low-energy diets	

- Patients with PCT respond to phlebotomy to reduce iron burden; chloroquine is used to form complexes with uroporphyrin.
- Treatment of erythropoietic protoporphyria includes administration of carotenoids for skin lesions.

Other Inborn Errors of Metabolism

HYPERAMMONEMIC SYNDROMES

- These syndrome have multiple causes: urea cycle enzyme deficiencies (e.g., ornithine transcarbamylase deficiency), transport defects of urea cycle intermediates, organic acidemias, fatty acid oxidation disorders, respiratory chain disorders, and disorders of pyruvate metabolism.
- The presentation varies with the age of the patient. Neonates with hyperammonemia have poor suck, lethargy, and even seizures or coma. Older children present more insidiously with failure to thrive and persistent vomiting or irritability. Episodes may be precipitated by processes that cause endogenous protein catabolism (e.g., excessive protein intake or infection).
- The diagnosis should be considered in any child with a family history of sudden infant death, Reye's syndrome, cyclic vomiting, ataxia, or unexplained failure to thrive.
- The diagnosis is made by blood ammonia levels, acid-base measurements, and serum glucose, lactate, pyruvate, ketone, and plasma amino acid levels. Determinations of urine organic and orotic acid excretion are essential in making the diagnosis and excluding other inborn errors of metabolism.
- Treatment: Ammonia removal is facilitated (dialysis, diversion of nitrogen from urea to other waste products with sodium benzoate); ammonia production is decreased (adequate intravenous glucose administration and antibiotics); LT may be lifesaving and corrects the metabolic abnormalities in urea cycle deficiencies; gene therapy for urea cycle defects is a possible future therapy.

DISORDERS CAUSING DAMAGE TO OTHER ORGANS (see also Chapter 23)

1. Crigler-Najjar syndrome type I
   - This autosomal recessive deficiency of hepatic uridine diphosphate–glucuronyl transferase results in the absence of bilirubin glucuronide conjugation in the liver and is characterized by unconjugated hyperbilirubinemia.

- The diagnosis is suggested by failure of phenobarbital to induce enzymatic activity to decrease bilirubin and serum bilirubin values in excess of 15 to 20 mg/dL, the absence of bilirubin conjugates in bile, and genotyping.
- Children who survive the neonatal period have an elevated risk of irreversible brain damage (kernicterus).
- Serum bilirubin levels increase with illness.
- Emergency treatment includes exchange transfusion and phototherapy (10 to 12 hours per day) to reduce serum bilirubin levels.
- Tin-protoporphyrin reduces serum bilirubin levels and may shorten the duration of daily phototherapy, but it increases photosensitivity.
- LT remains the only definitive treatment.

2. Primary hyperoxaluria (type I oxalosis)
   - This autosomal recessive inborn error of glyoxylate metabolism is caused by deficient or absent liver-specific peroxisomal alanine/glyoxylate aminotransferase.
   - The patient presents with recurrent urolithiasis or nephrocalcinosis that leads to end-stage kidney disease and, if untreated, death. This disorder does not cause liver disease.
   - Treatment includes a large fluid intake, low intake of calcium and oxalate, and supplementation with pyridoxine, alkali citrate, or phosphate.
   - Early recurrence of renal disease is common following isolated renal transplantation because the underlying metabolic defect in the liver remains unchanged.
   - Combined LT and renal transplantation is now advocated. It is essential to maintain a high urinary output immediately after LT until the renal oxalate load is greatly reduced.

3. Primary hypercholesterolemia
   - A homozygous mutation in the gene for the low-density lipoprotein receptor results in increased serum cholesterol levels. The incidence is 1 per million.
   - This disorder is a risk factor for myocardial ischemia and death within the first 3 decades of life.
   - The only effective treatment is LT; medications are not effective. Normalization of the metabolic defect before the development of atherosclerosis is the objective. Hepatocyte transplantation and gene therapy are being evaluated as definitive treatments.

FURTHER READING

Alwaili K, Alrasadi K, Awan Z, Genest J. Approach to the diagnosis and management of lipoprotein disorders. *Curr Opin Endocrinol Diabetes Obes* 2009; 16:132–140.

Colombo C. Liver disease in cystic fibrosis. *Curr Opin Pulm Med* 2007; 13:529–536.

Dhawan A, Mitry RR, Hughes RD. Hepatocyte transplantation for liver-based metabolic disorders. *J Inherit Metab Dis* 2006; 29:431–435.

Fairbanks KD, Tavill AS. Liver disease in alpha 1-antitrypsin deficiency: a review. *Am J Gastroenterol* 2008; 103:2136–2141:quiz 2142.

Farrell PM, Rosenstein BJ, White TB, et al. Guidelines for diagnosis of cystic fibrosis in newborns through older adults: Cystic Fibrosis Foundation consensus report. *J Pediatr* 2008; 153(Suppl):S4–S14.

Hansen K, Horslen S. Metabolic liver disease in children. *Liver Transpl* 2008; 14:391–411.

Harmanci O, Bayraktar Y. Gaucher disease: new developments in treatment and etiology. *World J Gastroenterol* 2008; 14:3968–3973.

Hoppe B, Beck BB, Milliner DS. The primary hyperoxalurias. *Kidney Int* 2009; 75:1264–1271.

Koeberl DD, Kishnani PS, Chen YT. Glycogen storage disease types I and II: treatment updates. *J Inherit Metab Dis* 2007; 30:159–164.

Lim-Melia ER, Kronn DF. Current enzyme replacement therapy for the treatment of lysosomal storage diseases. *Pediatr Ann* 2009; 38:448–455.

Martins AM, Valadares ER, Porta G, et al. Recommendations on diagnosis, treatment, and monitoring for Gaucher disease. *J Pediatr* 2009; 155(4 Suppl):S10–18.

Moyer K, Balistreri W. Hepatobiliary disease in patients with cystic fibrosis. *Curr Opin Gastroenterol* 2009; 25(3):272–278.

Scott CR. The genetic tyrosinemias. *Am J Med Genet C Semin Med Genet* 2006; 142C:121–126.

Taddei T, Mistry P, Schilsky ML. Inherited metabolic disease of the liver. *Curr Opin Gastroenterol* 2008; 24:278–286.

Thadani H, Deacon A, Peters T. Diagnosis and management of porphyria. *BMJ* 2000; 320:1647–1651.

CHAPTER 19

Budd–Chiari syndrome and other vascular disorders

Mack C. Mitchell Jr, MD

KEY POINTS

1 Hepatic vein occlusion, or Budd–Chiari syndrome, is an uncommon disorder characterized by hepatomegaly, ascites, and abdominal pain. The disorder most often occurs in patients with an underlying thrombotic diathesis including polycythemia vera, factor V Leiden mutation, protein C deficiency, paroxysmal nocturnal hemoglobinuria, tumors, and chronic inflammatory diseases.

2 The diagnosis is confirmed by visualization of thrombus or absent flow in hepatic veins on Doppler ultrasonography, three-phase computed tomography, or magnetic resonance imaging.

3 Budd–Chiari syndrome can be fatal without treatment. The approach to treatment should be stepwise, beginning with anticoagulation and followed by angioplasty or transjugular intrahepatic portosystemic shunt for portal decompression. Liver transplantation should be reserved for patients with advanced disease in whom other treatments fail. Improvements in treatment now offer 5-year survival rates of 85% to 90%.

4 Portal vein thrombosis (PVT) occurs in patients with an underlying thrombotic disorder or in patients with cirrhosis. Extension of hepatocellular carcinoma into the portal vein can also result in thrombosis. In the acute phase, anticoagulation is recommended. Band ligation of varices and beta blockers are used to prevent variceal bleeding in patients with chronic PVT.

5 Sinusoidal obstruction syndrome (veno-occlusive disease) of the liver is an occlusive disease of the small hepatic venules that mimics Budd–Chiari syndrome. It develops primarily in patients following allogeneic or autologous bone marrow transplantation, probably as a result of toxic injury to the endothelial cells caused by cytoreductive therapy. Treatment is largely supportive.

Budd–Chiari Syndrome

Budd–Chiari syndrome (BCS) results from obstruction to hepatic venous outflow and may be caused by either thrombotic or nonthrombotic occlusion.

CLASSIFICATION AND ETIOLOGY

1. BCS is classified according to the following:
   a. The duration of symptoms and signs of liver disease
      - Acute
      - Subacute
      - Chronic

  b. The site of obstruction
   - Small hepatic veins, excluding terminal venules
   - Large hepatic veins
   - Hepatic inferior vena cava (IVC)
  c. The cause of obstruction
   - Membranous web
   - Direct infiltration by tumor or metastasis along veins
   - Thrombosis

2. Most patients with BCS present within 3 months of the onset of symptoms. Most have subacute or chronic disease at the time of presentation, a finding suggesting that thrombosis of intrahepatic veins leads subsequently to occlusion of large collecting veins.
3. Membranous occlusion of the hepatic veins (MOHV) is a common cause of BCS in Asia but is rarely seen in the United States. The pathogenesis is the subject of controversy; many investigators have assumed that webs are congenital, but the onset of symptoms in the fourth decade of life and the pathologic features are more suggestive of a post-thrombotic event.
4. Most patients with BCS have an underlying thrombotic diathesis. In less than 20% of cases is the disorder idiopathic. Disorders associated with BCS include the following:
   a. Hematologic disorders
    - Polycythemia rubra vera
    - Myeloproliferative disorder associated with Janus kinase 2 (JAK2) mutation *V617F*
    - Paroxysmal nocturnal hemoglobinuria
    - Antiphospholipid syndrome
   b. Inherited thrombotic diathesis
    - Factor V Leiden mutation
    - Protein C deficiency
    - Prothrombin gene mutation (G20210A)
    - Protein S deficiency (rare)
    - Antithrombin deficiency (rare)
   c. Pregnancy or high-dose estrogen (oral contraceptives) use
   d. Chronic infections of the liver
    - Aspergillosis
    - Amebic abscess
    - Hydatid cysts
    - Tuberculosis
   e. Tumors
    - Hepatocellular carcinoma
    - Renal cell carcinoma
    - Leiomyosarcoma
   f. Chronic inflammatory diseases
    - Behçet's disease
    - Inflammatory bowel disease
    - Sarcoidosis

CLINICAL AND LABORATORY FEATURES

1. The classic triad of hepatomegaly, ascites, and abdominal pain is seen in most patients but is nonspecific.
   - Splenomegaly may develop in almost half of patients.
   - Peripheral edema suggests the possibility of thrombosis or compression of the IVC.
   - Jaundice is rare.

2. The natural history of untreated BCS is progression of symptoms often resulting in death caused by complications of portal hypertension. Untreated, the mortality rate is greater than 50%, except in some patients with membranous webs, in whom symptoms develop slowly.
3. Routine biochemical and hematologic parameters are as follows:
   - Little value in differential diagnosis
   - Abnormal but nonspecific
   - No distinctive pattern of abnormalities
4. Ascitic fluid characteristics are useful clues to the diagnosis:
   - High protein concentration (greater than 2.0 g/dL)
   - White blood cell count usually lower than 500/mm^3
   - Serum-ascites albumin gradient usually 1.1 or higher
5. Differential diagnosis includes the following:
   - Right-sided heart failure
   - Constrictive pericarditis
   - Metastatic disease involving the liver
   - Hepatocellular carcinoma
   - Alcoholic liver disease
   - Granulomatous liver disease

DIAGNOSIS

1. A high index of suspicion is necessary for diagnosis because clinical manifestations and laboratory results are nonspecific.
2. Imaging techniques for visualizing hepatic veins are as follows:
   a. **Ultrasonography**
      - Color-flow Doppler ultrasonography is better than duplex ultrasound, which is superior to real-time ultrasonography.
      - It provides cost-effective confirmation of low or absent hepatic venous blood flow.
      - It occasionally can visualize thrombus within hepatic veins.
      - The sensitivity of color-flow Doppler is 85% to 90%, with similar specificity.
   b. **Magnetic resonance imaging (MRI)** with gadolinium contrast or pulsed sequencing
      - It can visualize thrombus and detect absent hepatic venous blood flow.
      - It costs more than Doppler ultrasonography.
      - Sensitivity and specificity are approximately 90%.
   c. **Three-phase computed tomography (CT)** provides 85% to 90% sensitivity and specificity. It can also detect multifocal regenerative nodules (some larger than 2 cm) that develop in some patients.
3. Hepatic venography
   - Thrombus within hepatic veins
   - "Spider-web" pattern of collateral vessels
   - Inability to cannulate the hepatic vein orifices
   - Unnecessary if characteristic findings are noted on noninvasive imaging
   - Usually performed in conjunction with therapeutic intervention such as transjugular intrahepatic portosystemic shunt (TIPS)
4. Pathologic findings on liver biopsy specimens
   - Evidence of high-grade venous congestion
   - Centrilobular liver cell atrophy
   - Thrombi within terminal hepatic venules rarely seen
   - Heterogeneous involvement of liver occasionally problematic (i.e., sampling error)

5. **The diagnostic approach to a patient suspected of having hepatic vein occlusion should begin with color Doppler ultrasonography, followed by three-phase CT or MRI. If imaging is equivocal for BCS, then hepatic venography with inferior vena cavography should be performed to confirm the diagnosis. Liver biopsy may be of value to define the extent of fibrosis but is usually unnecessary.**

TREATMENT

1. **Medical therapy** provides short-term symptomatic benefit and is recommended as a first step.
    - Diuretics are useful for relieving ascites but do not alter the long-term outcome.
    - Anticoagulation with heparin followed by warfarin is recommended in all patients, because it prevents repeat thromboses; however, anticoagulation is beneficial in relieving symptoms long-term in less than 25% of patients. Anticoagulation is critical in patients with a defined thrombotic disorder.
    - Thrombolytic therapy has been used successfully in a few reported cases, although the long-term benefit is unclear.
2. Minimally invasive approaches
    a. Rationale
    - Hepatocellular injury may result from microvascular ischemia caused by congestion.
    - Portosystemic shunting provides a low-pressure path to decompress the congested liver.
    b. **Angioplasty** of short-segment obstructions such as webs or short hepatic vein stenoses. Relief of obstruction is temporary, and repeated treatment is required for long-term management.
    - Placement of a metal stent in the hepatic vein following angioplasty of a short-segment stenosis has been used to improve long-term patency.
    - Placement of a stent in the vena cava provides relief of compression from an enlarged caudate lobe of the liver and can be followed by a side-to-side portacaval or mesocaval shunt, if necessary.
    c. **TIPS** can be performed in more than 90% of patients despite occlusion of hepatic veins.
    - The mortality rate is less than 2%; complication rates are 15% to 20%.
    - The liver transplant-free 5-year survival rate is approximately 85%.
    - Coated stents have better long-term patency rates than noncoated stents.
    - Refractory encephalopathy develops in less than 10% of patients; it may require liver transplantation.
3. **Liver transplantation**
    - This corrects some underlying clotting disorders and restores hepatocellular function.
    - The actuarial 3-year survival rate is 80%, and the 5-year survival rate is approximately 70%; significant improvements have been made in survival in the Model for End-stage Liver Disease (MELD) era (see Chapter 9).
    - Liver transplantation is recommended in patients in whom minimally invasive procedures fail and in selected patients with liver failure or partial portal vein thrombosis (PVT).
    - BCS can recur in the post-transplant liver.
4. **Transcardiac membranotomy** has been used to relieve membranous obstruction of the IVC and rarely the hepatic veins. Other surgical procedures have been used in small numbers of patients with BCS from other causes. The results have been variable and are subject to the bias of reporting successes more often than failures.
5. **Portosystemic shunt surgery** was the mainstay of treatment for BCS before less invasive procedures such as TIPS were used widely; surgical portosystemic shunts remain an option but are no longer the preferred approach to management because of the high rate of complications.

    a. Options include the following:
- Side-to-side portacaval shunt
- Mesocaval shunt
- Mesoatrial shunt
- Side-to-side portacaval with cavoatrial shunt

    b. Success of portosystemic shunting depends on the following:
- Experience of the surgeon with a particular shunt
- The underlying disease
- Host factors including the extent of fibrosis or the presence of cirrhosis
- Hepatic function at the time of operation

    c. Shunt patency rates of 65% to 95% depend on the following:
- The duration of disease: the longer the duration, the lower the patency.
- The presence of fibrosis or cirrhosis lowers patency rates.
- The type of shunt: rates for mesoatrial shunts are slightly lower than those for mesocaval shunts.
- Continued thrombotic diathesis from the underlying disease is a factor.

    d. Survival (rates of 38% to 87% at 5 years) depends on the following:
- Continued graft patency
- Degree of fibrosis
- Type of shunt

ALGORITHM FOR EVALUATION AND MANAGEMENT OF BCS

1. The diagnosis of BCS should be suspected in any patient with ascites and hepatomegaly, particularly if evidence of a thrombotic diathesis is present. A high ascitic protein concentration or high serum-ascites albumin gradient is a clue to the diagnosis. Anticoagulation should be considered in those patients with a defined thrombotic disorder.
2. Color Doppler or duplex ultrasonography should be used to visualize the hepatic veins and determine the patency of the IVC. If doubt exists, three-phase CT or MRI is indicated.
3. If the patient has evidence of hepatic vein outflow obstruction, angioplasty or TIPS should be considered to provide portal decompression. An IVC stent can be placed to relieve compression temporarily by an enlarged caudate lobe. **All patients should undergo early portosystemic decompression.**
4. **If TIPS fails and cirrhosis is absent, surgical portosystemic shunt surgery should be considered.** Hepatic venography and vena cavography are required to determine the need for mesoatrial versus mesocaval shunting. Mesoatrial shunts are preferable in patients with a high pressure gradient across the hepatic vena cava, provided the surgeon is experienced in this operation. If the IVC is patent, mesocaval shunting with or without placement of an IVC stent is possible.
5. **If hepatic decompensation is present or if other interventions fail, liver transplantation is indicated.** Early portosystemic decompression with TIPS is desirable until a donor organ is available.

Portal Vein Thrombosis

CLASSIFICATION

1. **Acute PVT**
   - Symptoms less than 60 days before presentation
   - No evidence of underlying cirrhosis or portal hypertension on endoscopy or imaging

2. **Chronic PVT**
   - May develop in isolation or as a complication of cirrhosis
   - Presence of portal vein collaterals (portal cavernoma) and portal hypertension distinguish the chronic from the acute phase
3. **Splenic vein thrombosis**
   - May develop in isolation from thrombosis within the main portal vein
   - Leads to splenomegaly and isolated gastric varices without esophageal varices

ETIOLOGY

1. **As many as 70% of patients with PVT have an underlying thrombotic disorder.**
   - PVT is associated with the same disorders that are associated with BCS, listed earlier.
2. The following infections within the abdomen presumably result from pylephlebitis (septic phlebitis of the portal vein):
   - Acute appendicitis
   - Acute cholecystitis or cholangitis
   - Pancreatitis
3. Isolated thrombosis of the splenic vein may develop as a consequence of the following:
   - Chronic pancreatitis
   - Direct trauma to the abdomen
4. PVT in cirrhosis probably results from a combination of these factors:
   - Diminished blood flow within the portal vein
   - Reduced levels of protein C and protein S
   - Hepatocellular carcinoma, which can lead to PVT either through a procoagulant pathway or by direct invasion of the portal vein

CLINICAL FEATURES

1. Acute PVT
   - Abdominal pain and nausea
   - Intestinal ischemia, which may result particularly when thrombosis also involves the superior mesenteric vein
   - Intestinal infarction, which is uncommon but can be fatal
2. Chronic PVT
   - Gastroesophageal varices
   - Splenomegaly
   - Thrombocytopenia
   - Variceal bleeding, which is often well tolerated in the absence of cirrhosis
   - Ascites, which is rare in the absence of cirrhosis

DIAGNOSIS

1. Doppler ultrasonography has high sensitivity (greater than 70%) and specificity (greater than 80%) for diagnosing PVT.
2. CT and MRI can often identify thrombus within the portal vein and are helpful when Doppler ultrasonography results are equivocal. Sensitivity and specificity approach 98%. Occasionally, recanalization of the portal vein may cause problems in interpretation.
3. Liver biochemical test levels are normal except in patients with underlying chronic liver disease.

4. A thorough evaluation for an underlying thrombotic disorder and hepatocellular carcinoma is warranted.

TREATMENT

1. Acute PVT
   a. Anticoagulation with heparin or low-molecular-weight heparin is indicated in the acute phase.
      - It may promote recanalization if carried out within the first 30 days.
      - It reduces the risk of complications such as bowel infarction.
      - The need for long-term anticoagulation is based on the presence of an underlying thrombotic disorder.
   b. Thrombolysis is associated with a high rate of bleeding.
   c. Surgical thrombectomy is not recommended because of the unacceptable rate of complications, except possibly when resection of infarcted bowel is required.
2. Chronic PVT
   a. Long-term use of a beta-receptor blocker has been reported to reduce the risk of variceal bleeding.
   b. Band ligation of varices is safe and is as effective as in patients with other causes of varices (see Chapter 10).
   c. Surgical portosystemic shunts can be tried in patients in whom less invasive methods of treating varices fail.
   d. Splenectomy is effective in treating gastric varices resulting from isolated thrombosis of the splenic vein.
   e. The role of long-term anticoagulation in patients with underlying cirrhosis:
      - It has not been proven effective.
      - It is probably safe if patients are carefully selected.

Sinusoidal Obstruction Syndrome

DEFINITION AND ETIOLOGY

1. Sinusoidal obstruction syndrome (SOS) was originally described by Chiari in 1899, and was further described as hepatic vein endophlebitis by Bras in 1954. Histologic features include the following:
   - Subendothelial sclerosis of terminal hepatic venules
   - Thrombosis secondary to sclerosis
   - Sinusoidal fibrosis, particularly in later stages and with chronic injury
   - Centrilobular hepatocyte necrosis (may be a primary event)
2. SOS (formerly referred to as **veno-occlusive disease**) is most often seen
   - in an **acute form** following bone marrow transplantation (BMT) or hematopoietic stem cell transplantation. It is thought to result from toxicity from the preparative regimen of high-dose cytoreductive therapy, with or without hepatic irradiation.
   - in a **chronic, more indolent form** following toxicity of pyrrolizidine alkaloids from plants of the *Crotalaria, Senecio,* and *Heliotropium* genera. The alkaloids are ingested in the form of herbal teas, hence the term Jamaican bush tea disease.
3. Using a definition of SOS based on clinical manifestations (see later), no single histologic feature is pathognomonic. A correlation exists between the number of histologic abnormalities and the clinical severity of SOS.

CLINICAL FEATURES

1. SOS following BMT has been defined as the occurrence of two or more of the following characteristics appearing within 20 days after transplantation:
   - Painful hepatomegaly
   - Sudden weight gain of more than 2% of baseline body weight
   - Total serum bilirubin level greater than 2.0 mg/dL (34.2 μmol/L)

2. The occurrence of SOS is significantly correlated with the subsequent development of renal insufficiency, pleural effusions, heart failure, pulmonary infiltrates, and bleeding requiring blood transfusions.
3. CT may be helpful in distinguishing SOS from graft-versus-host (GVH) disease. Patients with SOS have periportal edema, ascites, and a narrow right hepatic vein, whereas those with GVH disease often have thickening of the small bowel.
4. Using clinical definitions, up to 50% of patients with BMT develop SOS. The mortality rate for all patients with clinical evidence of SOS is 30% to 40%.
5. The more chronic form of SOS develops in persons who ingest pyrrolizidine alkaloids. Clinical features of this condition are similar to those of hepatic vein occlusion and include tender hepatomegaly, abdominal pain, ascites, and fatigue. The absence of specific features and the lack of noninvasive methods for detecting this condition make diagnosis difficult. Liver biopsy specimens usually show sinusoidal and perivenular fibrosis, as well as subendothelial sclerosis. Poisoning is most often inadvertent and can result from contamination of foodstuffs with pyrrolizidine-containing plants.

RISK FACTORS FOR ACUTE SOS FOLLOWING BMT OR HSCT

1. Risk factors for SOS occurring after BMT include the following:
   - Pretransplant elevation in serum aspartate aminotransferase (AST) or alanine aminotransferase (ALT) levels
   - Past history of viral or drug-induced hepatitis
   - Past history of abdominal radiation
   - Older or very young (less than 6.5 years) recipient age
   - Poor pretransplant performance status and reduced pulmonary diffusion capacity
2. More intensive myeloablative cytoreductive regimens are associated with an increased frequency of SOS:
   - Radiation dose greater than 12 Gy
   - Cyclophosphamide plus busulfan
   - Cyclophosphamide, carmustine (BCNU), and etoposide

PATHOGENESIS

1. Cytoreductive therapy is toxic primarily to endothelial cells, both sinusoidal and vascular. These cells are more susceptible to glutathione depletion in response to various agents, including dacarbazine, azathioprine, and monocrotaline.
2. Various cytokines including tumor necrosis factor alpha (TNF-α) are released in response to cytoreductive therapy. Patients with hepatic failure and multiorgan failure syndrome have been shown to have high circulating levels of TNF-α and other cytokines. TNF in particular exerts procoagulant effects on protein C and may be involved in the pathogenesis of thrombosis in SOS; however, much of the pathophysiology is speculative at present.

TREATMENT

1. Treatment of SOS following BMT is largely supportive:
   - Excessive fluid administration, which results in worsening of cardiac and pulmonary function, should be avoided.
   - Support with platelet and red blood cell transfusions is often necessary because of the profound cytopenias that accompany BMT.
   - Use of dopamine and other pressors is often necessary to maintain renal perfusion, particularly in the presence of a capillary leak syndrome.
   - Broad-spectrum antibiotics are used to treat presumptive infection, pending identification of a specific causative organism.
2. **Defibrotide**, a polydisperse mixture of single-stranded oligonucleotide, may be of benefit in treating severe SOS, with a complete remission rate of 30% to 60%.
   - Antithrombin may be of benefit in preventing progression of SOS if given early in the course of the illness.
   - Prostaglandin E, ursodeoxycholic acid, pentoxifylline, and heparin all have had limited success in preventing SOS.
   - TIPS is technically feasible and has been of benefit in a small number of patients with SOS.
3. Treatment of chronic SOS associated with ingestion of pyrrolizidine alkaloids often requires liver transplantation because of the extensive fibrosis that is usually present at the time of diagnosis. Early cases may be managed with a portosystemic shunt.

FURTHER READING

Beckett D, Olliff S. Interventional radiology in the management of Budd–Chiari syndrome. *Cardiovasc Intervent Radiol* 2008; 31:839–847.

Buckley O, O'Brien J, Snow A, et al. Imaging of Budd–Chiari syndrome. *Eur Radiol* 2007; 17:2071–2078.

Garcia-Pagan JC, Heydtmann M, Raffa S, et al. TIPS for Budd–Chiari syndrome: long-term results and prognostics factors in 124 patients. *Gastroenterology* 2008; 135:808–815.

Hernandez-Guerra M, Turnes J, Rubinstein P, et al. PTFE-covered stents improve TIPS patency in Budd–Chiari syndrome. *Hepatology* 2004; 40:1197–1202.

Janssen HLA, Garcia-Pagan JC, Elias E, et al. Budd–Chiari syndrome: a review by an expert panel. *J Hepatol* 2003; 38:364–371.

Janssen HLA, Meinardi JR, Vleggaar FP, et al. Factor V Leiden mutation, prothrombin gene mutation, and deficiencies in coagulation inhibitors associated with Budd–Chiari syndrome and portal vein thrombosis: results of a case-control study. *Blood* 2000; 96:2364–2368.

Kamath PS. Budd–Chiari syndrome: radiologic findings. *Liver Transplant* 2006; 12(Suppl):S21–S22.

Mentha G, Giostra E, Majno PE, et al. Liver transplantation for Budd–Chiari syndrome: a European study on 248 patients from 51 centres. *J Hepatol* 2006; 44:520–528.

Narayanan Menon KV, Shah V, Kamath PS. The Budd–Chiari syndrome. *N Engl J Med* 2004; 350:578–585.

Orloff MJ, Daily PO, Orloff SL, et al. A 27-year experience with surgical treatment of Budd–Chiari syndrome. *Ann Surg* 2000; 232:340–352.

Parikh S, Shah R, Kapoor P. Portal vein thrombosis. *Am J Med* 2010; 123:111–119.

Plessier A, Sibert A, Consigny Y, et al. Aiming at minimal invasiveness as a therapeutic strategy for Budd–Chiari syndrome. *Hepatology* 2006; 44:1308–1316.

Reiss U, Cowan M, McMillan Horn B. Hepatic venoocclusive disease in blood and bone marrow transplantation in children and young adults: incidence, risk factors, and outcome in a cohort of 241 patients. *J Pediatr Hematol Oncol* 2002; 24:746–750.

Segev DL, Nguyen GC, Locke JE, et al. Twenty years of liver transplantation for Budd–Chiari syndrome: a national registry analysis. *Liver Transplant* 2007; 13:1285–1294.

Valla DC. Primary Budd–Chiari syndrome. *J Hepatol* 2009; 50:195–203.

CHAPTER 20

The liver in heart failure

Rania Rabie, MD, FRCP(C) ■ Florence S. Wong, MD, FRACP, FRCP(C)

KEY POINTS

1. Liver involvement (cardiac hepatopathy) in either forward or backward heart failure is frequent.

2. Backward heart failure causes congestion of the liver with hepatomegaly and nonspecific liver biochemical test abnormalities.

3. Forward heart failure causes ischemic damage to the liver if the circulatory failure is severe and prolonged. The pattern of a very rapid rise and fall in serum aminotransferase levels is characteristic.

4. Alternative diagnoses should be considered if abnormal liver biochemical test values are unusually high in the absence of an acute setting and, in particular, if the alkaline phosphatase level is more than twice normal or if the alanine aminotransferase (ALT) is much higher than the aspartate aminotransferase (AST) level.

5. The frequency and severity of liver involvement depend on the severity of heart failure, which determines prognosis unless cardiac cirrhosis is present.

6. No specific treatment is available for the liver dysfunction. Improvement in cardiac function results in return of liver biochemical test results to normal, unless cardiac cirrhosis is already present.

7. Cardiac surgery, including heart transplantation, carries a high mortality rate in patients with cirrhosis.

Overview

1. Liver dysfunction (cardiac hepatopathy) has long been recognized as a complication of both severe acute and chronic congestive heart failure.
2. Heart failure usually results from pump failure leading to decreased cardiac output, venous congestion, and retention of extracellular fluid.
3. An understanding of the hepatic circulation and normal liver architecture is important to appreciate how the hemodynamic changes of heart failure affect the liver and lead to the associated clinical, biochemical, and histologic features.

Hepatic Circulation

HEPATIC BLOOD SUPPLY

1. The liver has a dual blood supply:
   - The portal vein supplies approximately 66% to 83% of the blood flow to the liver and brings nutrient-rich but relatively less well-oxygenated venous blood from the stomach, intestine, and spleen.

- The hepatic artery, a branch of the celiac axis, provides the remaining 17% to 34% of the liver's blood supply; the arterial blood supplies approximately 50% of hepatic oxygen.
2. A reduction in portal inflow or hepatic sinusoidal pressure results in a reflex increase in hepatic arterial blood flow and thereby ensures a constant sinusoidal pressure.
3. Primary changes in hepatic arterial blood flow are not associated with changes in portal venous blood flow.
4. A decrease in cardiac output usually results in reduced hepatic blood flow. The percentage of cardiac output received by the liver, however, remains relatively stable.
5. Decreased perfusion is usually compensated for by increased oxygen extraction, which can increase up to 95%.
6. Hypercapnia, if present, causes generalized vasodilatation that increases blood flow to the liver further.

HEPATIC VENOUS DRAINAGE

1. The liver is drained by the hepatic vein, which is formed by the right, middle, and left hepatic veins.
2. The hepatic vein, in turn, drains into the inferior vena cava and then into the right atrium.

HEPATIC MICROCIRCULATION

1. The portal vein and the hepatic artery divide into branches to the right and left lobes of the liver. These branches further subdivide five to six times until their terminal branches reach the portal triads.
2. The portal vein tributaries open directly into hepatic sinusoids. The hepatic artery branches open into some but not all sinusoids. The sinusoids anastomose freely at all levels between the portal vein tributaries and the terminal hepatic venules.
3. Hepatic sinusoids have the following characteristics:
   - They form a rich vascular network that converges toward the terminal hepatic venule.
   - They are lined by both endothelial cells and specialized macrophages called Kupffer cells. No basement membrane underlies the endothelial cells.
   - The porous nature of the sinusoids allows for low hydrostatic pressure and free flow between the sinusoids and the interstitial space, the space of Disse.
   - The diameter of a sinusoid is less than that of erythrocytes, which therefore have to squeeze through the lumen of the sinusoid.
4. Narrowing of the sinusoidal lumen can seriously compromise oxygenation of hepatocytes.

Liver Architecture

1. The **histologic** unit of the liver is the **lobule** (Fig. 20.1A):
   - Its boundaries are surrounded by connective tissue stroma and portal triads.
   - The center of the lobule is the terminal hepatic vein.
2. The **functional** unit of the liver is the **acinus** (Fig. 20.1B):
   - Liver parenchymal cells are grouped into concentric zones centered around the portal triad; zone 1 is nearest, whereas zones 2 and 3 are more distal to the afferent blood vessels.
   - The oxygen tension and nutrient level of the blood decrease from zone 1 to zone 3.
   - Zone 1 hepatocytes are first to receive oxygenated blood and last to undergo necrosis.
   - Zones 2 and 3 receive blood of considerably less oxygen and nutrient content and are more vulnerable to hepatotoxins and hypoxic injury.

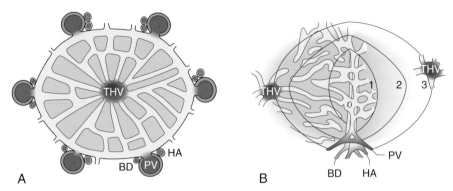

Fig. 20.1 **A,** The histologic unit of the liver: the lobule. **B,** The functional unit of the liver: the acinus. BD, bile duct; HA, hepatic artery; PV, portal vein; THV, terminal hepatic vein; 1, 2, 3, zones 1, 2, and 3 of Rappaport.

Pathophysiology

1. Hepatic ischemia develops when an imbalance occurs between hepatic oxygen supply and demand.
2. Forward failure of the heart leads to decreased cardiac output and hepatic blood flow.
3. Backward failure with venous engorgement causes hepatic congestion.
4. Both forward failure and backward failure of the heart lead to cellular hypoxia and liver damage.
5. Decreased arterial oxygen saturation also contributes to liver damage (Fig. 20.2).

CHRONIC PASSIVE CONGESTION

1. In heart failure with low cardiac output, total hepatic blood flow falls by approximately one third.
2. The increased systemic venous pressure is reflected as hepatic venous hypertension, which can cause hepatic cell atrophy as a result of sinusoidal congestion and expansion.
3. The accompanying perisinusoidal edema can result in decreased diffusion of oxygen and other metabolites to hepatocytes.
4. Collagenosis of the space of Disse from chronic congestion may play a minor role in impairing oxygen diffusion.
5. Low cardiac output and the consequent circulatory changes in the intestinal wall may allow increased diffusion of endotoxin into the portal blood and may augment damage to the liver.

DECREASED HEPATIC BLOOD FLOW

1. Increased oxygen extraction by the liver in states of low hepatic blood flow ensures constant oxygen consumption within wide limits of hepatic blood flow. The liver therefore does not suffer adverse effects of hypoxia as a result of decreased hepatic blood flow under basal conditions.
2. A greater than 70% reduction in hepatic blood flow decreases oxygen uptake, galactose elimination capacity, and adenosine triphosphate concentrations and increases the lactate/pyruvate ratio (an index of tissue hypoxia).
3. Hepatic arterial vasoconstriction with intense selective splanchnic vasoconstriction in states of significant hypoperfusion and shock causes hypoxic damage to the liver.

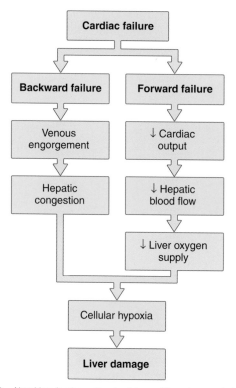

Fig. 20.2 Algorithm for the pathophysiology of liver damage in heart failure.

4. Hypoxic damage characteristically occurs in the area adjacent to the terminal hepatic vein (zone 3 of the acinus), the area farthest away from the oxygen-carrying blood supply.
5. Insufficient concentrations of substrates, accumulation of metabolites, and release of cytokines secondary to an inflammatory response all contribute to hypoxic damage even in the presence of systemic circulatory support.
6. Loss of mitochondrial oxidative phosphorylation, as a result of hypoxia, leads to impaired membrane function, disrupted intracellular ion homeostasis, and reduced protein synthesis.
7. Reperfusion injury can aggravate hepatic injury through the generation of reactive oxygen species once ischemic hepatocytes are reexposed to oxygen.
8. In acute heart failure, both reduced hepatic blood flow and increased central venous pressure contribute to the development of ischemic (or hypoxic) hepatitis.

Pathology

MACROSCOPIC

1. The liver is enlarged and purplish with rounded edges (Fig. 20.3).
2. Nodularity is inconspicuous, but if nodular regenerative hyperplasia (see later) or cardiac cirrhosis is present, nodules may be seen.

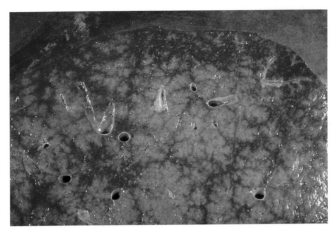

Fig. 20.3 Macroscopic appearance of the liver in heart failure.

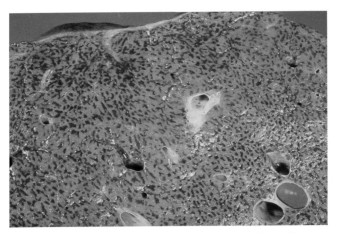

Fig. 20.4 Cut surface of the liver in heart failure showing the "nutmeg" appearance.

3. The cut surface shows prominent hepatic veins, which may be thickened.
4. A **"nutmeg" appearance** results from the contrasting combination of hemorrhagic central areas of the lobules and the normal yellow portal and periportal areas (Fig. 20.4).
5. Yellower than usual portal areas may be caused by an increase in portal fat.

MICROSCOPIC

1. The severity of hepatic histopathologic changes generally correlates with the clinical or biochemical severity of heart failure and with cardiac weight and chamber size.
2. Early in heart failure, the terminal hepatic veins become engorged and dilated. Sinusoids adjacent to the terminal hepatic veins are also dilated and are filled with erythrocytes for a variable extent toward the portal areas. In severe cases, the appearance is that of **peliosis hepatis** (blood lakes).

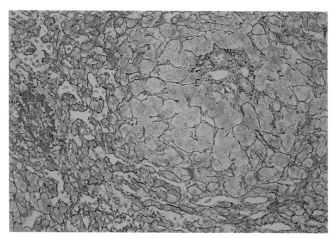

Fig. 20.5 Histopathology of the liver demonstrating collapse of the reticulin network around the terminal hepatic veins and nodular transformation in a patient with heart failure (Gordon & Sweet reticulin).

3. Also evident are compression and variable atrophy of the liver cell plates and an apparent increase in the amount of lipofuscin in the cytoplasm of liver cells.
4. Moderately severe heart failure can result in zone 3 liver cell necrosis. The cellular infiltrate is inconspicuous.
5. In acute severe hypotension and shock, midzone necrosis can also occur.
6. The necrotic hepatocytes are often packed with a brownish pigment, which probably is related to bilirubin degradation.
7. Liver cell necrosis progresses from zone 3 to the portal areas as the heart disease progresses. In the most severe form of liver congestion from heart failure, only a small area of normal-appearing hepatocytes remains in the periportal area.
8. The reticulin network condenses and may collapse around the terminal hepatic vein following loss of liver cells (Fig. 20.5).
   - Bridging can be seen extending from and joining adjacent terminal hepatic veins.
   - Ultimately, the unaffected portal areas are surrounded by rings of fibrous tissue, resulting in reverse lobulation.
9. True **cardiac cirrhosis** is rare. When present, it is associated with intimal fibrosis and thrombosis of small and medium-sized hepatic veins. The resulting ischemia is responsible for hepatocellular necrosis, and the stasis augments fibroblast activation and collagen deposition.
10. Regeneration of hepatocytes around the periportal area can occur, leading to liver cell plates that are many cells thick. These regenerating hepatocytes can reorganize into rounded periportal masses abutting compressed central hepatocytes and congested and dilated sinusoids. Such changes are best described as **nodular regenerative hyperplasia** (Fig. 20.6).
11. The wall of the terminal hepatic vein can undergo varying degrees of fibrous thickening called **phlebosclerosis** (Fig. 20.7).
12. Liver damage associated with heart failure is reversible once the heart failure is treated: hepatocytes regenerate, fibrous bands become narrower and acellular, and near-normal hepatic architecture is restored.

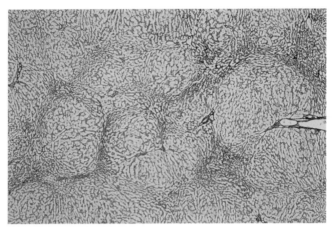

Fig. 20.6 Histopathology of the liver demonstrating nodular regenerative hyperplasia associated with heart failure (Gordon & Sweet reticulin).

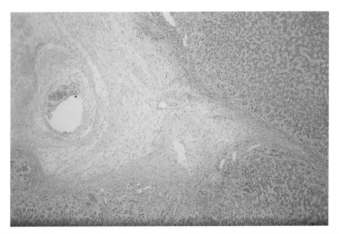

Fig. 20.7 Histopathology of the liver demonstrating phlebosclerosis in the wall of the terminal hepatic vein in a patient with heart failure (Masson trichrome).

Etiology (Table 20.1)

1. Left and right ventricular failure can often coexist, resulting in hepatic congestion.
2. Acute myocardial infarction with arrhythmia and cardiogenic shock can complicate coronary artery disease, with resulting ischemic hepatitis superimposed on the chronic hepatic congestion.
3. Rheumatic heart disease, with mitral stenosis and tricuspid regurgitation, appears to produce the most severe hepatic congestion.
4. The abrupt onset of atrial fibrillation or the development of bacterial endocarditis can decrease left ventricular output and can aggravate hypoxic liver damage.

TABLE 20.1 ■ **Causes of cardiac hepatopathy**

Cause	Percentage of total (%)
Cardiomyopathy	49
Valvular disease	23
Pericardial disease	17
Pulmonary disease	9
Mixed causes	2

Adapted from Myers RP, Cerini R, Sayegh R, *et al*. Cardiac hepatopathy: clinical, hemodynamic, and histologic characteristics and correlations. *Hepatology* 2003; 37:393–400.

5. Children with hypoplastic left heart syndrome and coarctation of the aorta are particularly prone to hepatic necrosis, possibly because of the combination of reduced systemic blood flow, a left-to-right shunt, and markedly elevated right ventricular pressure.
6. Conditions that cause both liver disease and heart failure include excess alcohol consumption, hemochromatosis, hepatitis C, infiltrative diseases such as amyloidosis, and vascular tumors of the liver such as hemangioendothelioma.
7. Some drugs used in cardiovascular disease can cause liver damage, such as steatosis and fibrosis, which may rarely progress to cirrhosis, as is the case with amiodarone.

Frequency

1. Liver involvement is common in severe heart failure.
2. As the incidence of rheumatic valve disease has declined, coronary artery disease with associated congestive cardiomyopathy has become an important cause of liver congestion.
3. The overall frequency of liver congestion in congestive cardiac failure depends on patient selection and the criteria used for defining liver involvement (clinical, biochemical, or histologic).
4. In patients with a cardiac index higher than 2 L/minute/m², only 20% to 30% of patients have minor elevations of serum liver enzyme levels. In contrast, in those with a cardiac index lower than 1.5 L/minute/m², up to 80% of patients have major liver biochemical abnormalities.

Clinical Features

CONGESTIVE HEPATOPATHY

1. In most patients, the clinical picture is dominated by symptoms and signs of right-sided heart failure, rather than those of liver disease (Table 20.2).
2. Stigmata of liver disease, such as palmar erythema, spider telangiectasias, and caput medusae are rare, unless the liver disease and heart failure have a common cause, such as hemochromatosis.
3. Right upper quadrant pain results from stretching of the liver capsule and is mediated by the phrenic nerve.

TABLE 20.2 ■ **Characteristics of patients with cardiac hepatopathy**

Characteristic	Acute heart failure (% of total)	Chronic heart failure (% of total)
Hepatomegaly	83	76
Jaundice	50	11
Ascites	42	68
Encephalopathy	25	2
Splenomegaly	8	15
Esophageal varices	0	8

Adapted from Myers RP, Cerini R, Sayegh R, *et al.* Cardiac hepatopathy: clinical, hemodynamic, and histologic characteristics and correlations. *Hepatology* 2003; 37:393–400.

4. The liver can return to normal size as fibrosis develops during the course of severe hepatic congestion, but it is never reduced in size.
5. Jaundice
   ■ Mild jaundice is common, but deep icterus is rare.
   ■ Jaundice increases with prolonged and repeated bouts of heart failure.
   ■ Hyperbilirubinemia may be in part unconjugated, related to infarcts of tissues, especially pulmonary infarcts. Jaundice may then be prolonged, with conjugated hyperbilirubinemia because of the inability of the hypoxic liver to handle the bilirubin load.
6. Patients with tricuspid regurgitation have a palpable systolic pulsation over the liver, related to the transmission of right atrial pressure to the hepatic vein.
7. Splenomegaly is frequent, but other features of portal hypertension are usually absent, except in severe cardiac cirrhosis associated with constrictive pericarditis.
8. Ascites is most likely related to increased sinusoidal pressure and permeability and increased leakage of lymph, rather than cirrhosis. As a result, the ascitic protein content is high (2.5 g/dL or higher), with a high serum-ascites albumin gradient (1.1 g/dL or higher).
9. Peripheral edema and pleural effusions probably reflect the cardiac disease, rather than the concomitant hepatic congestion.

ISCHEMIC HEPATITIS

1. This term refers to diffuse hepatic injury as a result of acute hypoperfusion.
   ■ The term *ischemic hepatitis* is a misnomer, because liver injury is characterized by centrilobular necrosis without inflammation.
   ■ Ischemic hepatitis as a result of low cardiac output may not be clinically obvious. A "shock" state is observed in only 50% of cases, and hypotension is not always documented; therefore, the left-sided heart failure may be subtle.
2. Usually, no specific symptoms result from liver injury, but occasional patients have symptoms of acute hepatitis (see Chapter 3).
   ■ Some patients have changes in mental status that more commonly reflect impaired cerebral perfusion than hepatic encephalopathy.
3. Hepatopulmonary syndrome develops in up to half of patients but is reversible.
4. Occasionally, functional renal failure (increased serum creatinine and potassium, low urinary sodium, and normal urinary sediment) occurs abruptly.

5. Fulminant hepatic failure with asterixis and coma as a complication of heart failure is rare. It usually develops 2 to 3 days after the circulatory failure. Serum aminotransferase levels can rise to more than 1000 U/L. Prognosis is poor; half of the patients die of the underlying cardiac disease.

CARDIAC CIRRHOSIS

1. Cardiac cirrhosis is rare, and the presentation is usually dominated by symptoms of right-sided heart failure.
2. Cardiac cirrhosis should be suspected in a patient with well-documented tricuspid regurgitation and absent hepatic pulsation.
3. Cardiac cirrhosis should also be considered in patients with the following:
   - Severe mitral stenosis
   - Constrictive pericarditis
   - Prolonged or recurrent severe congestive heart failure
   - Clinically severe passive congestion of the liver, yet a nonenlarged liver, with splenomegaly and ascites

COMMON CAUSES OF COMBINED LIVER DISEASE AND HEART FAILURE

- Hemochromatosis is suggested by an iron saturation greater than 50%, increased serum ferritin level, an increased hepatic iron index, and the *HFE* gene mutation (see Chapter 16).
- Long-term, excessive alcohol consumption can lead to alcoholic cirrhosis and alcoholic cardiomyopathy; the diagnosis is based on the patient's history (see Chapter 6).
- The metabolic syndrome is characterized by abdominal obesity, hypertension, diabetes mellitus, and dyslipidemia and is associated with nonalcoholic fatty liver disease and atherosclerosis (see Chapter 7).
- Hepatitis C is diagnosed by antibody to hepatitis C virus (anti-HCV) and by HCV RNA in serum (see Chapters 3 and 4).

Laboratory Features

CONGESTIVE HEPATOPATHY

The frequency of abnormal liver biochemical test levels in patients with heart failure varies widely in the published literature, most likely because of the heterogeneity of the patients described. No absolute correlation exists between the clinical severity of heart failure and abnormalities of liver biochemical test values. In general, however, patients with higher right atrial pressures and more profound clinical manifestations of heart failure tend to have more abnormal levels.

1. Bilirubin
- Increased serum bilirubin levels occur in 15% to 50% of patients with heart failure. **Jaundice is usually mild in heart failure**, with serum bilirubin levels generally less than 4.5 mg/dL (80 mmol/L).
- Approximately 50% to 60% of the serum bilirubin is unconjugated, because of a combination of mild hemolysis, reduced uptake, and decreased conjugation by hepatocytes.
- Markedly elevated serum bilirubin levels may be seen in acute right-sided heart failure. The hyperbilirubinemia appears to be related to hepatocellular dysfunction per se.

- Serum bilirubin levels may fall rapidly after improvement in hepatic congestion, with levels normalizing in 3 to 7 days.
- In patients with prolonged heart failure, serum bilirubin levels may not return to normal for many months after relief of the hepatic congestion because of covalent bonding of conjugated bilirubin with albumin to form *delta bilirubin*, which has a prolonged half-life of 21 days.
- An elevated total bilirubin level is an independent predictor of adverse cardiac outcome and death in patients with heart failure.
- In patients who undergo heart transplantation, direct and indirect bilirubin levels more than three times normal are significant negative predictors of survival after discharge.

2. Aminotransferases

- Levels are elevated in only 3% to 10% of patients with stable heart failure without decompensation. Levels are usually two to four times the upper limit of normal.
- **Markedly elevated levels** (more than 10 times the upper limit of normal) are seen in patients with acute worsening of severe chronic heart failure, hypotension, or shock, and indicate **ischemic hepatitis** (see later).
- **Aspartate aminotransferase (AST) levels tend to be higher than alanine aminotransferase (ALT) levels,** because of the AST-rich cardiac myocytes; the increase in AST generally appears earlier than the increase in ALT.
- Very high levels of AST can also be found in patients with drug-induced or viral hepatitis, but ALT levels are usually higher than AST levels in viral hepatitis (see Chapter 1).
- If the elevation of the AST level is caused by heart failure, the level can be expected to fall within a few days of circulatory improvement. In contrast, high levels of AST usually persist in cases of viral or drug-induced hepatitis and are independent of improvement in circulatory status.
- Moderate increases in AST levels can also be caused by myocardial infarction; consequent myocardial dysfunction and heart failure can complicate the interpretation of the elevated AST level. Simultaneous measurement of the troponin or the MB fraction of creatine kinase is helpful in diagnosing myocardial injury.
- A significant, albeit weak, correlation exists between the aminotransferase levels and both the right atrial pressure and the cardiac index. Improvement in cardiac function results in a return of serum aminotransferase levels toward normal in 3 to 7 days.

3. Alkaline phosphatase

- **Elevated alkaline phosphatase levels are uncommon in heart failure**. When present, the elevation is mild, usually not exceeding twice the upper limit of normal, unless the liver disease and heart failure have a common cause.
- The exact mechanism leading to an increased alkaline phosphatase level in patients with liver congestion is unknown. Both pressure-induced intrahepatic biliary obstruction and hepatic dysfunction may both play a role.
- When nodular regenerative hyperplasia complicates heart failure, the only abnormal liver biochemical test result may be an elevated serum alkaline phosphatase level.

4. International normalized ratio (INR)

- This value is **increased in more than 80% of patients** with heart failure.
- Prolongation of the prothrombin time is more common in acute than chronic hepatic congestion. In acute congestion, the prothrombin time may increase rapidly to twice normal, is not responsive to vitamin K administration, and may return to normal rapidly with successful treatment of the congestion.
- Affected patients are therefore very sensitive to the effects of warfarin.

- With successful treatment of chronic heart failure, the prothrombin time takes 2 to 3 weeks to return to normal.

5. Serum albumin

- This value is **moderately decreased in 30% to 50% of patients** with heart failure. Lower albumin levels are seen in patients with ascites and edema.
- The low serum albumin level may result in part from decreased hepatic synthesis and in part from a dilutional effect secondary to fluid retention.
- In general, the serum albumin level does not correlate with either the duration of heart failure or the extent of hepatic damage.
- The serum albumin level may require more than 1 month to improve following resolution of heart failure.

ISCHEMIC HEPATITIS

Changes in serum liver biochemical test levels in ischemic hepatitis are characteristic, and the diagnosis can be made by observing the following evolution of these changes:

- **Marked increases in aminotransferase levels with AST greater than ALT** (up to 100 times normal) occur within 24 to 48 hours of the acute circulatory failure.
- **A rapid return of the aminotransferase levels to normal** occurs in 3 to 11 days after treatment of acute heart failure.
- **A profound rise and fall in serum lactate dehydrogenase (LDH) levels,** moreso than the ALT, and an ALT/LDH ratio lower than 1.5 are more typical of ischemic hepatitis than of viral hepatitis.
- Alkaline phosphatase levels generally remain normal.
- Serum bilirubin levels may rise but are rarely greater than four times the upper limit of normal.
- INR is only mildly increased.

CARDIAC CIRRHOSIS

- No biochemical test distinguishes a congested noncirrhotic liver from one with cardiac cirrhosis.
- Therefore, **cardiac cirrhosis is a clinical and a histologic diagnosis.**

Radiologic Features

1. Doppler ultrasonography
   - Biphasic waveforms in the presence of cirrhosis
2. Contrast-enhanced computed tomography (CT)
   - Lobulated, patchy, and inhomogeneous pattern in a large liver
   - Irregular perivascular enhancement or delayed parenchymal enhancement
   - Distended inferior vena cava and early reflux of contrast medium into the inferior vena cava and hepatic veins
3. Transient elastography (Fibroscan)
   - A rapid and noninvasive measure of liver stiffness; a surrogate for liver fibrosis and validated in alcoholic liver disease and viral hepatitis
   - Apparently less reliable in heart failure because liver stiffness measurements are directly related to central venous pressure

Treatment

1. Treatment of liver congestion should be directed toward the primary problem, that is, heart failure.
2. Improvement in liver biochemical test levels usually follows clinical improvement unless cardiac cirrhosis is already present.
3. Management of established cardiac cirrhosis includes treatment of heart failure as well as paracentesis if refractory ascites is present.
   - Regular replacement of albumin after paracentesis is unnecessary because synthetic hepatic function is preserved.
   - No recommendations exist for screening for hepatocellular carcinoma (HCC) as in other causes of cirrhosis (see Chapter 27), but cases of HCC arising in cardiac cirrhosis have been reported.
   - Focal nodular hyperplasia nodules can also be found in patients with cardiac cirrhosis. The differential diagnosis includes macronodular regenerative nodules, dysplastic nodules, and HCC. Biopsy of the nodule may be required to make the diagnosis definitively.

CARDIAC SURGERY

1. Clinical improvement in cardiac function can be dramatic following definitive treatment of heart failure such as valve replacement, pericardiectomy for constrictive pericarditis, or correction of a congenital anomaly.
2. Cardiac cirrhosis with or without hepatic failure, however, results in a substantial rise in the perioperative mortality rate and may therefore be a contraindication to surgery (see Chapter 30).
   - Compensated Child class A patients appear to tolerate cardiac surgery satisfactorily, whereas Child class B and C patients have high rates of major postoperative complications and death.
   - A Child-Turcotte-Pugh score greater than 7 has a high sensitivity (86%) and specificity (92%) for predicting mortality after cardiac surgery with cardiopulmonary bypass and in one study performed better than the Model for End-stage Liver Disease (MELD) score in this setting (see Chapter 30).
   - Cardiopulmonary bypass may aggravate preexisting coagulopathy by leading to platelet dysfunction, fibrinolysis, and hypocalcemia. Limited evidence suggests that less invasive procedures such as angioplasty, valvuloplasty, and revascularization procedures without bypass are preferable in patients with cirrhosis.
3. Liver cirrhosis has generally been considered a contraindication to heart transplantation. In the few cases of heart transplantation performed in patients with liver cirrhosis, a 50% in-hospital mortality rate was reported.
   - Mortality was highest in patients with a cardiac diagnosis other than cardiomyopathy and in those with a previous sternotomy and massive ascites.
   - Combined heart and liver transplantation is feasible in carefully selected patients in expert centers.

Prognosis

1. The prognosis of liver dysfunction in the setting of cardiac disease is that of the underlying cardiac disease.

2. In chronic heart failure, the outcome will be favorable if the underlying cardiac condition is treated and the hepatic congestion resolves.
3. In ischemic hepatitis, the prognosis is often poor. Prolonged jaundice, especially if severe, is a poor prognostic sign.
4. Death in ischemic hepatitis is usually the result of heart failure. The hepatic disorder usually has little or no influence on the eventual outcome.
5. Cardiac cirrhosis in and of itself does not alter prognosis in general unless cardiac surgery is performed.

FURTHER READING

Allen LA, Felker GM, Pocock S, et al. Liver function abnormalities and outcome in patients with chronic heart failure: data from the Candesartan in heart failure. Assessment of reduction in mortality and morbidity (CHARM) program. *Eur J Heart Fail* 2009; 11:170–177.

Dichtl W, Vogel W, Dunst KM, et al. Cardiac hepatopathy before and after heart transplantation. *Transpl Int* 2005; 18:697–702.

Giallourakis CC, Rosenberg PM, Friedman LS. The liver in heart failure. *Clin Liver Dis* 2002; 6:947–967.

Henrion J, Schapira M, Luwaert R, et al. Hypoxic hepatitis: clinical and hemodynamic study in 142 consecutive cases. *Medicine (Baltimore)* 2003; 82:392–406.

Hsu RB, Chang CI, Lin FY, et al. Heart transplantation in patients with liver cirrhosis. *Eur J Cardiothorac Surg* 2008; 34:307–312.

Millonig G, Friedrich S, Adolf S, et al. Liver stiffness is directly influenced by central venous pressure. *J Hepatol* 2010; 52:206–210.

Myers RP, Cerini R, Sayegh R, et al. Cardiac hepatopathy: clinical, hemodynamic, and histologic characteristics and correlations. *Hepatology* 2003; 37:393–400.

Naschitz JE, Slobodin G, Lewis RJ, et al. Heart diseases affecting the liver and liver diseases affecting the heart. *Am Heart J* 2000; 140:111–120.

Raichlin E, Daly RC, Rosen CB, et al. Combined heart and liver transplantation: a single-center experience. *Transplantation* 2009; 88:219–225.

Shaheen AM, Kaplan GG, Hubbard JN, et al. Morbidity and mortality following coronary artery bypass graft surgery in patients with cirrhosis: a population-based study. *Liver Int* 2009; 29:1141–1151.

Shiffman ML. The liver in circulatory failure. In: Schiff ER, Sorrell MF, Maddrey WC, eds. *Schiff's Diseases of the Liver*. 10th edn. Philadelphia: Lippincott Williams & Wilkins; 2006:1185–1198.

Suman A, Barnes DS, Zein NN, et al. Predicting outcome after cardiac surgery in patients with cirrhosis: a comparison of Child-Pugh and MELD scores. *Clin Gastroenterol Hepatol* 2004; 2:719–723.

Teh SH, Nagorney DM, Stevens SR, et al. Risk factors for mortality after surgery in patients with cirrhosis. *Gastroenterology* 2007; 132:1261–1269.

Vandeursen VM, Damman K, Hillege HL, et al. Abnormal liver function in relation to hemodynamic profile in heart failure patients. *J Card Failure* 2010; 16:84–90.

Wanless IR, Liu JJ, Butany J. Role of thrombosis in the pathogenesis of congestive hepatic fibrosis (cardiac cirrhosis). *Hepatology* 1995; 21:1232–1237.

CHAPTER 21

The liver in pregnancy

Michelle Lai, MD, MPH ■ Jacqueline L. Wolf, MD

KEY POINTS

1 Liver diseases in pregnancy include those that occur exclusively in pregnancy and those that occur coincidentally in pregnancy or are present at the time of pregnancy.

2 Normal physiologic changes in pregnancy may alter the normal range for liver biochemical tests (Table 21.1).

3 Important clues to the diagnosis are found in the history and physical examination.

4 Laboratory findings with particular importance to diagnosing liver disease in pregnancy are proteinuria, hyperuricemia, elevated serum bile acid levels, thrombocytopenia, and anemia.

5 Abdominal ultrasonography may be helpful. Liver biopsy is rarely necessary, but it may be diagnostic for acute fatty liver of pregnancy.

6 Timely diagnosis and hence appropriate treatment are critical to outcome. Delivery of the infant is indicated for severe pre-eclampsia, eclampsia, acute fatty liver of pregnancy, and HELLP (hemolysis, elevated liver tests, low platelets) syndrome, and immunization is indicated in infants born to mothers with hepatitis B.

7 Although women with chronic liver disease may have more trouble conceiving, pregnancy has no adverse effect on the progression of liver disease.

Overview

1. Liver diseases in pregnancy consist of the following:
   - Those that occur exclusively during pregnancy
   - Those that occur coincidentally in pregnancy or are present at the time of pregnancy
2. The approach to the pregnant patient with abnormal liver biochemical test levels should include thorough history taking and physical examination.
3. Liver disorders unique to pregnancy include the following:
   - Hyperemesis gravidarum
   - Intrahepatic cholestasis of pregnancy (IHCP)
   - Acute fatty liver of pregnancy (AFLP)
   - Pre-eclampsia/eclampsia
   - HELLP (hemolysis, elevated liver tests, low platelets) syndrome
   - Hepatic rupture
4. Liver disorders that occur coincidentally with pregnancy include viral hepatitis, Budd–Chiari syndrome, cholelithiasis, and cholecystitis, Wilson disease, and autoimmune hepatitis (AIH).

TABLE 21.1 ■ Changes in liver biochemical test levels in normal pregnancy

Test	Change	Trimester of maximum change
Albumin	↓ 10%–60%	Second
Gamma globulins	None to slight ↓	Third
Fibrinogen	↑ 50%	Second
Transferrin	↑	Third
Bilirubin	None	—
Alkaline phosphatase	↑ Two- to fourfold	Third
AST	None	—
ALT	None	—
Cholesterol	↑ Twofold	Third

↑, increase; ↓, decrease; ALT, alanine aminotransferase; AST, aspartate aminotransferase.

From Olans LB, Wolf JL. Liver disease in pregnancy. In: Carlson KJ, Eisenstat SA, eds. *The Primary Care of Women,* 2nd edn. St. Louis: Mosby–Year Book; 2003:531–539.

Approach to the Pregnant Patient

HISTORY

1. Relation to time of gestation (Table 21.2)
2. Pruritus
   - Characteristic of IHCP
   - Affects palms of hands and soles of feet initially, then elsewhere
3. Nausea and vomiting
   - Occurs in 50% to 90% of all pregnancies
   - Key feature of hyperemesis gravidarum
   - When associated with headache and peripheral edema may indicate pre-eclampsia
   - When associated in late pregnancy with abdominal pain, with or without hypotension, may indicate hepatic rupture
4. Abdominal pain
   - The location, character, duration, and factors that induce or relieve pain should be noted
   - Right upper quadrant or midabdominal pain in late pregnancy may have ominous implications. Consider cholelithiasis, AFLP, hepatic rupture, and pre-eclampsia
5. Jaundice
   - Note the relation of jaundice to the onset of other symptoms
   - Jaundice follows pruritus in IHCP
6. Systemic symptoms
   - Headache, peripheral edema, foamy urine, oliguria, and neurologic symptoms may occur in pre-eclampsia
   - Fever, malaise, and a change in stools may indicate infection such as hepatitis
   - Easy bruisability may occur in HELLP syndrome
   - Weight loss or gain or dizziness may occur with liver disease in pregnancy
7. History of past pregnancy and birth control use
   - Note the time of onset of symptoms in previous pregnancies

TABLE 21.2 ■ **Differential diagnosis of elevated serum aminotransferase levels and/or jaundice according to trimester of pregnancy**

Trimester	Differential diagnosis
First	Hyperemesis gravidarum
	Gallstones
	Viral hepatitis
	Drug-induced hepatitis
	Intrahepatic cholestasis of pregnancy*
Second	Intrahepatic cholestasis of pregnancy
	Gallstones
	Viral hepatitis
	Drug-induced hepatitis
	Pre-eclampsia/eclampsia*
	HELLP syndrome*
Third	Intrahepatic cholestasis of pregnancy
	Pre-eclampsia/eclampsia
	HELLP syndrome
	Acute fatty liver of pregnancy
	Hepatic rupture
	Gallstones
	Viral hepatitis
	Drug-induced hepatitis

*Uncommon in this trimester.

HELLP, hemolysis, elevated liver tests, low platelets.

From Olans LB, Wolf J. Liver disease in pregnancy. In: Carlson KJ, Eisenstat SA, eds. *The Primary Care of Women*, 2nd edn. St. Louis: Mosby–Year Book; 2003:531–539.

- Note the outcome of previous pregnancies
- A history of jaundice with previous birth control use is a risk factor for IHCP
8. Relevant pregnancy-related factors
   - Multiple versus single gestation (Table 21.3)
   - Primiparous versus multiparous
   - Medications

PHYSICAL EXAMINATION

- Normal findings that occur in pregnancy include spider telangiectasias and palmar erythema
- Abnormal findings that occur with liver disease in pregnancy are jaundice, hepatomegaly, hepatic tenderness, friction rub or bruit, splenomegaly, Murphy's sign, and diffuse excoriations
- Systemic findings that may occur with liver disease in pregnancy are hypertension, orthostatic hypotension, peripheral edema, asterixis, hyperreflexia or other neurologic findings, ecchymoses, and petechiae

TABLE 21.3 ■ **Rates of recurrence of pregnancy-associated liver disease in subsequent pregnancies**

Disease	Rate of recurrence
Intrahepatic cholestasis of pregnancy	40%–70%
HELLP syndrome	4%–27%
Acute fatty liver of pregnancy	20%–70% in carriers of LCHAD mutation
Pre-eclampsia	2%–43%

HELLP, hemolysis, elevated liver tests, low platelets; LCHAD, long-chain 3-hydroxyacyl-coenzyme A dehydrogenase.

DIAGNOSTIC TESTS

- The only major restrictions compared with the nongravid state are radiation and gadolinium exposures
- Routine blood chemistry tests and a blood count are helpful. Uric acid levels are often elevated in AFLP and may be elevated in pre-eclampsia
- Hemolysis and a low platelet count occur in HELLP syndrome. Disseminated intravascular coagulation (DIC) with a low fibrinogen level, increased fibrin split products, and an elevated partial thromboplastin time may also occur in HELLP syndrome
- Elevations in the serum bile acid level occur before or are concurrent with the onset of IHCP
- Amylase and lipase levels should be checked in a patient with abdominal pain
- If viral hepatitis is suspected, serologic tests should be checked for the following: hepatitis A (immunoglobulin M [IgM] and IgG antibody to hepatitis A virus [anti-HAV]); hepatitis B (surface antigen [HBsAg] and antibody, core antibody, and, if HBsAg is positive, e antigen and antibody); hepatitis C (antibody to hepatitis C virus [anti-HCV] and possibly HCV RNA). If the patient has traveled to an endemic area, consider testing for hepatitis E (see Chapter 3)
- The benefits of endoscopy, including endoscopic retrograde cholangiopancreatography (ERCP), should be weighed against the risks in pregnancy. Risks include fetal hypoxia from sedative drugs or positioning. Sedative medications and radiation exposure should be minimized
- Abdominal ultrasonography is safe and useful
- Although abdominal computed tomography (CT) is more sensitive than abdominal ultrasonography for hepatic rupture and may yield more information, radiation exposure and the stability of the patient should be considered in decisions about the choice of imaging test
- Angiography is rarely needed for hepatic rupture
- Magnetic resonance imaging (MRI) is probably safe, although this is not conclusively proven. Gadolinium should not be used in pregnancy

Liver Disorders Unique to Pregnancy

See Table 21.4 for the laboratory findings associated with these disorders.

HYPEREMESIS GRAVIDARUM

1. **Definition:** Intractable vomiting in pregnancy that leads to dehydration, electrolyte disturbances, weight loss of 5% or more, and nutritional deficiencies.

TABLE 21.4 ■ **Results of laboratory tests in pregnancy-associated liver disease**

	Aminotrans-ferases*	Bile acids*	Bilirubin	Alkaline phosphatase*	Uric acid	Platelets	PT/PTT	Urine protein
Hyperemesis gravidarum	1–2×	Normal	<5 mg/dL	1–2×	Normal	Normal	Normal	Normal
Intrahepatic cholestasis of pregnancy	1–4×	30–100×	<5 mg/dL	1–2×	Normal	Normal	Normal	Normal
Acute fatty liver of pregnancy	1–5×	Normal	<10 mg/dL	1–2×	↑	±↓	±↑	±↑
Pre-eclampsia/eclampsia	1–100×	Normal	<5 mg/dL	1–2×	↑	±↓	±↑	↑
HELLP syndrome	1–100×	Normal	<5 mg/dL	1–2×	↑	↓	±↑	±↑
Hepatic rupture	2–100×	Normal	±↑	↑	Normal	±↓	±↑	Normal

*Results are indicated as times the upper limit of normal.

PT, prothrombin time; PTT, partial thromboplastin time.

2. **Epidemiology**
   - Most common in first trimester
   - Incidence: 0.3% to 2%
   - Risk factors: age less than 25 years, preexisting diabetes mellitus, hyperthyroidism, overweight, primiparity, multiple gestations, prior history of hyperemesis gravidarum, and molar pregnancy
3. **Etiology:** Thought to be multifactorial involving immunologic, hormonal, and psychological factors.
4. **Clinical and laboratory features**
   - Liver biochemical test abnormalities in 50% of patients
   - Serum alanine aminotransferase (ALT) elevations generally 1- to 3-fold but may reach 20 times the upper limit of normal
   - Occasional serum alkaline phosphatase and bilirubin elevations
   - Concomitant hyperthyroidism in 50%
5. **Diagnosis:** clinical.
6. **Treatment:** Supportive with rehydration, vitamin supplementation, small and frequent low-fat meals, and antiemetics (e.g., metoclopramide 10 to 30 mg orally four times daily or 10 mg intramuscularly or intravenously every 4 to 6 hours or ondansetron 4 to 8 mg orally every 8 hours or 8 mg intravenously every 4 to 8 hours); total parenteral nutrition possibly needed in severe cases.
7. **Outcome:** Observed lower rate of spontaneous abortion, but also lower birth weights and increased incidence of congenital hip dysplasia in infants.

INTRAHEPATIC CHOLESTASIS OF PREGNANCY

1. **Definition:** Reversible form of cholestasis characterized by intense pruritus in pregnancy, elevated serum ALT and fasting serum bile acid levels, and spontaneous relief of symptoms and signs within 4 to 6 weeks after delivery.
2. **Epidemiology**
   - More common in late second or third trimester, but can occur in any trimester
   - Incidence: 0.01% to 2%, with higher incidence in South Asian, South American, and Scandinavian populations; highest incidence (up to 27%) in Chilean Araucanian Indians
   - Risk factors: progesterone use in pregnancy, past medical or family history of IHCP, and personal history of intrahepatic cholestasis resulting from oral contraceptive or estrogen ingestion
3. **Etiology:** Multifactorial, including genetic, hormonal, and environmental factors. Theories include the following:
   - Gene variants of hepatocanalicular transport proteins (ATP-binding cassette [ABC] transporter B4 = phosphatidylcholine floppase, ABC transporter B11 = bile salt export pump, ABC transporter C2 = conjugated organic anion transporter, ATP8B1 = FIC1) and their regulators (e.g., the bile acid sensor farnesoid X receptor, FXR) found in some patients; incidence of IHCP increased in mothers of children with progressive familial intrahepatic cholestasis (PFIC) type 3
   - Inherited sensitivity to estrogens
   - Association with low serum selenium levels; decreasing incidence in Chilean population linked to increases in serum selenium levels
4. **Clinical and laboratory features**
   - Jaundice in 25% of patients and following the onset of pruritus
   - Elevated serum aminotransferase levels (up to four-fold), serum bile acid levels (30–100x), mono- or disulfated progesterone metabolites (particularly 3- and 5-alpha isomers), and occasionally serum cholesterol and triglyceride levels
   - Liver biopsy (not usually indicated) specimens reveal cholestasis with minimal hepatocellular necrosis
5. **Diagnosis:** clinical.
6. **Treatment**
   - Symptom management: sleeping in a cold room, topical alcohol and camphor menthol lotion, cholestyramine, and ursodeoxycholic acid (UDCA) 10 to 15 mg/kg body weight
   - Close monitoring and early delivery of fetus
7. **Outcome**
   - Mothers do well
   - Increased risk of preterm delivery (19% to 60%); meconium staining of amniotic fluid (24%); fetal bradycardia (14%); fetal distress (22% to 41%); fetal loss (0.4% on average; 4.1% in severe cases), particularly when fasting serum bile acid levels are greater than 40 μmol/L

ACUTE FATTY LIVER OF PREGNANCY

1. **Definition:** A rare life-threatening complication of pregnancy manifested by microvesicular fatty infiltration of the liver and progressive liver failure
2. **Epidemiology**
   - Onset in third trimester (usually after 35th week, but as early as 26 weeks; can occur in the immediate postpartum period)

- Incidence: 1 in 10,000 to 15,000 deliveries
- Risk factors: primiparity, multiple gestations, and male fetuses

3. **Etiology**
   - Defects in mitochondrial fatty acid beta-oxidation in the mother, caused by fetal deficiency in the long-chain 3-hydroxyacyl-coenzyme A dehydrogenase (LCHAD) enzyme. LCHAD is part of mitochondrial trifunctional protein (MTP) and catalyzes the third step in β-oxidation of long-chain fatty acids. Up to 70% of cases result from homozygous long-chain LCHAD deficiency in the fetus, with a heterozygous mother
   - Abnormal concentrations of fetal long-chain fatty acids enter the maternal circulation and have toxic effects in the mother
   - G1528C (E474Q mutation) in the MTP causes LCHAD deficiency
   - A second fatty-acid oxidation defect—hepatic carnitine palmitoyl transferase I deficiency—is also associated with maternal AFLP
   - Nutritional factors, alterations in lipoprotein synthesis, and enzyme deficiencies in the mitochondrial urea cycle are other proposed pathogenic factors

4. **Clinical and laboratory features**
   - Symptoms include headache, fatigue, malaise, nausea, vomiting, and abdominal pain
   - Jaundice may follow a prodrome
   - Progressive liver failure may occur, with coagulopathy, encephalopathy, or renal failure
   - 50% of patients have signs of pre-eclampsia
   - Serum aminotransferase levels are elevated (usually less than 500 U/L)
   - Serum alkaline phosphatase and bilirubin levels are mildly to moderately elevated
   - Hyperuricemia occurs in 80%

5. **Diagnosis**
   - Abdominal ultrasonography and CT are inconsistent in detecting fatty infiltration
   - If the disorder and a risk to delivering a premature infant are clinically suspected, then emergency liver biopsy should be done. The frozen liver biopsy specimen shows a microvesicular fatty infiltrate of liver detectable by Oil-Red-O stain

6. **Treatment**
   - Rapid delivery of the infant is critical. Most women improve, but fulminant hepatic failure may occur, and treatment with liver transplantation has been reported
   - Screening for a fatty acid oxidation defect is indicated in affected patients

7. **Outcome**
   - Maternal mortality rate of 8% to 18%
   - Fetal mortality rate of 18% to 23%

PRE-ECLAMPSIA/ECLAMPSIA

1. **Definition:** The triad of hypertension, proteinuria, and edema. Pre-eclampsia is a multisystem disease with renal, hematologic, hepatic, central nervous system, and fetal-placental involvement. Eclampsia is the presence of convulsions or coma in addition to the symptoms and signs of pre-eclampsia.

2. **Epidemiology**
   - More common in late second or third trimester, but may occur postpartum
   - Incidence: pre-eclampsia in 5% to 7% of pregnancies, eclampsia in 0.1% to 0.2%
   - Risk factors: insulin resistance, obesity, extremes of maternal age (age less than 20 or more than 45 years), primiparity, infection, family history of pre-eclampsia/eclampsia, multiple gestations, hydatidiform mole, fetal hydrops, polyhydramnios, and inadequate prenatal care

3. **Etiology:** Unknown. Proposed mechanisms include vasospasm, abnormal placental development, abnormal endothelial reactivity, activation of coagulation, and decreased nitric oxide synthesis. Levels of fms-like tyrosine kinase 1 (sFlt1; also known as soluble vascular endothelial growth factor) are high, and up-regulation of placental endoglin occurs. A mutation in the gene encoding STOX1 transcription factor has been proposed to cause susceptibility, but data are still not clear.

4. **Clinical and laboratory features**
   a. Hypertension
      ▪ Mild pre-eclampsia: blood pressure 140/90 mm Hg or higher but lower than 160/110 mm Hg
      ▪ Severe pre-eclampsia: blood pressure 160/110 mm Hg or higher
   b. Convulsions or coma in eclampsia
   c. Headaches, visual changes, abdominal pain, heart failure, respiratory distress, and oliguria are possible in severe disease

5. **Diagnosis**
   ▪ Clinical features suggest the diagnosis
   ▪ Serum aminotransferase levels are elevated in 90% of patients with eclampsia, 50% with severe pre-eclampsia, and 24% with mild pre-eclampsia
   ▪ Serum aminotransferase levels are elevated 5 to 100 times, with modest increases in serum bilirubin levels (up to 5 mg/dL)
   ▪ Thrombocytopenia and microangiopathic hemolytic anemia may occur
   ▪ Liver biopsy specimens, if available, may demonstrate periportal deposition of fibrin and fibrinogen associated with hemorrhage, with or without necrosis. In some cases, microvesicular fatty infiltration is seen, suggesting overlap with AFLP

6. **Treatment**
   ▪ Delivery of the infant is the preferred treatment of eclampsia and near-term pre-eclampsia. Management remote from term is controversial but may include bed rest, antihypertensive therapy, and magnesium sulfate
   ▪ The incidence of pre-eclampsia is **not** reduced with nutritional supplementation, including calcium, or with low-dose aspirin

7. **Outcome**
   ▪ Morbidity and mortality rates correlate with severity
   ▪ The most common cause of death is cerebral involvement
   ▪ The risk of hepatic rupture and HELLP syndrome is increased
   ▪ Risks to the fetus include prematurity, fetal growth retardation, abruptio placentae, and low birth weight
   ▪ Increased perinatal morbidity and mortality in the mother and fetus correlate with the severity of pre-eclampsia, preterm delivery, multiple gestations, and preexisting maternal medical conditions
   ▪ Postdelivery liver biochemical test abnormalities generally resolve

HELLP SYNDROME

1. **Definition:** Hemolysis, elevated liver tests, and low platelets
2. **Epidemiology**
   ▪ More common in the third trimester (usually at or after 32 weeks but as early as 25 weeks); 15% to 25% of cases occur postpartum (most within 2 days of delivery but can be later)
   ▪ Incidence: 0.2% to 0.6% of all pregnancies; 4% to 12% in women with pre-eclampsia/eclampsia

- May occur in patients with AFLP or de novo
- Risk factors: white race, multiparity, age greater than 25 years

3. **Etiology:** Unknown. Pathogenic factors may include abnormal vascular tone, vasospasm, coagulation, and LCHAD deficiency in the infant.
4. **Clinical and laboratory features**
   a. Epigastric pain (65%), nausea or vomiting (30%), headache (31%), hypertension (85%), visual changes, weight gain, edema
   b. Microangiopathic hemolytic anemia with increased serum lactate dehydrogenase and indirect bilirubin levels and decreased haptoglobin levels
   c. Elevated serum aminotransferase levels (from mild to 10 to 100 times)
   d. Decreased platelet count (may be lower than 10,000/mm^3)
   e. Proteinuria
   f. Positive D-dimer test is possibly predictive of HELLP syndrome in pre-eclamptic patients
   g. Postpartum resolution of the following:
      - Abnormal platelets, usually within the first 5 days
      - Hypertension or proteinuria, if present, up to 3 months
5. **Diagnosis:** Presence of hemolytic anemia, elevated serum aminotransferase levels, and low platelets
6. **Treatment**
   - Delivery of the infant is indicated in the presence of maternal or fetal distress or a rapidly dropping platelet count. Coexisting pre-eclampsia or AFLP may dictate early delivery
   - Hospitalization is indicated for treatment of hypertension, stabilization of DIC, seizure prophylaxis, and fetal monitoring
   - Corticosteroids are recommended if gestation is less than 34 weeks, to improve fetal lung maturity, but the use of corticosteroids to improve postpartum maternal outcome remains experimental
7. **Outcome**
   - Maternal mortality rate of 1%
   - Perinatal infant mortality rate of 7% to 22%
   - Complications: maternal DIC, abruptio placentae, eclampsia, ascites, subcapsular hematoma, hepatic rupture, wound hematoma, and renal, cardiopulmonary, or hepatic failure
   - Increased risk of infant prematurity, intrauterine growth retardation, DIC, and thrombocytopenia

HEPATIC RUPTURE

1. **Definition:** Rupture of the hepatic capsule
2. **Epidemiology**
   - Occurs in 1 in 45,000 to 1 in 250,0000 deliveries
   - Incidence: 0.9% to 2% in patients with HELLP syndrome
   - Most cases are associated with pre-eclampsia, eclampsia, AFLP, or HELLP
   - Also occurs with hepatocellular carcinoma, adenoma, hemangioma, and hepatic abscess
   - Recurrence is rare
3. **Etiology:** In HELLP and pre-eclampsia/eclampsia, hepatic rupture is usually preceded by severe intraparenchymal hepatic hemorrhage that progresses to subcapsular hematoma in patients with severe thrombocytopenia

4. **Clinical and laboratory features**
   - Usually occurs in last trimester or occasionally within 24 hours of delivery
   - Typical symptoms: sudden onset of abdominal pain, nausea, and vomiting followed by abdominal distention and hypovolemic shock
   - Usually involves the right lobe of liver but may occur in either or both lobes
   - Serum aminotransferase levels are increased 2 to 100 times and associated with anemia and consumptive thrombocytopenia, with or without DIC
5. **Diagnosis:** Abdominal ultrasonography, CT, MRI, and angiography are useful.
6. **Treatment**
   - Early recognition leads to prompt delivery and surgical or radiologic intervention
   - Surgical therapies include application of direct pressure, evacuation, packing or hemostatic wrapping, topical hemostatic agents, oversewing lacerations, hepatic artery ligation, partial hepatectomy, and liver transplantation
   - Angiographic embolization is an alternative option
7. **Outcome**
   - Maternal mortality rate of 50% (caused by hemorrhagic shock, hepatic failure, cerebral hemorrhage)
   - Fetal mortality rate of 10% to 60% (caused by placental rupture, prematurity, intrauterine asphyxia)

Pregnancy in Patients with Chronic Liver Disease

OVERVIEW

   - Patients have more difficulty conceiving
   - Pregnancy has no adverse effect on the progression of liver disease

CIRRHOSIS (see also Chapters 9 and 10)

1. **The risk of bleeding esophageal varices is increased** (more commonly in the second and third trimesters).
   a. Etiology: expanded maternal blood volume and fetal compression of maternal inferior vena cava and collateral vasculature
   b. Risk of esophageal bleeding
      - Cirrhosis: 18% to 32%
      - Known portal hypertension: 50%
      - Preexisting varices: 78%
   c. Treatment
      - Treatment of variceal bleeding is the same as in a nongravid patient and includes band ligation or sclerotherapy and, if necessary, transjugular intrahepatic portosystemic shunt placement or portosystemic shunt surgery
      - Screening endoscopy is recommended in patients with cirrhosis before pregnancy or early in the second trimester
      - Areas of controversy include the delivery method (elective caesarian section to avoid Valsalva maneuver during vaginal birth?) and primary prophylaxis of variceal bleeding with banding or beta blockers
   d. Outcome: maternal mortality rate of 18% to 50%

2. Other complications that occur in pregnant patients with cirrhosis are hepatic decompensation (24%), splenic artery aneurysm rupture (2.6%), postpartum uterine hemorrhage (7% to 10%), spontaneous abortion (30% to 40%), prematurity (25%), fetal stillbirth (13%), and neonatal mortality (4.8%).

3. Medications prescribed to manage the complications of cirrhosis should be reviewed carefully for safety in pregnancy (e.g., furosemide, spironolactone, beta blockers, fluoroquinolones, and rifaximin are pregnancy category C drugs according to the US Food and Drug Administration [FDA]; octreotide and lactulose are FDA category B drugs).

WILSON DISEASE (see also Chapter 17)

1. Impact on pregnancy: The disease may decrease fertility and increases the rate of recurrent spontaneous abortions.

2. Treatment: Pregnant patients should continue anticopper therapy (penicillamine, trientine, zinc) during pregnancy because serious adverse maternal outcomes, including death, can result if anticopper therapy is stopped.
   - Data in pregnancy are limited for all three anticopper drugs
   - Penicillamine is potentially teratogenic in animals and humans. Trientine is teratogenic in animals
   - Penicillamine is considered safe during pregnancy at relatively low doses (0.25 to 0.5 g/day). Trientine has appeared safe and effective based on limited data. Because of the potential teratogenic effects of penicillamine and trientine, zinc is recommended during pregnancy by some authorities

3. Special considerations: Genetic counseling should be offered.

AUTOIMMUNE HEPATITIS (see also Chapter 5)

1. Impact on pregnancy
   - The natural history of AIH is variable during pregnancy
   - Successful pregnancies can occur in women with well-controlled AIH
   - The rate of fetal loss is 19% to 24% (no different from that for other chronic diseases)

2. Treatment
   - Cessation of therapy during pregnancy is associated with relapse of disease
   - The use of azathioprine is controversial, but reports of experience in patients taking azathioprine following organ transplants or for inflammatory bowel disease have described good outcomes for mothers and infants
   - Patients should be monitored closely for flare-ups of AIH during pregnancy and in the early postpartum period

3. Special considerations: Women of childbearing age with AIH should be counseled to consider pregnancy only if the disease is well-controlled.

PRIMARY BILIARY CIRRHOSIS (see also Chapter 14)

1. Impact on pregnancy
   - Some data suggest that women with primary biliary cirrhosis may be able to have normal pregnancies
   - Antimitochondrial antibody titers and serum alkaline phosphatase, ALT, bile acid, bilirubin, and IgG and IgM levels improve during pregnancy
   - The risk of postpartum flare-up exists

2. Treatment: Continue UDCA, which is safe in pregnancy.

PRIMARY SCLEROSING CHOLANGITIS (see also Chapter 33)

1. Impact on pregnancy: The natural history in pregnancy is unknown.
2. Treatment: Continue UDCA, which is safe in pregnancy, improves maternal symptoms, and decreases the risk of fetal complications.

Viral Hepatitis and Herpes Simplex Virus Infections in Pregnant Women (see also Chapters 3 and 4)

OVERVIEW

- Of all the viral hepatitides, only the course of hepatitis E is affected by pregnancy
- Viral hepatitis may occur throughout pregnancy

HEPATITIS A

1. Epidemiology
   - This occurs in as many as 1 in 1000 pregnancies in the United States
   - Perinatal transmission is rare
   - Acute infection only occurs (no chronic disease)
2. Treatment
   - The course and management are unaffected by pregnancy
   - Prevention with immune globulin in an exposed mother is safe for mother and fetus
   - For infants of mothers infectious at or soon after delivery, the dose of immune globulin is 0.02 mL/kg intramuscularly (vaccination against HAV can be considered at age 2 years)

HEPATITIS B

1. Epidemiology
   - Acute disease occurs in 2 of 1000 pregnancies
   - Chronic disease occurs in 5 to 15 per 1000 pregnancies in the United States
2. Transmission to the infant may occur without immunoprophylaxis
   - When the mother is HBsAg positive and HBeAg negative, the chronic infection rate is 40%
   - When the mother is HBsAg and HBeAg positive, the chronic infection rate is 90%
   - The risk of transmission to the infant correlates with the mother's serum HBV DNA level
   - Following infection of the mother in the first trimester, 10% of neonates become HBsAg positive
   - Following infection of the mother in the third trimester, 80% to 90% of neonates become HBsAg positive
   - Transmission to the neonate is usually perinatal
3. Treatment: A combination of active (HBV vaccine) and passive (hepatitis B immune globulin) immunotherapy of the newborn is 85% to 95% effective in decreasing perinatal transmission to less than 10% (Table 21.5).

HEPATITIS C

1. Epidemiology
   - The overall rate of mother-to-infant transmission is generally low (4% to 10%). Higher rates of vertical transmission are reported when maternal viral titers are high (36% when

TABLE 21.5 ■ **Treatment of neonates born to mothers with hepatitis B**

Treatment	Age of administration to infant based on hepatitis B surface antigen status of mother		
	+	Unknown	–
Hepatitis B immune globulin 100 IU (0.5 mL IM)	≤12 hr	≤12 hr	Not administered
Hepatitis B vaccine, first dose 5.0 µg (0.5 mL IM)	≤12 hr	≤12 hr	≤1 wk
Subsequent hepatitis B vaccine doses:			
Recombivax HB 5 µg (0.5 mL)	1 mo	1–2 mo	1–2 mo
Engerix-B 10 µg (0.5 mL)	6 mo	6 mo	6–18 mo

IM, intramuscularly.

Adapted from American College of Obstetricians and Gynecologists. ACOG practice bulletin no. 86: viral hepatitis in pregnancy. *Obstet Gynecol* 2007; 110:941–956.

the maternal serum HCV RNA level is higher than 10^{10} copies/mL) and with human immunodeficiency virus coinfection
- HCV infection does not adversely affect pregnancy
- The course of HCV infection is not affected by pregnancy
2. Treatment
   - No effective prevention is available for infants
   - Treatment of chronic hepatitis C with pegylated interferon and ribavirin is **contraindicated** in pregnancy because ribavirin is teratogenic

HEPATITIS D

- Rare instances of vertical transmission have been reported
- Hepatitis B infection should be controlled to prevent the spread of hepatitis D virus

HEPATITIS E

- Jaundice is nine times more common in pregnant than nonpregnant women with hepatitis E
- Hepatitis E is the leading cause of fulminant hepatic failure in pregnancy
- The disease is more severe in the third trimester than at other times, with a maternal mortality rate of up to 27%, compared with 0.5% to 4% in nonpregnant patients. In patients with fulminant hepatic failure, the mortality rate is 65% in pregnant women compared with 23% in nonpregnant women
- The risk of abortion and intrauterine death is 12%
- Vertical transmission occurs in up to 33%
- No specific therapy during pregnancy exists

HERPES SIMPLEX VIRUS INFECTIONS

- Disseminated herpes simplex virus (HSV) infection during pregnancy is rare, but it has been reported, usually in the late second or third trimester
- The clinical presentation can include fulminant hepatitis (see Chapter 2)
- Fever, nausea, vomiting, abdominal pain, leukopenia, thrombocytopenia, coagulopathy, and markedly elevated serum aminotransferase levels are often present
- Liver biopsy specimens show extensive necrosis, often hemorrhagic, with typical intranuclear viral inclusion particles
- Hepatic necrosis, DIC, hypotension, and death can occur rapidly if antiviral therapy is not initiated promptly

Budd–Chiari Syndrome (see also Chapter 19)

1. Definition: Thrombosis of one or more of the three hepatic veins
2. Epidemiology
   - 20% of cases are associated with pregnancy and oral contraceptive use
   - Postpartum onset is rare and is associated with a poor prognosis
3. Etiology
   - A hypercoagulable state (e.g., factor V Leiden mutation) may play a role
   - It may be associated with antiphospholipid antibodies, pre-eclampsia, and ingestion of herbal teas
4. Clinical features
   - Symptoms are usually acute in pregnancy
   - Features include abdominal pain, hepatomegaly, and ascites
5. Diagnosis
   - MRI, ultrasonography, and liver biopsy are used
   - If possible, venography or angiography should be avoided until after pregnancy
6. Treatment: Same as in nonpregnant patients
7. Outcome: With acute onset in pregnancy, the maternal mortality rate is as high as 70%.

Cholelithiasis and Cholecystitis in Pregnant Women (see also Chapter 32)

1. Epidemiology
   - Symptomatic onset is most common in the second and third trimesters
   - The frequency in pregnancy is 18% to 19% in multiparous women and 7% to 8% in primiparous women. Symptomatic gallstones occur only in 0.1% to 0.3% of pregnancies
   - Risk factors include increasing age, increasing frequency and number of pregnancies, obesity, high serum leptin levels, insulin resistance, and low high-density lipoprotein levels
   - Frequency rates of new biliary sludge and gallstones in pregnancy are 14% and 2%, respectively, at the end of the second trimester and 31% and 2%, respectively, 2 to 4 weeks postpartum
   - Sludge disappears in 61% of patients at 3 months and in 96% at 12 months after delivery; gallbladder stones disappear in 13% to 28% of women by 1 year
2. Etiology
   - Increased estrogen levels lead to increased lithogenicity of bile in the second and third trimesters (increased cholesterol secretion and supersaturation of bile)

- Increased progesterone levels lead to larger gallbladder volume and decreased emptying time
3. Clinical features
   - Vomiting occurs in 32%, dyspepsia in 28%, and pruritus in 10%
   - Biliary pain occurs in 29% with preexisting stones and in 4.7% with sludge but generally does not occur in patients with new sludge or stones
4. Treatment
   a. Conservative medical management with intravenous fluids, correction of electrolytes, bowel rest, and broad-spectrum antibiotics is considered safe in pregnancy.
   b. Laparoscopic cholecystectomy should be performed in the second trimester if medical management fails or the patient has a relapse. Surgery should be avoided in the first trimester if possible.
      - A questionable increase in spontaneous abortions occurs when surgery is performed in the first trimester
      - Surgery in the third trimester is associated with premature labor in 40% of cases
   c. ERCP should be done for choledocholithiasis; it can be performed safely by shielding the fetus from radiation exposure and minimizing fluoroscopy time.

FURTHER READING

Aggarwal R, Naik S. Epidemiology of hepatitis E: current status. *J Gastroenterol Hepatol* 2009; 24:1484–1493.

American College of Obstetricians and Gynecologists. ACOG practice bulletin no. 86: viral hepatitis in pregnancy. *Obstet Gynecol* 2007; 110:941–956.

Badizadegan K, Wolf JL. Liver pathology in pregnancy. In: Odze RD, Goldblum JR, eds. *Surgical Pathology of the GI Tract, Liver, Biliary Tract, and Pancreas*. Philadelphia: Saunders Elsevier; 2009:1231–1243.

Brewer GJ, Johnson VD, Dick RD, et al. Treatment of Wilson's disease with zinc XVII: treatment during pregnancy. *Hepatology* 2000; 31:364–370.

Date RS, Kaushal M, Ramesh A. A review of the management of gallstone disease and its complications in pregnancy. *Am J Surg* 2008; 196:599–608.

Fang CJ, Richards A, Liszewski MK, et al. Advances in understanding of pathogenesis of aHUS and HELLP. *Br J Haematol* 2008; 143:336–348.

Glantz A, Marschall H-U, Mattsson L-Å. Intrahepatic cholestasis of pregnancy: relationships between bile acid levels and fetal complication rates. *Hepatology* 2004; 40:467–474.

Indolfi G, Resti M. Perinatal transmission of hepatitis C virus infection. *J Med Virol* 2009; 81:836–843.

Kondrackiene J, Beuers U, Kupcinskas L. Efficacy and safety of ursodeoxycholic acid versus cholestyramine in intrahepatic cholestasis of pregnancy. *Gastroenterology* 2005; 129:894–901.

Reck T, Bussenius-Kammerer M, Ott R, et al. Surgical treatment of HELLP syndrome–associated liver rupture: an update. *Eur J Obstet Gynecol Reprod Biol* 2001; 99:57–65.

Schramm C, Herkel J, Beuers U, et al. Pregnancy in autoimmune hepatitis: outcome and risk factors. *Am J Gastroenterol* 2006; 101:556–560.

Tan J, Surti B, Saab S. Pregnancy and cirrhosis. *Liver Transpl* 2008; 14:1081–1091.

Terrabuio DR, Abrantes-Lemos CP, Carrilho FJ, Cançado EL. Follow-up of pregnant women with autoimmune hepatitis: the disease behavior along with maternal and fetal outcomes. *J Clin Gastroenterol* 2009; 43:350–356.

United States Preventive Services Task Force: Screening for hepatitis B virus infection in pregnancy: U.S. Preventive Services Task Force reaffirmation recommendation statement. *Ann Intern Med* 2009; 150:869–873.

Urato AC. Maternal and neonatal herpes simplex virus infections. *N Engl J Med* 2009; 361:2678;author reply 2679.

CHAPTER 22

The liver in systemic disease

Jeremy F.L. Cobbold, PhD, MRCP ■ John A. Summerfield, MD, FRCP

KEY POINTS

1 Abnormalities in liver biochemical tests are associated with many different systemic diseases. These abnormalities are generally incidental, but in some systemic diseases the liver may be severely compromised (Table 22.1).

2 In evaluating patients with systemic disease and liver dysfunction, the challenge for the clinician is to distinguish among hepatic manifestations of the systemic disease, liver toxicity from drugs used to treat that disease, and a coexisting primary liver disorder.

3 Liver involvement can occur in heart failure, connective tissue diseases, endocrine disorders, granulomatous diseases, lymphoma, hematologic diseases, systemic infections, gastrointestinal disorders including celiac disease and inflammatory bowel disease, and amyloidosis.

Cardiac Disease (see Chapter 20)

HEART FAILURE

The liver may become congested secondary to right-sided heart failure; the following clinical, laboratory, and pathologic features related to the liver may be seen:

1. The patient has a dull ache in the right upper quadrant.
2. Hepatomegaly is noted in 50% of cases and is associated with splenomegaly or ascites in 10% to 20%. Other signs of right-sided heart failure include raised jugular venous pressure and peripheral edema (Table 22.2).
3. Abnormal liver biochemical test results seen are a raised bilirubin level in 25% to 75% of patients and normal or mildly elevated serum aminotransferase levels. The alkaline phosphatase (ALP) is usually (but not always) normal. Up to 75% of patients have a prolonged prothrombin time (PT).
4. Histopathologic examination shows an enlarged purplish liver with the cut surface having alternating patches of congested centrilobular regions and pale, less involved areas, the so-called **nutmeg** appearance.
5. Microscopically, the central veins and centrilobular sinusoids are dilated and engorged with blood; inflammation is not observed. Long-standing hepatic congestion can result in extensive fibrosis, so-called **cardiac cirrhosis**. Treatment of the underlying heart failure normally leads to an improvement in both clinical and laboratory parameters of liver function.

TABLE 22.1 ■ The liver in systemic disease

Disorder(s)	Hepatic manifestations	Liver biochemical test levels (most common abnormalities)
Cardiovascular		
Heart failure	Vascular congestion; hepatomegaly	↑Bil; ↑ALT; ↑PT
Ischemic hepatitis	Hepatocellular necrosis	↑↑↑ALT; ↑Bil
Connective Tissue		
Polymyalgia rheumatica and giant cell arteritis	Hepatocellular necrosis; portal inflammation	↑ALP; ↑ALT
Rheumatoid arthritis; Felty's syndrome; adult Still's disease	Nonspecific: portal inflammatory infiltrates and fibrosis; drug hepatotoxicity	↑ALP; ↑ALT
Systemic lupus erythematosus	Autoimmune hepatitis; autoimmune cholangiopathy; nodular regenerative hyperplasia; drug hepatotoxicity	↑↑ALP; ↑Bil; ↑↑ALT
Systemic sclerosis; Sjogren's syndrome	Budd–Chiari syndrome; antimitochondrial antibodies; primary biliary cirrhosis	↑↑ALP; ↑Bil; (↑)ALT
Endocrine and Metabolic		
Hyperthyroidism	Nonspecific inflammation and cholestasis	↑ALP; ↑ALT; ↑GGTP
Type 2 diabetes mellitus	Steatosis; steatohepatitis	↑ALT; ↑GGTP
Gastrointestinal and Nutritional		
Celiac disease (see Table 22.3)	Elevated aminotransferase levels; association with primary biliary cirrhosis, autoimmune hepatitis, and PSC; jaundice	↑ALT
Inflammatory bowel disease	Association with PSC, cholangiocarcinoma; hepatic steatosis; immunosuppressant medication hepatotoxicity; jaundice	↑ALT
Anorexia	Steatosis; liver failure	↑ALT
Obesity	Steatosis; steatohepatitis	↑ALT; ↑GGTP
Granulomatous		
Sarcoidosis	Epithelioid granulomas	↑↑ALP; ↑ALT
Hematologic		
Lymphomas, acute and chronic leukemias, myeloproliferative disorders (including myelofibrosis)	Hepatomegaly; infiltration; extrahepatic biliary obstruction	↑ALP; ↑Bil
Sickle cell disease	Hemolysis; ischemia; pigment cholelithiasis	↑↑Bil; ↑ALP; ↑ALT
Infections		
Sepsis	Intrahepatic cholestasis; ischemic hepatitis; drug hepatotoxicity	↑Bil; ↑ALP; ↑ALT
HIV infection	Hepatomegaly; coinfection with hepatitis B or C	↑ALT
Tuberculosis	Caseating granulomas; drug hepatotoxicity	↑ALT; ↑↑Bil; ↑ALP
Pneumonia	Nonspecific inflammatory changes	↑↑Bil; ↑ALP
Amyloidosis	Infiltration; vascular congestion	↑↑ALP; ↑ALT

ALT, alanine aminotransferase; ALP, alkaline phosphatase; Bil, bilirubin; GGTP, gamma glutamyltranspeptidase; HIV, human immunodeficiency virus; PSC, primary sclerosing cholangitis.

TABLE 22.2 ■ **Symptoms and signs of hepatic congestion in 175 patients with acute or chronic right-sided heart failure**

	Acute heart failure (%)	Chronic heart failure (%)
Any hepatomegaly (>11 cm span)	99	95
Marked hepatomegaly (>5 cm below right costal margin)	57	49
Peripheral edema	77	71
Pleural effusion	25	17
Splenomegaly	20	22
Ascites	7	20

Adapted from Richman SM, Delman AJ, Grob D. Alterations in indices of liver function in congestive heart failure with particular reference to serum enzymes. *Am J Med* 1961; 30:211–225.

ISCHEMIC HEPATITIS AND LEFT-SIDED HEART FAILURE

Hepatic damage associated with acute left ventricular failure is frequently termed ischemic hepatitis. It usually occurs in the setting of an acute myocardial infarction or cardiogenic shock but can result from an abrupt, severe decrease in cardiac output from any cause, as an effect of vasoactive drugs (e.g., cocaine, ergotamine overdosage), or from severe hypoxemia.

1. The major manifestations are biochemical: elevated serum levels of aspartate and alanine aminotransferase (AST, ALT) and lactate dehydrogenase (LDH) (predominantly hepatic fraction) to 25 or more times the upper limits. Values peak within 1 to 3 days of the inciting event and rapidly return to near normal, usually within 7 to 10 days. Serum bilirubin and ALP levels are generally normal or only mildly elevated. Liver failure and hepatic encephalopathy can occur.

2. Mortality rates in patients with ischemic hepatitis are high (40% to 50% in some series) but do not correlate with the degree of liver test abnormalities. The cause of death is related to the cause of the ischemic injury to the liver, not to liver failure. Treatment should be directed to correcting the underlying disease process.

Connective Tissue Diseases

POLYMYALGIA RHEUMATICA AND GIANT CELL ARTERITIS

1. Abnormalities in liver biochemical tests may be seen in both polymyalgia rheumatica and giant cell arteritis. Elevation of ALP levels occurs in approximately 30% of patients; elevated serum aminotransferase levels may also be observed.

2. Liver biopsy specimens demonstrate focal hepatocellular necrosis, portal inflammation, and scattered small epithelioid granulomas.

3. The liver abnormalities usually do not cause clinical problems and resolve within a few weeks of the initiation of corticosteroid therapy.

RHEUMATOID ARTHRITIS

1. Liver disease in rheumatoid arthritis (RA) is most commonly seen in patients with **Felty's syndrome** (splenomegaly and neutropenia in the setting of RA). These patients frequently have hepatomegaly, and approximately 25% have elevated serum aminotransferase and ALP levels. Liver biopsy findings are usually nonspecific: infiltration of portal areas with lymphocytes and plasma cells and mild portal fibrosis.
2. Some patients with RA develop **nodular regenerative hyperplasia** with atrophy and formation of regenerative nodules that may result in portal hypertension, ascites, and variceal hemorrhage (see Chapter 20). The pathogenesis of nodular regenerative hyperplasia has been proposed to be drug-induced or immune complex-induced obliteration of the portal venules.
3. Hepatotoxicity can be associated with salicylates, gold, and methotrexate.

ADULT STILL'S DISEASE

1. This multisystem inflammatory disorder of unknown origin is characterized by spiking fever, evanescent rash, arthritis, and multiorgan involvement.
2. Liver abnormalities including hepatomegaly and abnormal liver enzymes are seen in 50% to 75%; nonsteroidal anti-inflammatory drug use may be a significant cofactor.
3. After consideration of the possible contribution of medications to hepatic dysfunction, treatment of the underlying disorder with anti-inflammatory drugs, immunosuppressant medications, or biologic agents is indicated.

SYSTEMIC LUPUS ERYTHEMATOSUS

1. Liver biochemical test abnormalities are common in systemic lupus erythematosus (SLE), but clinically significant liver disease is uncommon.
2. Frequent abnormalities include elevated ALT and ALP levels, normally less than four times the upper limit of normal. A few patients (approximately 5%) develop jaundice.
3. Causes of liver biochemical abnormalities in SLE are as follows:
   - Steatosis (most common finding on liver biopsy)
   - Autoimmune hepatitis, either primary as a result of SLE or coexistent classic autoimmune hepatitis (see Chapter 5)
   - Autoimmune cholangiopathy, with an increase in ALP greater than ALT
   - Nodular regenerative hyperplasia (may be seen in all connective tissue diseases)
   - Coexistent viral hepatitis (in one study, 11% of patients with SLE were positive in serum for hepatitis C viral RNA)
   - Budd–Chiari syndrome, particularly in patients with antiphospholipid syndrome
   - Drugs, especially methotrexate and salicylates
4. Drugs suspected of causing abnormal liver biochemical test levels, particularly salicylates, should be withdrawn. Otherwise, the treatment of liver dysfunction in SLE depends on the cause. Most abnormal liver biochemical test results do not represent clinically significant liver disease.

SYSTEMIC SCLEROSIS (SCLERODERMA)

1. From 8% to 15% of patients with systemic sclerosis have **antimitochondrial antibodies**; these patients often have evidence of **primary biliary cirrhosis** on liver biopsy specimens (see Chapter 14). These changes are more frequent in patients with limited rather than diffuse forms of systemic sclerosis.

2. Nearly 5% of patients with primary biliary cirrhosis have symptoms of systemic sclerosis; which may antedate the diagnosis of primary biliary cirrhosis by many years.

SJÖGREN'S SYNDROME

1. From 5% to 10% of patients with Sjögren's syndrome and approximately 40% with both Sjögren's syndrome and RA have **antimitochondrial antibodies**; most of these patients also have elevated serum ALP levels.
2. Liver biopsy specimens in these patients frequently demonstrate changes of stage 1 primary biliary cirrhosis, even in the absence of liver biochemical test abnormalities.
3. The risk of clinical primary biliary cirrhosis in these patients is uncertain. Whether any early therapeutic intervention is of value is also unclear.

OTHER CAUSES OF VASCULITIS

1. Persons with **polyarteritis nodosa** often have chronic hepatitis B virus infection (see Chapters 3 and 4).
2. Persons with **cryoglobulinemia** often have chronic hepatitis C virus infection (see Chapters 3 and 4).

Endocrine and Metabolic Disorders

HYPERTHYROIDISM

1. Untreated hyperthyroidism is associated with abnormalities of liver biochemical test values, usually with a cholestatic picture. In severe cases, ischemic consequences of high-output heart failure may be observed.
2. Treatment with propylthiouracil may also lead to hepatotoxicity (see Chapter 8).

TYPE 2 DIABETES AND THE METABOLIC SYNDROME

1. Nonalcoholic fatty liver disease (NAFLD) may be considered the liver manifestation of the metabolic syndrome of obesity, insulin resistance, hypertension, and dyslipidemia (see Chapter 7). Approximately 60% of patients with type 2 diabetes mellitus have evidence of NAFLD, and the frequency increases to more than 90% in obese persons with type 2 diabetes mellitus.
2. A subset of patients will develop progressive disease, with an increased risk of the complications of cirrhosis, including hepatocellular carcinoma.
3. The most common cause of death in such patients remains cardiovascular disease.

Granulomatous Disease and Sarcoidosis (see Chapter 26)

1. Granulomatous diseases of the liver have numerous causes:
   - Systemic infections (e.g., tuberculosis)
   - Malignant disease (e.g., Hodgkin's lymphoma)
   - Drugs
   - Autoimmune disorders (e.g., autoimmune hepatitis)
   - Idiopathic conditions (e.g., sarcoidosis)

2. Abnormalities of liver biochemical test values are common in sarcoidosis but rarely require treatment. Typically, minor elevations of both aminotransferases and ALP levels are seen.
3. Rarer clinical manifestations include chronic intrahepatic cholestasis, portal hypertension, and Budd–Chiari syndrome.
4. Liver biopsy specimens demonstrate granulomas in the portal and periportal regions; cholestatic and necroinflammatory features may also be seen.
5. No treatment is required for patients with asymptomatic disease; ursodeoxycholic acid, corticosteroids, or methotrexate may be considered in patients with symptomatic disease.

Lymphoma and Hematologic Diseases

LYMPHOMA

1. The liver may be involved in 5% of patients with **Hodgkin's lymphoma** at presentation but in up to 50% of patients at autopsy. In addition, nonspecific inflammatory infiltrates or noncaseating granulomas are seen in the absence of direct hepatic involvement with lymphomas.
   ■ An elevated ALP level of 1.5 to 2.0 times the upper limit of normal is common even in the absence of direct liver involvement.
   ■ Jaundice is uncommon in Hodgkin's lymphoma and usually reflects hepatic infiltration with lymphoma, rather than extrahepatic biliary obstruction.
2. Hepatic involvement is observed in 25% to 50% of patients with **non-Hodgkin's lymphoma**; rarely, the liver may be the primary site of involvement. Typically, the lymphoma produces a nodular infiltrate of the portal areas. The clinical and laboratory presentation is similar to that of Hodgkin's lymphoma, except that extrahepatic obstruction, usually at the level of the porta hepatis, is much more common.

MALIGNANT HEMATOLOGIC CONDITIONS

1. **Systemic mastocytosis** may manifest with hepatosplenomegaly as well as with lymphadenopathy and skin lesions. Liver biopsy specimens show polygonal cells containing eosinophilic granules, predominantly in the portal tracts. Giemsa and toluidine blue staining allows detection of the characteristic metachromatic cytoplasmic granules. Periportal fibrosis may also be present. Cirrhosis develops in approximately 5% of patients.
2. Hepatomegaly is common in **acute lymphoblastic leukemia** and **acute myeloid leukemia** at diagnosis and is present in 95% and 75%, respectively, of cases post mortem. Liver biopsy is seldom performed because of the high risk of hemorrhage.
3. Most patients with chronic leukemias (e.g., **chronic lymphocytic leukemia, hairy cell leukemia**) also demonstrate evidence of liver infiltration at autopsy.
4. **Multiple myeloma** is rarely associated with clinically significant liver disease; hepatic manifestations may include diffuse sinusoidal or portal infiltration, nodular regenerative hyperplasia, jaundice, and complications of portal hypertension. Multiple myeloma is also associated with **amyloidosis** (see later).
5. Massive hepatomegaly is seen in **primary myelofibrosis** and other myeloproliferative disorders and is associated with extramedullary hematopoiesis and increased hepatic blood flow. The most common biochemical abnormality is an elevated ALP level, which may be associated with the severity of sinusoidal dilatation.

SICKLE CELL DISEASE

1. Although liver biochemical test abnormalities are common in patients with sickle cell disease, these abnormal values are frequently caused by other factors such as chronic viral hepatitis or heart failure.

2. **Hepatic crisis** usually occurs in the setting of sickle cell crisis and is marked by right upper quadrant pain, jaundice, and tender hepatomegaly.
   - Serum bilirubin levels are frequently as high as 10 to 15 mg/dL and may be as high as 40 to 50 mg/dL.
   - Serum AST and ALT levels are also elevated, usually up to 10 times normal.
   - The LDH level may be increased markedly, reflecting both liver dysfunction and hemolysis.
   - Hemolysis may contribute to rises in bilirubin and aminotransferase levels, whereas a raised ALP level is often of bone origin.
   - Liver biopsy specimens in hepatic crisis demonstrate sinusoidal distention, erythrocyte sickling, and phagocytosis of erythrocytes by Kupffer cells.
   - The differential diagnosis includes acute cholecystitis and cholangitis.
   - Treatment is supportive and usually results in clinical improvement in a few days, although fatal liver failure has been described.

3. **Pigment gallstones** have been reported in 40% to 80% of patients with sickle cell disease; choledocholithiasis has been described in 20% to 65% of patients at the time of cholecystectomy.
   - Abdominal ultrasonography or computed tomography (CT) may be helpful in establishing the diagnosis of cholecystitis.
   - Endoscopic retrograde cholangiopancreatography (ERCP) may be necessary to identify and treat stones in the bile duct.

Infections (see Chapter 29)

Many systemic infections may cause abnormalities in liver biochemical test results, either directly or indirectly. The abnormalities usually resolve on resolution of the underlying infection. Pneumonia is often accompanied by elevated liver enzymes. In particular, *Legionella pneumophila* (causing Legionnaire's disease), *Mycoplasma pneumoniae*, and *Pneumococcus* spp. infections may be associated with markedly raised aminotransferase levels and cholestasis.

SYSTEMIC INFECTION, SEPSIS, AND THE CRITICALLY ILL PATIENT

Elevated liver enzyme levels are often seen in patients with systemic sepsis. The causes and possible mechanisms are multiple; in most cases, the effect is multifactorial.

1. **Intrahepatic cholestasis** is common in sepsis, independent of the causative organism. Canalicular excretion of conjugated bilirubin is thought to be inhibited by high levels of proinflammatory cytokines, such as tumor necrosis factor-alpha and interleukin-6. Usually, no evidence of cholangitis is seen on liver biopsy specimens.

2. Biochemical findings include mildly raised serum ALP levels (one to three times the upper limit of normal) and increased serum bilirubin levels, although these levels may be discordant.

3. Antibiotics such as amoxicillin-clavulanic acid and flucloxacillin are associated with a cholestatic drug reaction (see Chapter 8).

4. Ischemic hepatitis (see earlier) may occur in a septic patient as a result of hemodynamic instability.

5. Parenteral nutrition is associated with hepatotoxicity and nonalcoholic steatohepatitis (see Chapters 7 and 8), which may be ameliorated by the addition of choline to the formula.

HUMAN IMMUNODEFICIENCY VIRUS
(HIV) INFECTION (see Chapter 25)

1. Approximately 70% of patients with the acquired immunodeficiency syndrome (AIDS) have clinical hepatomegaly, often with abnormal liver biochemical test levels.
2. The picture is usually hepatitic, with elevation of serum aminotransferases predominating, often related to coinfection with hepatitis B virus (HBV) or hepatitis C virus (HCV).

TUBERCULOSIS (see Chapters 26 and 29)

1. Miliary tuberculosis (TB) may affect the liver and may cause hepatitis and rarely jaundice. Liver biopsy specimens reveal multiple caseating granulomas.
2. Drug therapy, particularly with isoniazid and rifampin, may cause hepatitis with elevated serum aminotransferase levels and jaundice.
3. Coinfection with HIV or HCV is thought to be an independent risk factor for the development of antituberculous drug–induced hepatitis.

Gastrointestinal and Nutritional Disorders

CELIAC DISEASE

1. Serum aminotransferase levels are elevated (less than five times the upper limit of normal) in 40% of adults with celiac disease at the time of diagnosis. Histologic findings in the liver are seen in 66% of these patients but are usually mild and nonspecific.
2. Adherence to a gluten-free diet leads to normalization of serum aminotransferase levels in 75% to 95% of patients with celiac disease, usually within 1 year.
3. Autoimmune liver diseases are more prevalent in patients with celiac disease compared with the general population, including those with primary biliary cirrhosis, autoimmune hepatitis, and primary sclerosing cholangitis (PSC). The pathogenesis of these associations is unclear, but certain human leukocyte antigen (HLA) associations have been postulated. Adherence to a gluten-free diet has generally not been shown to provide benefit.
4. Other liver diseases associated with celiac disease are listed in Table 22.3.
5. Celiac disease may be associated with an increased risk of death from liver cirrhosis.

INFLAMMATORY BOWEL DISEASE

Liver abnormalities

1. Abnormal hepatic biochemistry values (mild elevations of serum aminotransferase and ALP levels) are common in patients with inflammatory bowel disease, with a frequency of approximately 30%.
2. In a large series, abnormal hepatic biochemistry was associated with increased mortality, but not with disease activity, although the reason for the increased mortality was unclear.
3. **Steatosis** is the most commonly observed abnormality on liver biopsy specimens. Additionally, **chronic hepatitis** characterized by either portal or lobular infiltrates of mononuclear inflammatory cells may be found. It is not clear whether hepatitis is a direct consequence of

TABLE 22.3 ■ Liver diseases associated with celiac disease

Isolated elevation of the aminotransferase levels (celiac hepatitis), reversible on gluten-free diet

Cryptogenic cirrhosis

Autoimmune liver disorders
  Primary biliary cirrhosis
  Autoimmune hepatitis: type 1 and type 2
  Autoimmune cholangitis
  Primary sclerosing cholangitis

Chronic hepatitis C

Hemochromatosis

Nonalcoholic fatty liver disease

Acute liver failure

Regenerative nodular hyperplasia

Hepatocellular carcinoma

Adapted from Rubio-Tapia A, Murray JA. The liver in celiac disease. *Hepatology* 2007; 46:1650–1165.

inflammatory bowel disease or a manifestation of **PSC** or another cause of liver disease such as **hepatitis C** or drugs. The frequency of **autoimmune hepatitis** is increased in patients with inflammatory bowel disease.

4. Patients with Crohn's disease infrequently develop hepatic **granulomas** or **amyloidosis.**

Biliary abnormalities

1. **PSC** is the most important hepatobiliary complication of inflammatory bowel disease; it occurs in 5% to 10% of patients with ulcerative colitis but in fewer than 1% of those with Crohn's disease (see Chapters 15 and 33).

2. The only sign of early PSC may be an elevated serum ALP level. Patients with more advanced disease may present with pruritus or jaundice.

3. Progression varies widely among affected persons, possibly related to an individual's HLA status. Most patients ultimately develop biliary cirrhosis with increasing serum levels of bilirubin and ALP and portal hypertension with ascites and variceal bleeding. Bacterial cholangitis may also be observed, particularly in patients who have undergone surgical or endoscopic intervention of the bile ducts.

4. Up to 20% of patients with PSC develop **cholangiocarcinoma.**

5. Diagnosis of PSC is made by visualization of the biliary tree by ERCP or magnetic resonance cholangiopancreatography (MRCP). The typical pattern is of multiple bile duct strictures with areas of beaded dilatation. Distinguishing benign strictures from cholangiocarcinoma by radiographic criteria is often difficult. Brush cytology and biopsy obtained at ERCP may be helpful (see Chapters 33 and 34).

6. Neither medical nor surgical treatment of the underlying inflammatory bowel disease alters the course of PSC. Treatment with ursodeoxycholic acid may result in some improvement in symptoms and liver biochemical test values. Patients with advanced liver disease secondary to PSC may be candidates for liver transplantation if they have not already developed cholangiocarcinoma, although PSC may recur in the graft.

OBESITY

1. The worldwide prevalence of obesity continues to rise and is closely associated with insulin resistance and NAFLD (see Chapter 7).
2. The mainstay of treatment is weight loss by dietary restriction. Bariatric surgery (gastric bypass or banding) reduces the severity of nonalcoholic steatohepatitis in obese patients.

ANOREXIA NERVOSA

1. Patients with anorexia nervosa may have elevated levels of liver biochemical test values, predominantly the aminotransferases.
2. Up to 30% of patients with moderately severe (body mass index 12 to 16) and 75% of those with severe (body mass index less than 12) anorexia nervosa have raised aminotransferase levels; marked increases are often a marker of impending multiorgan failure.
3. Transient increases in liver enzyme levels may occur during refeeding in patients with anorexia nervosa and other causes of starvation; generally, the abnormalities resolve completely when refeeding is completed.

Amyloidosis

Systemic amyloidosis is characterized by the extracellular deposition of fibrillar protein in many tissues. It may be classified as **AL (primary amyloid)** and **AA (secondary amyloid)**, accounting for approximately 90% of cases. The amyloid protein is seen as green birefringent extracellular material when stained with Congo red dye and viewed under polarized light.

1. In **primary amyloidosis** (approximately 80% of all cases), the amyloid consists of kappa or lambda immunoglobulin light chains produced by a monoclonal population of plasma cells. Bence Jones proteinuria may also be present, and approximately one third of patients have multiple myeloma.
2. In **secondary amyloidosis**, the amyloid is derived from serum amyloid A, secreted by the liver as an acute phase reactant in response to chronic infections or inflammatory processes such as tuberculosis, lepromatous leprosy, osteomyelitis, RA, Crohn's disease, or lymphoma.
3. The clinical presentation is usually nonspecific, and patients may present with symptoms related to deposition of amyloid in other organs: heart failure, nephrotic syndrome, intestinal malabsorption, peripheral or autonomic neuropathy, and carpal tunnel syndrome.
4. **Hepatic amyloidosis** should be suspected in patients with hepatomegaly in the setting of a chronic infectious or inflammatory process, particularly if it is associated with proteinuria or monoclonal gammopathy.
5. Hepatomegaly (passive congestion or infiltration) is found in up to 60% of affected patients; splenomegaly is much less common (approximately 5%).
6. Abnormalities of liver biochemical test values include a marked increase in serum ALP levels, with aminotransferases less than twice normal. The serum albumin level may be low, often secondary to proteinuria, which may be in the nephrotic range in 30% of patients.
7. Liver biopsy should be avoided, if possible, because of an increased risk of bleeding after biopsy.
8. The prognosis of patients with systemic amyloidosis is generally poor, with a median survival of less than 2 years. Mortality is usually the result of cardiac or renal disease and only rarely hepatic involvement. Treatment of predisposing chronic inflammatory conditions may improve the outcome.

FURTHER READING

Berry PA, Cross TJ, Thein SL, et al. Hepatic dysfunction in sickle cell disease: a new system of classification based on global assessment. *Clin Gastroenterol Hepatol* 2007; 5:1469–1476.

Carithers RL. Endocrine disorders and the liver. In: Gitlin N, ed. *The Liver and Systemic Disease*. London: Churchill Livingstone; 1997:59–72.

Chowdhary VR, Crowson CS, Poterucha JJ, Moder KG. Liver involvement in systemic lupus erythematosus: case review of 40 patients. *J Rheumatol* 2008; 35:2159–2164.

Csepregi A, Szodoray P, Zeher M. Do autoantibodies predict autoimmune liver disease in primary Sjögren's syndrome? Data of 180 patients upon a 5 year follow-up. *Scand J Immunol* 2002; 56:623–629.

Ebert EC, Hagspiel KD. Gastrointestinal and hepatic manifestations of systemic lupus erythematosus. *J Clin Gastroenterol* 2011; 45:436–441.

Ebert EC, Kierson M, Hagspiel KD. Gastrointestinal and hepatic manifestations of sarcoidosis. *Am J Gastroenterol* 2008; 103:3184–3192.

Ebert EC, Nagar M. Gastrointestinal manifestations of amyloidosis. *Am J Gastroenterol* 2008; 103:776–787.

Gertz MA, Kyle RA. Hepatic amyloidosis: clinical appraisal in 77 patients. *Hepatology* 1997; 25:118–121.

Giallourakis CC, Rosenberg PM, Friedman LS. The liver in heart failure. *Clin Liver Dis* 2002; 6:947–967.

Kyle V. Laboratory investigations including liver in polymyalgia rheumatica and giant cell arteritis. *Baillieres Clin Rheum* 1991; 5:475–484.

Mendes FD, Levy C, Enders FB, et al. Abnormal hepatic biochemistries in patients with inflammatory bowel disease. *Am J Gastroenterol* 2007; 102:344–350.

Pope JE, Thompson A. Antimitochondrial antibodies and their significance in diffuse and limited scleroderma. *J Clin Rheumatol* 1999; 5:206–209.

Rubio-Tapia A, Murray JA. The liver in celiac disease. *Hepatology* 2007; 46:1650–1658.

Walker NJ, Zurier RB. Liver abnormalities in rheumatic diseases. *Clin Liver Dis* 2002; 6:933–946.

Youssef WI, Tavill AS. Connective tissue diseases and the liver. *J Clin Gastroenterol* 2002; 35:345–349.

CHAPTER 23

Pediatric liver disease

Bernadette Vitola, MD ■ William F. Balistreri, MD

KEY POINTS

1 The liver is physiologically immature during the perinatal period, and significant maturational changes in hepatic metabolic processes occur during childhood; these metabolic processes affect the presentation of and reaction to viral and toxin exposures.

2 Acquired liver diseases that are seen in adults are rare in children. More commonly encountered in children are congenital or metabolic disorders.

3 Liver disease in children may manifest as hyperbilirubinemia, hepatomegaly, liver failure, cirrhosis, cystic disease of the liver, portal hypertension, or systemic disease resulting from the secondary effects of liver disease.

4 The secondary effects of liver disease may be life threatening and include the following:
- Metabolic derangements, such as hypoglycemia
- Coagulopathy secondary to low levels of vitamin K–dependent clotting factors that may result in intracranial hemorrhage in the infant
- Persistent endogenous "toxin" exposure, as may be seen in diseases such as galactosemia or fructosemia
- Sepsis as a cause of liver disease or as a result of secondary immunodeficiency from malnutrition
- Portal hypertension with potential gastrointestinal bleeding

Consequences of Physiologic Immaturity of the Liver

1. Altered metabolism and clearance of potentially toxic endogenous and exogenous toxic compounds:
   - Hepatic concentrations of cytochrome P-450 are low in infants. Similarly, activities of aminopyrine N-demethylase and aniline p-hydroxylase are low. Hepatic processes, such as clearance of certain drugs or bilirubin that depend on these systems, are inefficient. Therefore, potentially toxic serum levels of such compounds may be reached more rapidly in infants than in older persons.
   - Clearance of drugs that depend on metabolism by cytochrome P-450 is faster in older children than in adults. By puberty, an adult pattern of metabolism is established.
   - Lower levels of glutathione peroxidase and glutathione S-transferase (GST) are present in infants, thus making the infant liver potentially more prone to oxidant injury.
2. Bile acid pool size and composition may be altered. It is unclear whether the alterations are beneficial (some of the bile acids present may be more readily excreted in urine) or harmful (the atypical bile acids that are formed may exacerbate cholestasis).
3. **Physiologic jaundice: Up to one third of newborns develop unconjugated hyperbilirubinemia within the first week of life.** Breast-fed infants have a higher risk of developing

jaundice than do formula-fed infants. This occurrence is often referred to as *physiologic jaundice* and resolves spontaneously with no complications. Physiologic jaundice reflects the transition from clearance and metabolism of unconjugated bilirubin by the maternal system to that of the infant. The pathogenesis is likely multifactorial:

- Increased production of bilirubin: The newborn has a large red cell mass, and the cells have a shorter half-life than adult red cells.
- Inefficient serum protein binding of bilirubin: This affects hepatocellular uptake.
- Immature intracellular conjugation within the liver: This mechanism remains unproven, however, and is unlikely to be the sole cause.

4. Warning signs of pathologic jaundice are as follows:
- Elevated serum bilirubin level occurring before 3 days or lasting longer than 14 days of age
- Total serum bilirubin level greater than 15 mg/dL
- Conjagated serum bilirubin level greater than 2 mg/dL

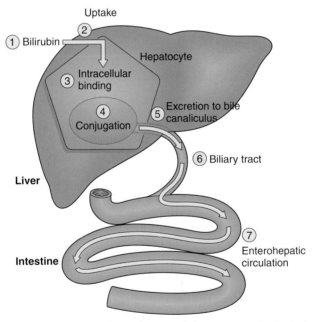

Fig. 23.1 Steps in bilirubin metabolism (see steps below corresponding to numbers in text).

Hyperbilirubinemia

PATHOPHYSIOLOGIC MECHANISMS

Alterations in any step of bilirubin metabolism may cause jaundice in excess of physiologic jaundice (Fig. 23.1; the numbers in the figure correspond to the numbers (1–7) in the following outline):

1. **Increased bilirubin production**: This can result from an increase in the release of heme from red blood cells, for the following reasons:
- Hemolysis due to Rh incompatibility, ABO incompatibility, or other minor blood group incompatibilities

- Increased fragility of erythrocytes in congenital spherocytosis, hereditary elliptocytosis, polycythemia, or red blood cell enzyme defects (glucose-6-phosphate dehydrogenase [G6PD]; pyruvate kinase [PK]; hexokinase [HK])
- Enclosed hematoma

2. **Decreased bilirubin uptake into the hepatocyte:**
    - This may be caused by hypothyroidism or gestational hormones that may inhibit the uptake of bilirubin across the hepatocyte membrane. Thyroxine is important for liver plasma membrane function.
    - A decrease in the amount of bilirubin bound to serum proteins also results in decreased uptake by hepatocytes. The reduction in bilirubin binding may be the result of hypoalbuminemia, generalized hypoproteinemia, or displacement of bilirubin from these proteins by drugs, including sulfonamides, salicylates, heparin, and caffeine.

3. **Abnormalities of intracellular binding or storage of bilirubin within hepatocytes:** These are rare disorders and include deficiencies or alteration in GST, the primary intracellular binding protein for bilirubin.
    - Treatment is not indicated, because no associated morbidity or mortality exists.

4. **Inefficient conjugation of bilirubin within the hepatocyte:** Within the hepatocyte, bilirubin is conjugated with glucuronic acid by bilirubin uridine diphosphate (UDP)-glucuronyl transferase to form bilirubin monoglucuronide or diglucuronide.
    - A decrease in UDP-glucuronyl transferase activity is seen in **Gilbert's syndrome**, resulting in benign elevations in serum unconjugated bilirubin levels, especially during stresses such as viral illnesses.
    - **Crigler–Najjar syndrome**, which localizes to chromosome 2q37, is characterized by the absence of bilirubin UDP-glucuronyl transferase that leads to severe hyperbilirubinemia with associated neurologic effects secondary to **kernicterus.**
    - Hepatic parenchymal disease can cause hyperbilirubinemia in the neonatal period, presumably secondary to hepatocyte damage (see later).

5. **Alterations in the excretion of bilirubin through the canalicular membrane into the biliary tract:** Bilirubin diglucuronide is excreted into the canaliculus by a carrier protein.
    - Alterations in this carrier protein are thought to be the cause of **Dubin–Johnson syndrome.** The genetic defect is on chromosome 10q24. Although this syndrome has no associated morbidity or mortality, it is characterized by elevated serum levels of conjugated and unconjugated serum bilirubin.
    - Hyperbilirubinemia is accentuated during pregnancy or with use of oral contraceptives.
    - The syndrome is likely an autosomal recessive disorder.
    - Affected persons have an increase in urinary coproporphyrin I levels.
    - Liver biopsy specimens show a characteristic melanin-like pigment deposited in hepatocytes but are otherwise histologically normal.
    - Because of the benign nature of this syndrome, no treatment is required.

6. **Structural abnormalities of the biliary tract** can prevent drainage of bile from the canaliculus into the intestine and can cause accumulation of bile and reflux of bilirubin into the systemic circulation:
    a. **Biliary atresia (BA)** is a progressive disease characterized by inflammation and fibrosis of the extrahepatic biliary tract resulting in partial or complete obliteration of the extrahepatic bile ducts.
        - BA typically manifests between 2 and 6 weeks of age as cholestasis (conjugated hyperbilirubinemia).
        - Liver biopsy specimens show fibrosis and bile duct proliferation.

- BA may be **syndromic** (in less than 15% of cases) and associated with cardiac anomalies, polysplenism, and malrotation or situs inversus, or **nonsyndromic** (majority of cases), origin unknown.
- This anomaly is treated initially with a Kasai **portoenterostomy**, which allows drainage of bile directly from the liver to the intestine. Although the procedure is not curative, it often delays the progression of disease.
- End-stage liver disease secondary to BA is the most common reason for liver transplantation in children.

b. **Intrahepatic cholestasis** is often associated with the histologic finding of **bile duct paucity**, defined as a reduced ratio of interlobular bile ducts to portal tracts (normal is 0.9 to 1.8; paucity is less than 0.5). Paucity of bile ducts may be **syndromic** (**Alagille's syndrome**, which is associated with peripheral pulmonic stenosis, butterfly vertebrae, and characteristic facies). Many forms of intrahepatic cholestasis do not exhibit bile duct paucity. Treatment for all forms is symptomatic, with special consideration given to management of malnutrition and pruritus. Liver transplantation may be required in some cases.

- **Progressive familial intrahepatic cholestasis, type I (PFIC-1)**, also known as **Byler's disease,** is caused by defects in the *FIC1* gene on chromosome 18q21–22. This P-type adenosine triphosphatase (ATPase) functions in transport of aminophospholipids across the hepatocyte canalicular plasma membrane. Patients characteristically have a low gamma glutamyltranspeptidase (GGTP) level. The average age of onset is 3 months, and progression to cirrhosis is variable. Watery diarrhea may occur, presumably secondary to intestinal absence of *FIC1*. Treatment is aimed at pruritus and poor growth. Liver transplantation is curative of the liver disease and typically is required in the first 2 decades of life. **Benign recurrent intrahepatic cholestasis (BRIC)** maps to the *FIC1* locus, but the disease does not progress.
- **Progressive familial intrahepatic cholestasis, type II (PFIC-2)**, is clinically similar to PFIC-1; both are associated with low serum GGTP levels. Watery diarrhea is typically not a component, and progression to cirrhosis may be more rapid than in PFIC-1. The syndrome results from defects in the hepatocyte bile salt export pump (BSEP) on chromosome 2q24.
- **Progressive familial intrahepatic cholestasis, type III (PFIC-3)** has a rapid progression to cirrhosis and liver failure. Elevated serum levels of GGTP characterize this syndrome. It is caused by mutations in *MDR3*, which encodes an active export pump involved with the translocation of phosphatidylcholine across the canalicular hepatocyte membrane.

c. **Choledochal cyst**, a cystic dilatation of the biliary tree, may be exclusively extrahepatic or include dilatations of the intrahepatic biliary tree.

- It appears to be most common in East Asia; more than 50% of the reported cases come from Japan.
- Most patients present in infancy with abdominal pain and jaundice, with or without a palpable abdominal mass.
- The diagnosis can be made by ultrasonography, computed tomography (CT), or endoscopic retrograde or magnetic cholangiopancreatography (ERCP; MRCP).
- Treatment is with surgical excision of the dilated segment, rather than bypass or drainage, because of the increased incidence of malignancy in the epithelium of the cyst.

7. **Alterations in the enterohepatic circulation** can produce an increase in reabsorption of bilirubin from the intestine. The cause may be intestinal obstruction, as in intestinal atresia or Hirschsprung's disease, or alterations in the bacterial flora by the use of antibiotics.

COMPLICATIONS

1. Unconjugated hyperbilirubinemia
   - Kernicterus (bilirubin encephalopathy) may result from elevated levels of unconjugated bilirubin. Populations at risk include neonates and individuals with Crigler–Najjar syndrome, type I.
   - Unconjugated bilirubin levels higher than 30 mg/dL are associated with development of encephalopathy.
   - Factors that increase the risk of kernicterus include hypoalbuminemia and bilirubin displacement from albumin by drugs or organic anions. Both conditions increase the serum concentration of unbound bilirubin able to diffuse into cells.
2. Cholestasis
   - Malnutrition secondary to fat malabsorption can lead to failure to thrive and fat-soluble vitamin deficiencies
   - Intractable pruritus
   - Xanthomatosis secondary to alterations in cholesterol metabolism

TREATMENT

a. Unconjugated hyperbilirubinemia
   - Double-volume exchange transfusion lowers the risk of kernicterus in the newborn by rapidly reducing the serum bilirubin concentration.
   - Phototherapy: Photoisomerization of bilirubin to a more polar compound allows excretion of bilirubin in the urine.
   - Faster bilirubin metabolism can be accomplished by administration of phenobarbital, which induces microsomal enzymes that facilitate bilirubin metabolism.
b. Cholestasis
   - Surgical correction of anatomic lesions may be effective.
   - Ursodeoxycholic acid, a choleretic bile acid, can be used to augment bile flow during cholestasis (15 mg/kg per day in divided doses).
   - Supplementation with fat-soluble vitamins is also necessary because absorption is poor without normal bile flow.
   - Liver transplantation may be necessary.

Hepatomegaly

The liver may increase in size because of cell swelling, venous congestion, infiltration with fat, or the accumulation of substances not normally present in the liver.

CAUSES

1. Cellular hyperplasia/hypertrophy
   - Hepatocytes
   - Kupffer cells
   - Inflammatory cells
2. Fibrosis
3. Venous congestion

4. Biliary tract dilatation
5. Accumulation of metabolic substances
   - Fat
   - Cholesterol
   - Glycogen
   - Sphingolipid
   - Sphingomyelin
   - Abnormal alpha-1 antitrypsin
   - Copper
6. Tumor infiltration

INFLAMMATORY CELL INFILTRATION AND KUPFFER CELL PROLIFERATION

- **Viral hepatitis** may manifest with tender hepatomegaly secondary to inflammation.
- The histologic features of **autoimmune hepatitis** include an intense inflammatory infiltrate, which may manifest as hepatomegaly on examination.

FIBROSIS

Congenital hepatic fibrosis may manifest with hepatomegaly and splenomegaly secondary to portal hypertension. Other diseases discussed in this section manifest with hepatomegaly secondary to infiltration of other substances or cells and result in fibrosis. As fibrotic material replaces the hepatocytes, the liver shrinks.

VENOUS CONGESTION

A **decrease in cardiac function** or **hepatic outflow obstruction (Budd–Chiari syndrome)** can result in passive congestion of the liver, which may manifest as hepatomegaly.

ACCUMULATION OF METABOLIC SUBSTANCES

1. Fat accumulation that causes hepatomegaly is seen in many disorders, the most common of which are obesity, malnutrition, and diabetes mellitus.
   a. **Diabetes mellitus** can cause hepatomegaly resulting from poor insulin control.
      - **Mauriac's syndrome** is characterized by the triad of poorly controlled diabetes mellitus, growth retardation, and hepatomegaly. Liver histology demonstrates fatty infiltration. This syndrome resolves with improvement in glycemic control.
   b. **Fatty acid oxidation defects** such as medium-chain acyl-coenzyme A (CoA) dehydrogenase deficiency (MCAD) and long-chain 3 hydroxyacyl-CoA dehydrogenase (LCHAD) deficiency manifest with hepatomegaly, hypoglycemia, and increased serum aminotransferase levels. These defects result in an inability to use fat, which builds up in the liver.
      - Decompensation is often precipitated by common childhood illnesses such as otitis media or acute gastroenteritis and is characterized by lethargy and severe hypoglycemia. Such episodes respond rapidly to fluid and glucose replacement.
      - The diagnosis is suggested by abnormal urine organic acids. The ratio of ketone bodies to dicarboxylic acid is low, signifying an inability to metabolize stored fats. Total serum carnitine is low, whereas the fraction of acylcarnitine is usually high.

    c. **Galactosemia** resulting from a deficiency of galactose-1-phosphate uridyltransferase usually manifests within the first few days of life. This deficiency leads to accumulation of galactose-1-phosphate and galactitol and in turn leads to fatty liver.
- The initial presentation may be with *Escherichia coli* sepsis in a neonate.
- If the disorder is not treated, affected infants will succumb to hepatic failure.
- Treatment is by removal of lactose (and galactose) from the diet, because lactose is broken down to glucose and galactose.

    d. **Oxidative phosphorylation defects,** as in **Alpers' syndrome,** result in profound **lactic acidosis.** This defect manifests as an elevated lactate-to-pyruvate ratio and an increase in 3-hydroxybutyrate.
- These disorders usually manifest with neurologic disease, myopathy, or seizures and progressive hepatic failure.
- It is frequently difficult initially to differentiate the side effects of seizure medications from Alpers' syndrome.

    e. **Reye's syndrome** (see later) may manifest with a rapidly enlarging liver resulting from triglyceride accumulation and hypertrophy of the smooth endoplasmic reticulum.
- The disorder is associated with a typical prodrome of viral illness, most commonly an upper respiratory tract infection or varicella, and has been linked to aspirin use.
- The presentation is with protracted vomiting, disorientation, and varying degrees of liver failure.
- Treatment is supportive.

2. Cholesterol accumulates in cholesteryl ester storage disease and Wolman's disease.
- Cholesteryl ester storage disease is otherwise asymptomatic.
- **Wolman's disease** is characterized by a decrease in the lysosomal enzyme acid lipase that results in decreased degradation of cholesterol. Poor nutritional status is also seen secondary to accumulation of lipid in the intestinal epithelium. Neurologic deterioration and death occur by 6 to 12 months of age. Treatment consists primarily of parenteral nutrition. Bone marrow transplantation, which may normalize acid lipase activity, has been proposed.

3. **Glycogen storage disease (GSD) type I and type IV** manifest with hepatomegaly secondary to accumulated glycogen in hepatocytes (see also Chapter 18).
- In **GSD I,** activity of glucose-6-phosphatase is absent or abnormal; therefore, gluconeogenesis cannot proceed. Patients develop profound hypoglycemia after short periods of fasting with lactic acidosis, hyperuricemia, hypophosphatemia, and hyperlipidemia. Treatment includes a high-starch diet often in the form of cornstarch or continuous feedings to provide a continuous source of glucose. Patients are also at increased risk of hepatic adenomas.
- **GSD IV** is rare and manifests in infancy with hepatosplenomegaly and poor weight gain caused by a debranching enzyme deficiency. Like GSD I, GSD IV results in defective gluconeogenesis and accumulation of glycogen. Treatment is with liver transplantation.

4. Sphingolipid accumulation is characteristic of **Gaucher's disease,** which results from an autosomal recessive deficiency of glucocerebrosidase, the lysosomal enzyme responsible for degrading sphingolipids (see also Chapter 18). Three forms are recognized:
- Type I typically manifests with hepatosplenomegaly and is a chronic non-neuropathic form of the disease.
- Type II also manifests with hepatosplenomegaly but has neuropathic features and is often fatal by age 2 years.
- Type III is associated with hepatosplenomegaly and the later onset of neuropathic features.

5. **Niemann–Pick disease** is characterized histologically by lipid-laden "foam cells" and stored sphingomyelin in macrophages. This disorder is caused by decreased sphingomyelinase that

results in accumulation of sphingomyelin and cholesterol in the reticuloendothelial system in many organs, including the liver

6. **Alpha-1 antitrypsin deficiency** presents with hepatosplenomegaly resulting from intracellular accumulation of abnormal alpha-1 antitrypsin molecules along the endoplasmic reticulum. The abnormal homozygous PiZZ alpha-1 antitrypsin–deficient phenotype can be determined electrophoretically, Liver transplantation has been used to treat liver disease associated with this disorder (see Chapter 18).

7. Copper storage diseases (see Chapter 17)
   a. **Wilson disease** (WD) is a genetic disease of copper overload; the abnormal gene is located on chromosome 13.
      - The carrier rate is 1 in 90. Expression of the disease appears to be variable even within the same family.
      - Defective copper excretion results in excess accumulation in the liver with subsequent accumulation in the central nervous system and other organs.
      - Liver disease manifests in the second to fourth decades of life. Later presentation tends to be neurologic or psychiatric.
      - WD is diagnosed by a serum ceruloplasmin level less than 20 mg/dL, liver copper greater than 250 µg/g, and urinary copper greater than 100 µg/day.
      - Liver biopsy specimens show steatosis early in the course; the disease progresses to inflammation and fibrosis with cirrhosis. A copper stain of the liver may be helpful in the diagnosis but is not specific, and the absence of stainable copper does not exclude WD.
      - Without treatment, the disease is fatal as a result of hepatic failure; it is controllable with copper chelation. Penicillamine and trientine are chelators that increase urinary excretion of copper. Zinc, which blocks intestinal absorption of copper, has also been used.
      - Some patients present with fulminant hepatic failure; the only effective treatment option in this situation is liver transplantation, which is curative.
   b. **Indian childhood cirrhosis** is a copper storage disease seen in young children.
      - The origin is unknown and has been attributed to excessive copper intake as well as a defect in copper excretion.
      - The disorder manifests earlier than WD with hepatic failure leading rapidly to death within weeks to months of presentation; the disease is often fatal by age 4 years.
      - Patients present with nonspecific complaints of anorexia and irritability but develop hepatomegaly and jaundice followed by secondary manifestations of liver disease.
      - Hepatic copper content is often higher than 1000 µg/g. Copper accumulation appears to inhibit transport of intracellular proteins and thereby causes hepatocyte swelling.
      - Treatment, like that of WD, is with chelation therapy.

TUMOR INFILTRATION

Tumor infiltration of the liver can contribute to hepatomegaly.
- Primary tumors include embryonal rhabdomyosarcoma of the biliary tree, teratoma, hepatoblastoma, and hemangioendothelioma.
- Tumors that may secondarily infiltrate the liver include neuroblastoma, Wilms' tumor, and lymphoma.
- CT can identify these tumors initially as focal abnormalities rather than as diffuse infiltration. Diagnosis is by biopsy.
- Treatment depends on the tumor type.

Acute Liver Disease

Many of the previously discussed diseases manifest after an indolent course or with subtle findings. Acute liver diseases, such as viral hepatitis and Reye's syndrome, have a more sudden onset.

1. **Viral hepatitis** (see Chapter 3). The most common causes of viral hepatitis in children are **hepatitis A and hepatitis B viruses**. Although both infections may manifest as an acute febrile illness with jaundice and hepatomegaly, the courses may differ. Additionally, the presentations and courses can differ from those in adults.

    a. **Hepatitis A** is transmitted by the fecal-oral route, and outbreaks can often be traced to day-care centers where hygiene may be suboptimal. Adults who work with children in day-care centers are at an increased risk of contracting this disease.

        ■ The disease is often asymptomatic (75% to 95%) in children, whereas adults are more commonly symptomatic (75% to 95%); a few develop severe liver disease.

        ■ Administration of the hepatitis A vaccine to children and adults at high risk should decrease the frequency of hepatitis A.

    b. **Hepatitis B** is transmitted perinatally. Children exhibit a clinical course similar to that of adults.

        ■ Rarely, an associated immune complex–mediated extrahepatic disease, such as membranous glomerulonephritis or papular acrodermatitis of childhood (Gianotti–Crosti syndrome), occurs.

        ■ Infants born to mothers who are positive for hepatitis B surface antigen (especially those positive for hepatitis B e antigen) are at high risk of becoming chronic hepatitis B virus carriers and of developing hepatocellular carcinoma.

        ■ Administration of hepatitis B immune globulin within 4 to 6 hours of birth followed by the first dose of the hepatitis B vaccine and subsequent completion of the series can prevent this disease. Hepatitis B vaccination of newborns is now routine in the United States.

2. **Reye's syndrome** is a rare cause of fulminant failure in children

    ■ This disorder typically manifests following a prodromal febrile illness such as an upper respiratory tract infection or varicella and is often associated with aspirin treatment.

    ■ Protracted vomiting occurs 5 to 7 days after the onset of the initial illness, usually as the first illness is improving. Progression to hepatic failure with associated neurologic deterioration, seizures, and coma may occur quite rapidly.

    ■ Serum aminotransferase levels are typically more than three to four times normal. A significantly elevated ammonia level or a prolonged prothrombin time indicates a greater likelihood of progressive liver failure.

    ■ Liver histology demonstrates hepatocytes with foamy accumulation of triglyceride. Electron microscopy demonstrates alterations in mitochondria; similar alterations are seen in mitochondria in the brain.

    ■ Treatment is supportive and focuses on controlling intracranial pressure. Survival depends on early diagnosis; patients treated before severe neurologic involvement occurs have a greater chance of complete recovery.

3. **Cystic liver disease** (see Chapter 28) results from lack of normal embryonic development of the biliary tree. A spectrum of diseases is seen, depending on the size of the bile duct involved.

    ■ **Caroli's disease** is the name given to cystic liver disease involving the large intrahepatic bile ducts. Because of bile stasis in the cysts, affected patients are predisposed to recurrent cholangitis.

■ Caroli's disease, along with most of the other polycystic liver diseases, may be associated with extrahepatic disease, particularly cystic disease of the kidneys.

Systemic Diseases Affecting the Liver (see Chapter 22)

1. **Cystic fibrosis (CF):** a disease of altered chloride secretion, most commonly affecting the lungs and pancreas. Many patients with CF have associated **focal and multilobular biliary cirrhosis** and associated complications such as portal hypertension (see also Chapter 18).
   ■ The presence of liver disease does not appear to depend on the genotype of CF, nor is it related to the severity of pulmonary disease.
   ■ Patients present with hepatomegaly, which may be erroneously attributed to hyperinflation of the lungs.
   ■ Patients with CF are known to have a high incidence of biliary sludge, cholelithiasis, bile duct strictures, microgallbladder, and prolonged neonatal cholestasis.
   ■ Treatment with ursodeoxycholic acid has been shown to improve the abnormal laboratory findings associated with liver disease in CF; however, it is unclear whether prophylactic therapy with ursodeoxycholic acid is beneficial in all patients with CF.
2. **Sickle cell disease**
   ■ Patients with sickle cell disease commonly have hepatomegaly, apparently secondary to sinusoidal dilatation and Kupffer cell hyperplasia. The origin is unclear but may be related to chronic low-level hypoxia.
   ■ An increased incidence of cholelithiasis secondary to rapid hemoglobin turnover is seen in this population.
3. **Obesity**
   a. In children as well as adults, obesity can lead to hepatomegaly, which is associated with steatosis, mild inflammation, and Kupffer cell hyperplasia.
   b. **Nonalcoholic fatty liver disease** is estimated to affect 3% to 5% of the general pediatric population, with the fraction increasing 10- to 20-fold in the obese pediatric population.
   c. Progression from steatosis to steatohepatitis to advanced fibrosis and cirrhosis has been documented in children as in the adult population (see Chapter 7).
      ■ The presence of the metabolic syndrome and of impaired insulin sensitivity appears to be more important than obesity alone in the development of steatosis and steatohepatitis.
      ■ Ethnic background is also a risk factor; Hispanics and Native Americans are at highest risk and African Americans are at lowest risk.
   d. Treatment consists primarily of weight loss and control of hyperglycemia and hyperlipidemia, if applicable. Weight loss should not be rapid, because of the potential to aggravate hepatic inflammation; weight loss of 500 g/week has been advocated in children.
      ■ Therapy with vitamin E has demonstrated a beneficial effect in adults and is currently being studied in children and adolescents.
4. **Total parenteral nutrition (TPN)**
   ■ In children, especially neonates, TPN is associated with cholestasis, which may progress to cirrhosis and liver failure.
   ■ The precise pathogenesis of liver disease resulting from TPN is unknown. It is likely multifactorial, including toxic substrates in the TPN solution, nutrient and micronutrient deficiency, and toxic bacterial byproducts that cross the atrophic intestinal mucosal barrier.
   ■ The only effective treatment is administration of enteral feedings.

5. **Celiac disease**
   - Patients with celiac disease may present with serum aminotransferase elevations, a prolonged prothrombin time, or nonspecific liver histologic changes even in the absence of gastrointestinal symptoms.
   - Celiac disease has also been associated with autoimmune hepatitis, primary sclerosing cholangitis, and primary biliary cirrhosis.
   - Treatment with a gluten-free diet typically normalizes both laboratory and liver histologic abnormalities.

6. **Primary sclerosing cholangitis (PSC) and inflammatory bowel disease (IBD)** (see Chapters 22 and 23).
   - Patients with IBD, especially ulcerative colitis, frequently develop PSC.
   - The progression of PSC is unrealted to the duration or severity of the IBD and may precede intestinal symptoms.
   - Treatment of IBD with immunosuppression does not ameliorate the symptoms or evolution of PSC.

7. **Childhood histiocytic syndromes:** Abnormal activation of the reticuloendothelial system may result in liver disease.
   - **Langerhans' cell histiocytosis (LCH)** has an incidence of 4 to 5 cases per 100,000, with a median age at diagnosis of 30.2 months. Abnormally activated Langerhans' cells can infiltrate the liver, thereby resulting in elevated serum aminotransferase levels, hypoalbuminemia, prolongation of the prothrombin time, and hepatomegaly. Liver histology commonly demonstrates a portal tract inflammatory infiltrate composed of lymphocytes, neutrophils, and eosinophils. LCH may be apparent if liver tissue is immunostained for S-100 protein. Sclerosing cholangitis is the classic process ascribed to LCH. Patients who require liver transplantation may be at increased risk of acute cellular rejection and post-transplantation lymphoproliferative disease.
   - **Hemophagocytic lymphohistiocytosis (HLH)** has an incidence of 1.2 cases per 100,000 per year and a median age at diagnosis of 2.9 months. This multi-organ disease is caused by abnormal activation of non-malignant macrophages. The clinical presentation is variable and includes acute liver failure in infancy. Liver histology reveals portal infiltrates (with lymphocytes) of varying size. Diagnostic criteria include hypertriglyceridemia, splenomegaly, cytopenias, and fever. Treatment is with bone marrow transplantation.

8. **Muscular dystrophies:** These are not particularly associated with liver disease, but they often manifest with an elevated serum aspartate aminotransferase (AST) level that leads the clinician to believe that the liver is involved. Further evaluation reveals an elevated creatine kinase level, thus confirming that the origin of the AST is muscle.

9. **Inborn errors of glycosylation:** Carbohydrate-deficient glycoprotein syndromes comprise a group of multisystem disorders with defects in *N*-linked oligosaccharide assembly.
   - Type Ia is the most common and best described. It is caused by defects in the phosphomannomutase 2 gene and has an incidence of 1 in 80,000.
   - Infants have a high mortality risk from multisystem disease. Those surviving infancy often have profound psychomotor and mental retardation. Patients can present in infancy with variable degrees of liver dysfunction secondary to steatosis or fibrosis.
   - The diagnosis is made by abnormal electrophoretic isofocusing of serum transferrin.
   - Treatment with d-mannose may ameliorate hepatic and gastrointestinal symptoms.

FURTHER READING

Alisi A, Manco M, Vania A, Nobili V. Pediatric nonalcoholic fatty liver disease in 2009. *J Pediatr* 2009; 155:469–474.

Balistreri WF, Bezerra JA, guest eds. Whatever happened to "neonatal hepatitis"? Pediatric hepatology. *Clin Liver Dis* 2006; 10:27–53.

Kurbegov AC, Sokol RJ. Hepatitis B therapy in children. *Expert Rev Gastroenterol Hepatol* 2009; 3:39–49.

Leonis MA, Balistreri WF. Evaluation and management of end-stage liver disease in children. *Gastroenterology* 2008; 134:1741–1751.

Mieli-Vergani G, Heller S, Jara P, et al. Autoimmune hepatitis. *J Pediatr Gastroenterol Nutr* 2009; 49:158–164.

Shneider BL. Progressive intrahepatic cholestasis: mechanisms, diagnosis, and therapy. *Pediatr Transplant* 2004; 8:609–612.

Sokol RJ, Shepherd RW, Superina R, et al. Screening and outcomes in biliary atresia: summary of a National Institutes of Health workshop. *Hepatology* 2007; 46:566–581.

Suchy FJ, Sokol RJ, Balistreri WF, eds. *Liver Disease in Children*. 3rd edn. Cambridge: Cambridge University Press; 2007.

Sundaram SS, Bove KE, Lovell MA, Sokol RJ. Mechanisms of disease: inborn errors of bile acid synthesis. *Nat Clin Pract Gastroenterol Hepatol* 2008; 5:456–468.

CHAPTER 24

Liver disease in the elderly

Santiago J. Muñoz, MD, FACP, FACG ■ Vishal Patel, MD

KEY POINTS

1 The clinical presentation, prognosis, and management of several liver disorders can be different in older patients than in younger persons.

2 Hepatic blood flow, liver size, and hepatic regenerative capacity decrease with age; these changes result in decreased metabolism of certain medications and a reduced ability of the liver to recover promptly from diseases such as acute viral hepatitis.

3 Certain disorders, such as acute liver failure and drug-induced hepatitis, are more severe and have a worse prognosis in elderly patients than in younger patients.

4 The development of hepatocellular carcinoma (HCC) is directly related to the duration of cirrhosis; therefore, elderly patients with cirrhosis should be screened regularly for HCC.

5 Advanced age is not a contraindication to liver transplantation, which should be considered in selected elderly patients with irreversible end-stage liver disease. Conversely, livers can be accepted from elderly donors, albeit with some risk of poor graft function and more rapid and severe recurrence of hepatitis C virus infection in the allograft.

Cellular and Biochemical Aspects

OVERVIEW

1. The aging process affects the liver, but to a lesser degree than other organs.
2. Hepatic size decreases by 6.5% in men and 14.3% in women, and hepatic blood flow diminishes with advancing age; these changes may result in alterations in cellular function and biochemical pathways in the liver.
3. These age-related alterations are of considerable importance, given the aging of our population and the fact the elderly use approximately one third of all prescribed medications, many of which are metabolized by the liver.

CELLULAR AND BIOCHEMICAL CHANGES IN THE AGING LIVER

1. Aging of liver cells is characterized primarily by decreased production of hepatic proteins; some abnormal proteins accumulate in aging liver cells (Table 24.1).
2. Histopathologic changes seen in aging livers include increases in cell size, the number of abnormal nuclei, and the frequency of chromosomal abnormalities. Often, the number and size of lysosomes also increase. Mitochondria increase in volume but decrease in number and, together with decreased hepatic blood flow, may contribute to reduced metabolism of certain drugs.

TABLE 24.1 ■ **Proteins that accumulate in aging livers**

Glucose-6-phosphate dehydrogenase

Phosphoglycerate kinase

NADP cytochrome c reductase

Cathepsin D

Superoxide dismutase

Aminoacyl-tRNA synthetases

NAPD, nicotinamide adenine dinucleotide phosphate.

Adapted from Dice JF. Aging and the uncertain role of sirtuins. In: Arias IM, Wolkoff A, Boyer J, et al, eds. *The Liver: Biology and Pathobiology.* Singapore: Wiley-Blackwell; 2009:955–960.

3. Lipofuscin, the "wear-and-tear" pigment, is a common finding on liver biopsy specimens from elderly persons. Lipofuscin has been thought to represent extensive nonenzymatic glycosylation and cross-linking of heterogeneous cellular components, including nucleic acids, proteins, and lipids. Evidence suggests that lipofuscin may represent, at least in part, accumulation of retinyl palmitate. Although lipofuscin is thought to be biologically inert, it may interfere with intracellular biochemical reactions.

4. As individuals age, hepatocytes become less sensitive to insulin and corticosteroids. Protein breakdown and both transcriptional and translational processes decrease. The altered breakdown of cellular protein may have important consequences for the cell life cycle and may be a major feature of the aging process.

Pathophysiology of the Aging Liver

OVERVIEW

1. Serum levels of routine liver biochemical tests, such as albumin, aminotransferases, and bilirubin, do not change significantly as persons age.

2. Age-related changes include decreases in liver weight, hepatic blood flow, metabolism of drugs, and responsiveness to hormonal and growth factors and delayed regeneration.

CHANGES IN DRUG METABOLISM

1. The systemic clearance of many drugs that are metabolized by the hepatic cytochrome P-450 (CYP) system (e.g., midazolam, phenytoin, propranolol, acetaminophen) is decreased in the elderly. However, the enzymatic activities of CYP3A and CYP2E1 do not change with aging; this finding suggests that elderly persons may be just as susceptible as younger persons to the hepatotoxic effects of drugs such as acetaminophen and ethanol.

2. Other mechanisms must be present to explain the reduced hepatic clearance of the previously mentioned drugs. A 40% decrease in hepatic volume and a 50% reduction in liver blood flow in elderly persons account for the reduction in systemic clearance of drugs, such as propranolol, that have a high first-pass hepatic uptake. The decrease in liver volume is most likely responsible for impaired clearance of medications that do not undergo significant first-pass hepatic uptake.

3. The volume of distribution of water-soluble drugs is generally reduced in elderly patients because of an increase in the ratio of body fat to body water. Although the metabolism of ethanol is essentially unaltered by aging, elevated blood ethanol levels can be observed in elderly subjects after acute intake of ethanol as a result of a reduction in the volume of distribution.
4. The age-related reduction in hepatic blood mostly results from a decrease in portal blood flow. Sensitive Doppler techniques have shown that portal blood flow decreases from 740 ± 150 mL/minute in persons less than 40 years of age to 595 ± 106 mL/minute in healthy persons who are more than 71 years old. The reduction in portal vein blood flow may relate to atherosclerosis, with a resulting decrease in mesenteric arterial blood flow.

ALTERATIONS IN CHOLESTEROL METABOLISM

1. The cholesterol content of bile increases with advancing age, as does the lithogenic index, because of the combination of increased hepatic secretion of cholesterol and decreased bile acid production. The elderly gallbladder also may be less responsive to endogenous chole-cystokinin (CCK), with a resulting decrease in postprandial contraction of the gallbladder. Supersaturated bile is four times as frequent in elderly women as in younger women.
2. The frequency of gallstones increases with age. Approximately 40% to 60% of persons in their eighth decade have gallstones. Complications of gallstone disease are more severe in the elderly.

Hepatic Diseases in the Elderly

ACUTE VIRAL HEPATITIS (see Chapter 3)

In elderly patients, the course of acute viral hepatitis may be more prolonged, severe, and indolent than in younger patients, probably because of an increased likelihood of comorbid conditions, an aged-related decline in immune function, and the decreased regenerative ability of the aging liver.

1. Hepatitis A
   ■ Hepatitis A is relatively uncommon in the elderly because of a high rate of preexisting immunity. However, increasing proportions of elderly persons in Western countries are not immune to hepatitis A (30% in the US population who are more than 50 years of age).
   ■ The mortality of acute hepatitis A increases with advancing age. The mortality rate is 0.4% in patients between ages 15 and 39 years, 1.1% in those age 40 years and older, and 4% in those more than 65 years old.
   ■ Elderly persons who plan to travel to areas where hepatitis A is endemic should be tested for antibody to hepatitis A virus. If seronegative, they should receive the first dose of the hepatitis A virus vaccine at least 4 weeks before travel; other indications for hepatitis A vaccination, as recommended by the Advisory Committee on Immunizations Practices, apply to elderly persons as well.
2. Hepatitis B
   ■ Acute hepatitis B is less common in elderly persons than in younger persons.
   ■ The presentation is generally more cholestatic in the elderly, with less hepatocellular necrosis. However, patients are frequently symptomatic, sicker, and have a longer recovery interval.

- Although the clearance of the hepatitis B surface antigen (HBsAg) takes somewhat longer in the elderly than the young, the overall prognosis is similar in the two groups; however, the elderly are more likely to remain chronically infected with hepatitis B virus (HBV).
- The elderly do not respond as well as younger persons to hepatitis B vaccination, probably because of a decrease in the number of antibody-producing B cells. Higher vaccine doses or booster immunization may be necessary for successful hepatitis B vaccination of older persons.
3. Hepatitis C
   - The incidence of hepatitis C is reported to be similar in the young and old. As with acute hepatitis A and B, cholestasis may be a prominent feature.
   - Spontaneous clearance of newly acquired hepatitis C is less likely in the elderly.
   - Although no mandated upper age limit exists for treatment with pegylated interferon alpha and ribavirin, caution should be exercised when treating the elderly with these drugs. Adverse reactions such as cardiac, central nervous system, and systemic effects can be more severe in the elderly. Because the elderly are more likely to have decreased renal function, careful dose selection and monitoring of renal function are important.
4. Other causes of hepatitis
   - In immunosuppressed and debilitated patients with hepatitis, the possibilities of herpes virus or cytomegalovirus infection should be considered and appropriately investigated.
   - In the elderly patient who presents with apparent acute viral hepatitis, the differential diagnosis should include ischemic hepatitis, sepsis, hepatic metastases, drug-induced hepatitis, and obstructive jaundice (see Chapter 1).
   - Conversely, older patients with jaundice and elevated liver enzyme levels presumed to result from extrahepatic biliary obstruction require evaluation for acute viral hepatitis.

CHRONIC VIRAL HEPATITIS (see Chapter 4)

1. Chronic hepatitis B
   - The clinical presentation of chronic hepatitis B in the elderly is generally similar to that of younger patients. However, many elderly patients with chronic hepatitis B are hepatitis B e antigen (HBeAg) negative and have low levels of serum HBV DNA, findings indicating a lesser degree of viral replication and infectivity. This serologic profile generally indicates a long duration of the disease and is termed the *inactive carrier state.*
   - Persons with the inactive carrier state generally do not require antiviral therapy. However, older inactive carriers may progress to cirrhosis at an annual rate of 4%.
   - The main antiviral agents for HBV treatment include entecavir, tenofovir, and peginterferon alpha 2a; lamivudine, adefovir, and telbivudine are no longer considered first-line agents. Treatment with peginterferon alfa-2a or lamivudine has been showed to be equally effective in younger and older groups.
   - The dose of entecavir, tenofovir, and other nucleoside or nucleotide analogues must be reduced when the creatinine clearance is less than 50 mL/minute, as occurs frequently in the elderly.
   - Advanced age is associated with an increased risk of hepatocellular carcinoma (HCC) and requires vigilant surveillance for this malignant disease in the elderly.
2. Chronic hepatitis C
   - The clinical presentation of chronic hepatitis C is similar in both young and elderly patients.

- In developed countries, the frequency of chronic hepatitis C in the elderly is increasing (approximately 1% in the United States and Germany and 16% to 42% in Italy, Spain, France, and Japan).
- Pegylated interferon alpha in combination with ribavirin is currently approved for the treatment of chronic hepatitis C. The tolerability of this combination therapy is often reduced in the elderly, with an increased frequency of neuropsychiatric side effects and ribavirin-induced anemia. Rates of sustained virologic response to treatment are decreased in the elderly.
- Treatment decisions should take in account comorbid conditions, life expectancy, stage of liver disease, and probability of a durable treatment response.
3. An important complication of chronic hepatitis B and C is the development of HCC. Because the development of HCC correlates with the duration of chronic hepatitis, elderly patients with cirrhosis resulting from chronic hepatitis B or C should be screened twice yearly with ultrasonography of the liver and serum alpha fetoprotein testing (see Chapters 9 and 27).

DRUG-INDUCED HEPATOTOXICITY (see Chapter 8)

1. **The risk of drug-induced hepatotoxicity increases with advancing age.** Approximately 20% of cases of jaundice in the elderly are secondary to medications, compared with 2% to 5% of patients of all ages who require hospitalization for jaundice.
2. Increased drug toxicity is caused by altered distribution (decreased albumin levels causing an increased volume of drug distribution), decreased clearance secondary to reduced blood flow and volume and depressed enzymes systems (in particular cytochrome P-450), and decreased renal clearance.
3. Elderly patients are more likely to be taking multiple medications. A threefold higher frequency of adverse drug reactions has been reported in patients taking six medications compared with those taking a single agent. Such polypharmacy increases the chance that cytochrome P-450 activity will increase or decrease, thereby leading to drug–drug interactions and associated toxicity.
4. Drug-induced hepatotoxicity should be a major diagnostic consideration in elderly patients who present with elevated liver enzyme levels or jaundice. The most common classes of drugs known to cause toxicity in the elderly include antibiotics (e.g., amoxicillin-clavulanic acid), cardiovascular drugs (e.g., amiodarone), and analgesics/antipyretics (e.g., acetaminophen). Table 24.2 lists some drugs for which hepatotoxicity increases with age.

TABLE 24.2 ■ **Example of therapeutic agents for which the risk of hepatotoxicity increases with age**

Dantrolene
Floxacillin
Halothane
Isoniazid
Methyldopa
Sulindac

5. All unnecessary medications should be discontinued. Essential agents should be switched to a different class.

NONALCOHOLIC FATTY LIVER DISEASE AND NONALCOHOLIC STEATOHEPATITIS (see Chapter 7)

1. Nonalcoholic fatty liver disease (NAFLD) is present in 20% to 30% of the general population. The prevalence increases with age and reaches 60% in persons 46 to 75 years of age. Nonalcoholic steatohepatitis (NASH) is approximately one tenth as frequent; 10% to 15% of persons with NASH may progress to cirrhosis, liver failure, and HCC.
2. The prevalence of metabolic syndrome that includes insulin resistance, obesity, diabetes mellitus, hypertriglyceridemia, and hypertension increases with age and is almost universally present in patients with NAFLD.
3. Older age is an independent predictor of severe liver fibrosis in patients with NASH.

AUTOIMMUNE LIVER DISEASES

1. Autoimmune hepatitis (see Chapter 5)
   - This typically occurs in middle-aged women. However, 17% to 56% of patients present when they are more than 65 years old, and in these patients the male-to-female ratio is 1:9.
   - Elderly patients commonly present with symptoms of jaundice, fatigue, or drowsiness and are more likely than younger patients to present with ascites.
   - The management strategy is identical in all adults; however, treatment in the elderly can be difficult because of the adverse effects of long-term corticosteroid use in postmenopausal women already at high risk for osteoporosis, glaucoma, arterial hypertension, and obesity.
2. Primary biliary cirrhosis (see Chapter 14)
   - This affects middle-aged women primarily, with a median age at onset of 50 years; up to 50% of patients in some populations present for the first time after age 65 years.
   - Most patients are asymptomatic at presentation, and the elderly are significantly less likely to present with symptoms (pruritus, weight loss, fatigue) than are patients less than 65 years of age.
   - Evidence regarding whether advancing age is a poor prognostic indicator in patients with primary biliary cirrhosis is conflicting.
   - It is particularly important to screen elderly patients for decreased bone density and to treat those with low density appropriately.
3. Primary sclerosing cholangitis (see Chapter 15)
   - This usually occurs in the third or fourth decade; therefore, the diagnosis is unusual in an elderly patient. Increased age is an independent risk factor for a poor outcome.
   - In elderly patients presenting with cholestatic jaundice and a cholangiogram resembling primary sclerosing cholangitis, carcinoma of the biliary tract should be excluded (see Chapter 34).

ALCOHOLIC LIVER DISEASE (see Chapter 6)

1. Substantial proportions of patients with alcoholic liver disease present at or beyond the fifth and sixth decades.
2. An age-related decrease in ethanol metabolism leads to increased acetaldehyde levels in the liver, which underlies the steatosis that occurs in the elderly liver with decreased mitochondrial fatty acid oxidation.

3. Older patients are more likely than younger patients to have histologically advanced liver disease and to exhibit the classic signs of hepatic decompensation: ascites, jaundice, and lower extremity edema.

4. Overall mortality from alcoholic liver disease is higher in patients who are more than 60 years old: 34% at 1 year, compared with 5% in younger patients. In patients more than 70 years old, the 1-year mortality rate increases dramatically to 75%.

METABOLIC LIVER DISEASES

1. Hereditary hemochromatosis (HH) (see Chapter 16)
   - Most persons with HH present by middle age, but some first present at an advanced age with HCC or other complications of end-stage liver disease.
   - HH can manifest in old age. Men with the HFE gene mutation *C282Y* may live long lives without biochemical or histologic abnormalities.
   - Female patients typically become symptomatic approximately 1 decade after their male counterparts, because of the iron-depleting effects of regular menses and childbirth.
   - Common symptoms may include fatigue, diabetes mellitus, impotence, and arthritis, all of which are common in the elderly population. HH should also be considered in an elderly patient presenting with a neurologic disorder, because iron overload can manifest as a cerebellar syndrome.
   - A major cause of death in patients with cirrhosis due to HH is HCC; screening with ultrasonography and serum alpha fetoprotein testing should be done every 6 months (see Chapter 27).
   - Elderly patients may not tolerate intensive phlebotomy therapy and may require less frequent phlebotomies of smaller volumes than younger patients.

2. Alpha-1 antitrypsin deficiency (see Chapter 18)
   - Patients with homozygous alpha-1 antitrypsin deficiency (α-1 ATD) usually present before age 65 years.
   - Heterozygous α-1 ATD has been thought to be the cause of cirrhosis in approximately 5% of patients with cirrhosis who are more than 65 years old; however, heterozygous α-1 ATD is frequent in the overall population. No evidence indicates that intracellular α-1 ATD globular inclusions are hepatotoxic in heterozygotes.
   - Although no specific effective treatment for α-1 ATD-related liver disease exists, diagnosis is important so that heterozygous or affected family members can be advised to avoid behaviors such as alcohol intake, smoking, and intravenous drug use, which may jeopardize their hepatic and pulmonary function.

3. Wilson disease (see Chapter 17): De novo diagnosis of this entity is rare in elderly persons. Rare patients are first diagnosed after the age of 65 years.

LIVER ABSCESS (see Chapter 28)

1. Most patients with a pyogenic liver abscess in the Northern Hemisphere are more than 60 years old, with a reported mean age of 47 to 65 years.

2. The diagnosis is more difficult to make in the elderly than in younger patients, because the typical presentation of fever, jaundice, and right upper quadrant pain may be absent. Elderly patients are more likely to have nonspecific symptoms, such as epigastric pain, weakness, fatigue, and shortness of breath.

3. Although approximately half of infections originate from the biliary tract (most often as a result of ascending cholangitis), other intra-abdominal and gastrointestinal sources should be investigated, including the following:

- Penetrating gastric or duodenal ulcers
- Pancreatitis
- Perihepatic abscess
- Portal vein thrombosis
- Peritonitis (of any cause)
- Inflammatory bowel disease
- Colon cancer
- Diverticulitis or diverticular abscess
- Cryptogenic conditions (in some cases resulting from poor dentition)
4. Elderly patients are more likely to have gallstone-related disease or a malignant tumor and more often have polymicrobial infection.
5. Almost one third of elderly persons with a hepatic abscess at autopsy may be misdiagnosed in life as having a hepatic malignant disease. Confirmation of tumor by needle biopsy should be obtained, especially if a primary site of malignancy is not present.
6. As in younger persons, pyogenic abscesses can be treated successfully by percutaneous aspiration and drainage in conjunction with systemic intravenous antibiotics.

GALLSTONES (see Chapter 32)

1. Gallstones are an age-related phenomenon. The mortality of untreated biliary tract disease also increases with age. Cancer of the gallbladder is more likely to occur in older patients than in younger patients (see Chapter 34).
   - Age-related changes including increased lithogenicity of bile, deconjugation of bile pigments, increased bactobilia, and altered gallbladder motility all may contribute to increased gallstone formation.
   - The frequency of bile duct stones reaches 50% in patients with cholelithiasis who are more than 80 years old.
2. The management of biliary disease with respect to age is summarized in Table 24.3.
   - With the advent of laparoscopic cholecystectomy, early operative intervention brought the mortality and morbidity rates for younger and older patients closer together.
   - Morbidity and mortality rates for endoscopic retrograde cholangiopancreatography (ERCP) with sphincterotomy are not significantly different between old and young, despite a longer duration of hospitalization in the elderly.

TABLE 24.3 ■ **Management of biliary disease in the elderly**

Condition	Treatment
Acute or chronic cholecystitis	Early cholecystectomy (preferably laparoscopic); if cholecystectomy not possible, placement of percutaneous cholecystostomy tube followed by cholecystectomy when possible
Cholangitis with choledocholithiasis	ERCP with sphincterotomy and stone extraction
Choledocholithiasis with gallstones in the gallbladder	ERCP with sphincterotomy; if symptoms persist, cholecystectomy or percutaneous cholecystostomy with laparoscopic bile duct exploration
Asymptomatic gallstones	Observation generally preferred over prophylactic intervention

ERCP, endoscopic retrograde cholangiopancreatography.

- Incidental appendectomy during cholecystectomy should not be performed in elderly patients because of the risk of wound infection and the relatively low lifetime risk of acute appendicitis.

HEPATIC TUMORS (see Chapter 27)

1. HCC
   - Elderly patients with cirrhosis are at increased risk of HCC; a clear association exists between the development of HCC and the duration of cirrhosis; in the Western world, 50% of patients with cirrhosis who develop HCC are more than 60 years old, and 40% are more than 70 years old.
   - Because of its long natural history, hepatitis C virus (HCV)–related cirrhosis is the leading cause of HCC in the elderly (5% per year). Increasingly, NAFLD has been found as a cause of cirrhosis and HCC in the elderly.
   - Screening for HCC should be performed as described previously; early detection of small tumors may prolong survival.
   - Nonsurgical treatment of HCC in the elderly includes radiofrequency ablation, transcatheter arterial chemoembolization (TACE), microwave ablation, yttrium-90 locoregional radiation, and specific chemotherapy with sorafenib, with outcomes similar to those in younger patients.
   - Hepatic resection for HCC can be done safely in well-compensated cirrhotic patients 70 years of age or older, depending on the location and size of the tumor. The overall prognosis, however, is worse than for patients younger than 70 years, even when curative resection is achieved.
   - Older age correlates with recurrence of HCC and worse outcomes.
   - Liver transplantation (LT) may be a treatment option (see later).
2. Metastatic tumors
   - Metastasis is the most common malignant tumor found in the liver in the elderly.
   - The frequency of hepatic metastases is greatest for tumors of the colon, pancreas, and stomach arising within the drainage area of the portal vein, but other tumors, such as lung and breast cancer, can also metastasize to the liver.
   - Survival is directly correlated with the extent of hepatic involvement.
   - Therapy may prolong survival; 20% of patients who undergo surgical resection of a solitary hepatic metastasis may be alive 5 years after resection.

ACUTE LIVER FAILURE (see Chapter 2)

1. Regardless of the cause, acute liver failure (ALF) has a higher mortality rate in the elderly than in the young (Table 23.4).
2. ALF resulting from hepatitis A is particularly devastating in the elderly, with a mortality rate much higher than that in young persons (see earlier).
3. Age greater than 40 years is a negative prognostic indicator for non–acetaminophen-induced ALF (see Chapter 8).
4. The best treatment for ALF in the elderly is to prevent its occurrence, as follows:
   - Vaccination against hepatitis A and B should be considered in all susceptible elderly persons.
   - Isoniazid and other drugs with high hepatotoxicity potential should not be used in the elderly unless absolutely necessary.
   - Unintentional overdose of acetaminophen should be avoided by carefully reviewing an elderly patient's medication list (including use of supplements) at each office visit.

TABLE 24.4 ■ **Survival rates in acute liver failure**

	Age <60 yr (%)	Age ≥60 yr (%)
Acetaminophen-related		
Spontaneous	65	60
After liver transplantation	83	NA
Overall	73	60
Nonacetaminophen-related		
Spontaneous	31	25
After liver transplantation	91	80
Overall	68	48

NA, not available.

Adapted from Schiødt FV, Chung RT, Schilsky ML, et al, and the ALFSG. Acute liver failure in the elderly. *Liver Transplant* 2009; 15:1481–1487.

■ Periodic monitoring of liver enzyme levels should be performed in elderly patients who require treatment with medications known to have hepatotoxic potential.

PORTAL HYPERTENSION (see Chapter 10)

1. Elderly patients admitted with bleeding esophageal varices have short-term mortality rates similar to those of younger patients; however, their 1-year survival rate is less than that of their younger counterparts.
2. Continuous infusion of octreotide is preferable to vasopressin or terlipressin in the medical treatment of bleeding varices in the elderly.
3. Variceal band ligation, sclerotherapy, and beta blocker therapy can be used to prevent recurrent variceal bleeding. Some older patients may be unable to tolerate the adverse effects (e.g., fatigue, dizziness, depression) of beta blockers.
4. A transjugular intrahepatic portosystemic shunt (TIPS) or portacaval shunt can be used for recurrent variceal bleeding; however, the usefulness of a shunt is limited by the relatively high frequency of postshunt hepatic encephalopathy.
   ■ A small-caliber stent of 7 to 8 mm should be used in patients who are more than 60 years old, to decrease the risk of hepatic encephalopathy.
   ■ Lowering the hepatic venous pressure gradient to just below 12 mm Hg may also minimize the risk of post-TIPS hepatic encephalopathy in elderly cirrhotic patients.
5. Elderly patients with refractory ascites or recurrent variceal bleeding, who are otherwise in good physiologic condition, should be considered for LT evaluation (see the next section).

LIVER TRANSPLANTATION (see Chapter 31)

1. Advanced age is not a contraindication to LT. Some studies, but not all, have shown that in patients older than age 60 years, 10-year survival after LT is comparable to that of younger patients. In 1999, 16% of liver recipients in Europe were more than 60 years old, and in 2000, more than 10.7% of liver recipients in the United States were more than 65 years old.

The decision to proceed with LT should be based on the overall health of the patient, not on chronologic age.

2. Factors contributing to worse mortality in the elderly include pre-LT hospitalization and a higher Model for End-stage Liver Disease (MELD) score. **The most common cause of death in long-term LT recipients who are 60 years of age or older is malignant disease, whereas for those less than 60 years old it is infection.**

3. Donor livers from persons more than 50 years old can be used safely. The increasing demand for donor livers has led to the more frequent use of livers from elderly donors.
   - Several groups have reported that patient and graft outcomes are identical regardless of the age of the donor liver even though older livers have significantly increased steatosis and are more likely to be used in patients requiring urgent LT.
   - The function of an older liver may be slightly worse in the early postoperative period, as evidenced by higher peak serum alanine aminotransferase and bilirubin levels and slightly lower bile outputs.

4. A significant increase in the frequency of delayed function is observed in livers from donors who are more than 50 years old compared with donors who are less than 30 years old. Recipients experiencing delayed function are three times as likely to require repeat LT. Early recognition of delayed function and subsequent repeat LT lead to similar 1-year patient survival rates in both groups.

5. Currently, livers from donors who are more than 65 years old are used preferentially in patients who have HCC, have a high MELD score, or require urgent LT (e.g., for hepatorenal syndrome or ALF). Ischemic time should be kept to a minimum when an older donor liver is used, to lessen preservation injury and postoperative hepatic graft dysfunction.

6. That livers from older donors are able to withstand the often extreme physiologic conditions imposed by LT (harvesting, implantation, reperfusion, rejection, toxic effects of drugs, infection) and ultimately provide excellent function is a clear demonstration that the human liver is highly resilient to the aging process.

7. LT recipients with HCV infection who receive livers from donors who are more than 65 years old have been shown to have worse outcomes secondary to an increased rate and severity of recurrent HCV infection.

FURTHER READING

Cainelli F. Hepatitis C virus infection in the elderly: epidemiology, natural history and management. *Drugs Aging* 2008; 25:9–18.

Czaja AJ. Clinical features, differential diagnosis and treatment of autoimmune hepatitis in the elderly. *Drugs Aging* 2008; 25:219–239.

Frith J, Jones D, Newton JL. Chronic liver disease in an ageing population. *Age Ageing* 2009; 38:11–18.

Gentona B, D'Acremonta V, Furrerb H, et al. Hepatitis A vaccines and the elderly. *Travel Med Infect Dis* 2006; 4:303–312.

Gramenzi A, Conti F, Felline F, et al. Hepatitis C virus–related chronic liver disease in elderly patients: an Italian cross-sectional study. *J Viral Hepat* 2010; 17:360–366.

Huang J, Li B, Chen G, et al. Long-term outcomes and prognostic factors of elderly patients with hepatocellular carcinoma undergoing hepatectomy. *J Gastrointest Surg* 2009; 13:1627–1635.

Ikeda K, Arase Y, Kawamura Y, et al. Necessities of interferon therapy in elderly patients with chronic hepatitis C. *Am J Med* 2009; 122:479–486.

Junaidi O, Di Bisceglie AM. Aging liver and hepatitis. *Clin Geriatr Med* 2007; 23:889–903.

Kawaoka T, Suzuki F, Akuta N, et al. Efficacy of lamivudine therapy in elderly patients with chronic hepatitis B infection. *J Gastroenterol* 2007; 42:395–401.

Mindikoglu AL, Miller RR. Hepatitis C in the elderly: epidemiology, natural history, and treatment. *Clin Gastroenterol Hepatol* 2009; 7:128–134.

Oishi K, Itamoto T, Kobayashi T, et al. Hepatectomy for hepatocellular carcinoma in elderly patients aged 75 years or more. *J Gastrointest Surg* 2009; 13:695–701.

Onji M, Fujioka S, Takeuchi Y, et al. Clinical characteristics of drug-induced liver injury in the elderly. *Hepatol Res* 2009; 39:546–552.

Saneto H, Kobayashi M, Kawamura Y, et al. Clinicopathological features, background liver disease, and survival analysis of HCV-positive patients with hepatocellular carcinoma: differences between young and elderly patients. *J Gastroenterol* 2008; 43:975–981.

Seitz HK, Stickel F. Alcoholic liver disease in the elderly. *Clin Geriatr Med* 2007; 23:905–921.

CHAPTER 25

Hepatobiliary complications of HIV

Vincent Lo Re III, MD, MSCE ■ K. Rajender Reddy, MD, FACP

KEY POINTS

1 Approximately 10% of human immunodeficiency virus (HIV)–infected persons worldwide are chronically infected with hepatitis B virus. The choice of antiviral therapy depends on the need for HIV treatment.

2 Approximately 30% of HIV-infected persons are chronically coinfected with hepatitis C virus (HCV). Antiretroviral therapy may improve hepatic outcomes and survival among coinfected patients. Pegylated interferon alpha plus weight-based ribavirin can achieve sustained virologic response in up to 72% of HIV-infected patients infected with HCV genotype 2 or 3 and up to 35% of those infected with HCV genotype 1 or 4. The role of protease inhibitors active against HCV in this population is under study.

3 Infiltrative infections (mainly disseminated bacterial and fungal processes) may lead to hepatocellular necrosis or granulomatous inflammation in HIV-infected patients with advanced immunosuppression. *Mycobacterium avium* complex infection is most common.

4 Macrovesicular hepatic steatosis is identified in 40% to 69% of liver biopsy specimens in patients coinfected with both HIV and HCV, and steatosis is associated with more advanced hepatic fibrosis.

5 Virtually every antiretroviral medication has been associated with hepatotoxicity. In the setting of suspected hepatotoxicity, discontinuation of antiretroviral medications should be considered if (1) serum aminotransferase levels exceed 10 times the upper limit of normal, (2) overt jaundice is identified, (3) symptomatic hepatitis develops, or (4) findings consistent with drug hypersensitivity (e.g., rash, fever, eosinophilia) are observed.

7 Acquired immunodeficiency syndrome (AIDS) cholangiopathy is a syndrome of biliary obstruction resulting from infection-associated strictures of the biliary tract, typically seen in patients with a CD4+ cell count lower than 100/mm^3. *Cryptosporidium parvum* is the most commonly associated pathogen.

Viral Hepatitis and Other Viral Infections

HEPATITIS A VIRUS

1. Seroprevalence of antibody to hepatitis A virus (HAV) is high among HIV-infected persons, with a range of 40% to 70%.
2. The annual cumulative incidence of HAV infection is reported to be 5.8% per year among HIV-positive persons.
3. HAV viremia is prolonged in HIV-infected persons, and the level of HAV viremia is higher compared with those without HIV infection, even with relatively high CD4+ T lymphocyte counts.

4. No evidence indicates that antiretroviral therapy (ART) has a detrimental effect on the course of HAV infection.
5. Hepatitis A vaccination is recommended for all HIV-positive/HAV-seronegative persons, with standard doses given 6 to 12 months apart. Immune response is excellent (overall response rate, 78% to 94%), even in persons with CD4+ counts lower than 200 cells/mm³ (response rate, 64%).

HEPATITIS B AND D VIRUSES

1. Worldwide, 10% of HIV-infected persons are chronically infected with hepatitis B virus (HBV).
2. HIV adversely affects the natural history of HBV infection. Compared with those infected with HBV alone, HIV-coinfected persons have a higher rate of progression from acute to chronic HBV, higher HBV DNA levels, lower rates of spontaneous hepatitis B e antigen (HBeAg) to antibody to HBeAg (anti-HBe) seroconversion, increased frequency of reactivation episodes, faster progression to hepatic cirrhosis, and earlier development of and more aggressive hepatocellular carcinomas.
3. HIV coinfection may accelerate progression of hepatitis D virus (HDV)–associated liver disease.
4. All HIV/HBV-coinfected patients with active HBV replication should be considered for HBV antiviral therapy, which can potentially prevent development of liver-related complications and reduce HBV transmission.
5. The goals of HBV treatment in HIV-infected persons are suppression of HBV DNA to an undetectable level (as for persons without HIV infection), return of serum aminotransferase levels to normal, HBeAg seroconversion (not applicable to HBeAg negative–pre-core/core promoter mutant states [see Chapters 3 and 4]), and improvement in liver histology.
6. As of 2011, seven antiviral medications have been approved in the United States for chronic HBV treatment, and three of these have also been approved for HIV treatment (Table 25.1). The choice of therapy for HBV infection depends on the need for HIV treatment.
7. **When both HIV and HBV infections meet criteria for treatment**, combination oral nucleoside/nucleotide analogue therapy with tenofovir 300 mg daily plus either emtricitabine 200 mg daily or lamivudine 300 mg daily is preferred. Because replication of both viruses depends on reverse transcription, dual HIV/HBV therapy can use the same reverse transcriptase-inhibiting agents to treat both viruses.

TABLE 25.1 ■ **Antiviral medications for chronic hepatitis B**

Interferon alfa-2b

Peginterferon alfa-2a

Lamivudine*

Adefovir

Entecavir

Telbivudine

Tenofovir*

*Also approved to treat HIV infection. Tenofovir is also available in combination with emtricitabine (Truvada®).

8. When HBV infection requires treatment but HIV infection does not, treatment options include the following:
   - Medications with no capacity to induce HIV-resistance mutations, such as subcutaneous peginterferon alfa-2a or oral adefovir (10 mg daily), can be used.
   - Antiviral therapy that includes tenofovir plus emtricitabine (or lamivudine) is an option.
   - Entecavir in the absence of ART can reduce HIV RNA levels and select for HIV-resistance mutations, so it should not be used in an HIV-infected person without ART. Telbivudine does not have intrinsic activity against HIV in vitro, but it has been associated with declines in HIV RNA levels and can select for lamivudine-resistance mutations. It is not a recommended treatment for the HIV/HBV-coinfected patient at present.

9. Frequent toxicities and low rates of therapeutic success have limited peginterferon alfa-2a use as HBV therapy in HIV-infected persons, but it may be effective for HBeAg-positive persons with elevated serum aminotransferase levels and low HBV DNA levels.

10. Because lamivudine resistance occurs at a rate of 15% to 25% per year, lamivudine resistance may be present in HIV-infected patients who previously received lamivudine as part of an ART regimen. However, tenofovir remains active in patients with lamivudine-resistant HBV infection and can suppress HBV DNA to undetectable levels, because of the potency of tenofovir and the lack of cross-resistance between lamivudine and tenofovir.

11. For patients receiving combination tenofovir plus emtricitabine (or lamivudine) who fail to suppress HBV DNA by 24 to 48 weeks, adding entecavir 1 mg daily may be considered.

12. Because hepatocellular carcinoma can occur at any stage of chronic HBV infection, screening with abdominal ultrasonography and alpha fetoprotein testing is recommended every 6 to 12 months (see Chapter 27).

13. HBV vaccination is recommended in all HIV-positive/HBV surface antibody (anti-HBs) −negative persons. The presence in serum of isolated hepatitis B core antibody (anti-HBc) with no other HBV markers most likely reflects previous exposure and recovery, rather than a false-positive test, but not necessarily.

14. Anti-HBs titers should be evaluated after HBV vaccination in HIV-infected persons. Immune reactivity to the HBV vaccine is frequently suboptimal in these persons in terms of rate of response, antibody titers, and durability. A CD4+ count higher than 500 cells/mm^3 and an HIV viral load lower than 1000 copies/mL promote optimal vaccine responses. Revaccination should be instituted if the anti-HBs titer is less than 10 IU/L.

HEPATITIS C VIRUS

1. Among HIV-infected persons, 30% are chronically coinfected with hepatitis C virus (HCV).

2. The natural history of HCV infection is adversely influenced by HIV coinfection. Compared with persons infected with HCV alone, HIV-coinfected persons more commonly progress to chronic HCV; have higher HCV RNA levels; are at higher risk of cirrhosis, hepatic decompensation, and liver-related death; and have a shorter survival once end-stage liver disease develops.

3. HCV-related liver disease is now a leading cause of death in the HIV-infected population.

4. HIV/HCV coinfection increases the risk of hepatocellular carcinoma compared with HIV monoinfection persons but not HCV monoinfection.

5. Available data suggest that ART favorably affects the course of HIV disease in HIV-infected patients, decreases mortality from liver disease, and should not be withheld from HIV/HCV-coinfected persons on account of potential toxicity.

6. The stage of hepatic fibrosis can help guide HCV treatment decisions in HIV/HCV patients. The incidence rate of hepatic decompensation events or death is higher in coinfected patients with more advanced fibrosis at the time of staging.

7. The timing of HCV therapy depends on the need for HIV treatment. HCV treatment should be considered first if liver disease is advanced and HIV infection is at an early stage. If HIV infection requires treatment, ART should be initiated first, and once the HIV infection is controlled, HCV therapy can be considered.

8. Given accelerated progression to end-stage liver disease among HIV/HCV-infected patients, treatment of chronic HCV infection should be considered in all coinfected patients who do not have decompensated cirrhosis or other contraindications. **Peginterferon alfa-2a plus ribavirin for 48 weeks (regardless of HCV genotype) is the standard of care for treating chronic HCV infection in the setting of HIV infection.** The main goals of treatment are viral eradication (i.e., sustained virologic response) and reduction in the risk of liver-related complications (see Chapter 4).

9. Weight-based ribavirin (1000 mg daily if body weight is less than or equal to 75 kg and 1200 mg if body weight is more than 75 kg) in combination with peginterferon alfa-2a can achieve sustained virologic response in up to 72% of HIV-infected HCV genotype 2 or 3 patients and in up to 35% of HIV-infected HCV genotype 1 or 4 patients. Most clinical trials have used a lower dose of ribavirin (800 mg daily), but increased response rates can be expected with weight-based ribavirin. The role of protease inhibitors active against HCV in coinfected patients is under study.

10. **Avoid zidovudine**, which likely inhibits the hematopoietic response to ribavirin-induced hemolysis and is associated with greater declines in the hemoglobin level during HCV therapy. Consider switching to an alternative nucleoside analogue before starting HCV treatment.

11. **Avoid didanosine**, which increases the risk of hepatic decompensation when used in conjunction with ribavirin and should not be administered during HCV therapy.

12. Because abacavir and ribavirin are both guanosine analogues, abacavir may compete intracellularly with ribavirin and interfere with the effect of the drug on HCV. However, with weight-based ribavirin, use of abacavir (or other ART) is not associated with a reduced early or sustained virologic response, a finding that suggests that any competitive effect between abacavir and ribavirin can be overcome with optimal weight-based ribavirin dosing. Abacavir can therefore be continued in HIV/HCV-coinfected patients during HCV therapy.

13. Some adverse effects of HCV therapy are more prominent in the HIV/HCV-infected population. Pegylated interferon can reduce absolute CD4+ cell counts during treatment, although the percentage of CD4+ cells is typically unchanged. Weight loss is more common among HIV/HCV-coinfected than HCV-monoinfected patients during HCV therapy.

14. Maintenance pegylated interferon monotherapy does not slow progression of hepatic fibrosis among HIV/HCV-infected nonresponders to pegylated interferon alpha plus ribavirin.

OTHER VIRUSES

1. **Acute infection with HIV** may manifest with hepatitis as part of a mononucleosis-like illness with fever, malaise, and myalgias; hepatosplenomegaly on physical examination; and

elevations of serum aminotransferase and alkaline phosphatase levels. This presentation is referred to as the **acute retroviral syndrome**.

2. Several other common viral infections can secondarily affect the liver and cause acute hepatitis. **Adenovirus, Epstein-Barr virus, cytomegalovirus, herpes simplex virus, and varicella-zoster virus** are rare causes of acute viral hepatitis in HIV-infected persons.

Other Infections (see also Chapter 29)

DISSEMINATED *MYCOBACTERIUM AVIUM* COMPLEX INFECTION

1. The designation MAC refers to infections caused by one of two nontuberculous mycobacterial species, either *Mycobacterium avium* or *M. intracellulare*.
2. In patients with acquired immunodeficiency syndrome (AIDS), MAC infection usually presents as disseminated disease and may involve the liver.
3. Symptoms of disseminated MAC infection include fever, night sweats, abdominal pain (especially in the right upper quadrant), diarrhea, and weight loss. Hepatosplenomegaly may be identified on physical examination.
4. Laboratory abnormalities frequently include anemia and elevated serum alkaline phosphatase and lactate dehydrogenase levels.
5. The diagnosis may be confirmed by the following:
   - Isolation of MAC from cultures of blood, lymph node, or bone marrow
   - Histopathologic findings on a liver biopsy specimen showing granulomas with positive acid-fast bacilli stains
   - Mycobacterial growth from culture of liver tissue obtained by biopsy

PELIOSIS HEPATIS

1. *Bartonella henselae* can cause peliosis hepatis, a vascular proliferative hepatic infection in HIV-infected persons with advanced immunosuppression that is characterized by multiple blood-filled cystic spaces.
2. Patients may report fever, abdominal pain, nausea, vomiting, anorexia, and weight loss. Hepatosplenomegaly may be detected on physical examination. Increased serum alkaline phosphatase levels and thrombocytopenia or pancytopenia may be identified.
3. Abdominal computed tomography (CT) typically shows hepatosplenomegaly and hypodense lesions scattered throughout the hepatic parenchyma.
4. Positive *Bartonella* serology can be used as supportive information in the appropriate clinical setting, but the diagnosis is confirmed by isolation of *Bartonella* from cultures of blood or liver tissue or by Warthin-Starry staining of a biopsy specimen.
5. Oral erythromycin 500 mg four times daily or doxycycline 100 mg twice daily for 4 months is the recommended therapy for peliosis hepatitis. Oral azithromycin 500 mg daily or clarithromycin 500 mg twice daily for 4 months may be an option for patients who cannot tolerate erythromycin or doxycycline.

FUNGAL AND PROTOZOAL INFECTIONS

A number of fungi and protozoa may infiltrate the liver in patients with AIDS, usually as part of disseminated disease (Table 25.2).

TABLE 25.2 ■ **Selected causes of liver disease in HIV-infected patients**

Infections

Bacteria

Mycobacterium avium complex

Mycobacterium tuberculosis

Bartonella henselae (peliosis hepatis)

Viruses

Hepatitis A virus

Hepatitis B virus

Hepatitis C virus

Hepatitis D virus (with hepatitis B)

Other: adenovirus, Epstein-Barr virus, cytomegalovirus, human immunodeficiency virus, herpes simplex virus, varicella-zoster virus

Fungi

Candida albicans

Coccidioides immitis

Cryptococcus neoformans

Histoplasma capsulatum

Sporothrix schenckii

Penicillium marneffei

Pneumocystis jirovecii

Protozoa

Microsporidia spp.

Schistosoma spp.

Toxoplasma gondii

Malignant diseases

Hepatocellular carcinoma

Lymphoma

Kaposi's sarcoma

Nonalcoholic fatty liver disease

Medications and toxins

Acetaminophen

Alcohol

Nucleoside analogues: didanosine, stavudine, zidovudine

Non-nucleoside reverse transcriptase inhibitors: nevirapine

Antituberculosis drugs: isoniazid, rifampin

Antimicrobials: macrolides, trimethoprim-sulfamethoxazole

Malignant Diseases

LYMPHOMA (see also Chapter 22)

1. Non-Hodgkin's lymphoma accounts for most systemic AIDS-related lymphomas, and the liver is involved in approximately one third of cases.

2. Hepatic involvement may be clinically silent or associated with pain and "B" symptoms, including fever, weight loss, and night sweats. Jaundice may occur with intrahepatic or extrahepatic bile duct obstruction.
3. Radiographic imaging usually reveals solitary or multiple hepatic lesions and involvement of abdominal lymph nodes.
4. The diagnosis can be established by biopsy of the hepatic lesions or an involved lymph node.

KAPOSI'S SARCOMA

1. This is observed predominantly in men who have sex with men.
2. Typically, it involves the liver in the setting of cutaneous disease. Abdominal pain, hepatomegaly, and elevations of serum alkaline phosphatase levels may be observed.
3. Abdominal ultrasonography may reveal nonspecific, small (5- to 12-mm) hyperechoic nodules. CT of the liver may show enhancing lesions in capsular, hilar, and portal areas with invasion into liver parenchyma.

HEPATOCELLULAR CARCINOMA (see also Chapter 27)

1. This is increasingly recognized in HIV-infected patients with cirrhosis.
2. It may occur in the setting of chronic HBV infection in the absence of cirrhosis.
3. Patients typically have evidence of advanced liver disease, and they may have an elevated serum alpha fetoprotein level and one or more liver masses on abdominal imaging studies.

Nonalcoholic Fatty Liver Disease

1. Macrovesicular hepatic steatosis is a common histologic finding in patients coinfected with HIV and HCV and is identified in 40% to 69% of liver biopsy specimens.
2. Risk factors for hepatic steatosis among HIV/HCV-coinfected patients have included white race, increased body mass index, hyperglycemia, use of dideoxynucleoside analogues (i.e., didanosine and stavudine), and lower plasma levels of high-density lipoprotein cholesterol.
3. Steatosis/steatohepatitis has been associated with more advanced HCV-related hepatic fibrosis in HIV-infected persons.
4. The frequency of hepatic steatosis among HIV/HBV-coinfected persons and HIV-monoinfected persons remains unclear.
5. Most patients are asymptomatic. Hepatomegaly is a frequent finding.
6. Elevated serum aminotransferase or alkaline phosphatase levels may be identified. Evidence of fatty liver may be noted on abdominal ultrasonography or CT.

Antiretroviral-Induced Hepatotoxicity

1. Virtually every ART has been associated with elevations in liver biochemical test levels.
2. Four main mechanisms of ART-related hepatotoxicity occur in HIV-infected persons:
   ■ Mitochondrial toxicity
   ■ Hypersensitivity reactions involving the liver
   ■ Direct drug toxicity
   ■ Immune reconstitution following initiation of ART in the presence of hepatitis coinfection

3. No clinical finding is specific for ART-induced hepatotoxicity. Symptoms may be absent or may consist of abdominal discomfort, nausea, rash, anorexia, jaundice, or fever.
4. Hepatotoxicity is usually suggested by elevations in serum aminotransferase levels. Cholestasis is less frequent, and some cases are characterized by mixed hepatitis and cholestasis.
5. Based on the AIDS Clinical Trial Group liver toxicity scale, severe hepatotoxicity is defined as either a grade 3 (5.1 to 10 times the upper limit of normal) or grade 4 (more than 10 times the upper limit of normal) change in serum aminotransferase levels during ART or a more than 3.5-fold increase in these levels above baseline if aminotransferase levels are elevated at initiation of ART.
6. HBV infection and HCV infection increase the risk of ART-associated hepatotoxicity, and the risk among HIV/HCV-coinfected patients with advanced fibrosis or cirrhosis is increased further. Eradication of HCV with antiviral therapy has been shown to improve tolerance to ART.
7. Patients with aminotransferase elevations before the initiation of ART have an increased risk of hepatotoxicity. Alcohol and cocaine use can exacerbate ART-induced hepatotoxicity.
8. In the setting of suspected hepatotoxicity, discontinuation of ART medications should be considered in the following circumstances:
   ■ Serum aminotransferase levels exceed 10 times the upper limit of normal.
   ■ Overt jaundice with elevated direct bilirubin levels is identified.
   ■ Symptomatic hepatitis develops (increased risk of severe liver injury).
   ■ Findings consistent with drug hypersensitivity (e.g., rash, fever, eosinophilia) are observed.

A summary of hepatic disorders manifesting in patients with HIV infection is shown in Table 25.2.

AIDS-Related Biliary Tract Diseases

AIDS CHOLANGIOPATHY

1. This syndrome of biliary obstruction resulting from infection-associated strictures of the biliary tract is typically seen in patients with a CD4+ cell count lower than $100/mm^3$.
2. The incidence of AIDS cholangiopathy has declined substantially with the use of ART.
3. *Cryptosporidium parvum* is the most common pathogen associated with AIDS cholangiopathy, but MAC, cytomegalovirus, *Microsporidia* spp., and *Cyclospora cayatensis* have also been identified. Noninfectious causes include lymphoma or Kaposi's sarcoma infiltrating the biliary tree. No specific cause is found in 20% to 40% of cases.
4. This condition should be suspected in patients with advanced immunosuppression (CD4+ count lower than $100/mm^3$) who present with fever, right upper quadrant or epigastric abdominal pain, nausea, vomiting, diarrhea, jaundice, and hepatomegaly.
5. The severity of abdominal pain varies with the biliary tract lesion. Severe abdominal pain usually suggests papillary stenosis, whereas milder abdominal pain is often associated with intrahepatic and extrahepatic sclerosing cholangitis without papillary stenosis.
6. Serum aminotransferase, alkaline phosphatase, and total bilirubin levels are typically mildly elevated, but 20% of patients may have normal liver biochemical test levels.
7. Radiographic imaging may demonstrate intrahepatic or extrahepatic biliary tract dilatation or thickening of the bile duct.
8. Endoscopic retrograde cholangiopancreatography (ERCP) is the preferred approach because it may be diagnostic (ampullary biopsy) or therapeutic (sphincterotomy). Cholangiography reveals one of four patterns:
   ■ Sclerosing cholangitis and papillary stenosis (most common)
   ■ Sclerosing cholangitis alone

- Papillary stenosis alone
- Long, extrahepatic bile duct strictures with or without sclerosing cholangitis
9. Treatment is primarily endoscopic; the approach varies with the anatomic abnormality:
   - Papillary stenosis: Consider sphincterotomy.
   - Isolated or dominant bile duct stricture: Consider endoscopic stenting.
   - Isolated intrahepatic sclerosing cholangitis: Consider ursodeoxycholic acid 300 mg three times daily.
10. Empiric antimicrobial therapy directed against typical pathogens (e.g., *C. parvum*) does not affect symptoms or cholangiographic abnormalities.

ACALCULOUS CHOLECYSTITIS

1. This may occur in patients with AIDS cholangiopathy.
2. Typical causes include cytomegalovirus, *C. parvum, Microsporidia* spp., and *Isospora belli*. Less common causes are *Candida albicans, Klebsiella pneumoniae, Salmonella typhimurium,* and *Pseudomonas aeruginosa.*
3. The presentation may be similar to that of calculous cholecystitis, with severe right upper quadrant pain, fever, and Murphy's sign. Critically ill patients may present with unexplained fever or vague abdominal discomfort (see chapter 32).
4. Physical examination may reveal a palpable right upper quadrant mass and jaundice (20%).
5. Leukocytosis, hyperbilirubinemia, and elevations in serum alkaline phosphatase and aminotransferase levels may be observed.
6. Abdominal ultrasonography may demonstrate a thickened (more than 3 to 4 mm) gallbladder wall, pericholecystic fluid, stones, or ductal abnormalities. In stable patients in whom the diagnosis is unclear after ultrasonography, cholescintigraphy with a hepatobiliary iminodiacetic acid (HIDA) scan may be useful. The diagnosis is confirmed by demonstrating failure of the gallbladder to opacify.
7. Once acalculous cholecystitis is established, secondary infection with enteric pathogens is common. After blood cultures are obtained, broad-spectrum antibiotics (e.g., piperacillin-tazobactam, ampicillin-sulbactam, third-generation cephalosporin with metronidazole, or imipenem) should be initiated. Antibiotic therapy can be narrowed after microbiologic diagnosis.
8. Definitive therapy is cholecystectomy. If surgical intervention is contraindicated, consider drainage of the gallbladder through percutaneous cholecystostomy.

FURTHER READING

Amorosa VK, Slim J, Mounzer K, et al. The influence of abacavir and other antiretroviral agents on virologic response to hepatitis C virus therapy among antiretroviral-treated HIV-infected patients. *Antivir Ther* 2010; 15:91–99.

Chen XM, LaRusso NF. Cryptosporidiosis and the pathogenesis of AIDS-cholangiopathy. *Semin Liver Dis* 2002; 22:277–289.

Gandhi RT, Wurcel A, Lee H, et al. Response to hepatitis B vaccine in HIV-1–positive subjects who test positive for isolated antibody to hepatitis B core antigen: implications for hepatitis B vaccine strategies. *J Infect Dis* 2005; 191:1435–1441.

Laurence J. Hepatitis A and B immunizations of individuals infected with human immunodeficiency virus. *Am J Med* 2005; 118(Suppl):75S–83S.

Lo Re V 3rd, Kostman JR, Amorosa VK. Management complexities of HIV/hepatitis C virus coinfection in the twenty-first century. *Clin Liver Dis* 2008; 12:587–609.

Lo Re V 3rd, Kostman JR, Gross R, et al. Incidence and risk factors for weight loss during dual HIV/hepatitis C virus therapy. *J Acquir Immune Defic Syndr* 2007; 44:344–350.

McGovern BH, Ditelberg JS, Taylor LE, et al. Hepatic steatosis is associated with nucleoside analogue use and hepatitis C genotype 3 infection in HIV-seropositive patients. *Clin Infect Dis* 2006; 43:365–372.

Nunez M. Hepatotoxicity of antiretrovirals: incidence, mechanisms and management. *J Hepatol* 2006; 44(Suppl):S132–S139.

Pineda JA, Romero-Gomez M, Diaz-Garcia F, et al. HIV coinfection shortens the survival of patients with hepatitis C virus–related decompensated cirrhosis. *Hepatology* 2005; 41:779–789.

Soriano V, Puoti M, Garcia-Gasco P, et al. Antiretroviral drugs and liver injury. *AIDS* 2008; 22:1–13.

Soriano V, Puoti M, Peters M, et al. Care of HIV patients with chronic hepatitis B: updated recommendation from the HIV-Hepatitis B Virus International Panel. *AIDS* 2008; 22:1399–1410.

Sulkowski MS, Mehta SH, Torbenson M, et al. Hepatic steatosis and antiretroviral drug use among adults coinfected with HIV and hepatitis C virus. *AIDS* 2005; 19:585–592.

Sulkowski MS, Thomas DL. Hepatitis C in the HIV-infected person. *Ann Intern Med* 2003; 138:197–207.

Torriani FJ, Rodriguez-Torres M, Rockstroh JK, et al. Peginterferon alfa-2a plus ribavirin for chronic hepatitis C virus infection in HIV-infected patients. *N Engl J Med* 2004; 351:438–450.

Weber R, Sabin CA, Friis-Moller N, et al. Liver-related deaths in persons infected with the human immunodeficiency virus: the D: A:D study. *Arch Intern Med* 2006; 166:1632–1641.

CHAPTER 26

Granulomatous liver disease

Jay H. Lefkowitch, MD

KEY POINTS

1 Granulomas consist of activated macrophages (epithelioid macrophages) accompanied by T lymphocytes and other immune cells, which infiltrate liver tissue as nodular lesions in reaction to foreign or indigestible antigen or as a hypersensitivity reaction.

2 The major causes of hepatic granulomas include infectious agents (especially tuberculosis), sarcoidosis, primary biliary cirrhosis, drugs, systemic diseases (e.g., Crohn's disease), and neoplasms (e.g., Hodgkin's lymphoma).

3 An elevated serum alkaline phosphatase level is the most common abnormality in serum liver biochemical test levels.

4 The cause of hepatic granulomas may remain unknown in up to 50% of cases.

5 The workup of hepatic granulomas includes a complete history of therapeutic drug use, tests for antimitochondrial antibodies and angiotensin-converting enzyme, and staining liver specimens with acid-fast and silver stains for mycobacteria and fungi, respectively.

Pathogenesis of Granulomas

DEFINITION

1. Granulomas are rounded, 1- to 2-mm collections of activated macrophages, T lymphocytes, and other immune cells that infiltrate a host of tissues, including the liver, in response to a foreign or indigestible antigen or as a hypersensitivity reaction (Fig. 26.1).
2. The principal immune cells in granulomas are activated macrophages resembling epithelial cells (epithelioid macrophages), CD4$^+$ T cells (T-helper, or Th, lymphocytes), and sometimes multinucleated giant cells that develop from macrophage fusion.
3. The cause of the granuloma influences the constituent immune cells and secreted products: Th type 1 (Th1) cells and cytokines predominate in mycobacterial granulomas, whereas Th2 cells and cytokines predominate in schistosomal granulomas (Fig. 26.2).
4. Granulomas evolve by the elaboration of secretory products (cytokines and chemokines) by their constituent cells (interferon gamma and interleukin-2 from Th lymphocytes), expansion of macrophage and T-cell pools, and specialization of macrophages for antigen digestion (Fig. 26.3).
5. Granulomas ultimately either resolve or undergo fibrosis or calcification.

MORPHOLOGIC TYPES

Several types of granulomas are described in liver disease according to their histologic features and constituents (Table 26.1).

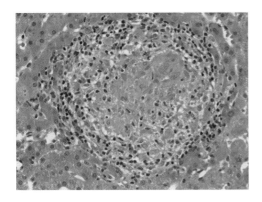

Fig. 26.1 Histopathology of a noncaseating hepatic granuloma in sarcoidosis. Epithelioid macrophages occupy the center of the granuloma with peripherally dispersed lymphocytes (hematoxylin and eosin [H&E]).

INCIDENCE AND LOCATION

1. Granulomas are found in **2.4% to 14.6% of liver biopsies**, although a figure of 10% is often quoted.
2. Granulomas are found in any of the following sites in the liver, alone or in combination with the following:
    - Lobular (tuberculosis, sarcoidosis, drugs)
    - Portal/periportal (sarcoidosis)
    - Periductal (primary biliary cirrhosis [PBC])
    - Perivenous (mineral oil lipogranulomas)
    - Periarterial/intra-arterial (phenytoin)

Causes of Hepatic Granulomas

The etiology is multifactorial, but the major causes and examples are shown in Table 26.2.

Clinical Features

SYMPTOMS AND SIGNS

They often include the following:
- Abdominal pain
- Weight loss
- Fatigue
- Chills
- Hepatomegaly
- Splenomegaly
- Lymphadenopathy
- Fever of unknown origin

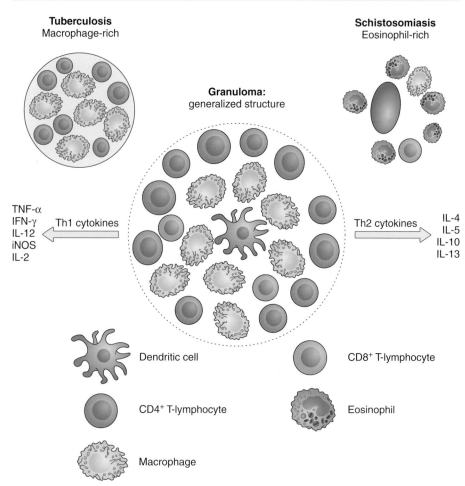

Fig. 26.2 Generalized and specialized structural and functional characteristics of hepatic granulomas. The cellular constituents of hepatic granulomas are diagrammed at the bottom. Note that tuberculosis macrophage-rich granulomas show a Th1-predominant lymphocytic response, with release of Th1 cytokines. In schistosomiasis, in contrast, enhanced numbers of eosinophils are present within the granulomas (mediated by secretion of interleukin-5 [IL-5]). In addition, release of interleukin-13 (IL-13) in schistosomiasis is an important factor resulting in portal fibrosis in the disease. IFN-γ, interferon gamma; IL-12, -2, -4, etc., interleukin-12, interleukin-2, interleukin-4, etc.; iNOS, inducible nitric oxide synthetase; Th1, T-helper type 1 lymphocyte; Th2, T-helper type 2; TNF-α, tumor necrosis factor alpha.

LIVER BIOCHEMICAL TESTS

1. The liver biochemical test pattern is that of **infiltrative disease**:
    ■ An elevated serum alkaline phosphatase level is typical: 3 to 10 times normal.
    ■ Serum aminotransferase levels are usually normal or only mildly raised.
2. Liver biochemical test levels may be normal.

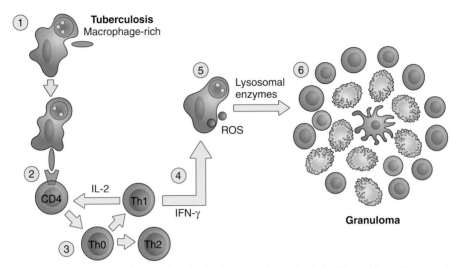

Fig. 26.3 Development of a granuloma (*red rods* represent mycobacteria). Step 1: Macrophage engulfs mycobacterium. Step 2: Macrophage presentation of mycobacterial protein product(s) to a receptor on CD4+ lymphocytes. Step 3: CD4+ lymphocytes differentiate to precursor T helper lymphocytes (Th0), later differentiating into Th1 or Th2 lymphocytes. Step 4: Th1 lymphocytes secrete interleukin-2 (IL-2), a clonal expander of CD4+ cells, as well as interferon gamma (IFN-γ), which up-regulates lysosomal enzymes and reactive oxygen species (ROS) in macrophages in step 5. Step 6: Further recruitment of macrophages and lymphocytes with ongoing digestion of mycobacteria.

TABLE 26.1 ■ **Types of granuloma**

Type	Histologic features	Cause(s)
Caseating	Peripheral macrophages with or without giant cells; central necrosis	Tuberculosis
Noncaseating	Cluster of macrophages with or without giant cells	Sarcoidosis Drugs
Lipogranuloma	Lipid vacuole(s) surrounded by macrophages and lymphocytes	Fatty liver Mineral oil
Fibrin-ring (doughnut granuloma)	Central lipid vacuole or empty space Macrophages and lymphocytes Ring of fibrin	Q fever Allopurinol Hodgkin's lymphoma

OTHER LABORATORY TESTS

1. The serum angiotensin-converting enzyme (ACE) level is elevated in sarcoidosis, PBC, silicosis, and asbestosis.
2. Serum globulin levels are elevated in sarcoidosis, berylliosis, and chronic granulomatous disease of childhood.
3. Peripheral blood eosinophilia may be present with drug- or parasite-related granulomas.

Specific Types of Granulomatous Liver Disease

SARCOIDOSIS (see also Chapter 22)

1. Sarcoid granulomas preferentially cluster in portal or periportal regions and are associated with hyaline fibrosis (Fig. 26.4).
2. Granulomas are noncaseating, may contain inclusions (asteroid and Schaumann's bodies), and can be located within lobular parenchyma as well as in or near portal tracts.
3. Other pathologic features may be seen:
   - Chronic intrahepatic cholestasis resulting from bile duct destruction
   - Bile duct damage resembling that seen in PBC
   - Periductal fibrosis resembling that seen in primary sclerosing cholangitis
   - Suppurative cholangitis
   - Granulomatous phlebitis

TABLE 26.2 ■ **Causes of hepatic granulomas**

Etiology	Specific cause(s)
Infections	Viral: cytomegalovirus infection, infectious mononucleosis, hepatitis C virus infection Bacterial: brucellosis, tuberculosis Rickettsial: Q fever Spirochetal: *T. pallidum* infection Fungal: histoplasmosis Parasitic: schistosomiasis
Primary biliary cirrhosis	Early stages most commonly
Foreign bodies	Suture, talc
Systemic disease	Sarcoidosis, Crohn's disease
Drugs	Allopurinol, phenytoin, penicillin
Neoplasia	Hodgkin's lymphoma

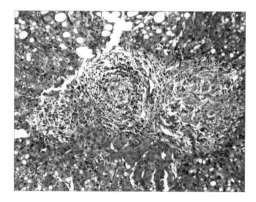

Fig. 26.4 Histopathology of clustered portal and periportal granulomas in a liver biopsy specimen from a patient with sarcoidosis. Sarcoid granulomas often result in hyaline fibrosis (shown here as increased blue-staining collagen fibers surrounding the granulomas) (trichrome).

- Hepatitis, including portal and lobular lymphocyte and plasma cell infiltrates with liver cell necrosis
- Cirrhosis, but rarely

TUBERCULOSIS (see also Chapter 29)

1. Caseation is seen in 29% of biopsy specimens and in 78% of autopsy specimens in patients with *Mycobacterium tuberculosis* infection (Fig. 26.5).
2. An acid-fast stain is infrequently positive (less than 10% of proven cases).
3. Tuberculous granulomas may be found throughout the liver parenchyma.
4. Rupture into bile ducts may result in tuberculous cholangitis.

SCHISTOSOMIASIS (see also Chapter 29)

1. The dense portal fibrosis seen grossly in advanced schistosomiasis is known as *Symmers' clay pipestem fibrosis.*
2. Schistosome eggs arrive in portal vein radicles where granulomas are formed, with a peripheral rim of eosinophils (Fig. 26.6).
3. Fine black hemozoin pigment (derived from hemoglobin breakdown by adult worms) may be seen microscopically in macrophages within granulomas, portal tracts, and sinusoids.

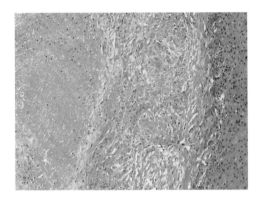

Fig. 26.5 Histopathology of a hepatic tuberculoma. Caseating necrosis is seen at the *far left,* at the center of the tuberculoma. Granulomas without necrosis surround the periphery of the lesion (H&E).

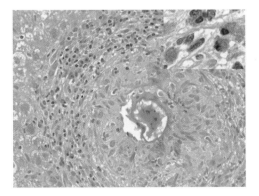

Fig. 26.6 Histopathology of a schistosomal granuloma. The center of the granuloma contains an ovum with miracidium, surrounded by abundant macrophages. The periphery of the granuloma shows lymphocytes and eosinophils. *Inset (upper right),* The eosinophil component is highlighted (H&E).

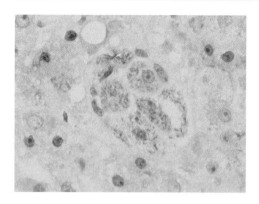

Fig. 26.7 Acid-fast stain of a liver granuloma in a patient with the acquired immunodeficiency syndrome and disseminated *Mycobacterium avium* complex infection. Abundant organisms are present in the granuloma (Ziehl-Neelsen).

4. Patients with schistosomiasis should be tested for hepatitis B and C viruses because of common endemicity and contributions of viral infection to comorbidity.

ACQUIRED IMMUNODEFICIENCY SYNDROME (AIDS) (see also Chapter 25)

1. Acid-fast and silver stains should be performed when granulomas are found in liver specimens from patients with AIDS.
2. Granulomas resulting from *Mycobacterium avium* complex infection in patients with AIDS characteristically show pale staining epithelioid macrophages containing linear structures (mycobacteria) on routine hematoxylin and eosin stain, with abundant, packed organisms in each macrophage on acid-fast stain (Fig. 26.7).
3. Cytomegalovirus hepatic infection occasionally results in small, noncaseating granulomas.
4. Other infections identified in hepatic granulomas in patients with AIDS include histoplasmosis, cryptococcosis, and toxoplasmosis.
5. Drugs used in AIDS therapy (e.g., sulfonamides, isoniazid) may cause hepatic granulomas (see Chapter 8).

PRIMARY BILIARY CIRRHOSIS (see also Chapter 14)

1. Granulomas may be seen in the livers of approximately 25% of patients with PBC.
2. Granulomas are usually seen in earlier stages of PBC, in portal tracts near damaged bile ducts (Fig. 26.8).
3. Occasionally, small, ill-defined histiocytic granulomas may be found within the lobular parenchyma (reported in 22.8% of PBC liver biopsy specimens by Drebber *et al* [2009]).

LIPOGRANULOMAS

1. These result from fatty liver or dietary mineral oil ingestion (in laxative or food products).
2. They consist of fat vacuoles, scattered lymphocytes and macrophages, and strands of connective tissue.
3. Mineral oil lipogranulomas are seen in portal tracts or near central veins (Fig. 26.9), or both.
4. This type of granuloma has no major clinical consequences.

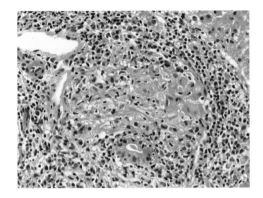

Fig. 26.8 Histopathology of a granuloma in primary biliary cirrhosis. The portal tract shown here contains a granuloma in the center of the field. Note that at 6 o'clock a damaged interlobular bile duct (florid bile duct lesion) infiltrated by mononuclear cells is visible. Granulomas arise near damaged bile ducts presumably because of release of antigenic material following duct injury (H&E).

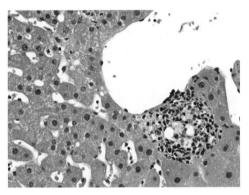

Fig. 26.9 Histopathology of a lipogranuloma adjacent to a central vein. Lipid vacuoles are surrounded by a mixture of macrophages and lymphocytes. Similar lesions may appear within portal tracts and are often related to exposure to mineral oil (H&E).

FIBRIN-RING ("DOUGHNUT") GRANULOMAS

1. These granulomas consist of a central vacuole or empty space, a surrounding pink ring of fibrin, epithelioid macrophages, and lymphocytes (Fig. 26.10).
2. Fibrin strands in these granulomas can be stained with the phosphotungstic acid–hematoxylin (PTAH) (Fig. 26.11) or Lendrum methods.
3. Fibrin-ring granulomas were first described in Q fever.
4. These granulomas have been considered nonspecific because of their association with diverse conditions:

   - Q fever
   - Hodgkin's lymphoma
   - Allopurinol ingestion
   - Cytomegalovirus infection
   - Epstein-Barr virus infection
   - Leishmaniasis
   - Toxoplasmosis
   - Hepatitis A
   - Systemic lupus erythematosus
   - Giant cell arteritis
   - Staphylococcal infection
   - Boutonneuse fever (*Rickettsia conorii*)

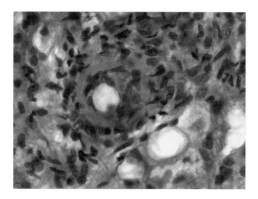

Fig. 26.10 Histopathology of a fibrin-ring granuloma in a patient with the acquired immunodeficiency syndrome and cytomegalovirus infection. This lesion (at the center of the field) is also called a "doughnut granuloma" because of the empty-appearing hole or lipid vacuole in the center, surrounded by a ring of fibrin and mononuclear cells (H&E)

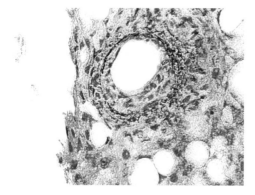

Fig. 26.11 Histopathology of a fibrin-ring granuloma. Fibrin strands are stained deep purple (phosphotungstic acid hematoxylin [PTAH]).

DRUG-RELATED GRANULOMAS

1. Approximately one third of hepatic granulomas may be caused by drugs.
2. Drug-related granulomas may be found throughout the hepatic parenchyma, contain eosinophils, and be accompanied by other evidence of drug hepatitis (cholestasis, fat, hepatocyte ballooning, and apoptosis).
3. The list of causative drugs is extensive (see Chapter 8).
4. Drug-related granulomas usually heal without sequelae.

MISCELLANEOUS GRANULOMATOUS CONDITIONS

1. In *children*, histoplasmosis is an important etiologic consideration, particularly in endemic geographic regions.
2. *Idiopathic granulomatous hepatitis* is seen in patients with fever of unknown origin and no established cause for the granulomas found on liver biopsy specimens.
3. Patients with *chronic hepatitis C* may have small, noncaseating granulomas in their liver biopsies; these may recur after liver transplantation.

Therapy

1. Therapy should be directed toward the causative agent, when known, including antibiotics for microbial infection, removal of the implicated drug in drug-related cases, and corticosteroids for sarcoidosis.
2. In idiopathic granulomatous hepatitis, disease may resolve spontaneously, with corticosteroid treatment, or with methotrexate.

FURTHER READING

Burt AD. Liver pathology associated with diseases of other organs or systems. In: Burt AD, Portmann BC, Ferrell L, eds. *MacSween's Pathology of the Liver.* 5th edn. Edinburgh: Elsevier Churchill Livingstone; 2007:881–932.

Denk H, Scheuer PJ, Baptista A, et al. Guidelines for the diagnosis and interpretation of hepatic granulomas. *Histopathology* 1994; 25:209–218.

Drebber U, Mueller JJM, Klein E, et al. Liver biopsy in primary biliary cirrhosis: clinicopathological data and stage. *Pathol Int* 2009; 59:546–554.

Ferrell LD. Hepatic granulomas: a morphologic approach to diagnosis. *Surg Pathol* 1990; 3:87–106.

Gaya DR, Thorburn KA, Oien KA, et al. Hepatic granulomas: a 10 year single centre experience. *J Clin Pathol* 2003; 56:850–853.

Knox TA, Kaplan MM, Gelfand JA, Wolff SM. Methotrexate treatment of idiopathic granulomatous hepatitis. *Ann Intern Med* 1995; 122:595-595.

Martin-Blondel G, Camara B, Selves J, et al. Etiology and outcome of liver granulomatosis: a retrospective study of 21 cases. *Rev Med Interne* 2010; 31:97–106.

Mert A, Tabak F, Ozaras R, et al. Hepatic granulomas in chronic hepatitis C. *J Clin Gastroenterol* 2001; 33:342–343.

Murphy E, Griffiths MR, Hunter JA, Burt AD. Fibrin-ring granulomas: a non-specific reaction to liver injury? *Histopathology* 1991; 19:91–93.

Portmann BC, Nakanuma Y. Diseases of the bile ducts. In: Burt AD, Portmann BC, Ferrell LD, eds. *MacSween's Pathology of the Liver.* 5th edn. Edinburgh: Elsevier Churchill Livingstone; 2007:517–582.

Sandor M, Weinstock JV, Wynn TA. Granulomas in schistosome and mycobacterial infections: a model of local immune responses. *Trends Immunol* 2003; 24:44–52.

Schneiderman DJ, Arenson DM, Cello JP, et al. Hepatic disease in patients with the acquired immune deficiency syndrome (AIDS). *Hepatology* 1987; 7:925–930.

Tjwa M, De Hertogh G, Neuville B, et al. Hepatic fibrin-ring granulomas in granulomatous hepatitis: report of four cases and review of the literature. *Acta Clin Belg* 2001; 56:341–348.

Vakiani E, Hunt KK, Mazziotta RM, et al. Hepatitis C–associated granulomas after liver transplantation: morphologic spectrum and clinical implications. *Am J Clin Pathol* 2007; 127:128–134.

CHAPTER 27

Hepatic tumors

Adrian M. Di Bisceglie, MD, FACP

KEY POINTS

1 Hemangioma of the liver is found in up to 7% of the normal population and is rarely of clinical consequence.

2 Other benign tumors of the liver are rare, including hepatic adenoma, which usually requires surgical resection because of the risks of rupture and the possible development of malignancy.

3 In the presence of cirrhosis, hepatocellular carcinoma (HCC) accounts for approximately 75% of all liver tumors. The most important risk factors for development of HCC are cirrhosis of any cause, hepatitis B virus infection, and hepatitis C virus infection with advanced fibrosis.

4 Although surgical resection offers the best chance of cure in HCC, few patients are suitable candidates for surgery. Liver transplantation is effective in selected patients.

5 Cholangiocarcinoma (CCC) is rising in incidence in the United States, probably in association with chronic liver disease. CCC of the central type is often associated with primary sclerosing cholangitis and has a poor prognosis.

Benign Tumors of the Liver

HEPATIC ADENOMA

- This is a benign proliferation of hepatocytes. It is a rare tumor that occurs largely in female patients. Its incidence has increased since the 1960s, probably related to the introduction and increased use of oral contraceptives.

- Studies have identified genetic abnormalities associated with adenoma, including hepatocyte nuclear factor (HNF)–1α inactivation and β-catenin activation.

- Patients typically present with pain or discomfort in the right upper quadrant, although occasional tumors are found incidentally. Adenomas may rupture, resulting in hemoperitoneum.

- Adenomas are usually single, but may be multiple, rarely with more than five lesions. The size is variable but typically greater than 5 cm in diameter at diagnosis and sometimes massive.

- Hepatic adenomatosis is a rare condition characterized by large numbers of adenomas in the liver with a high rate of recurrence.

- Histologic examination of hepatic adenoma shows benign hepatocytes organized in cords but with no portal triads.

- The presence of a mass in the liver may be confirmed by computed tomography (CT), ultrasonography, or magnetic resonance imaging (MRI). Technetium (^{99m}Tc) radioisotope scan may show a defect within the liver. The diagnosis may be confirmed by liver biopsy.

■ Treatment includes discontinuing the use of estrogens. **Surgical resection is usually advisable**, to obtain tissue to confirm the diagnosis and because of the risk of rupture. Liver transplantation may be considered for adenoma found in association with type I glycogen storage disease or hepatic adenomatosis because of the high risk of malignant transformation.

TUMOR-LIKE LESIONS OF HEPATOCYTES

1. **Focal nodular hyperplasia (FNH)** represents an abnormal proliferation of hepatocytes around an abnormal hepatic artery. The artery is usually embedded in a **characteristic central stellate scar.**
   - FNH is usually clinically silent and is typically found incidentally, often at the time of abdominal surgery for another reason.
   - In comparison with adenoma, FNH tends to be smaller and carries little risk of rupture. Multiple lesions are found in approximately 20% of patients.
   - A hepatic arteriogram may suggest the diagnosis if a tumor can be found surrounding a large hepatic artery.
   - The diagnosis may be difficult to make on needle biopsy. Excisional biopsy may be required and is usually curative.
2. **Nodular regenerative hyperplasia (NRH)** is characterized by the diffuse formation of nodules composed of hepatocytes throughout the liver. The pattern is similar to cirrhosis, except these nodules do not have a surrounding rim of fibrosis.
   - NRH is **often associated with identifiable systemic diseases** such as autoimmune disorders, rheumatoid arthritis (including Felty's syndrome), and myeloproliferative disorders (see Chapter 22).
   - The pathogenesis is unknown but often appears to be related to obliterative venopathy involving portal vein branches.
   - The incidence of NRH increases with age and is found most commonly in persons more than 60 years old.
   - NRH is often complicated by the development of presinusoidal portal hypertension. Patients may present with splenomegaly and hypersplenism or bleeding esophageal varices.
   - No specific therapy is available, but patients may require beta blocker therapy, endoscopic therapy, or rarely, portal decompression to prevent rebleeding from varices. Generally, patients with NRH tolerate variceal bleeding better than those with cirrhosis, presumably because they have relatively well-preserved hepatic synthetic function.
3. **Adenomatous hyperplasia** (macroregenerative nodule, dysplastic nodule)
   - This term is used for regenerative nodules of hepatocytes greater than 1 cm in diameter found in association with cirrhosis or, rarely, submassive hepatic necrosis. Adenomatous hyperplasia **represents a form of dysplastic nodule.**
   - In the context of cirrhosis, adenomatous hyperplasia is strongly associated with the development of HCC.
   - No specific therapy is needed. In patients with cirrhosis, the presence of adenomatous hyperplasia should signal the need for intensive surveillance for the development of HCC (see later).
4. **Partial nodular transformation:** This rare condition is characterized by the presence of nodules of hepatocytes located in the perihilar region and associated with portal hypertension.

HEMANGIOMA

- Hemangiomas of the liver are relatively common, identified in at least 7% of autopsies.
- They are composed of an endothelial lining on a thin fibrous stroma making up cavernous, blood-filled spaces.
- They are usually small; if larger than 10 cm in diameter, they are referred to as *giant or cavernous hemangiomas.*
- They are usually asymptomatic but, if large enough, may cause some abdominal discomfort. Occasionally, thrombosis within a giant hemangioma may result in consumption of platelets and thrombocytopenia, particularly in children (Kasabach–Merritt syndrome). Hemangiomas have been documented to increase in size over time but have no potential to become malignant.
- Hemangiomas usually do not require any specific therapy. They may be resected if they are associated with significant symptoms. Percutaneous needle biopsy should be avoided because of the risk of bleeding.

BENIGN HEPATIC TUMORS OF CHOLANGIOCELLULAR ORIGIN

1. **Bile duct adenoma:** This is typically a solitary subcapsular tumor, composed of a proliferation of small, round, normal-appearing bile ducts with cuboidal epithelium.
2. **Biliary microhamartoma** (von Meyenburg's complex): This is part of the spectrum of adult polycystic disease but may also be found together with polycystic disease (adult or childhood type), congenital hepatic fibrosis, or Caroli's disease (see Chapters 23, 28, and 33).
3. **Biliary cystadenoma:** This multiloculated cyst is analogous to mucinous cystadenomas of the pancreas. It has significant potential for development of malignancy.
4. **Biliary papillomatosis:** This rare condition consists of multicentric biliary tract adenomatous polypoid tumors that sometimes develop into adenocarcinoma (analogous to familial adenomatous polyposis).

BENIGN HEPATIC TUMORS OF MESENCHYMAL ORIGIN

These tumors are listed in Table 27.1.

TABLE 27.1 ■ **Benign hepatic tumors of mesenchymal origin**

Tumor	Comment
Mesenchymal hamartoma	Childhood tumor with a mixture of elements (bile ducts, vessels, and mesenchyma)
Infantile hemangioendothelioma	Tumor of infancy; may be complicated by thrombocytopenia, high-output heart failure; may require resection or ablation
Lipoma	Collection of lipocytes; distinct from focal fatty change within hepatocytes
Lymphangiomatosis	Masses of prominent, dilated lymphatic channels
Angiomyolipoma	Distinct radiographic appearance
Leiomyoma	Extremely rare
Fibroma	Solid fibrous tumor of the liver
Inflammatory pseudotumor	Chronic inflammation and fibrosis; may cause pain, fever
Myxoma	Myxomatous connective tissue

Malignant Tumors of the Liver

METASTATIC DISEASE

The liver is a common site of metastasis. **Metastases are by far the most common form of hepatic malignancy.** The most frequent sites of origin for hepatic metastases are lung, breast, and gastrointestinal and genitourinary tracts.

HEPATOCELLULAR CARCINOMA

HCC is a malignant tumor of hepatocytes.

1. **Epidemiology**
   - HCC is one of the most common malignant diseases worldwide. The incidence varies considerably around the world. High-incidence areas include China, Taiwan, Korea, and other parts of Southeast Asia, as well as most of sub-Saharan Africa, where the incidence may be as high as 120 per 100,000 population per year. Areas of intermediate incidence include Japan, the countries of southern Europe (particularly Italy and Spain), and the Middle East. Regions of low incidence include northern countries of Europe, the United States, and South America, where the rate may be as low as 5 per 100,000 population.
   - The incidence of HCC is rising in many developed Western countries.
   - The median age at diagnosis is in the fourth decade of life in high-incidence areas; it manifests at a somewhat older age in other regions, and it is much more common in men than in women.
2. **Risk factors**
   a. HCC is one of the few human cancers for which an etiologic factor can be identified in most cases. Known and possible risk factors are shown in Table 27.2.
   b. **Chronic hepatitis B virus (HBV) infection is the most common etiologic factor in high-incidence areas,** whereas chronic hepatitis C virus (HCV) infection plays the most important etiologic role in areas of intermediate incidence.
      - The precise mechanism by which chronic viral hepatitis results in HCC is not known but may be through liver regeneration and injury characteristic of cirrhosis.

TABLE 27.2 ■ **Known and possible risk factors in hepatocellular carcinoma**

Known	Possible
Cirrhosis (of any cause)	Alcohol (in absence of cirrhosis)
Chronic hepatitis B	Smoking
Chronic hepatitis C with cirrhosis	Anabolic or estrogenic steroids
Nonalcoholic steatohepatitis with cirrhosis	
Inherited metabolic disorders: Alpha-1 antitrypsin deficiency Hemochromatosis Hereditary tyrosinemia	
Carcinogens: Aflatoxin Thorotrast*	

*Thorotrast is a contrast agent that was used for arteriography for a period after World War II. It contains thorium dioxide, a low level emitter of alpha particles, which is retained in Kupffer cells.

- In addition, HBV is a DNA virus whose genome may become integrated within the genome of hepatocytes, thereby possibly influencing actions of oncogenes or tumor suppressor genes. The X protein of HBV is known to be a transactivator (i.e., it is capable of turning on DNA, again thereby possibly activating growth factors or oncogenes).
- HCV is an RNA virus that does not become integrated into the host genome. **Almost all cases of HCV-related HCC are associated with cirrhosis or advanced hepatic fibrosis**. Alcohol may be an important cofactor with HCV in the development of HCC.

c. Certain metabolic diseases may be associated with the development of HCC, but virtually always in the presence of cirrhosis (e.g., hemochromatosis, alpha-1 antitrypsin deficiency). Hereditary tyrosinemia is a rare inborn error of metabolism associated with severe liver injury and regeneration with development of HCC in childhood.

d. Environmental toxins play a role in the pathogenesis of HCC in some parts of the world. Aflatoxin is formed as a product of fungal contamination of stored foodstuffs. It is directly hepatocarcinogenic in rodents and, in humans, interacts with HBV to cause HCC.

e. Diabetes mellitus, obesity, and nonalcoholic steatohepatitis are emerging risk factors for HCC.

3. **Clinical features**

- Abdominal pain or discomfort and weight loss are the most frequent presenting symptoms. HCC may occasionally rupture, manifesting as an acute abdomen. Many patients diagnosed with HCC are asymptomatic, with the tumor detected incidentally or during screening of at-risk persons.
- HCC may also be associated with various paraneoplastic manifestations including hypoglycemia, erythrocytosis, hypercholesterolemia, and feminization.

4. **Diagnosis**

a. The use of imaging studies is critical. Ultrasonography, CT, and MRI are the mainstays of diagnosis.

   - Small HCCs are seen on ultrasonography as hypodense lesions. Tumors as small as 0.5 to 1 cm may be detected.
   - CT is useful in confirming the presence of tumors larger than 2 to 3 cm in diameter and in assessing the extent of tumor within the abdomen.

b. The use of multiphasic CT or MRI with multiphase images has greatly enhanced the sensitivity of detection.

   - **The diagnosis of HCC can be made with confidence if a lesion has a characteristic appearance with arterial enhancement and venous washout on multiphasic imaging.**

c. Serologic markers may be useful in diagnosis. Approximately 80% to 90% of patients with HCC have an elevated serum level of alpha fetoprotein (AFP), although most patients with a small tumor (less than 5 cm in diameter) have normal or minimally elevated levels.

   - AFP values may be raised in patients with chronic viral hepatitis and cirrhosis without HCC, thus causing diagnostic confusion.
   - AFP-L3 represents a lectin-bound fraction of AFP that may be more specific than AFP for HCC.

d. Liver biopsy may be required to confirm a diagnosis of HCC. The risk of bleeding after liver biopsy for HCC and other forms of malignancy is slightly higher than after liver biopsy for benign disease. Biopsy of the nontumorous portion of the liver is advisable to evaluate the severity of underlying liver disease, particularly if resection is contemplated.

e. **Fibrolamellar HCC** is a variant of HCC usually not associated with cirrhosis or any of the other known etiologic factors. It has a better prognosis than other forms of HCC.

5. **Treatment**
   - The overall outlook is poor. In Africa and Asia, where the diagnosis is often made when the tumor is at an advanced stage, HCC is associated with mean survival times measured in weeks to months.
   - Table 27.3 offers a scheme for the management of patients with HCC.
   - **Surgery:** Large resections of the liver are possible if cirrhosis is not present. However, only small resections, segmentectomy, or enucleation may be possible in a cirrhotic liver, so most patients are not amenable to surgery at the time of diagnosis because of the extent of the tumor or severity of the underlying liver disease. Rates of recurrence and development of new tumors after resection are high.
   - **Liver transplantation** appears to result in a survival rate similar to that of resection in patients with cirrhosis, but with a lower recurrence rate. HCC now represents an important indication for liver transplantation in developed Western countries. Unfortunately, liver transplantation is not available in all countries, and limitations of the supply of donor organs prevent widespread applicability of this form of treatment.
   - **Radiofrequency ablation** (RFA) is a technique that can be performed percutaneously and allows complete ablation of liver tumors with only one or two sessions.
   - **Injection of absolute ethanol** is associated with tumor necrosis and is easy to perform, with few side effects. Its use should be confined to tumors less than 4 cm in diameter. It may be most useful in patients with decompensated cirrhosis who will not tolerate surgery or in cases of recurrent HCC after surgery.
   - **Chemoembolization**, in which chemotherapeutic agents are injected into the hepatic artery, which is subsequently occluded, is effective in shrinking tumors and improves survival in selected patients.
   - **Targeted molecular therapies** appear promising in the treatment of HCC. **Sorafenib**, a multikinase inhibitor, has been shown to improve survival in patients with advanced HCC.
   - **Systemic chemotherapy** has not been as effective as regional chemotherapy (administered through the hepatic artery). Cisplatin, in combination with other agents, appears to be the most effective agent.
6. **Prevention**
   - **HCC is potentially a preventable form of cancer.** The widespread use of HBV vaccination is expected to decrease the rate of HCC in many high-incidence areas of the world. The incidence of HCV infection may also decline because of increased awareness and screening of donated blood.

TABLE 27.3 ■ **Treatment options for patients with hepatocellular carcinoma based on extent of tumor and underlying liver disease**

Extent of tumor	Cirrhosis	Treatment options
Confined to liver	No	Large-scale resection
Confined to liver	Yes, compensated	Segmentectomy; consider ethanol injection, RFA, chemoembolization, or liver transplantation
Confined to liver	Yes, decompensated	Liver transplantation
Spread beyond liver	Yes or no	Sorafenib

RFA, radiofrequency ablation.

■ At present, an effective vaccine is not available against HCV, although antiviral therapy to eliminate HCV infection appears to decrease the risk of HCC. Antiviral therapy of HBV infection with nucleos(t)ide analogues appears to decrease the risk of HBV-related HCC.

CHOLANGIOCARCINOMA (see also Chapter 34)

1. **Epidemiology**
   - Cholangiocarcinoma (CCC) is much less common than HCC and is distributed more evenly around the world. CCC tends to occur at an older age than HCC and has a more even sex distribution.
   - The risk of CCC appears to be increasing in the United States, probably in association with the increased prevalence of cirrhosis.
2. **Risk factors** (Table 27.4)
3. **Clinical features**
   - CCC is divided into two basic types: peripheral and central. They tend to have differing pathogeneses and clinical manifestations.
   - The peripheral type is rarely associated with primary sclerosing cholangitis. It often manifests with abdominal pain and weight loss.
   - The central type arises in major bile ducts and is often associated with chronic inflammation in bile ducts, as in primary sclerosing cholangitis. Klatskin's tumors arise in the bifurcation of the bile duct. Central-type CCC often manifests with obstructive jaundice.
4. **Diagnosis**
   - The diagnosis of peripheral-type tumors can be made by needle biopsy. Central tumors may be more difficult to diagnose because they arise in the presence of primary sclerosing cholangitis, so the bile ducts are already anatomically abnormal. Cytologic and histologic examination of material obtained by endoscopic brushing and biopsy, as well as direct cholangioscopy, may confirm the diagnosis. Elevated serum levels of CA 19–9 may also be useful in establishing the diagnosis.
   - CCC may be difficult to distinguish from other forms of adenocarcinoma, and the diagnosis may be confirmed only at laparotomy or autopsy. Mixed HCC/CCC may be found in association with cirrhosis.
5. **Treatment**
   - Peripheral CCC is sometimes amenable to resection. Central CCC may also be resected particularly when small, as with Klatskin's tumors.

TABLE 27.4 ■ **Risk factors for cholangiocarcinoma**

Primary sclerosing cholangitis

Chronic hepatitis C with cirrhosis

Clonorchis sinensis infestation

Intrahepatic lithiasis, cholelithiasis

Congenital anomalies (e.g., Caroli's disease)

Exposure to Thorotrast (see Table 27.2)

Benign cysts, von Meyenburg's complex

Inflammatory bowel disease

- With both types, however, the recurrence rate after resection is high, and survival is poor.
- Liver transplantation is currently not a viable therapeutic alternative in most patients because of the high post-transplant recurrence rate.

PEDIATRIC TUMORS OF THE LIVER (see also Chapter 23)

- Some tumors of the liver occur specifically in children. Furthermore, they often occur at specific ages, as shown in Figure 27.1.
- **Hepatoblastoma** is a malignant tumor of hepatocytes that occurs in children less than 2 years of age. It is not associated with cirrhosis. Virtually all patients have elevated serum AFP levels. Hepatoblastoma is considered potentially curable with a combination of surgery and chemotherapy.
- Although HCC is typically a disease of adults, it has been recorded in children as young as 4 years of age in association with HBV infection.

OTHER TUMORS OF THE LIVER

1. **Epithelioid hemangioendothelioma**
   - This tumor of vascular endothelial origin has low-grade malignant behavior. It may arise in organs other than the liver, particularly the lung.
   - Vascular invasion is a prominent feature. Malignant cells in this tumor stain positively for factor VIII. The tumor must be distinguished histologically from angiosarcoma and CCC.

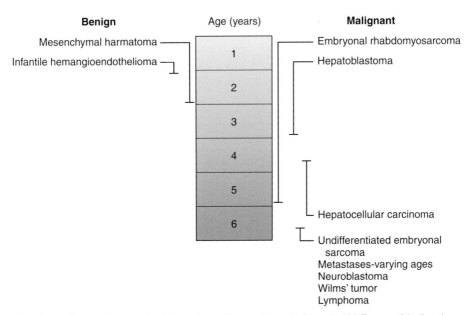

Fig. 27.1 Tumors that occur in children at specific ages. (From Di Bisceglie AM. Tumors of the liver. In: Feldman M, ed. *Atlas of the Liver,* 4th edn. Philadelphia: Springer; 2007. ©A. M. Di Bisceglie.)

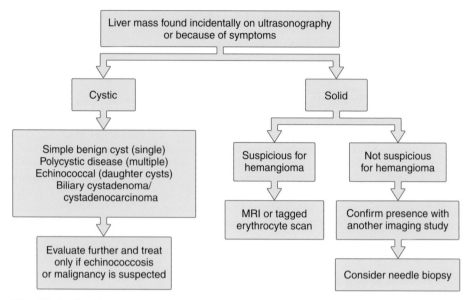

Fig. 27.2 Algorithm for the evaluation of a liver mass in a noncirrhotic patient. MRI, magnetic resonance imaging. (From Di Bisceglie AM. Tumors of the liver. In: Feldman M, ed. *Atlas of the Liver,* 4th edn. Philadelphia: Springer; 2007. ©A. M. Di Bisceglie.)

- Approximately one third of patients have metastases. Nonetheless, examples of prolonged survival with this tumor have been documented.
- This tumor is important to recognize because of its malignant behavior and because it is potentially curable with extensive resection or even liver transplantation.

2. **Primary hepatic lymphoma**
   - Although secondary involvement of the liver by lymphoma is common, primary lymphoma may also arise in the liver.
   - These tumors are often of B-cell origin and occur at increased frequency in patients with human immunodeficiency virus infection and acquired immunodeficiency syndrome.
   - These tumors respond poorly to chemotherapy and are associated with a poor prognosis.

3. **Angiosarcoma**
   - This is a high-grade malignant tumor of blood vessels arising within the liver.
   - Predisposing factors are exposure to vinyl chloride monomers and exposure to the intravenous contrast agent Thorotrast.
   - The tumor grows rapidly, responds poorly to radiation or chemotherapy, and has a poor prognosis.

Diagnostic Approach to Liver Masses or Tumors

The approach is different depending on whether the patient has cirrhosis. A scheme for evaluating the noncirrhotic patient is shown in Figure 27.2, and a scheme for evaluating the patient with cirrhosis is shown in Figure 27.3.

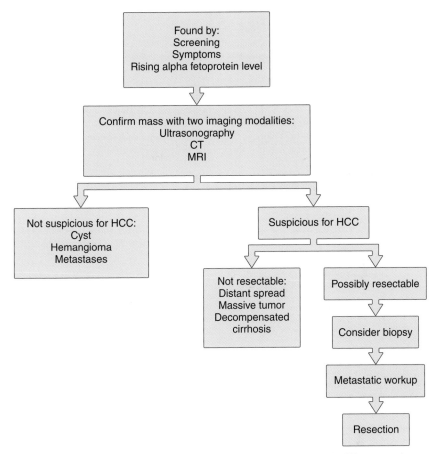

Fig. 27.3 Algorithm for the evaluation of a liver mass in a patient with cirrhosis. CT, computed tomography; HCC, hepatocellular carcinoma; MRI, magnetic resonance imaging. (From ©Di Bisceglie AM. Tumors of the liver. In: Feldman M, ed. *Atlas of the Liver*, 4th edn. Philadelphia: Springer; 2007. ©A. M. Di Bisceglie.)

FURTHER READING

Ang JP, Heath JA, Donath S, et al. Treatment outcomes for hepatoblastoma: an institution's experience over two decades. *Pediatr Surg Int* 2007; 23:103–109.

Di Bisceglie A, Lyra A, Schwartz M, et al. Hepatitis C-related hepatocellular carcinoma in the United States: influence of ethnic status. *Am J Gastroenterol* 2003; 98:2060–2063.

Bosetti C, Levi F, Boffetta P, et al. Trends in mortality from hepatocellular carcinoma in Europe, 1980–2004. *Hepatology* 2008; 48:137–145.

El-Serag H. Hepatocellular carcinoma: recent trends in the United States. *Gastroenterology* 2004; 127(Suppl):S27–S34.

Emre S, McKenna GJ. Liver tumors in children. *Pediatr Transplant* 2004; 8:632–638.

Heathcote E. Prevention of hepatitis C virus–related hepatocellular carcinoma. *Gastroenterology* 2004; 127(Suppl 1):S294–S302.

Hemming AW, Reed AI, Fujita S, et al. Surgical management of hilar cholangiocarcinoma. *Ann Surg* 2005; 241:693–699.

Jemal A, Siegel R, Ward E, et al. Cancer statistics, 2008. *CA Cancer J Clin* 2008; 58:71–96.

Llovet J, Bruix J. Systematic review of randomized trials for unresectable hepatocellular carcinoma: chemoembolization improves survival. *Hepatology* 2003; 37:429–442.

Llovet JM, Burroughs A, Bruix J. Hepatocellular carcinoma. *Lancet* 2003; 362:1907–1917.

Llovet JM, Ricci S, Mazzaferro V, et al. Sorafenib in advanced hepatocellular carcinoma. *N Engl J Med* 2008; 359:378–390.

Marrero J, Fontana R, Fu S, et al. Alcohol, tobacco and obesity are synergistic risk factors for hepatocellular carcinoma. *J Hepatol* 2005; 42:218–224.

Marrero JA, Fontana RJ, Su GL, et al. NAFLD may be a common underlying liver disease in patients with hepatocellular carcinoma in the United States. *Hepatology* 2002; 36:1349–1354.

Omata M, Tateishi R, Yoshida H, Shiina S. Treatment of hepatocellular carcinoma by percutaneous tumor ablation methods: ethanol injection therapy and radiofrequency ablation. *Gastroenterology* 2004; 127:S159-S66.

Tanaka H, Imai Y, Hiramatsu N, et al. Declining incidence of hepatocellular carcinoma in Osaka, Japan, from 1990 to 2003. *Ann Intern Med* 2008; 148:820–826.

Tan JCC, Coburn NG, Baxter NN, et al. Surgical management of intrahepatic cholangiocarcinoma: a population-based study. *Ann Surg Oncol* 2008; 15:600–608.

Welzel TM, Graubard BI, El-Serag HB, et al. Risk factors for intrahepatic and extrahepatic cholangiocarcinoma in the United States: a population-based case-control study. *Clin Gastroenterol Hepatol* 2007; 5:1221–1228.

CHAPTER 28

Hepatic abscesses and cysts

Helen M. Ayles, MBBS, MRCP, DTM&H, PhD ■ Sarah Lou Bailey, BSc, MBChB, MRCP

KEY POINTS

1   Hepatic abscesses may be amebic or pyogenic.

2   Diagnosis of hepatic abscess relies on good history taking and simple imaging.

3   The differentiation between amebic and pyogenic hepatic abscess relies on an adequate history (including travel history), imaging pattern, culture results, and serologic testing.

4   A history of dysentery or diarrhea is present in only 20% of patients with an amebic liver abscess. Amebic liver abscess is readily treated by antibiotics and luminal amebicides.

5   Pyogenic liver abscess is a life-threatening condition, resulting from infected blood or bile. Abscesses are frequently polymicrobial and include anaerobic organisms. Treatment is with appropriate antibiotics and drainage.

6   The most common infective cause of hepatic cysts worldwide is *Echinococcus granulosus*, the agent of hydatid disease; other noninfective causes include simple cysts, tumors, congenital biliary diseases, and polycystic disease.

Amebic Liver Abscess

OVERVIEW

1. Worldwide, 480 million people are infected with *Entamoeba histolytica*.
2. Amebic infection may be asymptomatic or may manifest as dysentery, hepatic amebic abscess, or other (rarer) manifestations.
3. The diagnosis and management of hepatic amebic abscess have been revolutionized by advances in imaging and interventional radiology.
4. Treatment now relies almost entirely on drug therapy.

PARASITOLOGY

1. Amebic liver abscess is caused by the protozoan *E. histolytica*. The reservoir of infection is human (Fig. 28.1).
2. The infective form is the cyst (12 μm in diameter), which is ingested. Excystation occurs in the small intestine. The trophozoite (10 to 60 μm) infects the colon and may cause inflammation and dysentery. Amebae spread to the liver through the portal circulation.
3. The cyst is able to survive outside the body for weeks or months, whereas the trophozoite degenerates in minutes.

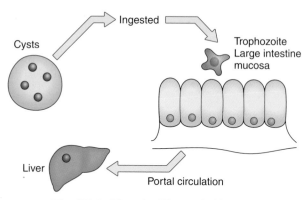

Fig. 28.1 Life cycle of *Entamoeba histolytica*.

4. Amebae may be pathogenic or nonpathogenic. The nonpathogenic form has been reclassified as *Entamoeba dispar*. Pathogenic species can be differentiated from nonpathogenic species by the following:
    ■ Zymodene analysis: 22 distinct isoenzyme patterns (zymodenes) on electrophoresis have been isolated
    ■ RNA and DNA probes

EPIDEMIOLOGY

1. **Infection with *E. histolytica* affects 10% of the world's population**; 40 to 50 million people develop amebic colitis or amebic liver abscess, and 40,000 to 100,000 deaths occur per year.
2. The prevalence of infection varies from less than 1% in industrialized countries to 50% to 80% in some tropical regions, and it has been found to be 100% in an area of The Gambia.
3. Spread is by the fecal-oral route and is increased by the following:
    ■ Poor sanitation
    ■ Contamination of food by flies
    ■ Unhygienic food handling
    ■ Unclean water
    ■ Use of human feces as fertilizer

4. High-risk groups are as follows:
    ■ Persons of lower socioeconomic status in endemic areas
    ■ Immigrants from endemic areas
    ■ Institutionalized populations (e.g., inpatients of psychiatric hospitals)
    ■ Men who have sex with men
    ■ Travelers
    ■ Persons who are immunosuppressed, including those with human immunodeficiency virus (HIV) infection

PATHOGENESIS

1. In the liver, *E. histolytica* lyses the host's tissue with proteolytic enzymes contained in cytoplasmic vacuoles.

2. The hepatic lesion is a well-demarcated abscess consisting of necrotic liver and usually affecting the right lobe. The initial host response to the ameba is neutrophil migration, but the ameba can also lyse neutrophils, thus releasing their enzymes and assisting in the process of tissue destruction.
3. The abscess contains acellular debris; amebic trophozoites are found only at the periphery of the lesion, where they can invade further.

4. The following host factors contribute to the severity of disease:
   - Age (children more than adults)
   - Pregnancy
   - Malnutrition and alcoholism
   - Corticosteroid use
   - Malignant disease

CLINICAL FEATURES

- Amebic liver abscess manifests with amebic colitis in only 10% of cases.
- Among patients, 20% have a past history of diarrhea or dysentery.
- *E. histolytica* can be isolated from the stool in approximately 50% of cases.

1. History: socioeconomic and demographic
   - Emigrant from or resident in an endemic area
   - Traveler to an endemic area
   - Men more than women (3 to 10 times)
   - Young adults more than children or elderly persons
2. Symptoms
   - Fever, rigors, night sweats
   - Nausea, anorexia, malaise
   - Right upper quadrant abdominal discomfort
   - Weight loss
   - Chest symptoms: dry cough, pleuritic pain
   - Diaphragmatic irritation: shoulder tip pain, hiccups
3. Physical examination
   - Fever
   - Tender hepatomegaly
   - Chest signs: dull right base (usually from raised hemidiaphragm); crackles at right base; pleural rub
   - Jaundice and peritonitis or pericardial rub: rare; poor prognostic signs

DIAGNOSIS

1. Laboratory findings (Table 28.1)
   - Increased serum bilirubin level is uncommon.
2. Diagnostic imaging
   a. Chest radiograph:
      - Elevation of right hemidiaphragm
      - Blunting of right costophrenic angle
      - Atelectasis

TABLE 28.1 ■ **Laboratory findings in amebic liver abscess**

Laboratory finding	Frequency (%)
Leukocytosis	80
Elevated serum alkaline phosphatase level	80
Anemia	>50
Increased erythrocyte sedimentation rate	Common
Proteinuria	Common
Elevated serum aminotransferase levels	Poor prognostic sign

    b. Ultrasonography
- Round or oval single lesion (sometimes multiple)
- Lack of significant wall echoes, so the transition from abscess to normal liver is abrupt
- Hypoechoeic appearance compared with normal liver; diffuse echoes throughout abscess
- Peripheral location, close to liver capsule
- Distal enhancement

    c. Computed tomography (CT)
- Well-defined lesions, round or oval, mostly single (sometimes multiple)
- Low density compared with surrounding liver tissue
- Nonhomogeneous internal structure

    d. Magnetic resonance imaging (MRI)
- Abscess characterized by low signal intensity on T1-weighted images and high signal intensity on T2-weighted images

    e. Radionuclide imaging
- Amebic liver abscess appears as a cold spot, apparently distinguishing it from pyogenic abscess; this modality has not been researched extensively for this use

3. Serologic tests: **The detection of antibodies is the mainstay of diagnosis of invasive amebiasis**. Available assays include the following:

    a. Indirect hemagglutination
- Sensitivity of 90% to 100%
- Raised titers may persist for more than 2 years.

    b. Latex agglutination
- Rapid results

    c. Indirect immunofluorescence
- Positivity may persist for more than 6 months after treatment.

    d. Gel diffusion
- Useful for differentiating recent from past infection because result remains positive for only 6 to 12 months after the onset of infection

    e. Counterimmunoelectrophoresis
- Cellulose acetate precipitation test (CAP) is highly sensitive and specific; becomes negative quickly after successful treatment; regarded as a reference test for amebic serology

    f. Complement fixation

    g. Enzyme-linked immunosorbent assay
- Sensitivity and specificity as high as 97.9% and 94.8%, respectively

    h. These tests are positive in *all* forms of invasive amebic disease (including dysentery). Combined testing may be necessary for accurate diagnosis.

■ Positive serologic tests are found in 95% to 100% of patients with amebic liver abscess.

4. **Aspiration of abscess** (when diagnosis is uncertain or for imminent rupture)
   ■ Yellow to dark brown "anchovy sauce"
   ■ Odorless
   ■ "Pus" consisting mainly of acellular debris; most amebae found in abscess wall

COMPLICATIONS

1. Rupture of abscess into the following:
   a. Chest, causing
      ■ Hepatobronchial fistula (± expectoration of "anchovy" pus)
      ■ Lung abscess
      ■ Amebic empyema
   b. Pericardium, causing
      ■ Heart failure
      ■ Pericarditis
      ■ Cardiac tamponade (often fatal; may be followed by constrictive pericarditis)
   c. Peritoneum, causing
      ■ Peritonitis
      ■ Ascites
2. Secondary infection is usually iatrogenic following aspiration.
3. Other complications (rare):
   ■ Fulminant hepatic failure
   ■ Hemobilia
   ■ Inferior vena cava obstruction
   ■ Budd–Chiari syndrome
   ■ Hematogenous spread causing cerebral abscess

4. Factors predisposing to complications:
   ■ Age greater than 40 years
   ■ Concomitant corticosteroid use
   ■ Multiple abscesses
   ■ Large abscess more than 10 cm in diameter
   ■ Erythrocyte sedimentation rate (ESR) and C-reactive protein level are reported to be very high in patients who present with or go on to develop systemic complications.

TREATMENT AND PROGNOSIS

Treatment of amebic liver abscess is usually with drugs alone.

1. Commonly used regimens (administered orally):
   ■ Metronidazole 750 mg three times daily for 5 to 10 days (pediatric, 35 to 50 mg/kg per day in three divided doses for 5 days), or
   ■ Tinidazole 2 g/day (pediatric, 50 to 60 mg/kg daily for 5 days) for 3 days, or
   ■ Chloroquine 1 g loading dose for 1 to 2 days, then 500 mg/day (pediatric, 10 mg/kg base) for 20 days. Luminal amebicides must **always** be used following the aforementioned regimens:

  - Diloxanide furoate 500 mg three times daily (pediatric, 20 mg/kg per day in three divided doses) for 10 days, or
  - Diiodohydroxyquin 650 mg three times daily (pediatric, 30 to 40 mg/kg per day in three divided doses; maximum 2 g/day) for 20 days, or
  - Paromomycin sulfate 25 to 35 mg/kg/day in three divided doses (pediatric, 25 to 35 mg/kg per day in three divided doses) for 5 to 10 days

2. Optimal management
   ■ Patients with suspected amebic abscess should be started on therapy while awaiting serologic confirmation. Response is usually rapid, with defervescence occurring in 48 to 72 hours.
   ■ Critically ill patients, those with left lobe abscess, or those who do not respond to initial drug therapy may require radiologically guided fine-needle aspiration to avoid rupture and to exclude a pyogenic abscess.
   ■ Complications such as rupture of the abscess may be managed medically but often require percutaneous drainage (Fig. 28.2). Surgical drainage is seldom required.

3. Prognosis
   a. Amebic liver abscess is an eminently treatable condition.
   b. The mortality rate is less than 1% in uncomplicated disease.
   c. Delay in diagnosis may result in abscess rupture, with a higher mortality rate:
      ■ Rupture into chest or peritoneum: 20% mortality rate
      ■ Rupture into pericardium: 32% to 100% mortality rate

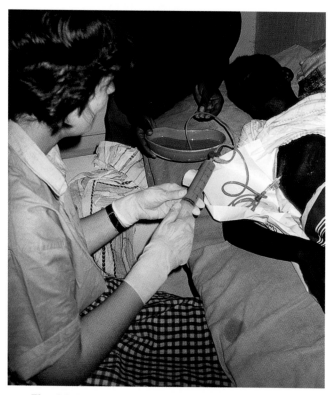

Fig. 28.2 Drainage of an amebic liver abscess in rural Africa.

Pyogenic Liver Abscess

OVERVIEW

1. Pyogenic liver abscess is a life-threatening condition.
2. The incidence varies but is estimated to be 8 to 20 per 100,000 hospital admissions in the United States.
3. Improvements in prognosis have been seen in the 2000s, but delays in diagnosis or failure to recognize this condition can result in high morbidity and mortality rates.
4. This is often associated with other medical conditions.

MICROBIOLOGY

Cultures of blood or abscess contents are positive in most cases.
- Lesions are **often polymicrobial.**
- *Klebsiella* species (particularly *Klebsiella pneumoniae*) have overtaken *Escherichia coli* as the most commonly reported causative bacteria.
- Microaerophilic organisms, particularly *Streptococcus milleri*, are increasingly common causes but need careful cultivation to isolate.
- Anaerobic organisms are commonly isolated from polymicrobial abscesses.
- Unusual organisms include *Salmonella, Haemophilus,* and *Yersinia* spp. Tuberculosis, actinomycosis, and melioidosis also occur, especially in patients with defective immunity (e.g., HIV infection, post-transplantation status).

EPIDEMIOLOGY

1. Pyogenic liver abscess is rare; population-based studies report 11 cases per million per year.
2. It is more common in middle-aged and older people.
3. Liver abscess often occurs in patients with a predisposing medical condition:
   - Biliary disease
   - Hypertension
   - Malignant disease
   - Previous abdominal surgery or endoscopic procedure
   - Diabetes mellitus
   - Cardiovascular disease
   - Crohn's disease
   - Diverticulitis
   - History of trauma

4. The gender distribution is equal.
5. No geographic or racial differences are noted.

PATHOGENESIS

1. Pyogenic infection is carried to the liver through the blood or bile. Frequently, no infective source is found (cryptogenic liver abscess); however, when one can be identified, common sources include the following:
   - Cholangitis, secondary to biliary stricture, stones, or endoscopic intervention
   - Intra-abdominal sepsis (e.g., diverticulitis, peritonitis)

- Generalized septicemia
- Dental infection
- Trauma, including liver biopsy or surgery
- Secondary infection of a preexisting liver cyst, neoplasm (including after ablative therapy), or rarely an amebic abscess

2. The right lobe of the liver is the most frequently involved.
3. Abscesses may be single or multiple; those caused by hematogenous spread are frequently multiple.
4. The abscess contains polymorphonuclear neutrophils and necrotic liver cells surrounded by a fibrous capsule.

CLINICAL FEATURES

1. History
   - Table 28.2 shows the results of a retrospective study of 79 patients.
2. Physical examination
   - Fever
   - Finger clubbing (rare)
   - Jaundice (in 33%)
   - Tender hepatomegaly
   - Classic triad of **fever, jaundice, and tender hepatomegaly** found in less than 10% of patients

DIAGNOSIS

1. Laboratory findings (Table 28.3)
2. Diagnostic imaging
   a. Chest radiograph abnormal in 50%:
      - Elevation of right hemidiaphragm
      - Blunting of right costophrenic angle
      - Atelectasis

TABLE 28.2 ■ **Presenting symptoms found in a retrospective study of 79 patients with pyogenic liver abscess**

Symptom	Frequency (%)
Fever	89.6
Right upper quadrant pain	72.2
Chills	69.0
Nausea	43.1
Vomiting	32.3
Weight loss	26.1
Jaundice	21.4
Headache	17.5
Myalgias	11.9
Diarrhea	10.7

From Rahimian J, Wilson T, Oram V, Holzman RS. Pyogenic liver abscess: recent trends in etiology and mortality. *Clin Infect Dis* 2004; 39:1654–1659.

- If a gas-forming organism is the cause of abscess, fluid levels may be visible below the diaphragm
  b. Ultrasonography
  - Round, oval, or elliptoid lesion
  - Irregular margin
  - Hypoechoic with variable internal echoes
  c. CT
  - Highly sensitive; detects up to 94% of lesions
  - Lesions show reduced attenuation and possibly enhance with contrast
  d. MRI
  - More sensitive at detecting small lesions than CT
  - Lesions have low signal intensity on T1-weighted images and very high signal intensity on T2-images; lesions enhance with gadolinium
  e. Radioisotope study
  - Gallium is avidly taken up by abscesses
3. Microbiology
  - Blood cultures should be taken before initiation of antibiotic therapy.
  - Positive blood cultures occur in 50% to 100%.
  - Aspiration of the abscess increases the yield of a positive microbiologic diagnosis.
  - In polymicrobial abscesses, all the causative organisms may not be present in the blood.

COMPLICATIONS

- Septicemia
- Metastatic abscess
- Septic shock
- Acute respiratory distress syndrome
- Renal failure
- Rupture

TREATMENT AND PROGNOSIS

1. Treatment
  a. In the past, standard treatment involved open surgical drainage of the abscess in combination with broad-spectrum antibiotics. Studies since the 1990s have shown improved

TABLE 28.3 ■ **Laboratory features in pyogenic liver abscess**

Feature	Frequency (%)
Increased erythrocyte sedimentation rate	100
Leukocytosis	75
Anemia	50
Elevated serum bilirubin level	Common
Elevated serum alkaline phosphatase level	Common
Increased serum aminotransferase levels	Common
Prolonged prothrombin time	Common
Decreased serum albumin level	Poor prognostic sign

results with either percutaneous drainage or aspiration in combination with antibiotics. Some patients can be managed medically without surgery or aspiration.

b. It is usually possible to combine diagnostic and therapeutic aspiration in these patients.

c. Complications of drainage include hemorrhage, perforation of a viscus, infection from the drain, and catheter displacement.

d. Antibiotic therapy should include coverage against gram-negative organisms as well as microaerophilic and anaerobic organisms. Empiric first-line regimens are as follows:

- Suspected biliary source: ampicillin + gentamicin + metronidazole
- Suspected colonic source: third-generation cephalosporin + metronidazole

e. Antibiotic therapy is usually intravenous initially. The duration of intravenous antibiotic therapy and the decision to change to oral therapy are governed by the individual clinical response. Antibiotic use for a total duration of 2 to 3 weeks is recommended.

f. Surgical intervention may be required if the patient fails to respond rapidly to therapy; a flexible approach must be adopted.

2. Prognosis
   - Untreated pyogenic liver abscess has a mortality rate approaching 100%.
   - Case series in the 2000s have reported mortality rates as low as 2.5% but usually 10% to 30%, depending on the underlying cause of the abscess and associated medical conditions. Improved mortality rates are thought to result from advanced imaging and diagnostic techniques and the use of percutaneous drainage.

Hepatic Cysts

OVERVIEW

Causes of cystic lesions in the liver are diverse.

1. Congenital
   a. Polycystic disease
      - **Infantile polycystic disease** is a rare autosomal recessive condition that results in cyst formation in the liver and kidneys. Hepatomegaly is often present at birth. Renal damage is usually the cause of reduced life span.
      - **Adult polycystic disease** is an autosomal dominant condition predominantly affecting the kidneys but with hepatic cysts in 33% of patients.
        - It is rarely associated with liver dysfunction.
        - Treatment should be considered only in the presence of symptoms. The optimal management is debated but depends on cyst morphology, severity of cystic disease, comorbidity, and recurrence rates; options include cyst unroofing, liver resection, and, for those with end-stage disease, liver transplantation.
   b. Choledochal cysts (see also Chapter 33)
      - Many disease entities manifest with cystic dilatation of the biliary tract. **Caroli's disease** is one of these conditions in which nonobstructive dilatation of intrahepatic bile ducts occurs.

2. Acquired
   a. Benign tumors (e.g., hamartomas)

b. Simple cysts
- Most are small and incidental.
- Treatment is indicated only for symptomatic cysts: aspiration combined with sclerosis, open surgery, or laparoscopic cyst unroofing, which is considered to be the optimal standard of care.

c. Infective, most commonly hydatid disease (caused by *Echinococcus granulosus*, discussed in the next section)

Hydatid Disease of the Liver (Fig. 28.3)

OVERVIEW

- Hydatid cystic disease has a worldwide distribution and is endemic in many sheep- and cattle-rearing regions of the world.
- Hydatid disease is a chronic and potentially dangerous condition that is often overlooked as a cause of abdominal pain and hepatic disease.

PARASITOLOGY

Hydatid cystic disease is caused by *Echinococcus granulosus*.

- *E. granulosus* is a 3- to 6-mm tapeworm.
- A carnivorous host, usually a dog, becomes infected by eating the viscera of infected sheep that contain hydatid cysts.
- Scolices from the cysts adhere to the small intestine of the dog and develop into the tapeworm.
- The tapeworm produces up to 500 ova in the host bowel.
- Infected dogs excrete *Echinococcus* eggs in feces. Eggs are viable in the environment for several weeks.
- Eggs are ingested by humans, either from contamination of soil and foodstuffs or from the dog's coat, and they hatch in the intestine to form oncospheres that invade tissue to enter the portal circulation.

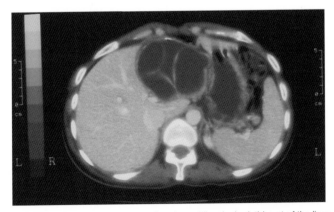

Fig. 28.3 Computed tomography of a multilocular hydatid cyst of the liver.

- Each oncosphere matures into a vesicle and subsequently a cyst, the metacestode.
- Cysts can form in any organ, most commonly the liver (50% to 70%). Cysts consist of a germinal layer that buds asexually to form daughter cysts, which contain protoscolices, the infective forms that are ingested by the definitive host (Fig. 28.4).

EPIDEMIOLOGY

Infections with *E. granulosus* occur worldwide. The scale of human disease is not fully documented, but rural communities face a significant health problem from infection.
Areas with a documented high prevalence of disease include the following sheep farming areas:

- Mediterranean countries
- Northern Kenya (Turkana district)
- Areas of South America
- Wales
- New Zealand

A case-control study conducted in Spain found that long-term coexistence with dogs is a major risk factor for the development of *E. granulosus* infection, especially coexistence with dogs with the opportunity to eat potentially infected offal.

PATHOGENESIS

1. Spread of oncospheres is through the bloodstream, usually the portal circulation, and results in hepatic disease in 50% to 70% of cases. Other sites of disease are as follows:
   - Lung (20% to 30%)
   - Bone (less than 10%)
   - Brain
   - Heart

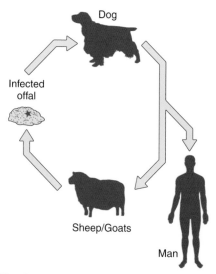

Fig. 28.4 Life cycle of *Echinococcus granulosus*.

2. Cysts enlarge slowly and cause tissue damage directly or by compromising the blood supply. The parasite causes a host response to form a collagenous capsule around the germinal layer. This capsule may calcify. Often, no host inflammatory response occurs.

CLINICAL FEATURES

1. Symptoms (Table 28.4)
   - Cysts may be asymptomatic and often become symptomatic only after decades, because of their slow growth. Symptoms are caused by pressure effects.
   - Symptoms may follow cyst rupture or leakage.
   - The presentation of a secondary infection of a hydatid cyst resembles the presentation of a pyogenic abscess.
2. Physical examination
   - Tender mass
   - Chest signs, especially at the right base
   - Fever
   - Jaundice

DIAGNOSIS

1. Laboratory findings
   - Elevated serum alkaline phosphatase level
   - Peripheral eosinophilia (>7%) in 30% of patients, usually indicating leakage or rupture of cyst
   - Elevated serum bilirubin level (uncommon)
2. Diagnostic imaging
   a. Chest x-ray
      - Elevation of the right hemidiaphragm
      - Cysts may be visible in the lung
      - Calcification of hepatic cyst may be visible below the diaphragm
   b. Ultrasonography
      - Cysts may be anechoic
      - Typically round
      - Septate or daughter cysts are often visible

TABLE 28.4 ■ **Clinical features of 650 patients with a liver hydatid cyst**

Feature	Number (%)
Abdominal pain	435 (66.9%)
Fullness in the upper abdomen and dyspepsia	234 (36.0%)
Hepatomegaly	201 (30.9%)
Asymptomatic	182 (28.0%)
Jaundice	104 (16.0%)
Mass in the right upper quadrant	39 (6.0%)
Acute abdomen	13 (2.0%)

From Tekin A, Kücükkartallar T, Kartal A, et al. Clinical and surgical profile and follow up of patients with liver hydatid cyst from an endemic region. *J Gastrointestin Liver Dis* 2008; 17:33–37.

- Separation of germinal membrane: "water-lily sign"
- Collapsed cysts may be visible
- Calcification of wall
- Hydatid "sand"

  c. CT
  - Germinal layer seen clearly
  - Daughter cysts readily visualized
  - Lesion of low attenuation: 3 to 30 Hounsfield units

  d. MRI
  - Characteristic low-intensity rim 4 to 5 mm thick, best seen on T2-weighted images
  - Lesion center nonhomogeneous
  - Lesion is hypointense on T1-weighted images, hyperintense on T2-weighted images

3. Serologic tests: Indirect haemagglutination (IHA) and enzyme-linked immunosorbent assay (ELISA) are 75% to 94% sensitive. Specificity is lower, necessitating a confirmatory test (e.g., molecular biologic methods or immunoblotting).
4. Molecular biologic tests: Polymerase chain reaction (PCR)–derived probes allow diagnosis and species differentiation.

COMPLICATIONS

1. Leakage or rupture of cyst (sometimes iatrogenic from aspiration of undiagnosed hydatid cyst) may result in the following:
   - Allergic reaction, including anaphylaxis (may be fatal)
   - Dissemination of disease
   - Cholangitis if cyst ruptures into the biliary tract
   - Hemoptysis and secondary infection if bronchial rupture
2. Secondary infection of cyst behaves like a pyogenic abscess.

TREATMENT AND PROGNOSIS

1. **Surgery remains the mainstay of treatment.**
   - Regardless of the type of surgical technique employed, the combination of surgery with chemotherapy is the safest and most effective approach.
   - Hydatid cysts manifesting with secondary infection should be treated as pyogenic abscesses; however, aspiration of an infected hydatid cyst is more hazardous than is aspiration of a pyogenic abscess.
2. Drug therapy includes the following:
   a. Albendazole 10 to 14 mg/kg/day orally for 3 months initially (may continue for 1 year) or
   b. Mebendazole 30 to 70 mg/kg/day orally for 3 months (may require up to 200 mg/kg per day)
      - These benzimidazole agents act on the germinal layer.
   c. Praziquantel (40 mg/kg orally per day for 14 days) has been used as a protoscolicide and, as such, has an important role preoperatively.
3. Surgical and radiologic options include the following:
   - Radical surgery: pericystectomy or hepatic resection
   - Conservative surgical treatment through unroofing and management of the residual cavity
   - Laparoscopic procedures
   - Percutaneous techniques, including puncture, aspiration, injection, reaspiration (PAIR)

The technique chosen depends on the condition of the patient, characteristics of the cyst, and experience of the surgeon or radiologist. The complication rate of surgery may be high. For example, 57% in a series of 59 patients had dissemination of infection, secondary infection, fistula formation, or complications from seepage of scolicidal agents into the biliary tract (causing a syndrome resembling sclerosing cholangitis).

4. Prognosis
   ■ Hydatid cysts may remain asymptomatic throughout a person's life.
   ■ Cyst rupture or infection is associated with considerable mortality.

Diagnostic Approach to Hepatic Abscesses and Cysts

A diagnostic approach to distinguishing liver abscesses from cysts is summarized in Figure 28.5. Key features include the following:
   ■ Important clues to the diagnosis are found in a carefully taken history from the patient.
   ■ The geographic history is of vital importance.

SEROLOGIC TESTS AND BLOOD CULTURES

   ■ Serologic tests are positive in 90% to 100% of cases of amebic liver abscess.
   ■ Serologic tests are positive in 75% to 95% of cases of hepatic hydatid disease.
   ■ Blood cultures should be performed on all febrile patients; amebic and hydatid cavities may become superinfected.
   ■ Blood cultures alone are positive in at least 50% of patients with a pyogenic liver abscess.

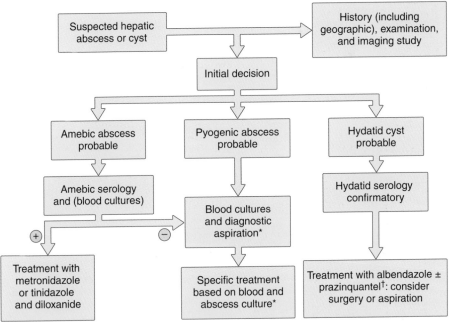

Fig. 28.5 Algorithm for the diagnostic approach to a suspected hepatic abscess or cyst. *Presumptive treatment is usually begun on the basis of clinical suspicion pending test results. †Indications for diagnostic aspiration: diagnosis of pyogenic abscess, critically ill patient requiring urgent diagnosis, failure of initial therapy.

IMAGING

- Imaging confirms the diagnosis of a cyst or abscess.
- **Ultrasonography is the investigation of choice** because of high sensitivity, lack of radiation, low cost, and ready availability.
- CT may provide further information, especially in pyogenic liver abscess (contrast enhanced) and hydatid disease.
- MRI may be more sensitive than ultrasonography and CT for detecting small lesions.

ASPIRATION

- This is required for diagnosis and treatment in cases of suspected pyogenic abscess.
- It gives a microbiologic diagnosis in more than 80% of patients with pyogenic abscess. Combined aspiration and blood cultures positively identify the causative organism in more than 85% of cases.
- It may be performed in cases of suspected amebic abscess if the abscess is large and rupture is imminent or if the diagnosis is in doubt. Usually, aspiration is *not* required for diagnosis.
- Aspiration should *not* be carried out in cases of suspected hydatid disease. It may be indicated if the cyst appears to be infected. In the event of aspiration of a hydatid cyst, efforts should be taken to prevent leakage of cyst contents, which has potentially serious sequelae. Aspiration should be performed by an experienced operator under imaging guidance through as thick a rim of normal liver as possible.

Table 28.5 lists the differences between hepatic abscesses and cysts.

TABLE 28.5 ■ Comparison of amebic and pyogenic liver abscess and hydatid cyst

Parameter	Amebic liver abscess	Pyogenic liver abscess	Hydatid cyst
Age	Any, mostly younger	Any, mostly older	Any, mostly older
Sex	Male > female	Equal	Equal
Epidemiologic features	Residence or travel in endemic area; poverty, poor hygiene	None; occasional association with helminth infection	Residence in endemic area; farm animal exposure
Associated medical conditions	Rare	Common (e.g., surgery; biliary tract disease; diverticulitis)	Rare
Significant jaundice	Rare	Common	Rare
Multiple abscesses (cysts)	Infrequent	Common	Septate and daughter cysts
Liver biochemical test levels	Mildly abnormal	More markedly abnormal	Mildly abnormal
Amebic serology	Positive	Negative	Negative
Hydatid serology	Negative	Negative	Positive
Blood cultures	Negative; positive result indicates superinfection	Frequently positive	Negative; positive result indicates superinfection
Abscess contents	Thick fluid; variable color, yellow-brown, odorless	Pus; creamy yellow, foul smelling	Aspiration not recommended; thin fluid
Effectiveness of medical therapy	Almost always	Often	Usually in combination with surgery
Surgery required	Hardly ever	Sometimes	Usually

FURTHER READING

Campos-Bueno A, Lopez-Abente G, Andres-Cercadillo AM. Risk factors for *Echinococcus granulosus* infection: a case-control study. *Am J Trop Med Hyg* 2000; 62:329–334.

Dziri C, Haouet K, Fingerhut A. Treatment of hydatid cyst of the liver: where is the evidence? *World J Surg* 2004; 28:731–736.

Gottstein B, Reichen J. Echinococcosis/hydatidosis. In: Cook GC, Alimuddin Z, eds. *Manson's Tropical Diseases*. 22nd edn. London: Elsevier; 2008:1549–1568.

Kershenobich D, Olivera-Martinez MA. Liver abscess. In: Schiff ER, Sorrell MF, Maddrey WC, eds. *Schiff's Diseases of the Liver*. 10th edn. Philadelphia: Lippincott Williams & Wilkins; 2006:1351–1358.

Kurland JE, Brann OS. Pyogenic and amebic liver abscesses. *Curr Gastroenterol Rep* 2004; 6:273–279.

Lodhi S, Sarwari AR, Muzammil M, et al. Features distinguishing amoebic from pyogenic liver abscess: a review of 577 adult cases. *Trop Med Int Health* 2004; 9:718–723.

Lok KH, Li KF, Li KK, Szeto ML. Pyogenic liver abscess: clinical profile, microbiological characteristics, and management in a Hong Kong hospital. *J Microbiol Immunol Infect* 2008; 41:483–490.

Mergen H, Genç H, Tavusbay C. Assessment of liver hydatid cyst cases: 10 years experience in Turkey. *Trop Doct* 2007; 37:54–56.

Prousalidis J, Kosmidis C, Anthimidis G, et al. Forty-four years' experience (1963–2006) in the management of primarily infected hydatid cyst of the liver. *HPB (Oxford)* 2008; 10:18–24.

Rahimian J, Wilson T, Oram V, Holzman RS. Pyogenic liver abscess: recent trends in etiology and mortality. *Clin Infect Dis* 2004; 39:1654–1659.

Santi-Rocca J, Rigothier MC, Guillén N. Host-microbe interactions and defense mechanisms in the development of amoebic liver abscesses. *Clin Microbiol Rev* 2009; 22:65–75.

Tekin A, Kücükkartallar T, Kartal A, et al. Clinical and surgical profile and follow up of patients with liver hydatid cyst from an endemic region. *J Gastrointestin Liver Dis* 2008; 17:33–37.

van Doorn HR, Hofwegen H, Koelewijn R, et al. Use of rapid dipstick and latex agglutination tests and enzyme-linked immunosorbent assay for serodiagnosis of amebic liver abscess, amebic colitis, and *Entamoeba histolytica* cyst passage. *J Clin Microbiol* 2005; 43:4801–4806.

Wells CD, Arguedas M. Amebic liver abscess. *South Med J* 2004; 97:673–682.

Yagci G, Ustunsoz B, Kaymakcioglu N, et al. Results of surgical, laparoscopic, and percutaneous treatment for hydatid disease of the liver: 10 years experience with 355 patients. *World J Surg* 2005; 29:1670–1679.

CHAPTER 29

Other infections involving the liver

Wolfram Goessling, MD, PhD ■ Raymond T. Chung, MD

Bacterial Infections Involving the Liver

Bacterial infections can affect the liver directly and often give a clinical picture of acute hepatitis.

LEGIONELLA PNEUMOPHILA

- Pneumonia is the predominant clinical manifestation; abnormal liver biochemical test levels are frequent, usually without jaundice and without affecting the clinical outcome.
- Liver histologic features are nonspecific, with portal infiltration, microvesicular steatosis, and focal necrosis; occasional organisms are seen.
- Initial treatment is with a fluoroquinolone or macrolide antibiotic.

STAPHYLOCOCCUS AUREUS (TOXIC SHOCK SYNDROME)

- This multisystem disease is caused by the staphylococcal toxic shock syndrome toxin (TSST-1) and has a mortality rate of 8%. Originally described in association with tampon use, it is now more frequently a complication of *Staphylococcus aureus* infections in surgical wounds, mostly in women.
- Typical findings include fever, a scarlatiniform rash, mucosal hyperemia, vomiting, diarrhea, and hypotension, with rapid development of multiorgan failure. Hepatic involvement is

almost always present, results from hypoperfusion and circulating toxins, and is marked by deep jaundice and high serum aminotransferase levels.

- Liver histologic findings include microvesicular steatosis, necrosis, and centrilobular cholestasis.
- The diagnosis is confirmed by culture of toxigenic *S. aureus* from vaginal swabs, blood, or other body sites or by demonstration of TSST-1.
- Treatment is with intravenous clindamycin plus nafcillin for methicillin-sensitive isolates or vancomycin or linezolid for methicillin-resistant isolates; intravenous immune globulin may be beneficial for cases of toxic shock syndrome caused by *Streptococcus pyogenes*.

CLOSTRIDIUM PERFRINGENS

- This is usually a mixed anaerobic infection that results in rapid development of local wound pain, abdominal pain, and diarrhea; it is associated with myonecrosis or gas gangrene.
- Jaundice may develop in up to 20% of patients with gas gangrene and is predominantly a consequence of massive intravascular hemolysis caused by the bacterial exotoxin, with resulting unconjugated hyperbilirubinemia.
- Liver involvement may include abscess formation and gas in the portal vein. Hepatic involvement does not appear to worsen mortality rates, which average 60%.
- Treatment is with intravenous penicillin and clindamycin.

LISTERIA MONOCYTOGENES

- This is characterized by meningoencephalitis and pneumonitis; hepatic involvement in adult human infection is rare.
- Neonates and patients with underlying chronic liver disease or immune deficiency are most commonly affected.
- Serum aminotransferase levels are typically very high.
- Patients may present with a single abscess, multiple microabscesses, or diffuse or granulomatous hepatitis; the outcome is worse with multiple abscesses.
- Treatment consists of abscess drainage and the combination of (amino) penicillins and aminoglycosides, typically for 3 to 4 weeks.

NEISSERIA GONORRHOEAE

- Half of all patients with disseminated gonococcal infection have abnormal liver biochemical test levels, mainly elevated serum alkaline phosphatase levels and elevated aspartate aminotransferase (AST) levels. Jaundice is uncommon.
- Perihepatitis **(Fitz-Hugh–Curtis syndrome)** is a common complication of gonococcal infection that affects women almost exclusively. It is believed to result from direct spread of infection from the pelvis and does not affect overall outcome. It can also be caused by infection with *Chlamydia trachomatis*.
- The sudden onset of sharp right upper quadrant pain, often following lower abdominal pain as an indicator of long-standing pelvic inflammatory disease, is typical. It may be confused with acute cholecystitis or pleurisy.
- This can be distinguished from gonococcal bacteremia by a characteristic friction rub over the liver and negative blood cultures. The diagnosis is made by vaginal cultures for *N. gonorrhoeae*.

Laparoscopy may show characteristic "violin-string" adhesions between the liver capsule and the anterior abdominal wall.

- Treatment is with intravenous ceftriaxone.

BURKHOLDERIA PSEUDOMALLEI (MELIOIDOSIS)

- This soil- and water-borne gram-negative bacterium that causes melioidosis is found predominantly in Southeast Asia and India. The clinical spectrum ranges from asymptomatic infection to fulminant septicemia.
- Severe disease involves the lung, gastrointestinal tract, and liver, with hepatomegaly and jaundice; liver histologic changes include inflammatory infiltrates, multiple small and large abscesses, and focal necrosis.
- Chronic disease is characterized by granulomas with central necrosis resembling tuberculous lesions. Organisms are rarely seen on Giemsa stains of liver biopsy specimens. The diagnosis can be made by serologic testing using an indirect hemagglutination assay.
- Initial antibiotic therapy consists of intravenous ceftazidime, imipenem, or meropenem.

SHIGELLA AND SALMONELLA SPP.

- Cholestatic hepatitis can be attributable to enteric infection with *Shigella* species; liver histologic findings include portal and periportal polymorphonuclear infiltration, focal necrosis, and cholestasis.
- **Typhoid fever** caused by *Salmonella typhi* frequently involves the liver. Some patients may present with acute hepatitis, characterized by fever and tender hepatomegaly. Cholangitis, cholecystitis, and liver abscesses may occur.
- Mild to moderate elevations of serum bilirubin (up to 16% of cases) and aminotransferase (up to 60%) levels are common in typhoid fever and should not prompt a search for a separate diagnosis.
- Hepatic damage appears to be mediated by bacterial endotoxin, which can produce nonspecific reactions, such as sinusoidal and portal inflammation, necrosis, hypertrophy of Kupffer cells, and non-necrotizing granulomas.
- Hepatic abnormalities do not appear to affect outcome and typically remit after 2 to 3 weeks of treatment with fluoroquinolones, third-generation cephalosporins, or ampicillin.

YERSINIA ENTEROCOLITICA

- This infection manifests as ileocolitis in children and terminal ileitis and mesenteric adenitis in adults.
- Patients with hepatic involvement have underlying comorbidities such as diabetes mellitus, cirrhosis, or hemochromatosis; excess tissue iron appears to be a predisposing factor.
- The subacute septicemic form of the disease resembles typhoid fever or malaria. Multiple abscesses are diffusely distributed in the liver and spleen. The mortality rate approaches 50%.
- The granulomatous form produces noncaseating granulomas.

COXIELLA BURNETII (Q FEVER)

- This is characterized by relapsing fevers, headache, myalgias, malaise, pneumonitis, and culture-negative endocarditis; the liver is commonly affected. The predominant abnormality is an elevated serum alkaline phosphatase level.

- The hepatic histologic hallmark is the intra-acinar granuloma with a central fat vacuole surrounded by a fibrin ring and macrophages, the "fibrin-ring granuloma" or "doughnut lesion."
- The diagnosis is confirmed by serologic testing for complement-fixing antibodies.
- Doxycycline is the treatment of choice.

RICKETTSIA RICKETTSII (ROCKY MOUNTAIN SPOTTED FEVER)

- Mortality caused by this systemic tick-borne illness has decreased considerably as a result of early recognition; a few patients present with multiorgan manifestations and have a high mortality rate.
- Hepatic involvement is frequent in multiorgan Rocky Mountain spotted fever, predominantly as jaundice; pathologic examination reveals portal perivascular inflammation and vasculitis.
- Treatment with tetracycline should be initiated when infection is suspected.

ACTINOMYCES ISRAELII (ACTINOMYCOSIS)

- *Actinomyces israelii* is found worldwide in soil.
- Cervicofacial infection is the most frequent manifestation of actinomycosis, but gastrointestinal involvement is common (13% to 60% of cases).
- Hepatic involvement is present in 15% of cases of abdominal actinomycosis, most often as abscesses, and is thought to result from metastatic spread from other abdominal sites through the portal vein. The course is more indolent than that of other causes of pyogenic hepatic abscess (see Chapter 28). Abscesses may be multiple and in both lobes of the liver.
- The diagnosis is based on aspiration of an abscess cavity and visualization of characteristic "sulfur granules" or a positive anaerobic culture.
- Most abscesses resolve with a prolonged course of intravenous penicillin or oral tetracycline.

BARTONELLA BACILLIFORMIS (BARTONELLOSIS, OROYA FEVER)

- This is endemic to Colombia, Ecuador, and Peru and is transmitted by infected sandflies.
- This acute febrile illness is accompanied by jaundice, hemolysis, hepatosplenomegaly, and lymphadenopathy.
- Centrilobular necrosis of the liver and splenic infarction may occur.
- Mortality rates resulting from sepsis or hemolysis approach 40%, but prompt treatment with chloramphenicol, fluoroquinolones, or tetracycline prevents fatal complications.

BRUCELLA SPP. (BRUCELLOSIS)

- This may be acquired from infected pigs (*Brucella suis*), cattle (*B. abortus*), goats (*B. melitensis*), or sheep (*B. ovis*).
- It manifests as an acute febrile illness with arthralgias, headaches, and malaise or as subacute or chronic disease.
- Hepatomegaly and abnormal liver biochemical test levels are common; jaundice may be present in severe cases. Typically, liver histologic examination shows multiple noncaseating granulomas and, less often, focal portal tract infiltration or fibrosis.
- The diagnosis is confirmed by serologic testing in combination with an animal exposure history.
- Imaging reveals lesions with central calcification and a necrotic rim.
- A prolonged course of combination antimicrobial therapy with streptomycin, rifampin, and doxycycline is most effective.

Spirochetal Infections of the Liver

LEPTOSPIRA SPP. (LEPTOSPIROSIS)

1. This is among the most common zoonoses in the world, with a wide range of domestic and wild animal reservoirs. Human-to-human transmission is uncommon. Up to 80% of the population has been exposed in some tropical countries; it is uncommon in the United States. Human disease can occur as one of two syndromes: anicteric leptospirosis and Weil's disease.
2. **Anicteric leptospirosis** accounts for more than 90% of cases. It is characterized by a self-limited biphasic course. A few patients have elevated serum aminotransferase and bilirubin levels with hepatomegaly.
    ■ The first phase begins abruptly, with viral illness–like symptoms associated with fever, leptospiremia, and characteristic conjunctival suffusion (an important diagnostic clue) and lasts 4 to 7 days; leptospires are present in the blood or cerebrospinal fluid (CSF).
    ■ The second or immune phase, lasting 4 to 30 days, follows 1 to 3 days of improvement and is characterized by myalgias, nausea, vomiting, abdominal tenderness, and aseptic meningitis in up to 80% of patients.
3. **Weil's disease** is a severe icteric form of leptospirosis and constitutes 5% to 10% of all cases. Complications are mainly the result of direct vascular damage by the *Leptospira*. The two phases of disease are less distinct:
    ■ The first phase is often marked by jaundice, which may last for weeks.
    ■ During the second phase, fever may be high, and hepatic and renal manifestations predominate. Jaundice is marked, with serum bilirubin levels approaching 30 mg/dL. Aminotransferase levels usually do not exceed five times the upper limit of normal, and thrombocytopenia is common. Acute tubular necrosis, which can lead to renal failure, cardiac arrhythmias, and hemorrhagic pneumonitis, are common. Mortality rates range from 5% to 40%.
4. The diagnosis of leptospirosis is made on clinical grounds in conjunction with positive cultures of blood or CSF in the first phase or urine in the second phase. Isolation of the organism is difficult and may require many weeks. Microagglutination testing and serologic testing by enzyme-linked immunosorbent assay (ELISA) may confirm the diagnosis in the second phase.
5. Liver histologic examination reveals individual hepatocyte damage and canalicular cholestasis with mild portal inflammation.
6. Doxycycline 200 mg per day is given in mild cases (effective only if given early) and as prophylaxis after exposure. Severe cases require intravenous penicillin, with a risk of a Jarisch-Herxheimer reaction. Most patients recover without residual organ impairment.

TREPONEMA PALLIDUM (SYPHILIS)

1. **Congenital syphilis**
    ■ Liver involvement may result from immunologic mechanisms and is worsened by penicillin treatment.
    ■ Newborns have characteristic mucocutaneous lesions and osteochondritis, as well as hepatosplenomegaly and jaundice.
    ■ Liver histologic examination reveals diffuse hepatitis with spirochetes seen mostly in the spaces of Disse.
2. **Secondary syphilis**
    ■ Liver involvement is characteristic (up to 50% of cases) and usually manifests with non-specific symptoms. Jaundice, hepatomegaly, and right upper quadrant tenderness are less common. Nearly all patients exhibit generalized lymphadenopathy.

- Biochemical testing generally reveals low-grade elevations of serum aminotransferase and bilirubin levels, with a disproportionate elevation of the serum alkaline phosphatase level.
- Liver histologic examination reveals focal necrosis, especially in the periportal and centrilobular regions, or granulomas and portal vasculitis. Spirochetes may be demonstrated by silver staining in up to half of patients.
- Liver dysfunction may be worsened by the Jarisch-Herxheimer reaction as a response to treatment, which can occur with treatment of all spirochete infections.

3. **Tertiary (late) syphilis**
   - Hepatic lesions are common but typically silent. Occasionally, tender hepatomegaly and nodularity may raise the suspicion of metastatic cancer (hepar lobatum).
   - If hepatic involvement is unrecognized, hepatocellular dysfunction and complications of portal hypertension can ensue.
   - The characteristic lesions in tertiary syphilis are single or multiple gummas with central necrosis, often surrounded by granulation tissue consisting of a lymphoplasmacytic infiltrate with endarteritis obliterans. Exuberant deposition of scar tissue can ensue. Treponemes are rarely found.
   - Treatment consists of benzathine penicillin G.

BORRELIA BURGDORFERI (LYME DISEASE)

- This multisystem disease is caused by the tick-borne spirochete *Borrelia burgdorferi*. Predominant manifestations are dermatologic, cardiac, neurologic, and musculoskeletal. Hepatic involvement occurs in 20% of affected patients and usually manifests as hepatomegaly with increased serum aminotransferase and lactate dehydrogenase levels.
- In early stages, the spirochetes disseminate hematogenously from the skin and multiply in the organs of the reticuloendothelial system, including the liver. The clinical picture is suggestive of acute hepatitis and often accompanies erythema chronicum migrans, the sentinel rash.
- Liver histologic examination reveals hepatocyte ballooning, marked mitotic activity, microvesicular fat, hyperplasia of Kupffer cells, a mixed sinusoidal infiltrate, and intraparenchymal and sinusoidal spirochetes on Warthin-Starry stain.
- The diagnosis is confirmed by serologic testing in a patient with a typical clinical history.
- Hepatic involvement does not appear to affect overall outcome, which is excellent in primary disease after antibiotic treatment with doxycycline or penicillin.

Parasitic Diseases that Involve the Liver (Table 29.1)

PROTOZOAL INFECTIONS

1. **Amebic liver abscess** (see Chapter 28)
2. **Malaria**

Malaria is one of the most important public health problems worldwide, annually infecting about 300 to 500 million persons in more than 100 countries and causing at least 1 million deaths.

   a. Life cycle (Fig. 29.1)
      - The liver is affected during two stages of the malarial life cycle; the pre-erythrocytic phase and the erythrocytic phase, during which symptoms are noted.

TABLE 29.1 ■ Parasitic infections of the liver

Disease (Organism)	Endemic Areas	Predisposition	Pathophysiology	Presentation	Diagnosis	Treatment
Protozoans						
Amebiasis (*Entamoeba histolytica*)	Worldwide, especially Africa, Asia, Mexico, South America	Poor sanitation, sexual transmission	Hematogenous spread and tissue invasion, abscess formation	Fever, right upper quadrant pain, peritonitis, elevated right hemidiaphragm	Cysts in stool, serology, imaging	Metronidazole 750 mg t.i.d. × 7–10 days or tinidazole 2 g daily × 5 days, then iodoquinol 650 mg PO t.i.d. × 20 days or paromomycin 25–35 mg/kg/day PO in 3 doses × 7 days
Malaria (*Plasmodium falciparum, P. malariae, P. vivax, P. ovale*)	Africa, Asia, South America	Mosquito bites	Sporozoite clearance by hepatocytes, exoerythrocytic replication in liver	Tender hepatomegaly, splenomegaly, jaundice hepatic failure rare (with viral hepatitis or *P. falciparum*)	Parasite on thick/thin smear	Quinidine or quinine for sensitive species only; atovaquone/proguanil or quinine + doxycycline or tetracycline or clindamycin for *P. falciparum*; primaquine for hepatic stage of *P. vivax* and *P. ovale*
Visceral leishmaniasis (*Leishmania donovani*)	Mediterranean, Middle East, Asia, Africa, Central and South America	Immunosuppression	Infection of reticuloendothelial cells	Fever, weight loss, hepatosplenomegaly, secondary bacterial infection, hyperpigmentation	Amastigotes on spleen, liver or bone marrow aspirate	Liposomal amphotericin B, sodium stibogluconate, or miltefosine
Toxoplasmosis (*Toxoplasma gondii*)	Worldwide	Intrauterine infection, immunosuppression	Hepatic inflammation and necrosis due to replication of parasite	Fever, lymphadenopathy, hepatosplenomegaly, atypical lymphocytosis	Serology, organism in tissue	Pyrimethamine, folinic acid, and sulfadiazine × 3–4 wk
Nematodes						
Ascariasis (*Ascaris lumbricoides*)	Tropical climates	Ingestion of raw vegetables	Migration of larvae to the liver, invasion of bile ducts by adult worm	Abdominal pain, fever, jaundice, biliary obstruction	Ova in stool, worms in stool or on imaging, pathology with perioval granulomas	Albendazole 400 mg × 1; mebendazole 100 mg b.i.d. × 3 days; or ivermectin 150–200 µg/kg × 1

Disease	Distribution	Exposure/Risk	Mechanism	Clinical	Diagnosis	Treatment
Toxocariasis (Toxocara canis, T. cati)	Worldwide	Exposure to dogs or cats	Migration of larvae in liver (visceral larva migrans)	Granulomas with eosinophilia	Larvae on biopsy, serology	Albendazole 400 mg b.i.d. × 5 days or mebendazole 100–200 mg b.i.d. × 5 days
Hepatic capillariasis (Capillaria hepatica)	Worldwide	Rodent exposure	Migration of larvae to the liver with inflammatory reaction due to eggs	Acute or subacute hepatitis, tender hepatomegaly, occasionally splenomegaly, eosinophilia	Worms or eggs on liver biopsy	Mebendazole 200 mg b.i.d. × 20 days or albendazole 400 q.d. × 10 days
Strongyloidiasis (Strongyloides stercoralis)	Asia, Africa, South America, Southern Europe, United States	Immunosuppression, especially HTLV-1-associated leukemia	Penetration of larvae from the intestine to the liver	Hepatomegaly, jaundice	Larvae in stool or duodenal aspirate; larvae in portal tract or lobule	Ivermectin 200 µg/kg × 2 days or albendazole 400 mg b.i.d. × 7 days
Trichinosis (Trichinella spiralis)	Temperate climates	Ingestion of raw or undercooked meet	Hematogenous dissemination to all organs, including liver	Occasionally jaundice, biliary obstruction	History, eosinophilia, fever, biopsy with larvae in muscle or hepatic sinusoids	Corticosteroids for allergic symptoms; albendazole 400 mg b.i.d. × 8–14 days or mebendazole 200–400 mg t.i.d. × 3 days, then 400–500 t.i.d. × 10 days
Trematodes						
Schistosomiasis (Schistosoma mansoni, S. japonicum)	Asia, Africa, South America, Caribbean	Exposure to fresh water	Fibrogenic host immune response to eggs in portal vein	Acute: eosinophilic infiltrate Chronic: hepatosplenomegaly, presinusoidal hypertension	Ova in stool, on rectal or liver biopsy with perioval granuloma	Praziquantel 40 mg/kg in two doses × 1 day or oxamniquine 15 mg/kg × 1. Acute toxemia: praziquantel 75 mg/kg
Fascioliasis (Fasciola hepatica)	Worldwide	Cattle or sheep raising; ingestion of contaminated watercress	Migration of larvae through the liver	Acute: fever, abdominal pain, jaundice, hemobilia Chronic: hepatomegaly	Ova in stool, worms in bile duct on ERCP	Triclabendazole 10 mg/kg × 1–2; bithionol 30–50 mg/kg q.o.d. × 10–15 doses; or nitazoxanide 500 mg b.i.d. × 7 days

(Continued)

TABLE 29.1 ■ Parasitic infections of the liver—*cont'd*

Disease (Organism)	Endemic Areas	Predisposition	Pathophysiology	Presentation	Diagnosis	Treatment
Clonorchiasis, opisthorchiasis (*Clonorchis sinensis, Opisthorchis viverrini, O. felineus*)	Southeast Asia, China, Japan, Korea, Eastern Europe	Ingestion of freshwater fish	Migration through ampulla with egg deposition in bile ducts	Biliary hyperplasia and obstruction, choledocholithiasis, cholangiocarcinoma	Ova in stool, worms detected in bile ducts at ERCP	Praziquantel 75 mg/kg in 3 doses × 2 days or albendazole 10 mg or kg × 7 days
Cestodes						
Echinococcus (*Echinococcus granulosus, E. multilocularis, E. vogeli*)	Worldwide	Ingestion of vegetables contaminated with dog feces	Migration of larvae to liver with cyst formation	Tender hepatomegaly, fever, eosinophilia, biliary obstruction	Serology, imaging, potentially aspiration	Surgery or PAIR procedure + albendazole 400 mg b.i.d. × 4 wk

b.i.d., twice daily; ERCP, endoscopic retrograde cholangiopancreatography; HTLV-1, human T-cell lymphotrophic virus type I; PAIR, puncture, aspiration, injection, reaspiration; PO, orally; q.d., daily; q.o.d., every other day; t.i.d., three times daily.

Adapted from Chung RT, Friedman LS. Liver abscess and bacterial, parasitic, fungal, and granulomatous liver disease. In: Feldman M, Friedman LS, eds. *Gastrointestinal and Liver Disease: Pathophysiology/Diagnosis/Management*, 7th edn. Philadelphia: Saunders; 2002:1343–1363.

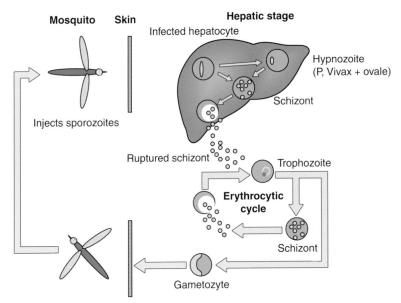

Fig. 29.1 Life cycle of *Plasmodium* species.

- Malarial sporozoites injected by an infected female *Anopheles* mosquito circulate to the liver, enter hepatocytes, and mature to schizonts. When the schizont ruptures, merozoites are released into the bloodstream and invade erythrocytes. The four major species of *Plasmodium* responsible for malaria differ with respect to the number of merozoites released and the maturation times.
- Infection by *Plasmodium falciparum* or *P. malariae* is not associated with a residual liver stage after release of merozoites, whereas infection by *P. vivax* or *P. ovale* has an exo-erythrocytic stage, the hypnozoite, which persists in the liver and can divide and mature into schizont forms again.
- The extent of hepatic injury varies with malarial species (most severe with *P. falciparum*) and severity of infection. Unconjugated hyperbilirubinemia is most commonly seen as a result of hemolysis, but occasional hepatocyte dysfunction can be seen, leading to conjugated hyperbilirubinemia as well as a prolonged prothrombin time.
- Reversible reductions of portal venous blood flow during the acute phase of falciparum malaria may be a consequence of micro-occlusion of portal venous branches by parasitized erythrocytes.
b. Histopathology
  - In an acute attack of falciparum malaria, large quantities of malarial pigment, hemozoin (an iron porphyrin protein complex resulting from hemoglobin degradation by the parasite) accumulates in Kupffer cells, which hypertrophy and phagocytose erythrocytes. Sinusoidal dilatation also occurs.
  - Later, one often sees a mild portal infiltrate and portal pigment deposition. All abnormalities reverse with successful treatment.
c. Clinical features
  - Only the erythrocytic stage of malaria is associated with clinical illness. Symptoms develop 30 to 60 days after exposure to an infected mosquito and include cyclical fever,

malaise, anorexia, nausea, vomiting, diarrhea, and myalgias. Tender hepatomegaly and splenomegaly, as well as jaundice caused by hemolysis, are common in adults, especially with heavy infection by *P. falciparum.*

- Hepatic failure is generally seen only in association with concomitant viral hepatitis or with severe *P. falciparum* infection.

d. Diagnosis

- The differential diagnosis includes hepatotropic and nonhepatotropic viral hepatitis, gastroenteritis, amebic liver abscess, yellow fever, typhoid fever, tuberculosis, leptospirosis, and brucellosis.
- The diagnosis of acute malaria rests on clinical history, physical examination, and identification of parasites on peripheral thick or thin blood smears. Because the number of parasites in the blood may be small, repeated smear examinations should be performed when the index of suspicion is high.
- Serologic assays are less useful for acute than for chronic infection.

e. Treatment

- Treatment depends on the species and the pattern of chloroquine resistance for falciparum infection. In general, chloroquine is effective for *P. malariae, P. vivax, P. ovale,* and *P. falciparum* in areas endemic for chloroquine-sensitive species. Resistant falciparum infections can be treated with atovaquone/proguanil, or quinine in combination with doxycycline, tetracycline, or clindamycin, or artemether/lumefantrine, or artesunate alone.
- For *P. vivax* and *P. ovale* infections, treatment with primaquine (in persons without glucose-6-phosphate dehydrogenase deficiency) is indicated to eliminate the exoerythrocytic hypnozoites in the liver.

f. Hyperreactive malarial splenomegaly (tropical splenomegaly syndrome)

- Repeated exposure to malaria may lead to an aberrant immunologic response with overproduction of immunoglobulin M (IgM) malarial antibody and high levels of IgM aggregates, dense hepatic sinusoidal lymphocytosis (similar to that seen in Felty's syndrome), hyperplasia of Kupffer cells, and massive splenomegaly.
- Severe anemia resulting from hypersplenism, especially in women of childbearing age, can result; variceal bleeding is uncommon.
- Treatment consists of lifelong antimalarial therapy and supportive care of anemia with blood transfusions.

3. Babesiosis

- This is caused by *Babesia* species and is transmitted by the deer tick *Ixodes dammini/scapularis.* This malaria-like illness is endemic to the Northeast and Midwest of the United States.
- Patients present with fever, anemia, hepatosplenomegaly, and abnormal liver biochemical test levels.
- Immunocompromised or asplenic patients are often affected more severely.
- Combination therapy with atovaquone 750 mg twice daily and azithromycin 500 mg followed by 250 mg once daily or with clindamycin 600 mg three times daily and quinine 650 mg three to four times daily for 7 days is recommended.

4. Leishmaniasis

Visceral leishmaniasis is caused by *Leishmania* species, mostly *L. donovani,* and is endemic in the Mediterranean, the Middle East, Asia, Africa, and Latin America.

a. Life cycle

- The parasite multiplies in the gut of the female sandfly as a flagellated promastigote and migrates to the pharynx. Following injection into the human host, promastigotes are phagocytosed by macrophages in the reticuloendothelial system, where they multiply as amastigotes and are taken up with the next blood meal of the sandfly.

b. Clinical features

- Among early infections, 60% to 95% are subclinical.
- Visceral infection begins with a papular or ulcerative skin lesion at the site of the sandfly bite (similar to the cutaneous form of the disease). Following an incubation period of 2 to 6 months, twice daily fevers, weight loss, diarrhea (of bacillary, amebic, or leishmanial origin), and progressive painful hepatosplenomegaly develop, often accompanied by pancytopenia and polyclonal hypergammaglobulinemia. Liver biochemical test levels are typically normal.
- Secondary bacterial infections resulting from infiltration and suppression of reticuloendothelial cell function include pneumonia, pneumococcal infection, and tuberculosis and are important causes of mortality.
- Physical findings include often massive hepatomegaly, soft and nontender splenomegaly, jaundice, or ascites in severe disease, as well as generalized lymphadenopathy and muscle wasting. Cutaneous gray hyperpigmentation, which prompted the name **kala-azar** ("black fever"), is characteristically seen in India. Oral and nasopharyngeal nodules resulting from granuloma formation can be seen in Africa.

c. Histopathology

- Organisms are found in macrophages of the liver and spleen, bone marrow, and lymph nodes. Kupffer cells containing amastigotes proliferate. Occasionally, parasite-bearing cells aggregate within noncaseating granulomas.
- Hepatocyte necrosis is mild compared with that seen in cutaneous leishmaniasis. Healing is accompanied by fibrous deposition similar to that seen in congenital syphilis, and occasionally the liver looks cirrhotic (Rogers' cirrhosis); complications of cirrhosis are rare.

d. Diagnosis

- This is based on history, physical examination, and demonstration of tissue amastigotes.
- The demonstration of parasites or parasitic DNA in tissue is diagnostic. The highest yield comes from aspiration of the spleen, with parasites seen in 95% of cases. Liver aspiration is safer and has 70% to 85% sensitivity, as does bone marrow aspiration. Lymph node aspiration has 60% sensitivity.
- Serologic testing by ELISA or direct agglutination can be used to support a presumptive diagnosis of visceral leishmaniasis with 95% sensitivity and specificity. The leishmanin skin test (Montenegro test) is typically negative and unhelpful in acute visceral disease.

e. Treatment

- No specific measures are necessary to treat hepatic involvement. Treatment of secondary bacterial infections is essential, and specific antileishmanial chemotherapy should be initiated promptly.
- Liposomal amphotericin B is approved for treatment. Sodium stibogluconate (Pentostam) is available through the Centers for Disease Control and Prevention (CDC) under an investigational protocol. Alternative agents include paromomycin and pentamidine, which has significant toxicity.
- Patients with acquired immunodeficiency syndrome (AIDS) and leishmaniasis often fail to respond or relapse following treatment with conventional regimens.

4. Toxoplasmosis

Infection caused by *Toxoplasma gondii* is found worldwide. In the United States, serologic surveys suggest that 20% to 40% of the population have been exposed to *T. gondii*, resulting in chronic or latent infection. Toxoplasmosis causes clinical disease either when transmitted congenitally or as an opportunistic infection complicating AIDS.

   a. Life cycle
      ■ Cats are the definitive hosts; humans and other animals are incidental hosts that become infected by ingestion of oocysts.
      ■ The oocysts mature in the intestinal tract of humans to become sporozoites, which penetrate the intestinal mucosa, become tachyzoites, and circulate systemically, thus invading a wide array of cell types. They can form tissue cysts, containing many bradyzoites, which are responsible for latent infection.
      ■ Hepatic involvement has been observed in severe, disseminated infection.
   b. Clinical features
      ■ Acquired toxoplasmosis can manifest as a mononucleosis-like illness with fever, chills, headache, and lymphadenopathy. Uncommonly, hepatomegaly, splenomegaly, and minimal elevations of serum aminotransferase levels are present.
      ■ Infection of immunocompromised hosts can result in encephalitis, chorioretinitis, pneumonitis, myocarditis, and, uncommonly, hepatitis.
      ■ Atypical lymphocytosis, an otherwise unusual feature of parasitic disease, may occur.
   c. Diagnosis
      ■ This is best made by detecting specific IgM or IgG antibody using indirect immunofluorescence or an enzyme immunoassay (EIA) and isolation of *T. gondii* from blood, body fluids, or tissue.
   d. Treatment
      ■ Antibiotic therapy (pyrimethamine 25 to 100 mg daily and sulfadiazine 1 to 1.5 g four times daily), plus folinic acid to minimize hematologic toxicity, for 3 to 4 weeks, should be administered to immunocompetent persons with severe infection and immunocompromised or pregnant patients.

HELMINTHIC INFECTIONS: ROUNDWORMS (NEMATODES)
(see Table 29.1)

1. Ascariasis

Ascaris lumbricoides is estimated to infect approximately 25% of the world's population, especially in tropical countries and areas of lower socioeconomic standing.

   a. Life cycle
      ■ Humans are infected by ingesting embryonated eggs, usually in raw vegetables. The larvae hatch in the duodenum and migrate to the cecum, where they penetrate the mucosa, enter the portal circulation, and reach the liver, pulmonary artery, and lungs. The larvae grow in the alveolar spaces, are regurgitated and swallowed, and become mature adults in the intestine 2 to 3 months after ingestion, eventually reaching 15 to 35 cm, whereupon the cycle repeats itself.
   b. Clinical features
      ■ Most infected persons are asymptomatic or minimally symptomatic during larval migration. Symptoms are generally proportionate to the worm burden.
      ■ Cough, fever, dyspnea, wheezing, and substernal chest discomfort have been reported in the first 2 weeks of infection, as has hepatomegaly, when the larvae pass through the liver.
      ■ Chronic infection is more frequently characterized by episodic epigastric or periumbilical pain. If the worm burden is particularly heavy, small bowel obstruction, intussusception, volvulus, perforation, or appendicitis may occur.

■ Fragments of disintegrating worms within the biliary tree can serve as a nidus for biliary calculus formation. Preexisting disease of the biliary tract or pancreatic duct can predispose to worm migration into the bile ducts, with resulting obstructive jaundice, cholangitis, cholecystitis, pancreatitis, or pylephlebitis and intrahepatic abscesses.

c. Diagnosis
■ In the absence of a history of worm passage or regurgitation, the diagnosis is made definitively by identification of characteristic eggs in stool specimens. Larvae have also been identified in sputum and gastric washings. Liver biopsy specimens may show granulomas surrounding typical eggs.
■ Patients with biliary or pancreatic symptoms can be evaluated by ultrasonography or by endoscopic techniques, either retrograde cholangiopancreatography (ERCP) or direct choledochoscopy, which may identify the parasite and permit extraction of the worm.

d. Treatment
■ Infected persons may be treated with a single dose of albendazole 400 mg, mebendazole 100 mg twice daily for 3 days, or ivermectin 200 μg/kg × 1 dose.
■ In patients with intestinal obstruction, piperazine citrate may be used (75 mg/kg for 2 days to a maximum of 3.5 g in adults and 2 g in children under 20 kg). This agent paralyzes the worm and facilitates excretion.
■ Intestinal or biliary obstruction may require surgical or endoscopic intervention and removal of the worm. In the absence of intestinal perforation or ischemia, conservative management may be attempted first for up to 24 hours.

2. Toxocariasis
Toxocara canis and *T. cati* infect dogs and cats, respectively; in other hosts, the development of the parasite larvae is arrested. Infection occurs worldwide, especially in children.

a. Life cycle
■ Infection is acquired when soil or food containing eggs is ingested. The eggs hatch in the small intestine and release larvae, which penetrate the intestinal wall, enter the portal circulation, and reach the liver and systemic circulation. The immature worms bore through the vessel walls and migrate through the tissues, thus leading to secondary inflammatory responses. They do not return to the intestinal lumen; therefore, neither eggs nor larvae appear in the feces.
■ When larvae become trapped in tissue, they provoke granuloma formation with a predominance of eosinophils. The liver, brain, and eye are the most frequently affected organs.

b. Clinical features
■ Most infections are asymptomatic. Two major clinical syndromes are recognized:
  – Occult infections are associated with nonspecific symptoms, including abdominal pain, anorexia, fever, and wheezing.
  – **Visceral larva migrans** is seen most commonly in children with a history of pica. Findings include fever, hepatomegaly, urticaria, and leukocytosis with persistent eosinophilia, hypergammaglobulinemia, and elevated blood group isohemagglutinins. Pulmonary, cardiac, neurologic, and ocular manifestations are often seen.

c. Diagnosis
■ The diagnosis should be considered in persons with a history of pica, exposure to dogs or cats, and persistent eosinophilia.
■ Stool studies are not useful because the larvae do not mature to produce eggs in humans and do not remain in the gastrointestinal tract.
■ A definitive diagnosis is made by identification of the larvae in affected tissues, although blind biopsies are low in yield and are not routinely recommended. Ultrasound-guided

liver biopsy may be necessary to differentiate visceral larva migrans from hepatic capillariasis.
- A strongly positive ELISA result using excretory-secretory larval antigens provides supportive evidence of infection.

d. Treatment
- Albendazole 400 mg twice daily for 5 days or mebendazole 100 to 200 mg twice daily for 5 days is the treatment of choice. Significant pulmonary, cardiac, ophthalmologic, or neurologic manifestations may warrant the use of systemic corticosteroids. The disease is rarely fatal,

3. **Hepatic capillariasis**

Capillariasis is a worldwide zoonosis, and infection with *Capillaria hepatica* is acquired by ingestion of eggs in contaminated soil, food, or water, especially by children under poor hygienic conditions.

a. Life cycle
- Larvae released in the cecum penetrate the intestinal mucosa, enter the portal venous circulation, and become lodged in the liver, where adult worms develop within 3 weeks to a size of 20 mm. As the female worm dies, it releases eggs into the hepatic parenchyma and produces an intense granulomatous and fibrosing reaction.

b. Clinical features
- The features may be similar to those of visceral larva migrans, but it manifests as acute or subacute hepatitis. Patients may have tender hepatomegaly and, occasionally, splenomegaly, prominent eosinophilia, mild elevations of serum aminotransferase, alkaline phosphatase, and bilirubin levels, anemia, and an elevated erythrocyte sedimentation rate.

c. Diagnosis
- Adult worms or eggs can be detected in liver biopsy or autopsy specimens. Associated histologic findings in the liver include necrosis, fibrosis, eosinophilic infiltrate, and granuloma formation. Finding of *C. hepatica* ova in stool likely reflects passage of infected animal material and is not helpful.

d. Treatment
- Treatment is generally unsuccessful. Mebendazole 200 mg twice daily for 20 days is the drug of choice; alternatively, albendazole 400 mg daily for 10 days may be used.

4. **Strongyloidiasis**

Strongyloides stercoralis is prevalent in the tropics and subtropics, southern and Eastern Europe, and the United States. Infection is usually asymptomatic.

a. Life cycle
- Humans are infected by the filariform larvae, which penetrate intact skin, are carried to the lungs, migrate through the alveoli, and are swallowed to reach the intestine, where maturation ensues. Worms are typically found in the duodenum and proximal jejunum.
- Autoinfection can occur if the rhabditiform larvae transform into infective filariform larvae in the intestine, thus causing persistent infection even decades after exposure; reinfection occurs by penetration of the bowel wall or perianal skin and entry into the portal circulation and then the liver.
- Symptomatic infection results from a heavy infectious burden or infection in an immunocompromised person, especially in patients with human T-cell lymphotrophic virus-1, but not in patients with human immunodeficiency virus (HIV) infection. A **hyperinfection syndrome** may result from dissemination of filariform larvae into any organ, including the liver, lung, and brain, which is not ordinarily in the life cycle of the nematode.

b. Clinical features

- As with other helminthic infections, acute infection can lead to a pruritic eruption followed by fever, cough, wheezing, abdominal pain, diarrhea, and eosinophilia.
- When the liver is affected, cholestatic liver biochemical abnormalities can be seen. Liver biopsy specimens may show periportal inflammation, and larvae may be observed in intrahepatic bile canaliculi, lymphatic vessels, and small branches of the portal vein.

c. Diagnosis

- The diagnosis is based on the identification of larvae in the stool or intestinal biopsy specimens. Immunodiagnostic tests may be indicated if the organism cannot be demonstrated. The presence of an obstructive hepatobiliary picture in a person with established strongyloidiasis suggests possible dissemination.

d. Treatment

- For acute infection, the drug of choice is ivermectin 200 µg/kg daily for 2 days; alternatively albendazole can be used. Retreatment with a second course may be necessary in immunocompromised patients or those with disseminated disease.
- Hyperinfection syndrome requires longer courses of treatment.
- Treatment options are limited following dissemination, and mortality rates are as high as 85%.

5. Trichinosis

a. Life cycle

- Humans may be infected with *Trichinella spiralis* by consuming raw or undercooked pork bearing larvae, which are released in the upper gastrointestinal tract, enter the small intestine, penetrate the mucosa, and disseminate through the systemic circulation. Larvae can be found in myocardium, CSF, brain, and, less commonly, liver and gallbladder. In the small bowel, the larvae develop into adult worms, which release larvae that migrate to striated muscle, where they become encapsulated.

b. Clinical features

- Clinical manifestations occur when the worm burden is high and include diarrhea, fever, myalgias, periorbital and facial edema, conjunctivitis, and leukocytosis with marked eosinophilia. Jaundice may result from biliary obstruction. Severe complications include myocarditis, central nervous system involvement, and pneumonitis.

c. Diagnosis

- This is based on a characteristic history in association with fever and eosinophilia. Serologic studies for antibody to *Trichinella* may not be helpful in the acute phase of infection. Muscle biopsy can confirm the diagnosis.
- Rarely, hepatic histologic examination may demonstrate invasion of hepatic sinusoids by larvae.

d. Treatment

- Corticosteroids are used to relieve allergic symptoms, followed by antihelminthic treatment with albendazole 400 mg twice daily for 8 to 14 days or, alternatively, mebendazole 200 to-400 mg three times a day for 3 days, followed by 400 to 500 mg three times a day for 10 days.

HELMINTHIC INFECTIONS: FLATWORMS (TREMATODES)
(see Table 29.1)

1. Schistosomiasis

Schistosomiasis (bilharziasis) is caused by trematodes (blood flukes) of the genus *Schistosoma*. Approximately 200 million persons are infected worldwide, with approximately 200,000 deaths annually. An estimated 400,000 people, mostly immigrants from endemic areas, are infected in the United States. Humans and mammals are the definitive hosts (see Table 29.1).

a. Life cycle (Fig. 29.2)

- The infectious cycle is initiated by penetration of the skin by free-swimming cercariae released from snails to fresh water. Within 24 hours, the cercariae reach the peripheral venules and lymphatics and the pulmonary vessels. They pass through the lungs and reach the liver, where they lodge, develop into adults 1 to 2 cm long, and mate.

- Mated adult worms then migrate to their ultimate destinations in the inferior mesenteric venules (*Schistosoma mansoni*), superior mesenteric venules (*S. japonicum*), or the veins around the bladder (*S. hematobium*). These locations correlate with the clinical complications associated with each species. The eggs are deposited in the terminal venules and eventually migrate into the lumen of the involved organ, after which they are excreted in the stool or urine.

- Eggs remaining in the organ provoke a robust granulomatous response. Excreted eggs hatch immediately in fresh water and liberate early intermediate miracidia, which infect their snail hosts. The miracidia transform into cercariae within the snails and are then released into the water, from which they may again infect humans.

b. Clinical features

- The severity of clinical symptoms is related to the total worm burden in the host and possibly genetic susceptibility factors and is caused by the host reaction to the schistosomes.

- **Acute toxemic schistosomiasis (Katayama's syndrome)** is believed to result from immune complex formation as a consequence of the host immunologic response to the antigenic challenge by the adult worms and eggs and occurs 4 to 8 weeks after exposure. Manifestations include headache, fever, chills, cough, diarrhea, myalgias, arthralgias, tender hepatomegaly, splenomegaly, and eosinophilia.

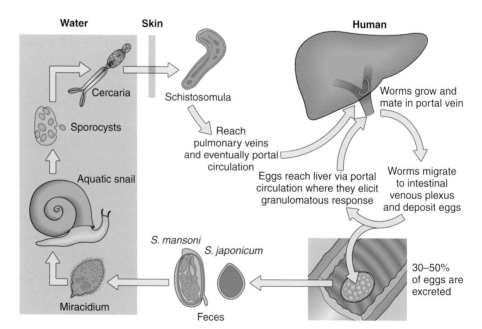

Fig. 29.2 Life cycle of *Schistosoma* species.

- Untreated acute schistosomiasis invariably progresses to chronic disease over many years. Mesenteric infection leads to hepatic complications, including periportal fibrosis, presinusoidal occlusion, and, ultimately, presinusoidal portal hypertension, as a result of the inflammatory reaction to eggs deposited in the liver. With severe schistosomal infection, portal hypertension becomes progressive, leading to ascites, gastroesophageal varices, and splenomegaly.
- Chronic schistosomal infection may be complicated by increased susceptibility to *Salmonella* infections. Hepatitis B and C infections are also common in persons living in endemic areas and may accelerate the progression of liver disease and the development of hepatocellular carcinoma.
- Laboratory findings in chronic schistosomiasis include anemia from recurrent gastrointestinal bleeding or hypersplenism, eosinophilia, an elevated erythrocyte sedimentation rate, and increased serum IgE levels. Liver biochemical test levels are generally normal until the disease is advanced.

c. Diagnosis

The diagnosis of acute schistosomiasis should be considered in a patient with an exposure history to fresh water who has abdominal pain, diarrhea, and fever. Multiple stool examinations for ova using the Kato-Katz thick smear may be required to confirm the diagnosis, because results are frequently negative in the early phases of disease.

- Serologic testing has proved useful in facilitating earlier diagnosis. Sigmoidoscopy or colonoscopy may reveal rectosigmoid or transverse colonic involvement and may be useful in chronic disease when few eggs pass in the feces.
- Ultrasonography and liver biopsy are useful for demonstrating periportal (or "pipestem") fibrosis but not for diagnosing acute infection.

d. Treatment

- Praziquantel 40 mg/kg given for 1 day in two divided doses is the treatment of choice for infection caused by *S. hematobium, S. mansoni, and S. intercalatum*; cure rates are 60% to 90%. The recommended dose for *S. japonicum* and *S. mekongi* is 60 mg/kg divided into 2 or 3 doses.
- Treatment of acute toxemic schistosomiasis requires praziquantel 75 mg/kg for 1 day in three divided doses and, in some cases, prednisone for the prior 2 to 3 days to suppress immune-mediated helminthicidal or drug reactions.
- Periodic treatment of patients in endemic areas will keep the burden of infection low and will minimize chronic complications.
- Noncirrhotic, presinusoidal portal hypertension may lead to variceal bleeding requiring band ligation or sclerotherapy. Advanced chronic schistosomal liver disease can be managed with a distal splenorenal shunt with or without splenopancreatic disconnection or esophagogastric devascularization with splenectomy. Since the advent of praziquantel, complicated schistosomal liver disease has become uncommon.

2. Fascioliasis

Fascioliasis, caused by the sheep liver fluke *Fasciola hepatica*, is endemic in many areas of Europe and Latin America, North Africa, Asia, the Western Pacific, and some parts of the United States, and it causes 2 million infections worldwide.

a. Life cycle (Fig. 29.3)

- The life cycle is spent between herbivores and intermediate aquatic snail hosts. Eggs passed in the feces of infected mammals into fresh water give rise to miracidia that penetrate snails and emerge as cercariae, which encyst as metacercariae on aquatic plants such as watercress. Hosts become infected when they consume plants bearing the encysted organisms, which bore into the intestinal wall, enter the abdominal cavity,

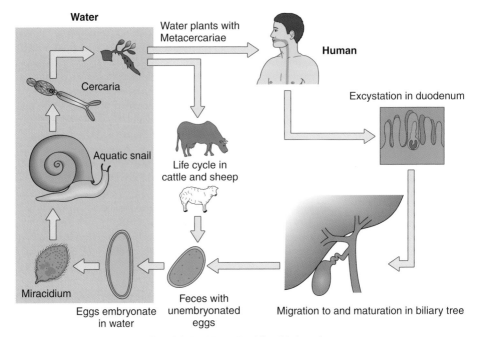

Fig. 29.3 Life cycle of *Fasciola hepatica.*

penetrate the hepatic capsule, and settle in the bile ducts, where they develop into adults within 3 to 4 months and reach a length of 20 to 30 mm.

b. Clinical features
- Fascioliasis is divided into three phases corresponding to three syndromes:
  - **Acute:** migration of young flukes through the liver. This phase is marked by fever, right upper quadrant pain, and eosinophilia. Urticaria with dermatographia and non-specific gastrointestinal symptoms are common. Physical examination often reveals fever and a tender, enlarged liver. Splenomegaly is reported in up to 25% of cases, but jaundice is rare. Eosinophilia can be profound (occasionally more than 80%). Abnormalities of liver biochemical tests are minimal.
  - **Latent:** corresponds to the settling of the flukes into the bile ducts and lasts months to years. Affected persons are mostly asymptomatic but may experience vague gastrointestinal symptoms. Eosinophilia persists, and fever can occur.
  - **Chronic obstructive:** consequence of intrahepatic and extrahepatic bile ductal inflammation and hyperplasia evoked by the presence of adult flukes. This phase may be marked by recurrent biliary pain, cholangitis, cholelithiasis, and biliary obstruction. Blood loss may result from epithelial injury, and rare cases of overt hemobilia have been described. Liver biochemical testing commonly demonstrates a cholestatic pattern. Long-term infection may lead to biliary cirrhosis and secondary sclerosing cholangitis, but no convincing association with malignancies of the liver or biliary tract exists.

c. Diagnosis
- This diagnosis should be considered in patients with prolonged fever, abdominal pain, diarrhea, tender hepatomegaly, and eosinophilia. Because eggs are not passed during the acute phase, the diagnosis depends on the detection of antibodies to excretory-secretory proteins by EIA. In the latent and chronic phases, the diagnosis is made definitively by

detection of eggs in stool, duodenal aspirates, or bile. Occasionally, ultrasonography or ERCP demonstrates the flukes in the gallbladder and bile duct.

- Hepatic histologic findings include necrosis and granuloma formation with eosinophilic infiltrates and Charcot–Leyden crystals. Eosinophilic abscesses, epithelial hyperplasia of the bile ducts, and periportal fibrosis may also be seen.

d. Treatment
- Unlike other liver fluke infections, praziquantel is not effective for fascioliasis.
- A single dose of triclabendazole 10 mg/kg once or twice (Egaten, available only directly from the manufacturer) is effective; alternatively, bithionol 30 to 50 mg/kg every other day for 10 to 15 doses, which is available directly from the CDC, or nitazoxanide 500 mg twice daily for 7 days can be used.

3. **Clonorchiasis and opisthorchiasis**
Clonorchis sinensis, Opisthorchis viverrini, and *O. felineus* are trematodes (liver flukes) of the family Opisthorchioidea. *C. sinensis* and *O. viverrini* are widespread in East and Southeast Asia and affect 7 and 1.7 million people, respectively, mostly of lower socioeconomic status. *O. felineus* infects humans and domestic animals in Eastern Europe. All three trematodes have similar life cycles and clinical features.

a. Life cycle
- All require two intermediate hosts, an aquatic snail and freshwater fish. Eggs are passed in the feces into fresh water, are consumed by snails, and hatch as free-swimming cercariae, which seek and penetrate fish or crayfish and encyst in skin or muscle as metacercariae. The mammalian host is infected when it consumes raw or undercooked fish. The metacercariae excyst in the small bowel and migrate into the ampulla of Vater and bile ducts, where they mature into 10- to 20-mm adult flukes. Infection can be maintained for 2 decades or longer.

b. Clinical features
- Infection is clinically silent or has nonspecific features, with fever, abdominal pain, and diarrhea.
- Chronic manifestations correlate with the fluke burden and are dominated by fever, right upper quadrant pain, tender hepatomegaly, and eosinophilia. With a heavy worm burden in the bile ducts, chronic or intermittent biliary obstruction can ensue, with frequent development of cholelithiasis, cholecystitis, jaundice, and, ultimately, recurrent pyogenic cholangitis (see Chapter 33).
- Serum alkaline phosphatase and bilirubin levels are elevated, and mild to moderate elevations of serum aminotransferase levels are also seen. Long-standing untreated infection leads to exuberant inflammation resulting in periportal fibrosis, marked biliary epithelial hyperplasia and dysplasia, and a substantially increased risk of cholangiocarcinoma.
- **Cholangiocarcinoma** resulting from clonorchiasis or opisthorchiasis tends to be multicentric and arises in the secondary biliary radicles of the hilum of the liver. The diagnosis should be suspected in infected persons with weight loss, jaundice, epigastric pain, or an abdominal mass.

c. Diagnosis
- The diagnosis is based on detection of characteristic fluke eggs in the stool. Stool examination is usually positive except late in the disease, when biliary obstruction supervenes. In these cases, the diagnosis is made by identifying flukes in the bile ducts or gallbladder at surgery or in bile obtained by postoperative drainage or percutaneous aspiration.
- Endoscopic or intraoperative cholangiography reveals slender, uniform filling defects within intrahepatic ducts that are alternately dilated and strictured and that may mimic sclerosing cholangitis.
- Serologic testing is generally not helpful.

d. Treatment
- All patients with clonorchiasis or opisthorchiasis should be treated with praziquantel, which is uniformly effective in a dose of 75 mg/kg in three divided doses for 2 days. Side effects are uncommon and include headache, dizziness, and nausea. Alternatively, albendazole 10 mg/kg for 7 days can be used. After treatment, dead flukes may be seen in the stool or biliary drainage.
- When the burden of infecting organisms is high, the dead flukes and surrounding debris or stones may cause biliary obstruction necessitating endoscopic or surgical drainage.

HELMINTHIC INFECTIONS: CESTODES (TAPEWORMS)

Echinococcosis (see also Chapter 28 and Table 29.1)

Fungal Liver Disease

CANDIDIASIS

Candida species are found worldwide and are common commensal organisms. They may cause invasive systemic infection in persons who are severely immunocompromised. The liver can become infected by *C. albicans* in the setting of disseminated, multiorgan disease.

1. Conditions that can predispose to disseminated candidiasis include pregnancy, immunologic defects, HIV infection, diabetes mellitus, and severe zinc or iron deficiency.
2. Most cases of disseminated infections, especially **hepatosplenic candidiasis**, occur in leukemic patients undergoing high-dose chemotherapy and become manifest during the period of recovery from severe neutropenia. In leukemic patients, the frequency is as high as 51% to 91%. The disease is often overwhelming, with a high mortality rate.
   - A less frequent presentation in the compromised host is isolated or focal hepatic candidiasis, thought to result from colonization of the gastrointestinal tract by *Candida*, which disseminates locally following the onset of neutropenia and mucosal injury caused by high-dose chemotherapy. Resulting fungemia of the portal vein seeds the liver and leads to hepatic microabscesses and macroabscesses.
   a. Clinical features
      - In either focal or disseminated candidiasis involving the liver, clinical features include high fever, right upper quadrant abdominal pain and distention, nausea, vomiting, diarrhea, anorexia, and tender hepatomegaly. The serum alkaline phosphatase level is nearly invariably elevated, with variable elevations in serum aminotransferase and bilirubin levels.
   b. Diagnosis
      - CT of the abdomen is the most sensitive test to detect hepatic or splenic granulomas or abscesses, which are often multicentric.
      - In most cases, liver biopsy specimens reveal macroscopic nodules, portal and periportal necrosis with microabscesses, and granulomas surrounding neutrophilic abscesses, as well as characteristic yeast and hyphal forms of *Candida*. Cultures of biopsy material are negative in most cases.
      - Polymerase chain reaction testing has been used for diagnosis.
      - Laparoscopy may also be employed to confirm the diagnosis.
   c. Treatment
      - If hepatic candidiasis is diagnosed in its focal form, response rates to therapy with intravenous amphotericin B 0.5 to 1.0 mg/kg/day are better (nearly 60%) than in

disseminated disease. Liposomal amphotericin can be used to reduce the frequency of side effects, especially nephrotoxicity. Other options include a combination of amphotericin B with flucytosine, itraconazole, or fluconazole. Caspofungin has been shown to be effective in patients with hepatosplenic candidiasis resistant to amphotericin B.

■ Occasionally, surgical resection (e.g., splenomegaly in focal disease) may be attempted. Despite all efforts, mortality rates remain high.

HISTOPLASMOSIS

Infection with *Histoplasma capsulatum* is acquired through inhalation in an endemic area. Most patients are asymptomatic. Most symptomatic patients have disease confined to the lungs. Severely immunocompromised persons (e.g., with AIDS) in endemic regions are predisposed to disseminated histoplasmosis, affecting mainly those organs rich in macrophages.

a. Clinical features
   ■ The liver can be invaded in both the acute and chronic forms of progressive disseminated histoplasmosis. Fever, weight loss, oropharyngeal ulcers, hepatomegaly, and splenomegaly may be present in chronic disease.
   ■ In children with acute hepatic disease, marked hepatosplenomegaly is universal and is associated with high fever and lymphadenopathy.
   ■ Hepatosplenomegaly is present in 30% of adults with acute disease (often the AIDS-defining illness). Serum aminotransferase and alkaline phosphatase levels are often elevated.

b. Diagnosis
   ■ Yeast forms are small (3 to 4 μm) but can be identified in sections of liver biopsies on standard hematoxylin and eosin staining and are best seen with a Grocott silver stain either diffusely infiltrating the sinusoids or in granulomas. The organism is difficult to culture and hardly ever grows from biopsy specimens.
   ■ Serologic testing for complement-fixing antibodies is helpful in confirming the diagnosis. In immunocompromised persons, who may not be capable of mounting a significant antibody response, detection of *H. capsulatum* antigens in urine and serum can be useful. The histoplasmin skin test indicates prior sensitization and has no diagnostic value.

c. Treatment
   ■ Disseminated histoplasmosis should be treated with intravenous amphotericin B.
   ■ Itraconazole is used in mild to moderate infections or to complete therapy after successful response to amphotericin.

FURTHER READING

Albrecht H. Bacterial and miscellaneous infections of the liver. In: Zakim DS, Boyer TD, eds. *Hepatology*. Philadelphia: Saunders; 2003:1109–1124.

Bryan RT, Michelson MK. Parasitic infections of the liver and biliary tree. In: Surawicz C, Owen RL, eds. *Gastrointestinal and Hepatic Infections*. Philadelphia: Saunders; 1995:405–454.

Canto MIF, Diehl AM. Bacterial infections of the liver and biliary system. In: Surawicz C, Owen RL, eds. *Gastrointestinal and Hepatic Infections*. Philadelphia: Saunders; 1995:355–389.

Diaz-Granados CA, Duffus WA, Albrecht H. Parasitic diseases of the liver. In: Zakim DS, Boyer TD, eds. *Hepatology*. Philadelphia: Saunders; 2003:1073–1107.

Drugs for parasitic infections. *Med Lett* 2007; 5(Suppl):e1–e15.

Hay RJ Fungal infections affecting the liver. In: Bircher J, Benhamou JP, McIntyre N et al, eds. *Oxford Textbook of Clinical Hepatology*. Oxford: Oxford University Press; 1999:1025–1032.

Kibbler CC, Sanchez-Tapias JM. Bacterial infection and the liver. In: Bircher J, Benhamou JP, McIntyre N, et al, eds. *Oxford Textbook of Clinical Hepatology*. Oxford: Oxford University Press; 1999:989–1016.

Kim AY, Chung RT. Bacterial, parasitic, and fungal infections of the liver, including liver abscess. In: Feldman M, Friedman LS, Brandt LJ, eds. *Gastrointestinal and Liver Disease: Pathophysiology/Diagnosis/Management*. 9th edn. Philadelphia: Saunders Elsevier; 2010:1359–1370.

Lucas SB, Other viral and infectious diseases and HIV-related liver disease. In: MacSween RNM, Burt AD, Portmann BC, et al, eds. *Pathology of the Liver*. London: Churchill Livingstone; 2002:363–414.

Maguire JH. Disease due to helminths. In: Mandell GL, Bennet JE, Dolin R, eds. *Mandell, Douglas, and Bennett's Principles and Practice of Infectious Diseases*, 7th edn. Philadelphia: Churchill Livingstone Elsevier; 2009:3573–3575.

Palomo AM, Warell DA, Francis N, et al. Protozoal infections. In: Bircher J, Benhamou JP, McIntyre N, et al, eds. *Oxford Textbook of Clinical Hepatology*. Oxford: Oxford University Press; 1999:1033–1058.

Warren KS, Bresson-Hadni S, Miguet JP, et al. Helminthiasis. In: Bircher J, Benhamou JP, McIntyre N, et al, eds. *Oxford Textbook of Clinical Hepatology*. Oxford: Oxford University Press; 1999:1059–1086.

CHAPTER 30

Surgery in the patient with liver disease and postoperative jaundice

Jacqueline G. O'Leary, MD, MPH ■ Lawrence S. Friedman, MD

KEY POINTS

1. Minor liver biochemical test abnormalities are common after surgery; overt liver dysfunction is uncommon but more likely if the patient has preexisting liver disease.

2. Hepatic blood flow is reduced by anesthesia, blood loss, and other hemodynamic derangements.

3. Operative mortality is increased in patients with acute hepatitis, alcoholic hepatitis, severe chronic hepatitis, and Child-Pugh class B and C cirrhosis; when using the Child-Pugh classification, additional risk factors include emergency surgery, biliary surgery, cardiac surgery, liver resection, ascites, and hypoxemia.

4. The Model for End-stage Liver Disease (MELD) score predicts operative mortality with greater granularity than the Child-Pugh classification and is remarkably linear for MELD scores higher than 8. American Society of Anesthesiologists (ASA) class IV adds an additional 5.5 MELD points, and age greater than 70 years adds an additional 3 MELD points.

5. Postoperative jaundice may result from an increased pigment load as a result of transfusions or hemolysis, hepatocellular dysfunction as a result of reduced hepatic blood flow, drug toxicity, infection, or, rarely, biliary obstruction.

Effects of Anesthesia and Surgery on the Liver

OVERVIEW

1. Surgical procedures, whether performed using general or local (i.e., spinal or epidural) anesthesia, are often followed by changes in liver biochemical test results.

2. Postoperative elevations of serum aminotransferase, alkaline phosphatase, or bilirubin levels are generally minor and transient, and in patients without underlying cirrhosis, these changes are not clinically significant.

3. Clinically significant hepatic dysfunction can occur in patients with preexisting acute liver disease or cirrhosis and is more common in patients with compromised hepatic synthetic function.

EFFECTS OF ANESTHETIC AGENTS ON THE CIRRHOTIC LIVER

1. At baseline, hepatic arterial and venous perfusion of the cirrhotic liver is decreased because of the following:
   ■ Portal hypertension that decreases portal blood flow

403

- Impaired autoregulation that decreases arterial blood flow
- Arteriovenous shunting around the liver
- Reduced splanchnic inflow

2. Decreased hepatic perfusion at baseline makes the cirrhotic liver more susceptible to hypoxemia and hypotension in the operating room; induction causes a reduction in hepatic blood flow by 30% to 50%.

OTHER INTRAOPERATIVE FACTORS

Intraoperative factors that may decrease hepatic oxygenation by further decreasing hepatic blood flow or increasing splanchnic vascular resistance are as follows:
- Hypotension caused by hepatorenal syndrome or shock
- Hemorrhage
- Hypoxemia caused by ascites, hepatic hydrothorax, hepatopulmonary syndrome, portopulmonary hypertension, or aspiration
- Hypercapnia
- Heart failure
- Vasoactive drugs
- Intermittent positive pressure ventilation
- Pneumoperitoneum during laparoscopic surgery
- Traction on abdominal viscera: reflex dilatation of splanchnic capacitance vessels

HEPATIC METABOLISM OF ANESTHETIC AGENTS

1. Inhalational anesthetic agents are lipid-soluble compounds that require hepatic transformation to more water-soluble compounds for biliary excretion.
2. Consequences of hepatic metabolism:
   a. Prolonged anesthetic action in patients with liver disease (also caused by hypoalbuminemia and impaired biliary excretion)
   b. Formation of toxic intermediates or reactive oxygen species, especially in the presence of hypoxia or reduced hepatic blood flow
      - Halothane → hepatitis (rare)
      - Enflurane → hepatitis (even rarer)
3. **Isoflurane, desflurane, sevoflurane, and nitrous oxide** are preferable in patients with liver disease because these agents undergo the least hepatic metabolism and hepatic arterial blood flow alterations, and resulting hepatitis is rare.
4. Propofol is an excellent anesthetic choice in patients with liver disease; although it is metabolized by hepatic glucuronidation, its serum half-life remains short even in patients with cirrhosis, and it does not precipitate hepatic encephalopathy.

OTHER AGENTS IN LIVER DISEASE

1. Narcotics and sedatives are generally well tolerated in patients with compensated liver disease.
   a. These drugs have a prolonged duration of action in decompensated liver disease.
      - Narcotics have high first-pass extraction by the liver:
         - Blood levels increase as hepatic blood flow decreases.
         - Bioavailability is increased because of portosystemic shunting.
         - Preferred agents are fentanyl and sufentanil, which have similar durations of action in healthy persons and in patients with cirrhosis.

- Benzodiazepines have low first-pass extraction by the liver:
  - Those eliminated by glucuronidation (oxazepam, lorazepam) are not affected by liver disease.
  - Those not glucuronidated (diazepam, chlordiazepoxide) have enhanced sedative effects in liver disease and should be avoided.
  b. They may precipitate hepatic encephalopathy in patients with severe liver disease.
  c. Smaller than standard doses are indicated for those drugs whose metabolism is affected by liver disease.
2. Muscle relaxants
  a. Succinylcholine should be avoided. Resistance occurs in patients with liver disease in part because of decreased hepatic pseudocholinesterase production. The large doses required in patients with liver disease may cause difficulty in reversing their effect postoperatively.
  b. The volume of distribution for nondepolarizing muscle relaxants is increased. Larger doses may be required.
  - Atracurium and cisatracurium are preferred because neither the liver nor the kidney is required for elimination.
  - Doxacurium is preferred for longer cases such as liver transplantation and is metabolized by the kidney.

EFFECT OF SURGERY

1. The nature and extent of surgery may be more important determinants of postoperative hepatic dysfunction than anesthesia.
2. Perioperative risk is increased with biliary tract and open abdominal surgery and is greatest with cardiac surgery and liver resection.
  a. In patients with cholecystitis, laparoscopic cholecystectomy is permissible in patients in Child-Pugh class A and selected patients in Child-Pugh class B without portal hypertension; however, in patients with more advanced cirrhosis with portal hypertension, cholecystostomy is preferable.
  b. Risk factors for hepatic decompensation after cardiac surgery include total time on cardiopulmonary bypass, use of pulsatile as opposed to nonpulsatile bypass, and need for perioperative vasopressor support; cardiopulmonary bypass may exacerbate coagulopathy.
  c. Less invasive cardiovascular procedures (e.g., angioplasty, valvuloplasty, endovascular aneurysm repair) are preferred to open surgery in patients with advanced cirrhosis. Occasionally, however, major cardiac surgery (including heart transplantation) may be performed at the same time as liver transplantation.

Estimation of Operative Risk in Patients with Liver Disease

Absolute contraindications to surgery (other than liver transplantation) are listed in Table 30.1.

PROBLEMS IN ESTIMATING OPERATIVE RISK

- Large prospective studies and randomized controlled trials are lacking.
- Data on acute and chronic hepatitis are limited.
- The effects of comorbid conditions on surgical risk are difficult to quantitate.

TABLE 30.1 ■ **Contraindications to elective surgery in patients with liver disease**

Acute liver failure

Acute viral hepatitis

Alcoholic hepatitis

Acute renal failure

Severe cardiomyopathy

Hypoxemia

Severe coagulopathy (despite treatment)

American Society of Anesthesiologists class V

ACUTE HEPATITIS (see Chapter 3)

1. Causes include the following:
   - Viruses (e.g., hepatitis A, B, C, D, E viruses, cytomegalovirus, Epstein–Barr virus)
   - Drugs (including herbal preparations and over-the-counter medications)
   - Toxins (including alcohol)
   - Autoimmune liver disease
   - Genetic disorders (e.g., Wilson disease)
   - Ischemic hepatitis
   - Hepatic vein thrombosis
2. Acute hepatitis of any cause increases operative risk.
3. Elective surgery can usually be avoided in patients with acute hepatitis. In the past, exploratory laparotomy was often performed to differentiate viral hepatitis from cholestatic disorders. Currently, such a distinction is made by a combination of serologic testing, radiologic imaging, cholangiography, and/or percutaneous liver biopsy.
4. Acute hepatitis is almost always self-limited or treatable. It is best to postpone elective surgery until liver dysfunction is investigated and the course of the disease is observed. Elective surgery can be undertaken when the patient improves.

CHRONIC HEPATITIS (see Chapters 4 and 5)

1. Chronic hepatitis is defined as persistent liver inflammation for more than 6 months. Surgical risk appears to correlate with clinical, biochemical, and histologic severity of disease.
   - Elective surgery is contraindicated in active, symptomatic disease, particularly when synthetic or excretory function is impaired or portal hypertension is present.
   - Surgery in patients with autoimmune hepatitis who are receiving corticosteroid therapy requires "stress" doses.
2. Hepatitis B or C virus carrier
   a. These patients have no increased surgical risk.
   b. In general, antiviral therapy should not be interrupted in the perioperative period.
   c. A risk exists that the patient may infect medical and surgical personnel (the higher the viral load, the higher the risk). Control measures include the following:
      - Universal precautions should be used when contacting any bodily fluid.
      - Hepatitis B vaccine should be administered to all personnel at risk

- Immediate hepatitis B immune globulin and the vaccine series should be given to unvaccinated personnel who sustain an exposure to hepatitis B.
- No postexposure prophylaxis is recommended for hepatitis C.

ALCOHOLIC LIVER DISEASE AND NONALCOHOLIC FATTY LIVER DISEASE (see Chapters 6 and 7)

1. Alcoholic fatty liver
   - Elective surgery is not contraindicated in the presence of normal liver function.
   - It may be desirable to postpone surgery until nutritional deficiencies are corrected or the acute effects of alcohol have resolved.
2. Alcoholic hepatitis
   - A spectrum of severity exists, but surgical risk is increased.
   - Severe alcoholic hepatitis is a contraindication to elective surgery.
   - Abstinence from alcohol and supportive therapy for at least 12 weeks are generally required before elective surgery.
3. Alcoholism is associated with additional perioperative risks independent of liver disease:
   - Drug metabolism is altered (e.g., acetaminophen toxicity may occur after standard doses in alcoholic patients).
   - Patients should be observed for signs and symptoms of withdrawal.
4. Nonalcoholic fatty liver disease (NAFLD)
   - NAFLD has increased in frequency as the prevalence of obesity has increased in the population.
   - At the time of bariatric surgery, approximately 3% of patients are found incidentally to have cirrhosis.
   - Hepatic steatosis of more than 30% may increase mortality and morbidity after major hepatic resection.
   - Bariatric surgery is not contraindicated in patients with compensated cirrhosis; however, clinically significant portal hypertension increases surgical risk.
   - NAFLD improves after bariatric surgery in more than 90% of cases.

CIRRHOSIS (see Chapter 9)

1. Cirrhosis is a pathologic diagnosis characterized by nodular regeneration and vascular distortion leading to portal hypertension.
2. Decompensated cirrhosis is a clinical diagnosis characterized by the presence of one or more of the following:
   - Ascites
   - Hepatic encephalopathy
   - Varices
   - Hepatorenal syndrome
   - Synthetic dysfunction (hypoalbuminemia or prolonged prothrombin time [PT])
3. Difficulties in detection or diagnosis:
   - Multiple causes
   - Wide spectrum of severity
   - Lack of correlation between the presence of cirrhosis and biochemical tests of liver function
   - Importance of careful history and physical examination (e.g., cutaneous spiders, palmar erythema, splenomegaly)

TABLE 30.2 ■ **Child–Turcotte–Pugh scoring system and Child-Pugh classification**

	1	2	3
Ascites	None	Easily controlled	Poorly controlled
Encephalopathy	None	Mild	Advanced
Albumin (g/dL)	>3.5	2.8–3.5	<2.8
Bilirubin (mg/dL)	<2.0	2.0–3.0	>3.0
Prothrombin time (sec prolonged)	≤4	4–6	>6
Child–Turcotte–Pugh score	5–6	7–9	10–15
Child–Pugh Class	A	B	C

4. Important consequences in the postoperative period:
   - Fluid and electrolyte disturbances, renal failure
   - Hypoxemia (right-to-left shunts)
   - Altered drug metabolism
   - Increased susceptibility to infection (abdominal abscess, sepsis)
   - Nutritional wasting
   - Portal hypertension (ascites, variceal hemorrhage)
   - Hepatic encephalopathy

Use of the Child-Pugh Classification to Assess Surgical Risk (Table 30.2)

1. Various **risk factors** have been identified in several, relatively small, retrospective studies of nonportosystemic shunt surgery: emergency surgery, upper abdominal (especially biliary) surgery, low serum albumin, prolonged PT or partial thromboplastin time (PTT), elevated serum bilirubin, anemia, ascites, encephalopathy, malnutrition, postoperative bleeding, portal hypertension, hypoxemia, infection, and Child-Pugh class (Table 30.3).
2. Difficulties in interpreting individual studies:
   - Small numbers of patients
   - Retrospective: selection bias
   - Arbitrary choices of parameters examined
3. Child-Pugh classification (see Table 30.2) reliably predicted operative mortality in independent studies over a 27-year span (Garrison *et al* [1984]; Mansour *et al* [1997]; Neff *et al* [2011]).
   - Child-Pugh class A mortality: 10%
   - Child-Pugh class B mortality: 17 to 30%
   - Child-Pugh class C mortality: 63% to 82%
4. Problems with the use of the Child-Pugh classification:
   - Definition of terms (e.g., "no ascites" means clinically or sonographically absent?)
   - Subjective parameters (e.g., encephalopathy: "mild" versus "advanced")
   - Assignment of overall class based on components in different classes (Child–Turcotte–Pugh score uses point system to add greater precision; see Table 30.2)
5. **Child-Pugh classification** has been the most widely used predictor of surgical risk. Its usefulness has been demonstrated in retrospective, but not prospective, studies. It correlates with postoperative mortality and morbidity (liver failure, encephalopathy, bleeding, sepsis, ascites, renal failure, and pulmonary failure). Morbidity rates are even higher than mortality rates.

TABLE 30.3 ■ **Risk factors for surgery in patients with cirrhosis**

Patient characteristics	Anemia
	Ascites
	Child-Pugh class B and C
	Encephalopathy
	Hypoalbuminemia
	Hypoxemia
	Infection
	Malnutrition
	Higher MELD score
	Portal hypertension
	Prolonged INR >1.5 that does not correct with vitamin K
	Higher American Society of Anesthesiologist class
Type of surgery	Cardiac surgery
	Emergency surgery
	Hepatic resection
	Open abdominal surgery

INR, international normalized ratio; MELD, Model for End-stage Liver Disease.

When using the Child-Pugh classification, additional risk factors predictive of perioperative mortality include the following:
- Emergency surgery
- Biliary tract surgery: marked vascularity of the gallbladder bed in patients with portal hypertension
- Hepatic resection: generally contraindicated in decompensated cirrhosis but feasible in Child-Pugh class A cirrhosis (risk of morbidity and mortality correlates with preoperative portal hypertension and the amount of liver resected)
- Additional risk factors for hepatic resection: active hepatitis, thoracotomy, pulmonary disease, diabetes mellitus, malignancy, and fatty liver
- Cardiac surgery (see earlier)
- Hypoxemia (Po_2 less than 60 mm Hg): e.g., as a result of hepatopulmonary syndrome or portopulmonary hypertension
- Risk of surgery on the respiratory tract: increased in patients with chronic obstructive pulmonary disease and cirrhosis
- Ascites: risk of abdominal wall herniation and wound dehiscence

Use of the Model for End-stage Liver Disease Score to Assess Surgical Risk

1. The Model for End-stage Liver Disease (MELD) was developed to predict outcomes following insertion of a transjugular intrahepatic portosystemic shunt (TIPS). It is used to prioritize candidates for liver transplantation and is increasingly used to predict surgical risk in patients with cirrhosis. The MELD is a linear regression model based on serum bilirubin, international normalized ratio (INR), and serum creatinine.

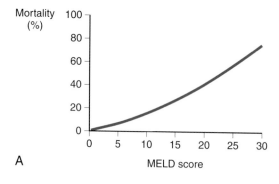

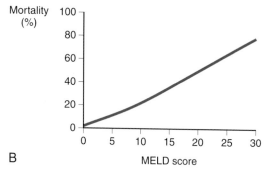

Fig. 30.1 The association between operative mortality and Model for End-stage Liver Disease (MELD) score in patients with cirrhosis undergoing surgery. **A,** 30-day mortality. **B,** 90-day mortality. *(From Teh SH, Nagorney DM, Stevens SR, et al. Risk factors for mortality after surgery in 772 patients with cirrhosis.* Gastroenterology 2007; 132:1261–1269.)

2. Advantages of MELD score over the Child-Pugh classification:
   - Objective
   - Weighs the variables
   - Does not rely on arbitrary cutoff values

   The result is increased precision in predicting postoperative mortality.
3. Results of the largest retrospective study of MELD as a predictor of perioperative mortality (Teh *et al* [2007]) are as follows:
   a. MELD score up to 7: Mortality rate was 5.7%.
   b. MELD score of 8 to 11: Mortality rate was 10.3%.
   c. MELD score of 12 to 15: Mortality rate was 25.4%.
   d. The increase in risk of death was almost linear for MELD scores higher than 8 (Fig. 30.1).
   e. Limitations:
      - Median MELD score was 8; few patients had a MELD score higher than 15.
      - Most patients had a platelet count higher than 60,000/mm^3 and an INR lower than 1.5.
4. When using the MELD score to predict surgical risk, additional risk factors predictive of perioperative mortality include the following:
   a. ASA class (Table 30.4):
      - In ASA class IV, patients add 5.5 MELD points.
      - ASA class V is a contraindication to surgery, except liver transplantation; 100% mortality is expected.
   b. Older age; in patients whose age is greater than 70 years, add 3 MELD points.
5. To calculate 7-day, 30-day, 90-day, and 1-year surgical mortality based on the MELD score, ASA class, and age, use the algorithm at http://www.mayoclinic.org/meld/mayomodel9.html

TABLE 30.4 ■ **American Society of Anesthesiologists classification**

Class	
I	Healthy patient
II	Patient with mild systemic disease without functional limitation
III	Patient with severe systemic disease with functional limitation
IV	Patient with severe systemic disease that is a constant threat to life
V	Moribund patient not expected to survive >24 hr with or without surgery
E	Emergency nature of surgery (added to classification I–V above)

6. In patients with a MELD score ≥15, a serum albumin level ≤2.5 mg/dL has been shown to be associated with a much higher postoperative mortality rate (60%) than that associated with a serum albumin level >2.5 mg/dL (14%).

Obstructive Jaundice (see Chapters 33 and 34)

SURGICAL RISK

1. Mortality rate: 8% to 28%
2. Risk factors based on a multivariate analysis performed in 373 patients undergoing surgery for relief of biliary obstruction:
   a. Initial hematocrit value lower than 30%
   b. Initial serum bilirubin level greater than 11 mg/dL
   c. Malignant cause of obstruction
      ■ All three present → mortality rate 60%
      ■ All three absent → mortality rate less than 5%
3. Additional risk factors for morbidity and mortality after surgery for obstructive jaundice: azotemia, hypoalbuminemia, cholangitis
4. Risk factors for surgery of bile duct stones:
   ■ Serum bilirubin level
   ■ Other medical illnesses (however, not a risk factor for endoscopic sphincterotomy)
   ■ Preoperative endoscopic sphincterotomy
5. Situations in which endoscopic sphincterotomy for bile duct stones is preferable to surgery:
   ■ Patients at high operative risk
   ■ Retained stones after cholecystectomy
   ■ Severe acute cholangitis

PERIOPERATIVE COMPLICATIONS IN PATIENTS WITH OBSTRUCTIVE JAUNDICE

These are presumed to result from increased circulating levels of endotoxin caused by impaired bile salt delivery to bowel and decreased hepatic reticuloendothelial function.

1. Renal failure
   ■ Decreased glomerular filtration rate in 60% to 75% (versus less than 1% of anicteric surgical patients)
   ■ Frank renal failure in 8% with a mortality rate higher than 50%

2. Disseminated intravascular coagulation
3. Gastric stress ulcers and bleeding
4. Delayed wound healing, wound dehiscence, and incisional hernias
5. Strategies to reduce potential complications:
    ■ Reduction or prevention of endotoxemia: experimental—oral bile salts, oral antibiotics, or lactulose
    ■ Preoperative intravenous antibiotic administration to prevent wound infection
    ■ Adequate perioperative hydration: possibly a critical factor
    ■ Avoidance of aminoglycosides and nonsteroidal anti-inflammatory drugs because these drugs may precipitate renal failure

PREOPERATIVE BILIARY DECOMPRESSION

1. Endoscopic or percutaneous biliary drainage is preferable to surgery for benign conditions in cirrhotic patients.
    ■ Sphincterotomy is associated with an increased risk of bleeding in patients with coagulopathy or thrombocytopenia; in these patients, balloon dilatation is preferable.
2. Routine biliary decompression before surgery for malignant obstruction does not reduce subsequent operative mortality and increases morbidity:
    ■ No decrease in mortality occurs.
    ■ Complications of transhepatic biliary drainage include cholangitis, sepsis, dehydration, and catheter displacement.
    ■ Routine preoperative endoscopic internal biliary drainage increases the rate of morbidity and does not decrease the rate of mortality in patients undergoing pancreatic cancer resection and therefore is not recommended unless surgery is delayed and the patient has cholangitis or pruritus.
3. Endoscopic biliary decompression is a useful alternative to surgery for palliation of patients with inoperable malignancy or poor surgical risk; however, it does not generally prolong survival. Endoprosthesis insertion may also be a reasonable alternative to operative bypass in selected patients; endoscopic stenting is associated with fewer early complications and surgery with fewer late complications.

Hepatic Resection (see Chapter 27)

1. Hepatocellular carcinoma is a common complication of cirrhosis; it has an occurrence rate of 1% to 4% per year.
2. MELD is the best predictor of morbidity and mortality in patients with cirrhosis who undergo liver resection.
    ■ In a large study of 1017 patients, a MELD score higher than 8 was associated with a mortality rate of 4% and a morbidity rate of 16%, although most patients underwent small resections and had a mean MELD score of 6.
    ■ In another study, the postoperative mortality rate for patients with a MELD score of 9 or higher was 29% versus 0% for those with a MELD score lower than 9.
3. Alternatives to hepatic resection in patients with hepatocellular carcinoma include radiofrequency ablation, percutaneous ethanol injection, transarterial chemoembolization, doxorubicin- or yttrium-90–impregnated microsphere embolization, external beam radiation with CyberKnife, and liver transplantation; disease-free survival is greatest in patients after liver transplantation.

4. Postresection liver failure is defined by the "50-50" rule:
   - The PT index (patient's PT relative to control PT) is less than 50% (the INR is greater than 1.7).
   - The serum bilirubin level is higher than 50 μmol/L (2.9 mg/dL).
   - The mortality rate is 59% when these criteria are met versus 1.2% when they are not met.

Preoperative Evaluation and Preparation

GENERAL MEASURES

1. History and physical examination:
   - Patients should be screened for unrecognized liver disease (routine liver biochemical tests in asymptomatic healthy patients are not required).
   - Patients with cirrhosis can have normal laboratory test results; screening laboratory testing cannot replace a through history and physical examination.
   - The status of patients with known liver disease should be assessed (determine Child-Pugh class, MELD score, ASA class).
   - A careful medication and alcohol history should be included.
   - Physical examination findings in cirrhosis may include palmar erythema, spider angiomas, abnormal hepatic size or contour, splenomegaly, hepatic encephalopathy, ascites, testicular atrophy, and gynecomastia.
2. Liver biochemical tests: aspartate aminotransferase (AST), alanine aminotransferase (ALT), alkaline phosphatase, bilirubin, and albumin
   a. Of unclear cost effectiveness in healthy, asymptomatic patients
   b. Indicated in patients who drink alcohol regularly and those with a remote history of hepatitis or risk factors for hepatitis (e.g., injection drug use); check hepatitis B surface antigen and antibody to hepatitis C virus
   c. Further investigation of any patient with clinical or biochemical evidence of liver disease:
      - Hepatocellular dysfunction: biochemical and serologic testing for viral hepatitis, autoimmune liver disease, and metabolic disorders; possible liver biopsy
      - Cholestasis: radiologic or endoscopic imaging (abdominal ultrasonography, possibly magnetic resonance, endoscopic, or transhepatic cholangiography), with or without liver biopsy

TREATMENT OF COAGULOPATHY

1. Impaired hemostasis in liver disease
   a. Vitamin K deficiency: decreased levels of factors II, VII, IX, and X
   b. Decreased hepatic protein synthesis: decrease in levels of all factors except VIII, which may be increased
   c. Low-grade disseminated intravascular coagulation causing increased fibrinolysis
   d. Pattern of hemostatic abnormalities:
      - Prolonged PT
      - Normal or increased PTT
      - Prolonged thrombin time
      - Low plasma fibrinogen level
      - Decreased plasma levels of antithrombin, protein C, and protein S
   e. Thrombocytopenia: result of hypersplenism or alcohol-induced bone marrow suppression

    f. The degree of prolongation of the PT does not correlate with the patient's risk of bleeding because of changes in levels of both procoagulant and anticoagulant factors in the plasma of patients with cirrhosis.

2. Preoperative preparation
- Vitamin K 10 mg intravenously (one to three doses): corrects hypoprothrombinemia related to malnutrition or intestinal bile salt deficiency, not hepatocellular disease
- Fresh frozen plasma in patients with hepatocellular dysfunction: aim for an INR lower than 1.5 (large volumes, short half-life limit efficacy)
- Platelet transfusions: 8 to 10 U when count is lower than 50,000/mm^3
- Surgical risk and bleeding risk in patients with INR greater than 1.5 or platelets lower than 50,000/mm^3 are unknown because they have not been studied
- Adjunctive therapy considered only when active bleeding does not respond to standard measures: 1-deamino-8-D-arginine vasopressin (DDAVP, factor VIII stimulant, shortens bleeding time, clinical usefulness uncertain), antifibrinolytic agents (ε-aminocaproic acid, tranexamic acid, value uncertain), recombinant factor VIIa (expensive, short half-life, of unproven benefit)

TREATMENT OF ASCITES (see Chapter 11)

1. Derangements in liver disease
    a. Factors contributing to development of ascites with or without hepatic hydrothorax in cirrhosis:
- Portal hypertension
- Decreased plasma oncotic pressure (hypoalbuminemia)
- Increased hepatic lymph
- Secondary hyperaldosteronism
- Peripheral vasodilatation → stimulation of renin-angiotensin system → renal vasoconstriction → avid sodium retention

    b. Associated electrolyte abnormalities:
- Hyponatremia (impaired free water clearance)
- Hypokalemic alkalosis

2. Management
    a. Diagnostic paracentesis in patients with new or worsening ascites: to exclude infection or malignancy and to differentiate spontaneous from secondary (surgical) bacterial peritonitis
    b. Control of ascites before abdominal surgery to reduce risk of postoperative wound dehiscence or herniation:
- Rigid salt restriction (2-g sodium diet)
- Combination diuretics: spironolactone 100 → 400 mg/day + furosemide 40 → 160 mg/day, if necessary
- Preoperative TIPS: may lower surgical risk in patients with low MELD scores, no encephalopathy, and refractory ascites or large varices who require intra-abdominal surgery
- Monitoring of patient's weight, intake and output, urinary sodium concentration (greater than 25 mEq/L if diuretics are effective); if necessary, central venous pressure monitoring
- 1L fluid restriction if hyponatremia (sodium lower than 125 mEq/L) present

    c. When intraoperative volume expansion is needed, blood products, intravenous 25% salt-poor albumin, and (in the absence of hyponatremia) 5% dextrose in water (D5W) can be administered; crystalloid should be avoided if possible

TREATMENT OF RENAL DYSFUNCTION (see Chapter 12)

1. Decompensated cirrhosis leads to increased levels of endogenous vasodilators, peripheral vasodilatation, chronic hyperdynamic circulation, and low blood pressure.
   - Serum creatinine may overestimate renal function because of muscle wasting and decreased urea synthesis.
   - Serum creatinine and blood urea nitrogen (BUN) should be monitored perioperatively.
2. The following nephrotoxic drugs should be avoided:
   - Aminoglycosides
   - Nonsteroidal anti-inflammatory drugs
   - Intravenous contrast agents
3. The differential diagnosis of acute kidney injury in patients with cirrhosis includes the following:
   - Volume depletion
   - Drug nephrotoxicity
   - Acute tubular necrosis
   - Hepatorenal syndrome
4. **Hepatorenal syndrome** is characterized by a serum creatinine level >1.5 mg/dL despite diuretic withdrawal and volume expansion with intravenous salt-poor albumin in the setting of cirrhosis and ascites and the absence of parenchymal kidney disease and nephrotoxic drug use.
   a. It may be precipitated by sudden volume loss (e.g., bleeding, rapid diuresis, paracentesis), infection (e.g., spontaneous bacterial peritonitis), or a decrease in cardiac output.
   b. Potential treatments are as follows:
      - Oral midodrine (an alpha agonist), subcutaneous octreotide, and intravenous albumin (not approved by the US Food and Drug Administration [FDA])
      - Intravenous norepinephrine (titrated to increase mean arterial pressure 10 mm Hg) and intravenous albumin (not approved by FDA for this indication)
      - Intravenous terlipressin (under study but not available in the United States) and intravenous salt-poor albumin

TREATMENT OF HEPATIC ENCEPHALOPATHY (see Chapter 13)

1. Pathophysiology: This state of disordered central nervous system function is characterized by disturbances in consciousness, behavior, and personality. Pathogenic factors include the following:
   - Shunting of portal venous blood into the systemic circulation
   - Hepatic dysfunction resulting in failure to detoxify neurotoxic agents such as ammonia
2. Diagnosis
   a. Obvious in patients with confusion or stupor, asterixis, and elevated blood ammonia level
   b. Possibly subtle:
      - Sleep disturbances such as day-night reversal
      - Personality changes
      - Tremor
      - Hyperreflexia
   c. Importance of preoperative recognition: high frequency in the postoperative period of precipitating or exacerbating factors:
      - Gastrointestinal bleeding
      - Constipation
      - Azotemia

- Hypokalemic alkalosis
- Sepsis
- Hypoxia
- Use of central nervous system depressant drugs (e.g., narcotics or benzodiazepines)

3. Treatment
   a. Control of clinically overt encephalopathy preoperatively (preemptive therapy is of unproven benefit)
   b. Correction of precipitating factors
   c. Lactulose: oral unabsorbable disaccharide in dose needed to achieve three bowel movements per day:
      - Converts intestinal ammonia (NH_3) to unabsorbable ammonium (NH_4^+)
      - Enhances growth of nonammoniagenic intestinal bacteria
   d. Oral antibiotics should be added when lactulose has not achieved adequate control (e.g., rifaximin 550 mg twice daily)

MISCELLANEOUS ISSUES

1. Risk of hypoglycemia in acute hepatic failure and to a lesser extent in cirrhosis: When this risk is present, an intravenous infusion of 10% dextrose in water (D10W) should be administered.
2. Gastroesophageal varices: Primary prophylaxis with nonselective beta blockers or endoscopic band ligation to prevent variceal bleeding is indicated.
3. All cirrhotic patients are at high risk of protein-energy malnutrition; mortality is increased after surgery in malnourished patients.
   - When time permits, preoperative enteral nutritional supplementation improves immunocompetence and short-term prognosis.
   - Percutaneous gastrostomy is contraindicated in patients with ascites or coagulopathy.

POSTOPERATIVE MONITORING FOR SIGNS OF HEPATIC DECOMPENSATION

- Onset of jaundice, encephalopathy, ascites
- Rise in serum bilirubin, prolongation of PT, worsening renal function, hypoglycemia

Postoperative Jaundice

Postoperative jaundice can occur in patients with or without underlying liver disease. Pathophysiologic mechanisms in the postoperative period are often multiple (see Table 30.5).

1. **Increased pigment load** (predominantly indirect hyperbilirubinemia)
   - Resorption of hematoma or hemoperitoneum
   - Transfusion: 10% of erythrocytes in a unit of 14-day-old bank blood undergoing hemolysis within 24 hours of transfusion
   - Hemolysis (rare): usually in setting of congenital erythrocyte defect, such as glucose-6-phosphate dehydrogenase (G6PD) deficiency or sickle cell disease
   - Postcardiac surgery status: risk factors include preoperative elevations of serum bilirubin level and right atrial pressure, valve replacement (and number of valves replaced), and use of intra-aortic balloon counterpulsation; in this setting, hyperbilirubinemia is a marker of increased mortality rate

TABLE 30.5 ■ **Causes of postoperative jaundice**

Increased bilirubin load
Hemolysis after transfusion
Hematoma resorption
Underlying hemolytic anemia
Gilbert's syndrome*

Impaired hepatocellular function
Anesthesia drugs: halothane, enflurane, rarely isoflurane, desflurane, sevoflurane
Other drugs: e.g., phenothiazines, isoniazid, methyldopa, androgens, estrogens
Antibiotics: tetracycline, chloramphenicol, erythromycins, sulfonamides, nitrofurantoin
Total parenteral nutrition
Viral hepatitis
Ischemic hepatitis
Sepsis
Benign postoperative intrahepatic cholestasis

Extrahepatic obstruction
Bile duct stone
Cholecystitis, cholangitis, abscess
Biliary stricture, leak, tumor
Pancreatitis

*Unconjugated hyperbilirubinemia resulting from congenital defect in the hepatocyte uptake of bilirubin.

■ Inherited disorder of bilirubin metabolism (e.g., Gilbert's syndrome): may be coincidentally diagnosed after a surgical procedure

2. **Impaired hepatocellular function**
   a. Benign postoperative intrahepatic cholestasis: hepatocyte dysfunction from various stresses, such as hypoxemia, anesthesia, hemorrhage, sepsis, extensive transfusions; often occurs in the setting of prolonged, difficult surgery with postoperative multiorgan failure:
      ■ Peak serum bilirubin of up to 40 mg/dL on postoperative day 2 to 10 with variable elevation of alkaline phosphatase and no more than mild elevation of aminotransferases
      ■ May mimic extrahepatic obstruction
      ■ Prognosis depends on the overall condition of the patient, not liver status; liver function returns to normal if and when patient recovers
   b. Hyperbilirubinemia of sepsis triggered by bacterial infections, especially gram-negative sepsis and pneumococcal pneumonia
   c. Viral hepatitis:
      ■ Hepatitis C: historically the most common cause of post-transfusion hepatitis (up to 90% to 95% of cases); now rare; acute hepatitis occurs 6 to 7 weeks after transfusion
      ■ Hepatitis B: also uncommon with contemporary serologic screening of donated blood; incubation period 12 to 14 weeks
      ■ Rarely Epstein–Barr virus, cytomegalovirus, or hepatitis D (with B)
   d. Drug-related hepatitis:
      ■ Halothane: rare, with frequency of 1 in 35,000 exposures; onset of fever within 2 to 10 days of exposure; pathophysiologic mechanism involves immune sensitization to trifluoroacetylated liver proteins formed by oxidative metabolism of halothane by cytochrome P-450 2E1 in persons with a possible genetic predisposition
      ■ Enflurane: less common cause of hepatitis than halothane

- Other drugs (e.g., erythromycin, sulfonamides, phenytoin, isoniazid, amoxicillin-clavulanate [Augmentin]); some drugs may cause of intrahepatic cholestasis (e.g., chlorpromazine, anabolic steroids).

  e. Ischemic hepatitis (shock liver): in setting of trauma, shock, hyperthermia; typically associated with marked elevations of serum aminotransferase levels (often to more than 5000 U/L), as well as lactate dehydrogenase levels, that fall abruptly with stabilization of the patient; delayed rise in bilirubin up to 20 mg/dL often seen

  f. Total parenteral nutrition: possible associated with hepatomegaly, minor elevations of serum aminotransferase levels, fatty infiltration (presumably from high glucose load or possibly carnitine or choline deficiency), or intrahepatic cholestasis and nonspecific peri-portal inflammation (presumably from intravenous amino acids or fat emulsions and possibly toxic bile salts such as lithocholic acid); fatty liver possibly reversible with a decrease in the percentage of glucose or lecithin or choline supplementation

3. **Extrahepatic obstruction** (uncommon cause of jaundice in postoperative period)
   - Unrecognized bile duct injury with biloma formation, usually during cholecystectomy
   - Cholangitis, subphrenic or subhepatic abscesses secondary to biliary obstruction
   - Choledocholithiasis, biliary or pancreatic tumor
   - If biliary obstruction is suspected, evaluation with ultrasonography or computed tomography and cholangiography (magnetic resonance cholangiopancreatography or ERCP) may be required

FURTHER READING

Azoulay D, Buabse F, Damiano I, et al. Neoadjuvant transjugular intrahepatic portosystemic shunt; a solution for extrahepatic abdominal operation in cirrhotic patients with severe portal hypertension. *J Am Coll Surg* 2001; 193:46–51.

Dixon JM, Armstrong CP, Duffy SW, et al. Factors affecting morbidity and mortality after surgery for obstructive jaundice: a review of 373 patients. *Gut* 1983; 24:845–852.

Fernandes NR, Schwesinger WH, Hilsenbeck SG, et al. Laparoscopic cholecystectomy and cirrhosis: a case-control study of outcomes. *Liver Transpl* 2000; 6:340–344.

Garrison RN, Cryer HM, Howard DA, et al. Clarification of risk factors for abdominal operations in patients with hepatic cirrhosis. *Ann Surg* 1984; 199:648–655.

Hsu KY, Ghau GY, Lui WY, et al. Predicting morbidity and mortality after hepatic resection in patients with hepatocellular carcinoma: the role of Model for End-Stage Liver Disease score. *World J Surg* 2009; 33:2412–2419.

Lee KK, Kim DG, Moon IS, et al. Liver transplantation versus liver resection for the treatment of hepatocellular carcinoma. *J Surg Oncol* 2010; 101:47–53.

Mansour A, Watson W, Shayani V, Pickleman J. Abdominal operations in patients with cirrhosis: still a major surgical challenge. *Surgery* 1997; 122:730–736.

Merli M, Nicolini G, Angeloni S, et al. Malnutrition is a risk factor in cirrhotic patients undergoing surgery. *Nutrition* 2002; 18:978–986.

Mummadi RR, Kasturi KS, Chennareddygari S, et al. Effect of bariatric surgery on nonalcoholic fatty liver disease: systematic review and meta-analysis. *Clin Gastroenterol Hepatol* 2008; 6:1396–1402.

Neeff H, Miriaskin D, Spangenberg H-C, et al. Perioperative mortality after non-hepatic general surgery in patients with liver cirrhosis: an analysis of 138 operations in the 2000s using Child and MELD scores. *J Gastrointest Surg* 2011; 15:1–11.

Northup PG, Wanamaker RC, Lee VD, et al. Model for End-Stage Liver Disease (MELD) predicts non-transplant surgical mortality in patients with cirrhosis. *Ann Surg* 2005; 242:244–251.

O'Leary JG, Yachimski PS, Friedman LS. Surgery in the patient with liver disease. *Clin Liver Dis* 2009; 13:211–231.

Teh SH, Christein J, Donohue J, et al. Hepatic resection of hepatocellular carcinoma in patients with cirrhosis: Model of End-Stage Liver Disease (MELD) score predicts perioperative mortality. *J Gastrointest Surg* 2005; 9:1207–1215.

Teh SH, Nagorney DM, Stevens SR, et al. Risk factors for mortality after surgery in patients with cirrhosis. *Gastroenterology* 2007; 132:1261–1269.

Telem DA, Schiano T, Goldstone R, et al. Factors that predict outcome of abdominal operations in patients with advanced cirrhosis. *Clin Gastroenterol Hepatol* 2010; 8:451–457.

Tripodi A, Primignani M, Chantarangkul V, et al. An imbalance of pro- vs anti-coagulation factors in plasma from patients with cirrhosis. *Gastroenterology* 2009; 137:2105–2111.

van den Broek MA, Olde Damink SW, Dejong CH, et al. Liver failure after partial hepatic resection: definition, pathophysiology, risk factors and treatment. *Liver Int* 2008; 28:767–780.

van der Gaag NA, Rauws EA, van Eijck CH, et al. Preoperative biliary drainage for cancer of the head of the pancreas. *N Engl J Med* 2010; 362:129–137.

Ziser A, Plevak DJ, Wiesner RH, et al. Morbidity and mortality in cirrhotic patients undergoing anesthesia and surgery. *Anesthesiology* 1999; 890:42–53.

CHAPTER 31

Liver transplantation

Stevan A. Gonzalez, MD, MS ■ Emmet B. Keeffe, MD, MACP

KEY POINTS

1 Liver transplantation is an important treatment option in patients with end-stage liver disease and is associated with a significant survival benefit.

2 Advances in immunosuppressive drug therapy have led to improved long-term survival in liver transplant recipients based on a decreased rate of allograft rejection and fewer side effects of therapy.

3 Assessment of the severity of liver disease and evaluation of the benefit of liver transplantation relative to expected survival are key factors in the timing of referral for liver transplant evaluation and assessment of transplant candidacy.

4 The use of partial allograft transplants, including living donor liver and split liver transplants, as well as the use of marginal allografts, has increased as a response to the major imbalance between the need for donor organs and the number of patients awaiting liver transplantation.

5 Long-term post-transplant care involves treatment of complications and strategies to decrease the risk of sequelae associated with the use of immunosuppressive drugs.

Overview

1. Liver transplantation has a major survival benefit in patients with end-stage liver disease (ESLD) who would otherwise have a high short-term mortality rate.
2. More than 16,000 patients are currently listed for liver transplantation in the United States, and approximately 6000 persons undergo liver transplantation annually.
   - The number of patients on the transplant waiting list remained stable during the late 2000s.
   - Approximately 2000 patients die every year while awaiting liver transplantation.
3. Advances in surgical techniques and post-transplant care have led to improved long-term survival of liver transplant recipients.
   - Overall adjusted survival rates following deceased donor liver transplantation is approximately 87% at 1 year, 73% at 5 years, and 59% at 10 years.
   - Survival among transplant recipients varies based on the pretransplant diagnosis.
   - The 5-year survival rates following transplantation are greatest in patients with cholestatic liver disease or metabolic disorders, whereas patients with noncholestatic liver diseases such as chronic viral hepatitis, alcoholic liver disease, and autoimmune hepatitis have lower survival rates.

TABLE 31.1 ▦ **Indications for liver transplantation in adults**

Category	Disease
Noncholestatic or inflammatory	Chronic hepatitis C
	Chronic hepatitis B
	Alcoholic liver disease
	Autoimmune hepatitis
	Cryptogenic cirrhosis
	Nonalcoholic fatty liver disease
	Drug-induced liver injury
	Sarcoidosis
Cholestatic	Primary biliary cirrhosis
	Primary sclerosing cholangitis
	Secondary biliary cirrhosis
	Idiopathic adulthood ductopenia
	Cystic fibrosis
	Familial intrahepatic cholestasis syndromes
Metabolic	Alpha-1 antitrypsin deficiency
	Hereditary hemochromatosis
	Wilson disease
	Glycogen storage disease
Malignant	Hepatocellular carcinoma
	Neuroendocrine tumors
	Epithelioid hemangioendothelioma
	Fibrolamellar hepatocellular carcinoma
Extrahepatic	Familial amyloidosis
	Primary hyperoxaluria
	Homozygous familial hypercholesterolemia
Miscellaneous	Acute liver failure
	Budd–Chiari syndrome
	Polycystic liver disease
	Giant cavernous hemangioma
	Noncirrhotic portal hypertension
	Retransplantation

Selection of Candidates

INDICATIONS FOR LIVER TRANSPLANTATION

1. Liver transplantation should be considered in patients with **irreversible liver failure** resulting from acute or chronic liver diseases, as well as **hepatocellular malignant diseases** (Table 31.1).
2. All forms of effective therapy should be explored before liver transplantation.
3. The severity of liver disease and the potential benefit of liver transplantation are important considerations in evaluating a patient's candidacy for transplantation.

ASSESSMENT OF LIVER DISEASE SEVERITY

An accurate assessment of the risk of morbidity and mortality associated with progressive ESLD is critical to determining the appropriate timing for referral to a liver transplant center and is a key factor in prioritization for transplantation.

TABLE 31.2 ■ **Child–Turcotte–Pugh scoring system and Child–Pugh Classification**

	Points		
	1	**2**	**3**
Ascites	None	Slight-moderate	Tense
Encephalopathy grade	0	1–2	3–4
Serum albumin level (g/dL)	>3.5	2.8–3.5	<2.8
Serum bilirubin level (mg/dL)	<2.0	2.0–3.0	>3.0
INR	<1.7	1.7–2.3	>2.3
(or PT above normal)	(<4)	(4 to 6)	(>6)

Child–Pugh class (Child-Turcotte-Pugh score)
A (5–6)
B (7–9)
C (10–15)

INR, International normalized ratio; PT, prothrombin time.

Adapted from Murray KF, Carithers RL Jr. AASLD practice guidelines: evaluation of the patient for liver transplantation. *Hepatology* 2005; 41:1407–1432.

1. Child–Turcotte–Pugh (CTP) score (Table 31.2)
   ■ This score was developed to predict operative mortality in persons with cirrhosis who required portacaval shunt surgery for variceal bleeding.
   ■ Child–Pugh classes B and C are associated with a survival benefit following liver transplantation.
   ■ This score was previously used for allocation of donor organs and is still widely used to predict the risk of perioperative mortality in cirrhotic patients undergoing surgery (see Chapter 30).
2. Model for End-stage Liver Disease (MELD)
   ■ The MELD was initially developed to predict 3-month mortality in patients undergoing transjugular intrahepatic portosystemic shunt (TIPS) placement.
   ■ The components—serum creatinine and total bilirubin levels and the international normalized ratio (INR) of prothrombin time—are key determinants of survival (Table 31.3).
   ■ It is superior to the CTP score in predicting short-term (3-month) mortality in patients with ESLD.
   ■ It was introduced in 2002 as the **basis for allocation of donor organs** in the United States.
3. The Baveno IV consensus workshop identified four clinical stages of ESLD, based on the development of complications, each of which may predict mortality (Table 31.4). The risk of clinical decompensation and progression from compensated ESLD to a more advanced stage is approximately 10% per year.

BENEFIT OF LIVER TRANSPLANTATION

Merion *et al* (2005) performed a survival analysis of more than 12,000 adult patients listed for liver transplantation in the United States. Survival in transplant recipients over a 1-year follow-up was compared with survival in patients who did not receive transplants:
   ■ Transplant recipients had a significant benefit in survival, with 79% lower mortality overall.

TABLE 31.3 ■ **Model for End-stage Liver Disease**

MELD score = 9.57 × log$_e$ (serum creatinine [mg/dL]) + 3.78 × log$_e$ (serum bilirubin [mg/dL]) + 11.20 × log$_e$ (INR) + 6.43

INR, international normalized ratio; MELD, Model for End-stage Liver Disease..

Adapted from Wiesner R, Edwards E, Freeman R, et al. Model for End-stage Liver Disease (MELD) and allocation of donor livers. *Gastroenterology* 2003; 124:91–96.

TABLE 31.4 ■ **Clinical stages of cirrhosis and mortality risk**

Stage	Complications	1-yr mortality risk (%)
1	No varices No ascites	1
2	Varices present No ascites	3.4
3	Ascites present	20
4	Variceal hemorrhage	57

Adapted from D'Amico G, Garcia-Tsao G, Pagliaro L. Natural history and prognostic indicators of survival in cirrhosis: a systematic review of 118 studies. *J Hepatol* 2006; 44:217–231.

■ Patients with a MELD score of 15 or higher benefited most from liver transplantation.
■ A MELD score lower than 15 was associated with a greater post-transplant mortality rate than the waitlist mortality rate, particularly with a MELD score lower than 11, in which the post-transplant mortality rate was more than three times greater than the waitlist mortality rate.

REFERRAL TO A LIVER TRANSPLANT CENTER

1. Referral to a liver transplant center should be considered for the following:
   ■ Patients with evidence of decompensated liver disease reflected in elevated MELD or CTP scores
   ■ Patients who develop complications such as hepatic encephalopathy, variceal bleeding, ascites with or without spontaneous bacterial peritonitis, or renal insufficiency
2. Priority of organ allocation in the United States is entirely based on an individual's MELD score, with no minimal listing criteria used.
3. Time spent on a transplant waitlist has not been a factor in prioritization since the MELD score was implemented; thus, early listing of patients has no advantage.

LIVER TRANSPLANT EVALUATION

In addition to hepatology and transplant surgery consultations, a liver transplant evaluation includes various laboratory tests, imaging studies, and other consultations (Table 31.5).

TABLE 31.5 ■ Liver transplant evaluation

Extensive laboratory testing for accurate assessment of current clinical status, evaluation of potential causes of underlying chronic liver disease, and screening for comorbid illnesses

Accurate assessment of renal function

Imaging for surveillance for HCC, assessment of hepatic vasculature, and evaluation of hepatic anatomy

Cardiopulmonary evaluation, which may include right or left heart catheterization, depending on risk factors

Psychosocial assessment

Age-appropriate screening tests including colonoscopy, mammogram, PSA level, and Pap test

HCC, hepatocellular carcinoma; PSA, prostate-specific antigen.

TABLE 31.6 ■ Contraindications to liver transplantation

Active uncontrolled infection or sepsis
Severe neurologic compromise, including brain death
Cardiovascular disease
   Severe or symptomatic coronary artery disease
   Heart failure
   Valvular disease
Pulmonary disease
   Chronic obstructive pulmonary disease with oxygen dependence
   Pulmonary fibrosis
   Severe pulmonary hypertension
Concurrent extrahepatic malignant disease
Lack of psychosocial support or inability to comply with treatment regimen
Active alcohol or substance abuse
Anatomic abnormalities precluding liver transplantation
Compensated cirrhosis without complications (Child–Pugh class A)
Acquired immunodeficiency syndrome

CONTRAINDICATIONS TO LIVER TRANSPLANTATION (Table 31.6)

1. **Relative contraindications** include poor nutritional status, high body mass index, poorly controlled chronic illnesses such as diabetes mellitus, portal and mesenteric thromboses, inadequate management of psychiatric disorders, and past history of malignant disease.
2. **Absolute contraindications** include severe cardiopulmonary disease, infection, and psychosocial concerns.

CLINICAL MANAGEMENT WHILE PATIENT IS ON WAITLIST

1. The MELD score and listing status should be updated at regular intervals.
2. Surveillance for hepatocellular carcinoma (HCC): A diagnosis of HCC has an impact on priority for transplantation (see Chapter 27).
3. The complications of ESLD should be treated.

Donor Selection

Selection of an appropriate donor organ for liver transplantation is critical to ensuring optimal post-transplant outcomes and is an important consideration in the use of partial allografts.

DONOR SELECTION CRITERIA

1. Adequate allograft volume, to prevent small-for-size syndrome:
   - Volume should be at least 35% to 40% of normal liver size for the recipient.
   - The minimum percentage of allograft to body weight is 0.8%.
2. ABO compatibility
3. Absence of significant liver fibrosis or steatosis (less than 20% to 30%)
4. Donor age less than 60 years
5. Confirmed brain death
6. Absence of evidence of bacterial or fungal infection
7. Absence of risk factors for, or evidence of, chronic viral hepatitis or human immunodeficiency virus (HIV) infection
8. Absence of significant comorbid conditions such as diabetes mellitus, obesity, or extrahepatic malignant disease

PARTIAL ALLOGRAFT TRANSPLANTS

1. **Living donor liver transplantation (LDLT)**
   a. LDLT is performed in approximately 200 to 300 patients annually in the United States and comprises less than 5% of transplantations.
   b. The distribution of age among LDLT recipients has changed significantly since 2000; approximately three fourths of LDLTs are now performed in adults.
   c. LDLT is generally not acceptable for patients with a high MELD score (>30), because post-transplant mortality in this group may be as much as threefold higher than that for recipients of deceased donor allografts.
   d. Risk to the donor is a major consideration:
      - The mortality rate is from 0.1% to as high as 0.5%.
      - The complication rate is approximately 30% to 40%.
      - The risk decreases with increased liver transplant program LDLT experience (threshold of more than 20 cases).
2. **Split liver transplants**
   - The donor organ is split between two recipients.
   - The most common technique involves division into grafts for one pediatric and one adult recipient.

EXTENDED-CRITERIA DONORS

1. Use of organs with characteristics associated with an increased risk of poor allograft function: (extended-criteria donors (ECDs)) has increased since 2000 in response to the need for donor organs (Table 31.7). Use of allografts from donors after cardiac death has increased and currently accounts for 5% of all liver transplantations.
2. Use of donor organs otherwise considered to be marginal may be beneficial in selected transplant candidates, particularly those with advanced liver disease who do not have sufficient MELD points to receive a deceased donor graft.

TABLE 31.7 ■ **Potential characteristics of extended-criteria donors**

Increased age >60 yr
Donation after cardiac death
Increased duration of intensive care hospitalization or use of vasopressors
Hepatic steatosis (>30%–40% of liver volume)
Elevated body mass index or obesity
Diabetes mellitus
Hypernatremia
Hepatitis B core antibody positivity
Hepatitis C antibody positivity
High-risk exposure to hepatitis B, hepatitis C, or human immunodeficiency virus
Human T-cell lymphotropic virus positivity
Extrahepatic malignant disease
Suboptimal allograft appearance
Prolonged warm or cold ischemia time
Organ sharing outside local area

3. Use of ECDs may have an impact on recurrent disease, particularly hepatitis C. Factors associated with fibrosis progression and reduced survival in recipients of an ECD allograft with chronic hepatitis C include the following:
   ■ Increased donor age
   ■ Prolonged warm or cold ischemia time
   ■ Donation after cardiac death
   ■ Allograft steatosis

Major Diseases Considered for Transplantation

VIRAL HEPATITIS (see Chapters 3 and 4)

1. Chronic hepatitis C
   a. Chronic hepatitis C, **the most common indication for liver transplantation,** accounts for 40% to 50% of all cases in the United States.
   b. Treatment with peginterferon alpha and ribavirin should be considered in all patients who are potential transplant candidates before liver transplantation; achievement of a sustained virologic response may avert the need for transplantation or eliminate the risk of disease recurrence if transplantation is required (see Chapter 4).
   c. Recurrence of hepatitis C virus infection is universal in patients with chronic hepatitis C and detectable viremia who undergo liver transplantation.
      ■ Up to 30% of patients develop recurrent liver disease that progresses to cirrhosis within 5 years.
      ■ A few patients (less than 5%) develop **fibrosing cholestatic hepatitis C**, characterized by jaundice, cholestasis, resistance to antiviral therapy, and a high risk of mortality within 1 year.
   d. Antiviral therapy may be considered following liver transplantation, although rates of sustained virologic response are low.
2. Chronic hepatitis B
   ■ Antiviral therapy with a nucleoside or nucleotide analogue is recommended for all cirrhotic patients with detectable hepatitis B virus (HBV) DNA in serum; oral agents with

high potency and a low rate of antiviral drug resistance, such as entecavir or tenofovir, are preferred.

- Use of an oral nucleoside or nucleotide analogue and hepatitis B immune globulin (HBIG) following liver transplantation has had a major impact on decreasing the rate of recurrent HBV infection and improving post-transplantation survival.

ALCOHOLIC LIVER DISEASE (see Chapter 6)

1. Abstinence in patients with decompensated alcoholic liver disease may result in significant clinical improvement in liver disease over time.
2. Most transplant centers require at least 6 months of abstinence before consideration of a patient for liver transplantation; extensive psychosocial evaluation is required.
3. Rates of recidivism following liver transplantation vary greatly and may be as high as 33%; however, recidivism does not appear to have an impact on overall graft or patient survival.

CRYPTOGENIC CIRRHOSIS (see Chapter 9)

1. Most patients diagnosed with cryptogenic cirrhosis have nonalcoholic steatohepatitis (NASH) and the metabolic syndrome (see Chapter 7).
2. Attention should be given to cardiovascular risk factors in patients with cryptogenic cirrhosis or NASH who are undergoing liver transplant evaluation.

CHOLESTATIC LIVER DISEASE

1. Primary biliary cirrhosis (PBC) (see Chapter 14)
   - The Mayo PBC risk score may be useful in assessing disease severity.
   - Therapy with ursodeoxycholic acid has the greatest survival benefit when initiated early in the natural history of PBC.
   - The benefit of ursodeoxycholic acid following liver transplantation is uncertain.
2. Primary sclerosing cholangitis (PSC) (see Chapter 15)
   - PSC is associated with an increased risk of cholangiocarcinoma, with a rate of 1.5% per year once jaundice develops; dominant strictures should be assessed for the presence of malignancy.
   - Roux-en-Y choledochojejunostomy is typically performed at the time of liver transplantation.
   - Close surveillance for colon cancer should be conducted before and after liver transplantation because of the association between PSC and inflammatory bowel disease, as well as the potential for colonic high-grade dysplasia or cancer.

HEPATOCELLULAR CARCINOMA (see Chapter 27)

1. The proportion of liver transplants performed for HCC has increased since 2000 and now accounts for approximately 13% of all liver transplants in the United States.
2. Patients with early-stage HCC who undergo liver transplantation have equivalent rates of survival compared with patients who do not have HCC. The **Milan criteria** define the tumor size that is acceptable for liver transplantation:
   - If one solitary lesion is found, it must be less than 5 cm in greatest diameter.
   - If two or three lesions are present, each must be less than 3 cm in greatest diameter.

■ The absence of vascular invasion of tumor and of evidence of extrahepatic metastases must be ascertained.

3. Patients with HCC who fulfill the Milan criteria are eligible for higher prioritization through MELD exception points.

4. Several groups have proposed expanded criteria in which tumor size may exceed the Milan criteria without sacrificing post-transplant survival; these proposed criteria have not yet been validated.

METABOLIC LIVER DISEASE

1. Alpha-1 antitrypsin deficiency (see Chapter 18)
   ■ Serum alpha-1 antitrypsin levels can be low in patients with ESLD; therefore, protease inhibitor (Pi) phenotypic analysis is required for diagnosis.
   ■ Liver transplantation results in conversion to the donor alpha-1 antitrypsin Pi phenotype, and levels of alpha-1 antitrypsin typically normalize quickly following liver transplantation.

2. Hereditary hemochromatosis (see Chapter 16)
   ■ Decreased post-transplant survival was reported in the past, likely because of associated nonhepatic disease, including an increased risk of heart failure and arrhythmias, but survival rates have improved with better patient selection.

3. Wilson disease (see Chapter 17)
   ■ All patients with ESLD who do not respond to chelation therapy should be considered for liver transplant listing.
   ■ Liver transplantation corrects the metabolic defect associated with excessive copper deposition.
   ■ Patients with fulminant Wilson disease are eligible for United Network for Organ Sharing (UNOS) status 1A classification because of the high mortality rate associated with this presentation.

AUTOIMMUNE HEPATITIS (see Chapter 5)

1. Liver transplantation may be required for patients who are refractory to immunosuppressive therapy and who develop decompensated ESLD.

2. **The risk of graft rejection may be increased following liver transplantation.**

ACUTE LIVER FAILURE (ALF) (see Chapter 2)

1. ALF is uncommon but is associated with a high risk of mortality.

2. Many patients who present with ALF ultimately require liver transplantation.

3. Status 1A is the category assigned to patients with ALF who receive top priority for liver allocation (Table 31.8).

Exceptional Conditions in Transplant Listing

Several complications of ESLD or individual diagnoses are associated with a significant risk of morbidity or mortality. In some cases, this additional risk may not be reflected in the MELD score, and providing MELD exception points may be considered, depending on regional organ allocation policy.

TABLE 31.8 ■ **Criteria for United Network for Organ Sharing (UNOS) Status 1A designation in acute liver failure**

Age >18 yr
Life expectancy without liver transplantation of <7 days
Onset of encephalopathy within 8 wk of the first symptoms of liver disease
Absence of preexisting liver disease
Admission to an intensive care unit and one of the following:
   Ventilator dependence
   Requirement for renal replacement therapy
   INR >2.0
Fulminant Wilson disease

INR, international normalized ratio.

RENAL FAILURE

Renal failure is common in patients with ESLD. An elevated serum creatinine level, reflected in the MELD score, is an independent predictor of pretransplant mortality.

1. Hepatorenal syndrome (HRS) (see Chapter 12)
   - Acute kidney injury occurs in up to 20% of patients hospitalized with ESLD.
   - Development of HRS is associated with a high mortality rate and occurs in up to 18% of patients with ascites after 1 year and 39% at 5 years.
   - The median survival of patients with type I HRS is as short as 2 weeks, and the median survival of those with type II HRS is approximately 6 months.
   - Patients who develop type I HRS (acute onset within 2 weeks) should be referred for expedited liver transplant evaluation.
2. Simultaneous liver–kidney (SLK) transplantation
   a. A dual liver and kidney transplant evaluation may need to be considered in some transplant candidates.
   b. The use of SLK transplantation has increased significantly since the introduction of the MELD system; the frequency of SLK varies widely among transplant centers.
   c. A consensus conference in 2008 proposed key factors that may identify SLK transplant candidates:
      - Established end-stage renal disease
      - Acute kidney injury requiring renal replacement therapy for more than 8 weeks
      - Histologic evidence of significant chronic kidney disease on a kidney biopsy specimen
      - Chronic renal insufficiency with a glomerular filtration rate lower than 30 mL/minute

HEPATOPULMONARY SYNDROME (see Chapter 9)

1. This syndrome is defined as the **triad of cirrhosis with portal hypertension, arterial hypoxemia (Po_2 less than 70 mm Hg), and intrapulmonary vasodilatation.**
2. Intrapulmonary shunting can be demonstrated by contrast ("bubble") echocardiography or technetium-99m (^{99m}Tc)–macroaggregated albumin scanning.
3. This syndrome is associated with a significantly increased risk of mortality without liver transplantation; the risk of mortality increases with the degree of hypoxemia.
4. MELD exception points may be given to patients with significant hypoxemia (Po_2 less than 60 mm Hg).
5. Complete resolution typically follows liver transplantation.

PORTOPULMONARY HYPERTENSION

1. This is characterized by the presence of cirrhosis with portal hypertension, normal pulmonary capillary wedge pressure, **elevated mean pulmonary arterial pressure (greater than 25 mm Hg),** and elevated pulmonary vascular resistance (more than 240 dynes/second/cm^5); right heart catheterization is required for diagnosis.
2. This disorder is associated with an increased mortality risk of up to 50% at 1 year; elevated mean pulmonary artery pressure greater than 35 mm Hg is associated with increased perioperative mortality and is a contraindication to liver transplantation.
3. All affected patients should be considered for vasodilator therapy.
4. Some reports indicate that liver transplantation may be safe with successful vasodilator therapy; however, data are limited.

OTHERS

Other diagnoses such as small-for-size syndrome, familial amyloidosis, cystic fibrosis, and primary hyperoxaluria may receive MELD exception points in an effort to decrease waitlist mortality, as well as limit extrahepatic disease. Policies regarding the use of MELD exception points are typically decided on locally by regional review boards.

Immunosuppression

CORTICOSTEROIDS

1. These drugs inhibit complement and antibody-mediated immunity as well as production of cytokines, including interleukin (IL)-1, IL-2, and interferon gamma.
2. They are an important component of liver transplant immunosuppression as induction agents, in maintenance therapy, or in the treatment of allograft rejection.
3. Side effects include diabetes mellitus, hypertension, hyperlipidemia, and increased risk of osteoporosis.

CYCLOSPORINE AND TACROLIMUS (CALCINEURIN INHIBITORS)

1. These agents block transcription and production of IL-2 and lead to inhibition of T-cell activation.
2. Introduction of cyclosporine in the 1980s led to a significant decline in allograft rejection.
3. Tacrolimus is the most common immunosuppressive agent used following liver transplantation.
4. Drugs are metabolized through the cytochrome P-450 system; therefore, blood levels are affected by medications that induce or inhibit cytochrome P-450 metabolism.
5. Side effects include nephrotoxicity, neurotoxicity, hypertension, diabetes mellitus, and hyperlipidemia.

MYCOPHENOLATE MOFETIL AND MYCOPHENOLIC ACID

1. These antimetabolites inhibit lymphocyte activation through disruption of purine synthesis.
2. They are typically used in maintenance regimens in combination with other agents.
3. Side effects include myelosuppression and gastrointestinal symptoms; no nephrotoxicity occurs.

SIROLIMUS

1   This agent inhibits cytokine-mediated signaling pathways and lymphocyte cell cycle progression and leads to decreased cellular activation and proliferation.
2. Side effects include hyperlipidemia, myelosuppression, gastrointestinal symptoms, delayed wound healing, and possibly hepatic artery thrombosis; no nephrotoxicity occurs.
3. It may be used as an alternative agent in patients with renal failure.

ANTIBODY THERAPY

1. Antithymocyte globulin is a polyclonal antibody directed against T cells that leads to their depletion and that may be used as induction therapy or in the management of acute allograft rejection.
2. OKT-3 is a monoclonal antibody that binds to CD3, inactivates the T-cell receptor, and leads to lymphocyte depletion.
3. Both antithymocyte globulin and OKT-3 can result in profound myelosuppression.
4. Monoclonal antibodies directed against the IL-2 receptor—daclizumab and basiliximab—are used increasingly as induction agents in corticosteroid-sparing regimens.

Post-transplant Complications

PRIMARY GRAFT NONFUNCTION

1. This occurs in the immediate postoperative period.
2. It is characterized by progressive elevations in serum aminotransferase levels and worsening coagulopathy in the absence of vascular abnormalities.
3. It may require repeat transplantation.

HEPATIC ARTERY THROMBOSIS OR STENOSIS

1. It is associated with biliary complications resulting from ischemic injury.
2. Ultrasonography may be useful in the diagnosis.
3. It may require surgical revision; hepatic artery stenosis may be amenable to angioplasty or stent placement.

BILIARY TRACT COMPLICATIONS

1. They occur in up to 25% of liver transplant recipients, typically within the first year.
2. Strictures are the most common biliary complication and may be classified as anastomotic or nonanastomotic based on location.
    - Most biliary strictures (80%) are anastomotic.
    - Nonanastomotic strictures are strongly associated with hepatic artery thrombosis.
3. Arterial patency should be assessed during the evaluation of a suspected biliary stricture.

ALLOGRAFT REJECTION

1. **Acute cellular rejection** is common, occurring in up to 40% of patients, and does not have a major impact on post-transplant survival, although it is associated with significant morbidity.

2. **Chronic rejection** is characterized histologically by ductopenia and may result in progressive allograft dysfunction and the potential need for repeat transplantation.

INFECTIONS

1. **Bacterial and viral infections** are common following liver transplantation as a consequence of immunosuppressive therapy; patients are also at increased risk of **fungal infection**.
2. **Cytomegalovirus (CMV) infection** is most common in CMV-seronegative recipients of CMV-seropositive allografts; infection may be associated with pancytopenia and may result in severe disseminated disease, hepatitis, enterocolitis, or pneumonitis.
3. **Herpes simplex virus** may become reactivated in the setting of immunosuppression.
4. **Epstein–Barr virus** is associated with the development of **post-transplant lymphoproliferative disorder**, which may occur in the setting of primary infection or reactivation.
5. Antimicrobial prophylaxis regimens and immunization are required following liver transplantation to minimize the risk of serious nosocomial, community-acquired, and opportunistic infections.

RENAL FAILURE

1. This is a common post-transplant complication.
2. It typically occurs as a result of long-term calcineurin inhibitor therapy.
3. Use of sirolimus may be beneficial in this setting because of the absence of nephrotoxicity.

RECURRENT DISEASE

1. Recurrent hepatitis C may result in allograft dysfunction, progressive fibrosis, and ultimately allograft failure; many liver transplant programs perform liver biopsies at regular intervals to assess for recurrent disease and the need for antiviral therapy.
2. Following liver transplantation for HCC, close surveillance should be considered, particularly in patients who exceed the Milan criteria, given the increased potential for recurrence.
3. Recurrent disease can also be seen following liver transplantation for autoimmune hepatitis, NAFLD with steatohepatitis, PBC, and PSC.

MALIGNANT DISEASE

1. Patients are at higher risk of de novo extrahepatic malignant diseases following liver transplantation, including post-transplant lymphoproliferative disorder and skin, colorectal, and gynecologic cancers.
2. Close surveillance with standard cancer screening tests is recommended.

POST-TRANSPLANT METABOLIC SYNDROME

1. The development of hypertension, hyperlipidemia, obesity, and diabetes mellitus are common following liver transplantation.
2. These complications result from the combined effects of corticosteroids and immunosuppressive medications.
3. The risk of cardiovascular events and associated mortality may be increased.

FURTHER READING

D'Amico G, Garcia-Tsao G, Pagliaro L. Natural history and prognostic indicators of survival in cirrhosis: a systematic review of 118 studies. *J Hepatol* 2006; 44:217–231.

Eason JD, Gonwa TA, Davis CL, et al. Proceedings of Consensus Conference on Simultaneous Liver Kidney Transplantation (SLK). *Am J Transplant* 2008; 8:2243–2251.

Freeman RB, Gish RG, Harper A, et al. Model for End-Stage Liver Disease (MELD) exception guidelines: results and recommendations from the MELD exception study group and conference (MESSAGE) for approval of patients who need liver transplantation with diseases not considered by the standard MELD formula. *Liver Transpl* 2006; 12(Suppl):S128–S136.

Kamath PS, Wiesner RH, Malinchoc M, et al. A model to predict survival in patients with end-stage liver disease. *Hepatology* 2001; 33:464–470.

Mazzaferro V, Regalia E, Doci R, et al. Liver transplantation for the treatment of small hepatocellular carcinomas in patients with cirrhosis. *N Engl J Med* 1996; 334:693–699.

Merion RM, Schaubel DE, Dykstra DM, et al. The survival benefit of liver transplantation. *Am J Transplant* 2005; 5:307–313.

Murray KF, Carithers RL Jr. AASLD practice guidelines: evaluation of the patient for liver transplantation. *Hepatology* 2005; 41:1407–1432.

Pomfret EA, Washburn K, Wald C, et al. Report of a national conference of liver allocation in patients with hepatocellular carcinoma in the United States. *Liver Transpl* 2010; 16:262–278.

Wiesner R, Edwards E, Freeman R, et al. Model for end-stage liver disease (MELD) and allocation of donor livers. *Gastroenterology* 2003; 124:91–96.

CHAPTER 32

Cholelithiasis and cholecystitis

Peter F. Malet, MD ■ Jay P. Babich, MD

KEY POINTS

1   The two main types of gallstones are cholesterol and pigment. The pathogenesis of cholesterol and pigment stones is different, but the clinical syndromes they cause are similar.

2   Most gallbladder stones are asymptomatic. When they become symptomatic, biliary pain is the most common manifestation. Hallmarks of biliary pain are its episodic nature and location in the upper abdomen, usually in the right upper quadrant. Other conditions may coexist with gallstones and account for symptoms attributed initially to the stones.

3   The treatment of choice for symptomatic gallbladder stones is laparoscopic cholecystectomy; when this approach is not feasible, open cholecystectomy is the alternative. Magnetic resonance cholangiopancreatography (MRCP) or endoscopic retrograde cholangiopancreatography (ERCP) may be used to investigate for bile duct stones preoperatively.

4   Acute cholecystitis is the most common complication of gallstones. Cholecystectomy is the treatment of choice. Consultation with the internist, gastroenterologist, and surgeon is warranted to arrive at the most efficient plan for care.

5   Acute acalculous cholecystitis requires a high index of suspicion for diagnosis; patients are usually quite ill, and rapid therapy is necessary.

Classification of Gallstones

1. Gallstones are common worldwide and, although mostly asymptomatic, can result in a wide spectrum of symptoms and presentations.
2. The two main types of gallstones are cholesterol and pigment.
3. Cholesterol and pigment stones have distinctly different compositions, pathogeneses, and clinical associations.
4. In the United States and other Western countries, most (generally 80% to 90%) stones in the gallbladder are cholesterol stones. Pigment stones comprise the remainder. In some South American countries, pigment stones are rare. In some East Asian countries, the proportion of pigment stones is significantly higher than that in Western countries.
5. The clinical syndromes caused by gallstones in the gallbladder are similar regardless of the type of stone involved.

CHOLESTEROL STONES

1. These stones are composed primarily of cholesterol (proportion varies, generally greater than 60%) and mucin, calcium salts of bilirubin, phosphate, carbonate, and palmitate, and small

amounts of various other substances. "Pure" (100%) cholesterol stones account for approximately 10% to 15% of all cholesterol stones.

2. Some stones contain less than 60% cholesterol but have the morphologic and microstructural features of typical cholesterol stones; these are termed *mixed stones.*

3. Major clinical associations with cholesterol stones are as follows:
   - Aging
   - Female gender
   - Obesity
   - Pregnancy
   - Rapid weight loss
   - Native American ethnicity
   - Genetic factors

PIGMENT STONES

1. These are composed mostly of pigment and calcium salts.
2. The two types of pigment stones are black and brown.
   a. **Black pigment stones**: black and composed primarily of calcium bilirubinate and other pigment, mucin, calcium salts of phosphate and carbonate, and small amounts of various other substances. These stones are found almost exclusively in the gallbladder and only rarely in the bile ducts (BDs). Most patients have no identifiable predisposing condition. The major known associated conditions are as follows:
      - Old age
      - Cirrhosis
      - Hemolysis (particularly sickle cell disease and hereditary spherocytosis)
      - Possibly total parenteral nutrition (TPN)
   b. **Brown pigment stones**: typically brown and composed primarily of calcium bilirubinate, cholesterol, calcium palmitate, and small amounts of various other substances These stones are found mostly in the BDs and, in East Asia, frequently in the gallbladder as well; in Western countries, brown stones in the gallbladder are unusual.
      - Most patients with brown stones in the BDs have stasis and/or infection as a predisposing condition. This type of stone may occur in patients many years after cholecystectomy.

Pathogenesis

CHOLESTEROL STONES

1. Supersaturation of bile with cholesterol (cholesterol saturation index [CSI] greater than 1.00) is a necessary but not sufficient condition. Also thought to be important are an absolute or relative increase in gallbladder mucin, other nucleating factors, and calcium ions and possibly a decrease in antinucleating factors. Gallbladder stasis plays a role in some cases.

2. Initial events in cholesterol stone formation involve the nucleation of cholesterol monohydrate crystals from biliary cholesterol-phospholipid vesicles and formation of a stone nidus by an aggregation of calcium salts, pigment, and/or mucin. The nucleation time of gallbladder bile (time to formation of cholesterol crystals) in patients with cholesterol stones is significantly shorter than that in normal controls.

PIGMENT STONES

1. **Black pigment**: Precipitation of calcium salts and pigment is the major pathophysiologic event. Failure to maintain calcium ions in solution is considered important, resulting in the precipitation of calcium bilirubinate, phosphate, and carbonate. Gallbladder mucin is thought to act as a nucleating factor, and other nucleating factors are postulated to be involved.

2. **Brown pigment**: Precipitation of calcium bilirubinate and calcium salts of fatty acids is the major pathophysiologic event. Beta glucuronidase from bacterial or tissue sources is important in deconjugating bilirubin and in causing its precipitation with calcium; an analogous process is thought to result in fatty acid precipitation. Biliary stasis and bacteria in bile are believed to be important for stone formation.

Diagnosis

1. Ultrasonography
   - Fast, readily available, noninvasive
   - Limited by operator skill
   - Limited in determining size or number of stones present
   - 95% sensitivity for detecting gallstones 1.5 mm or more in diameter
2. Computed tomography (CT)
   - Often provides more extensive information than ultrasonography
   - Not as sensitive as ultrasonography because some stones do not contain enough calcium to be detected
   - Some benefit in detecting BD stones
   - Useful in the diagnosis of suspected biliary pancreatitis
3. Magnetic resonance cholangiopancreatography (MRCP)
   - Not recommended for the diagnosis of gallbladder stones
   - Useful when the probability of BD stones is low to intermediate
   - Has replaced diagnostic endoscopic retrograde cholangiopancreatography (ERCP) for detection of BD stones
   - 85% sensitivity for detecting BD stones
4. Endoscopic ultrasonography (EUS)
   - Excellent for detecting ampullary stones
   - Excellent visualization of gallbladder and pancreatobiliary system without interference from bowel gas, liver, or subcutaneous tissue
   - Can detect presence of cholelithiasis in patients who have had negative ultrasonography results
   - More than 90% sensitivity for the diagnosis of gallbladder stones (Fig. 32.1) or BD stones

Natural History

ASYMPTOMATIC GALLSTONES

Increased use of ultrasonography in the evaluation of abdominal pain has led to the identification of incidental gallstones. **Most patients with gallstones are asymptomatic** and remain asymptomatic after decades of follow-up. The rate at which asymptomatic patients develop biliary

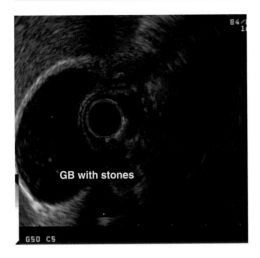

Fig. 32.1 Endoscopic ultrasonographic image of a gallbladder filled with gallstones. *(Courtesy of David M. Friedel, MD.)*

pain is approximately 1% to 2% annually. The risk of presenting initially with a complication rather than with biliary pain alone is low. **Because the rate of developing symptoms is low, the consensus is that asymptomatic patients with gallstones should not undergo prophylactic cholecystectomy.**

BILIARY PAIN

The term *biliary pain* is preferred to *biliary colic*, because biliary pain is not true colic. It is thought to arise from transient obstruction of the cystic duct by stones or sludge.

1. Features
   - Location in the right upper quadrant or epigastrium: It may radiate around to the right lower to middle back or occasionally to the right shoulder.
   - It may range from mild to severe and may be described as cramping, pressure-like, toothachy, stabbing, like childbirth, or like a heavy weight. Patients often state that they cannot find a comfortable position during an attack and may walk around waiting for the pain to end. Some patients may experience nausea during an episode, but vomiting is uncommon. Patients have no systemic signs of toxicity.

   - It usually has a definite onset with a duration of 15 to 30 minutes, lasting up to 3 to 4 hours. A duration longer than 12 hours is unusual unless acute cholecystitis is developing.
   - Episodic nature: The interval between episodes varies from daily to once every few months or even longer; some patients have only one episode every year or more. It is unusual for a patient to have only a single episode of biliary pain.

   - In many cases, biliary pain may not be as typical as just described.
   - The term *chronic cholecystitis* is still used by some clinicians to describe the condition in which a patient experiences repeated bouts of biliary pain. Strictly speaking, the term should be used to describe histologic changes in the gallbladder.
   - The correlation between the pathologic changes in the gallbladder and clinical symptoms is often inexact.

2. Differential diagnosis of right upper quadrant and epigastric abdominal pain
    - Peptic ulcer disease
    - Choledocholithiasis
    - Pancreatitis
    - Gastroesophageal reflux
    - Angina pectoris
    - Bowel obstruction
    - Liver-related conditions
    - Lower rib pain
    - Irritable bowel syndrome
    - Nephrolithiasis

3. Natural history
    - Approximately 75% of patients will have at least one additional attack within a 2-year period.
    - The risk of developing a serious complication (acute cholecystitis, pancreatitis, or cholangitis) in a patient who has experienced a first episode of biliary pain is approximately 1% to 2% per year.

Surgical Treatment

1. Clinicians generally agree that **cholecystectomy for asymptomatic gallstones is not warranted**, with few exceptions, subject to individual patient and physician preference. One exception is porcelain gallbladder (see later) because of the risk of cancer.
2. The threshold for performing cholecystectomy for abdominal symptoms atypical of biliary pain varies considerably among surgeons.

ELECTIVE SURGERY FOR BILIARY PAIN

1. **Laparoscopic cholecystectomy (LC)** is the treatment of choice for symptomatic gallstones.
2. **Approximately 5% to 10% of patients undergoing cholecystectomy will have stones in the BD, often asymptomatic.** The possibility of BD stones may have to be evaluated before elective cholecystectomy based on clinical, radiologic, and laboratory features (see Chapter 33).
3. Approximately 5% of planned LCs are converted to an open cholecystectomy at the surgeon's discretion, usually because of dense adhesions or other technical factors. Occasionally, an initial attempt at LC may be deemed inappropriate because of expected extensive right upper quadrant scarring related to previous surgery.

Medical Treatment

BILE SALTS (URSODEOXYCHOLIC ACID, OR URSODIOL)

1. This treatment is rarely used. It may be considered in patients with radiolucent stones who are at high surgical risk or who refuse surgery.
2. The overall dissolution rate for all patients is only 20% to 30%. The highest success rates (approximately 60% to 70%) are in patients with stones smaller than 5 mm in diameter. Oral dissolution therapy is not recommended for stones larger than 20 mm.

3. Patients with frequent or relatively severe biliary pain are not good candidates because treatment for 12 to 24 months is required for dissolution.
4. The recommended dose of ursodeoxycholic acid is 10 mg/kg per day.
5. After complete dissolution, stones recur in approximately 50% of patients within 5 years.

Acute Cholecystitis

Acute cholecystitis is the most common acute complication of gallbladder stones and is the leading indication for emergency cholecystectomy. Usually, the diagnosis is straightforward, but in some cases the presentation is atypical. In managing acute gallstone complications, the pace of the diagnostic evaluation, the number and type of diagnostic studies, and the threshold for therapeutic intervention are dictated by the patient's overall condition.

1. Pathogenesis
   - Cystic duct obstruction is the precipitating event, usually caused by a stone, but mucus, sludge, and viscous bile may also play a role.
   - Bacteria are not involved in the initial events, although the inflamed gallbladder may later become secondarily infected.
   - The release of intracellular enzymes and the activation of inflammatory mediators are consequences of bile stasis and lead to inflammation of the gallbladder mucosa.
2. Clinical features: range from deceptively mild to quite severe with systemic toxicity
   a. Up to 75% of patients with acute cholecystitis report prior attacks of biliary pain.
   b. Most patients present with moderate pain in the epigastrium or right upper quadrant, which may radiate to the right shoulder or scapula. The pain usually has been present for several hours, commonly 3 to 6 hours, before the patient seeks medical attention.
   c. Many patients have nausea and some have vomiting, although rarely severe. They may be febrile, but usually not with a temperature higher than 102°F; a higher fever suggests bacteremia or an abscess.
   d. Patients have right upper quadrant tenderness and often Murphy's sign (accentuated tenderness to palpation during inspiration).
   e. In some cases, it may be difficult to determine whether the patient has mild acute cholecystitis or prolonged biliary pain. Admission to the hospital for continued observation and testing is justified and usually resolves the issue.
   f. Variations in the presentation of acute cholecystitis include the following:
      - No or minimal pain and tenderness may be reported, particularly in an elderly or obtunded patient. Acute cholecystitis should be considered in all patients with unexplained bacteremia or sepsis, intra-abdominal abscess, or peritonitis.
      - Some patients present in a toxic manner with high fever, severe abdominal pain and tenderness, bacteremia, and marked leukocytosis. When a suppurative complication such as an abscess is suspected, CT is useful.
      - Some patients present with symptoms and signs typical of biliary disease and decompensation of one or more organ systems or multisystem organ failure. In such cases, stabilization of the patient's overall medical condition takes precedence over cholecystectomy, and drainage of the gallbladder through cholecystostomy may need to be considered.
3. Laboratory features
   - A white blood cell (WBC) count of 10 to 15,000/mm^3 is typical.
   - Serum aspartate aminotransferase (AST), alanine aminotransferase (ALT), alkaline phosphatase, and bilirubin levels may be normal or just slightly elevated.

- If the alkaline phosphatase level is disproportionately elevated relative to the aminotransferase levels, choledocholithiasis should be considered, and the diameter of the BDs should be determined by a radiologic study, such as ultrasonography or CT.

4. Diagnosis
   - The diagnosis of acute cholecystitis is based on the combination of characteristic clinical features and confirmatory radiologic studies.
   - Ultrasonography or radionuclide hepatobiliary scanning with iminodiacetic acid derivatives (hepatic 2,6-dimethyliminodiacetic acid [HIDA] or diisopropyl iminodiacetic acid [DISIDA]) may be used.

   a. Hepatobiliary scanning
      - This is performed by injecting a fasting patient with radiolabeled HIDA or DISIDA, which is taken up by the liver and excreted into bile. Normally, the radionuclide enters the gallbladder and is excreted into the duodenum within 1 to 2 hours. If the gallbladder does not fill by 1 hour, intravenous morphine may be administered to enhance gallbladder filling (morphine-augmented hepatobiliary scanning). In patients with acute cholecystitis, the radionuclide fails to enter the gallbladder but does enter the duodenum (except with high-grade BD obstruction).
      - A **positive** scan (read 3 to 4 hours after injection) reveals **nonfilling of the gallbladder** with excretion of the radionuclide into the small bowel.
      - The sensitivity and specificity of hepatobiliary scanning for acute cholecystitis are approximately 95% and 90%, respectively.
      - False-positive results may occur in patients with gallbladder stasis; this can present a diagnostic problem in patients with suspected acute acalculous cholecystitis (AAC; see later).

   b. Ultrasonography
      - Signs of acute cholecystitis include gallstones, a dilated gallbladder, a thickened gallbladder wall (thicker than 4 mm), edema within the gallbladder wall, and pericholecystic fluid.
      - Ultrasonography is more operator dependent than hepatobiliary scanning but provides more information, is more rapidly performed, and is generally available throughout the day and night. Dilatation of the BD can be readily detected on ultrasonography.
      - The sensitivity and specificity of ultrasonography for acute cholecystitis are 90% to 95% and 80%, respectively.

5. Treatment

   Measures to take within the first few hours after admission in patients with suspected acute cholecystitis include the following:
   - Complete blood count with differential
   - Comprehensive metabolic panel
   - Blood cultures
   - Ultrasonography or hepatobiliary scan
   - Surgical consultation

   a. Initial treatment
      - The usual practice is to administer antibiotics to all patients with acute cholecystitis. Coverage for enterococci and gram-negative aerobic organisms is usually sufficient. In patients who are extremely toxic, coverage for anaerobic organisms is also judicious.
      - Intravenous fluids must be started immediately.
      - Any electrolyte (particularly potassium, magnesium, calcium, and phosphorus) abnormality or acid-base imbalance should be corrected.

- Patients should take nothing by mouth; rarely, a nasogastric tube may be required if vomiting is severe.
- Mild analgesia may be necessary for pain, but symptoms and signs should not be masked.
- Medical treatment of associated medical conditions should be prompt and thorough, in anticipation of surgery.

  b. Course after hospital admission

- Most patients improve over 24 to 72 hours without surgical intervention. This allows time to optimize fluid and electrolyte status and to treat any other coexisting medical conditions before planned surgery.
- Some patients either do not improve after admission or worsen. In such cases, urgent surgical intervention must be strongly considered.
- If the patient has a seriously decompensated medical condition, such as heart failure or pulmonary insufficiency, attention must be directed to this condition before surgery or another intervention. In such patients, serious consideration must be given to either surgical or radiologically guided **cholecystostomy** as a temporizing measure for relieving cholecystitis.

6. Timing of surgery

Immediate surgical consultation should be obtained for patients with suspected acute cholecystitis.

7. Treatment options for acute cholecystitis

- LC
- Open cholecystectomy
- Cholecystostomy: Surgical or radiologically guided cholecystectomy may be performed as soon as the diagnosis is reasonably secure and the patient is stable enough to undergo the surgery. Generally, this is within the first 2 to 4 days after admission. In most cases, LC is appropriate.

- When a complication, such as an abscess, gangrenous wall, or perforation, has occurred or is suspected, open cholecystectomy is warranted.
- Patients with cirrhosis are at particularly high risk for surgery and require optimization of their medical status preoperatively. Transfusion of fresh frozen plasma may be necessary to correct severe coagulation defects (see Chapter 30).

Acute Acalculous Cholecystitis

Acute cholecystitis in the absence of gallstones in the gallbladder is termed acalculous cholecystitis (AAC). AAC accounts for less than 5% of all cases of acute cholecystitis and is most frequently encountered in already hospitalized patients but is also occasionally seen in outpatients.

1. Pathogenesis

- As with calculous disease, cystic duct occlusion is thought to be the principal pathophysiologic event in AAC. Ductal occlusion may result from sludge, microlithiasis, viscous bile, or mucus and mural inflammation and edema.
- Gallbladder stasis is also a factor.
- Gallbladder ischemia is considered to play an important role.

2. **Clinical associations: most common following nonbiliary tract surgery, severe burns, severe trauma, sepsis, or use of TPN.**

- Other associations include human immunodeficiency virus infection, vasculitis, allergic arteritis, and *Salmonella* infection.
- Sometimes, no identifiable underlying condition is present.

3. Diagnosis
   - A high index of suspicion for AAC is warranted because symptoms and signs may be less apparent than in calculous disease, particularly in hospitalized patients with serious underlying disorders and on mechanical ventilation. Some patients may present with fever and bacteremia alone.
   - Ultrasonography or hepatobiliary scanning should be performed immediately if AAC is suspected. Ultrasonography may show sludge in the gallbladder lumen, in addition to the ultrasonographic signs of cholecystitis seen with calculous disease. Hepatobiliary scanning results are positive in more than 90% of patients with AAC.
   - When diagnostic uncertainty exists despite hepatobiliary scanning and ultrasonography, particularly if the patient is septic, **diagnostic ultrasound-guided percutaneous puncture of the gallbladder** should be considered. If examination of the aspirated bile suggests infection, a catheter can be left in place for gallbladder drainage, thus providing therapy as well.
   - AAC has a high mortality rate, especially if treatment is delayed. Gangrene, perforation, and abscess of the gallbladder are more frequent than in calculous cholecystitis.
4. Treatment
   - Medical measures are the same as for calculous cholecystitis; broad antibiotic coverage is indicated.
   - Optimally, cholecystectomy should be performed without undue delay. An open approach is required more often than for calculous disease.
   - In patients too ill to undergo cholecystectomy, either surgical or radiologically guided cholecystostomy for gallbladder drainage may be performed.

Postcholecystectomy Problems

- The term *postcholecystectomy syndrome* has been used to describe persisting symptoms after cholecystectomy; it usually applies to patients who are past the immediate postsurgical period, to avoid confusion with immediate postsurgical incisional pain. The term is nonspecific, and its use should be discouraged (see Chapter 33).
- Most commonly, persisting symptoms after cholecystectomy are caused by a condition that the patient had preoperatively and that is not related to gallstones, such as gastroesophageal reflux, peptic ulcer, or irritable bowel syndrome.
- Retained BD stones may occur in a small percentage of patients after cholecystectomy. Elevated liver enzyme levels and a dilated BD on ultrasonography are usually found in these patients (see Chapter 33).

Biliary Sludge

The same symptoms and complications that can occur with gallstones may also occur with biliary sludge, although probably less frequently.

DEFINITION

- The term *sludge* is used to describe microscopic agglomerations of cholesterol crystals, mucin, calcium bilirubinate, and other pigment crystals. Sometimes, microspheroliths (microscopic gallstones) are also present.

PATHOGENESIS

- Sludge does not inevitably progress to stone formation.
- In most cases of sludge, no definable clinical association is apparent. Predisposing conditions include prolonged TPN, pregnancy, and use of the antibiotic ceftriaxone.
- The presumed mechanism for sludge formation is nucleation (precipitation) of cholesterol crystals in bile; gallbladder stasis probably plays a role in many cases. Factors that maintain calcium in solution may be disrupted and may contribute to the precipitation of calcium bilirubinate.

DIAGNOSIS

- On abdominal ultrasonography, sludge appears as mobile echogenic material within the lumen without acoustic shadowing.
- EUS can also detect sludge.

NATURAL HISTORY

- This is not well established; spontaneous resolution and reappearance of sludge may occur over time.
- Gallbladder sludge may be associated with acute cholecystitis, acute cholangitis, and probably acute pancreatitis.

TREATMENT

- This depends on the clinical setting and similar to the treatment of gallstones.
- In asymptomatic cases, observation alone is sufficient.

Other Less Common Syndromes Associated with Gallstones

1. **Porcelain gallbladder** (calcification in the gallbladder wall) may develop over many years and, if dense enough, may be detected on plain abdominal radiographs or, if less dense, by CT. Gallbladder carcinoma is found in a variable proportion of gallbladders with wall calcification, especially mucosal calcification. Prophylactic cholecystectomy has been recommended for patients with porcelain gallbladder.
2. **Mirizzi's syndrome** is the obstruction of the common hepatic duct as a result of extrinsic compression from a stone impacted in the cystic duct or the gallbladder neck. The patient usually presents with symptoms typical of acute cholangitis: fever, right upper quadrant pain, and jaundice.
   - Treatment is by cholecystectomy; preoperative ERCP is typically required for biliary decompression as well as to reduce operative risk to the BD.
3. **Cholecystoenteric fistula** results from erosion of a gallstone, usually large, through the gallbladder wall into an adjacent organ.
   - The most common sites of fistulization are into the duodenum, right side of the colon, stomach, and jejunum. Stones larger than 2.5 cm may produce bowel obstruction, commonly referred to as *gallstone ileus;* the terminal ileum is the most common site of obstruction.
   - Fistulae that are asymptomatic usually do not require intervention; those that are symptomatic require bowel closure along with cholecystectomy.

4. Emphysematous cholecystitis is characterized by clinical manifestations that are similar to, but more severe than, those of acute cholecystitis; gas-forming organisms have secondarily infected the gallbladder wall. Imaging demonstrates pockets of gas in the area of the gallbladder fossa. Urgent initiation of anaerobic coverage with appropriate antibiotics and early cholecystectomy are recommended.

FURTHER READING

Elwood DR. Cholecystitis. *Surg Clin North Am* 2008; 88:1241–1252.

Everhart JE, Yeh F, Lee ET, et al. Prevalence of gallbladder disease in American Indian populations: findings from the Strong Heart Study. *Hepatology* 2002; 35:1507–1512.

Glasgow RE, Mulvihill SJ. Treatment of gallstone disease. In: Feldman M, Friedman LS, Brandt LJ, eds. *Sleisinger and Fordtran's Gastrointestinal and Liver Disease: Pathophysiology/Diagnosis/Management*, 9th edn. Philadelphia: Saunders Elsevier, 2010:1121–1138.

Grundy SM. Cholesterol gallstones: a fellow traveler with metabolic syndrome? *Am J Clin Nutr* 2004; 80:1–2.

Halpert RD. Biliary system and gallbladder. In: *Gastrointestinal Imaging*. 3rd edn. St. Louis: Mosby Elsevier; 2006: 221–260.

Harinck F, Bruno MJ. Endosonography in the management of biliopancreatic disorders. *Best Pract Res Clin Gastroenterol* 2009; 23:703–710.

Napolean B, Markoglou C, Lefort C, Durivage G. EUS in bile duct, ampullary and gallbladder lesions. In: Hawes RH, Fockens P, eds. *Endosonography*. Philadelphia: Saunders Elsevier; 2006:217–238.

Paumgartner G, Greenberger NJ. Gallstone disease. In: Greenberger NJ, Blumberg R, Burakoff R, eds. *Current Diagnosis and Treatment: Gastroenterology, Hepatology, and Endoscopy*. New York: McGraw-Hill; 2009:537–546.

Portincasa P, Moschetta A, Palasciano G. Cholesterol gallstone disease. *Lancet* 2006; 368:230–239.

Ryu JK, Ryu KH, Kim KH. Clinical features of acute acalculous cholecystitis. *J Clin Gastroenterol* 2003; 36:166–169.

Sakorafas GH, Milingos D, Peros G. Asymptomatic cholelithiasis: is cholecystectomy really needed? A critical reappraisal 15 years after introduction of laparoscopic cholecystectomy. *Dig Dis Sci* 2007; 52:1313–1325.

Tse F, Liu L, Barkun AN, et al. EUS: a meta-analysis of test performance in suspected choledocholithiasis. *Gastrointest Endosc* 2008; 67:235–244.

Wang DQ-H, Afdhal NH. Gallstone disease. In: Feldman M, Friedman LS, Brandt LJ, eds. *Sleisinger and Fordtran's Gastrointestinal and Liver Disease: Pathophysiology/Diagnosis/Management*. 9th edn. Philadelphia: Saunders Elsevier; 2010:1089–1120.

Yosoff IF, Barkun JS, Barjun AN. Diagnosis and management of cholecystitis and cholangitis. *Gastroenterol Clin North Am* 2003; 32:1145–1168.

CHAPTER 33

Diseases of the bile ducts

Ira M. Jacobson, MD ■ Douglas M. Weine, MD

Bile Duct Stones

COMPOSITION

1. Most BD stones are cholesterol stones that have formed in the gallbladder.
2. Black pigment stones are formed in the gallbladder and are associated with hemolytic disorders such as sickle cell disease. They are also common in persons with cirrhosis.
3. Brown pigment stones make up the majority of BD pigment stones, form within the BD, and are associated with chronic biliary stasis, biliary strictures, and recurrent pyogenic cholangitis.

CLINICAL FEATURES

1. Presenting features of BD stones are as follows:
   - Pain
   - Cholangitis
   - Pancreatitis
   - Jaundice
2. Pain from BD stones resembles pain of gallbladder origin.
   - Epigastric or right upper quadrant pain is present.
   - Abdominal tenderness is greater with cholecystitis than with BD stones.
   - Obstructive jaundice from BD stones is usually accompanied by pain.
   - Jaundice associated with malignancy is more likely to be painless.
3. Features of cholangitis include the following:
   - **Charcot's triad**, consisting of abdominal pain, fever, and jaundice: Each feature may not be present in all patients with cholangitis.
   - **Reynolds' pentad** consists of Charcot's triad plus hypotension and altered mental status.
   - Fever may be accompanied by severe rigors.
   - Cholangitis is more frequent with BD stones than with malignant BD obstruction.
   - Severe cholangitis must be considered life-threatening and requires urgent intervention.
4. The timing of presentation with BD stones is variable:
   - Before cholecystectomy
   - During intraoperative cholangiography (IOC)
   - Shortly after cholecystectomy
   - Months to years or decades after cholecystectomy
5. Gallstone pancreatitis (see later)
   - Small gallstones pose a greater risk of pancreatitis than do large stones (they migrate more easily through the cystic duct).

LABORATORY FEATURES

1. Elevations in serum liver biochemical test levels include alanine aminotransferase (ALT), aspartate aminotransferase (AST), alkaline phosphatase, gamma glutamyltranspeptidase (GGTP), and bilirubin.
   - **Marked elevations in serum ALT and AST levels may occur,** even levels higher than 1000 U/L transiently, especially with cholangitis.
   - Levels fall rapidly, even as the alkaline phosphatase level rises if stone impaction persists.
   - This condition can be confused with hepatitis.
2. Elevations in serum amylase and lipase levels suggest concomitant acute pancreatitis.
3. Elevations in the white blood cell (WBC) count occur with cholangitis or pancreatitis.
4. Positive blood cultures can be found with cholangitis.

IMAGING STUDIES

1. Ultrasonography
   - Excellent for detecting gallbladder stones; less sensitive for BD stones
   - May be limited by obesity, gas in the intestine
   - Sensitive for detecting BD dilatation
   - More sensitive for BD stones when the duct is dilated
   - Absence of BD dilatation or detectable stones does not exclude BD stones

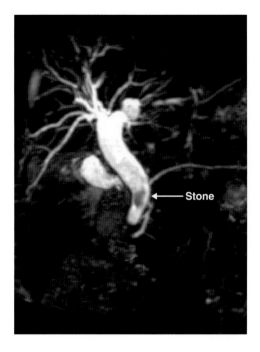

Fig. 33.1 Magnetic resonance cholangiographic image showing a large stone in the distal bile duct.

2. Computed tomography (CT)
   - Sensitivity lower than 50% for BD stones
   - Detection depends on the presence of calcifications in stones
   - Sensitivity similar to that of ultrasonography for detecting a dilated BD
   - Need to avoid oral contrast agents on initial images (can obscure BD stones)
3. Magnetic resonance cholangiopancreatography (MRCP) (Fig. 33.1)
   a. Detection of BD stones depends on T2-weighted images
   b. Contrast provided by fluid in the ducts
   c. Sensitivity and specificity greater than 90%
   d. Sensitivity lower for small stones
   e. Limited availability and high cost; contraindications include pacemakers, defibrillators, or certain other metallic implants
      - Feasibility should be checked with the radiologist regarding compatibility with orthopedic implants.
4. Endoscopic ultrasonography (EUS) (Fig. 33.2)
   - Sensitivity and specificity rival those of endoscopic retrograde cholangiopancreatography (ERCP)
   - Less risk than ERCP but still an endoscopic procedure requiring sedation
   - Most suitable for choledocholithiasis when EUS and ERCP can be performed at the same session
5. ERCP (Fig. 33.3)
   - Has been the "gold standard"
   - Can miss small stones, especially in dilated ducts
   - Most often done when therapeutic intervention is anticipated
   - Risks of ERCP include pancreatitis, bleeding (usually from sphincterotomy), retroperitoneal perforation, and anesthesiology-related complications.

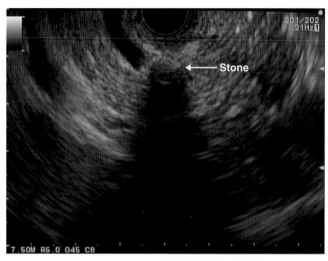

Fig. 33.2 Endoscopic ultrasonographic image of a bile duct stone.

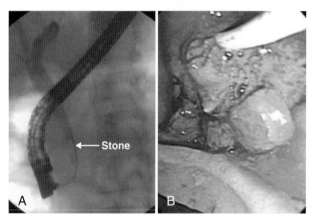

Fig. 33.3 **A,** Endoscopic retrograde cholangiogram (ERC) showing a distal bile duct stone (arrow) before stone extraction. **B,** Stone adjacent to the sphincterotomy site after balloon extraction.

6. Percutaneous transhepatic cholangiography (THC)
   - Seldom used for evaluation or treatment of BD stones, except with acute cholangitis when ERCP is unavailable or fails or is anatomically impossible because of prior surgery
   - Occasionally used to facilitate a "rendezvous procedure" (combined THC and ERCP) when ERCP alone fails

TREATMENT

1. **ERCP and endoscopic sphincterotomy**: treatment of choice at most centers
   - Successful clearance of BD in more than 90% of patients
   - Definitive treatment of BD stones in postcholecystectomy patients

- Most common treatment of BD stones when laparoscopic cholecystectomy is planned and BD stones are documented or strongly suspected
- Permits leaving gallbladder intact after ERCP in patients at high risk for surgery; need for subsequent cholecystectomy is 10% to 20% within 5 to 10 years

2. Role of preoperative versus postoperative ERCP
   a. ERCP has no routine preoperative role.

   b. Risk factors for BD stones are as follows:
      - Elevated liver biochemical test levels
      - BD dilatation on imaging
      - BD stones seen on imaging
      - Initial presentation with cholangitis

   c. Preoperative ERCP is appropriate when the suspicion for BD stones is high.
   d. Postoperative ERCP is effective therapy if BD stones are confirmed on IOC.
   e. Unsuccessful postoperative ERCP may result in a second operation (should seldom occur in experienced centers).

3. Laparoscopic cholecystectomy plus extraction of BD stones
   - High success rates (80% to 90%) are reported by expert surgeons when IOC results are positive for BD stones.
   - The usual approach is the transcystic duct route.
   - Laparoscopic choledochotomy is also possible.
   - Surgical expertise is still not widely available.
   - Many surgeons prefer preoperative or postoperative ERCP.

4. Open choledochotomy
   - This was standard care before ERCP in the 1970s; it is seldom performed currently except for large retained stones not extractable by other methods.
   - It is performed either at the time of cholecystectomy or after a patient presents with symptomatic choledocholithiasis.
   - If the gallbladder contains stones, laparoscopic cholecystectomy after ERCP extraction of BD stones is usually performed, but leaving the gallbladder intact is an option in high-risk patients.

5. ERCP techniques for the treatment of choledocholithiasis
   - Guidewire cannulation of BD using a sphincterotome is a common technique; the sphincterotome is advanced over a guidewire into the BD.
   - Needle-knife precut sphincterotomy is performed when cannulation of the BD is difficult.

6. Large stones: may require more advanced ERCP techniques
   - Mechanical lithotripsy with a large basket
   - Extracorporeal shock wave lithotripsy (rarely used in the United States)
   - Laser lithotripsy through choledochoscopy: "baby scope" inserted into the BD through the channel of a side-viewing endoscope
   - Electrohydraulic lithotripsy through a "baby scope"

7. Complications of ERCP and sphincterotomy
   a. **Pancreatitis** occurs in 5% of patients. It may result either from the diagnostic portion of the procedure or from cautery-induced injury to the pancreatic duct orifice.
      - Symptoms of pancreatitis may not occur until 6 to 12 hours following the procedure.
      - Management of post-ERCP pancreatitis is similar to that of other forms of pancreatitis.
      - No pharmacologic means of proven efficacy exist to prevent ERCP-related pancreatitis.
      - Pancreatitis is more common in patients with a difficult cannulation, suspected or proven sphincter of Oddi dysfunction (SOD), or a needle-knife precut sphincterotomy.

- Temporary placement of a stent in the pancreatic duct appears to reduce the risk, as well as the severity, of post-ERCP pancreatitis.
  b. **Bleeding** occurs in 2% to 3% and is usually self-limited.
    - It may occasionally require blood transfusions and even angiographic embolization or surgery.
    - Epinephrine injection, balloon tamponade, or electrocautery at the time of ERCP may stop bleeding.
  c. **Perforation** (usually retroperitoneal) occurs in 1%.
    - It often responds to nonsurgical management with nasogastric decompression, nasobiliary drainage (if the complication has been recognized during ERCP), and intravenous broad-spectrum antibiotics.
    - Surgery is required if signs of infection cannot be controlled with antibiotics.
  d. **Infection** may occur when adequate drainage is not provided following ERCP.
    - An endoprosthesis should be placed to provide drainage until the BD can be cleared.
8. Long-term stent placement
   - It is reserved for patients in whom stone extraction is not accomplished.
   - It is most appropriate for frail or elderly patients.
   - Cholangitis occurs in 10% to 40% in ensuing years.
9. Ursodeoxycholic acid in addition to endoprosthesis placement reportedly can result in significant shrinkage or even dissolution of retained duct stones, thus facilitating subsequent attempts to clear the duct after a stent has been placed.
10. Oral dissolution therapy with bile salts is not appropriate as the sole treatment of BD stones.
11. Surgery should be performed for otherwise unextractable BD stones in good operative candidates.
12. Urgent ERCP in combination with intravenous broad-spectrum antibiotics (e.g., piperacillin/tazobactam or metronidazole plus a fluoroquinolone), pending blood culture results, is indicated in patients with severe cholangitis.

GALLSTONE PANCREATITIS

1. This is related to impaction of a stone in the ampulla of Vater with occlusion of the pancreatic duct orifice.

2. Clinical features at presentation
   - Epigastric pain radiating through to the back
   - Nausea and vomiting
   - Low-grade fever
   - Tachycardia
   - Hypotension, if sequestration, or "third-spacing," of fluid is significant

3. Laboratory features
   - Leukocytosis
   - Elevated liver biochemical test levels (usually to a greater degree than in alcoholic and other causes of pancreatitis)
   - Elevated serum amylase and lipase levels
   - Elevated blood urea nitrogen and creatinine levels if third-spacing is sufficient to compromise renal blood flow
   - Hypocalcemia in moderate to severe cases
   - Hyperglycemia

■ Hypoxemia in severe cases resulting from pulmonary capillary leak, which may result in acute respiratory distress syndrome

4. **Ranson's criteria:** This is the most commonly used of the many classification systems to predict the severity of an episode of acute pancreatitis. On admission, the following are noted:
   ■ Age greater than 55 years
   ■ Blood glucose level higher than 200 mg/dL
   ■ WBC count higher than 16 000/mm^3
   ■ Serum lactate dehydrogenase (LDH) level higher than 350 IU/L
   ■ Serum AST level higher than 250 U/L
   At 48 hours, the following are noted:
   ■ Decrease in hematocrit value by more than 10%
   ■ Serum calcium level lower than 8 mg/dL
   ■ Base deficit greater than 4 mmol/L
   ■ Blood urea nitrogen level increase greater than 5 mg/dL
   ■ Estimated fluid sequestration greater than 6 L
   ■ Arterial oxygen tension lower than 60 mm Hg
   The presence of fewer than three criteria indicates mild pancreatitis.
   Three or more criteria are associated with more severe pancreatitis and higher mortality rates.
   A simpler scoring system is **BISAP** (blood urea nitrogen > 25 mg/dL, impaired mental status, systemic inflammatory response, age >60 years, pleural effusion), which is under study.

5. Medical treatment: similar to that for other forms of pancreatitis
   ■ Strictly nothing by mouth initially; trend toward earlier enteral feeding during recovery
   ■ Intravenous hydration
   ■ Careful recording of intake and output
   ■ Use of antibiotics to prevent infection in severe acute pancreatitis (controversial)
   ■ Monitoring of laboratory data, including blood counts and electrolytes
   ■ Serial contrast-enhanced CT to monitor patients with moderate or severe pancreatitis for the development of pancreatic necrosis, pseudocysts, or abscesses

6. Published randomized studies on the role of ERCP in gallstone pancreatitis:
   ■ ERCP has no benefit in mild gallstone pancreatitis unless clear evidence of a retained BD stone exists.
   ■ One study demonstrated a reduced risk of local and systemic complications and shorter hospitalizations in severe pancreatitis.
   ■ Another study showed a reduced risk of cholangitis.
   ■ A third study showed no benefit to urgent ERCP.
7. Concomitant pancreatitis and cholangitis comprise a strong indication for urgent ERCP and sphincterotomy.

Postcholecystectomy Problems

DEFINITION

Postcholecystectomy syndrome is a term used for the persistence of gastrointestinal symptoms, usually biliary-type pain, in a patient who has undergone a cholecystectomy.
1. Causes are numerous and are often unrelated to cholecystectomy or the biliary tract.
2. Soon after cholecystectomy, postsurgical complications such as a bile leak must be excluded.

DIFFERENTIAL DIAGNOSIS

In addition to BD stones, the following nonbiliary entities should be considered:
- Irritable bowel syndrome
- Gastroesophageal reflux disease
- Esophageal spasm
- Peptic ulcer
- Chronic pancreatitis

SPHINCTER OF ODDI DYSFUNCTION

1. A possible cause of postcholecystectomy syndrome
2. Clinical criteria for diagnosis
   - Biliary-type pain
   - BD dilatation
   - Elevated serum aminotransferase or alkaline phosphatase levels on repeated occasions during episodes of pain
3. Diagnosis
   - The gold standard for the diagnosis of SOD is an elevated sphincter of Oddi (SO) pressure (greater than 40 mm Hg) at SO manometry during ERCP.
   - SO manometry is not available at all centers that perform ERCP.
   - SO manometry may add to the risk of pancreatitis during ERCP
   - Noninvasive imaging techniques such as nuclear hepatobiliary scanning may be useful.
4. Type 1 SOD
   - All three clinical criteria are met.
   - SOD is almost always present, and SO manometry is not required
5. Type 2 SOD
   - The patient meets one or two clinical criteria.
   - This type accounts for about half of patients with SOD.
   - Only patients with abnormal SO manometry results have a good long-term response to sphincterotomy.
6. Type 3 SOD
   - Patients have biliary pain alone.
   - None of the clinical criteria are present.
   - SO manometry is abnormal in up to half of patients.
   - The response to sphincterotomy has not been well studied.
   - Treatment decisions should be individualized.
7. SOD can occur in patients with an intact gallbladder:
   - Some clinicians recommend empiric cholecystectomy, not biliary endoscopy, as initial therapy for patients with unexplained biliary-type right upper quadrant pain, even without cholelithiasis.

Postoperative Bile Duct Injuries and Leaks

OVERVIEW

1. These disorders are reported in roughly 0.2% of cholecystectomies.
2. Bile leaks can cause acute illness resulting from intraperitoneal bile collections.

3. The most dreaded complication is major BD injury leading to a stricture, which may result in recurrent cholangitis, liver atrophy, or secondary biliary cirrhosis.
4. Bile leaks or injuries may occur as complications of liver transplantation (see Chapter 31).

CLASSIFICATION

1. Types of biliary tract injuries during cholecystectomy:
   - Bile leak without interruption of ductal continuity
   - Injury to one or more ducts with impairment or complete interruption of bile flow but without a bile leak
   - Combined bile leak and damage to a duct resulting in interrupted flow
2. Classification system proposed by Strasberg *et al* (1995):
   - **Type A:** bile leak from a minor duct with preservation of continuity between the liver and duodenum (examples of type A leaks include injury to the cystic duct remnant or the duct of Luschka, an accessory duct connecting the gallbladder to the liver bed)
   - **Type B:** occlusion of the right hepatic duct or one of its branches (occurs because the right hepatic duct is mistaken for the cystic duct during cholecystectomy as a result of an anatomic variation in which the cystic duct joins the right hepatic duct rather than the BD)
   - **Type C:** transection rather than occlusion of an aberrant right hepatic duct, resulting in a bile leak
   - **Type D:** lateral injury to an extrahepatic duct with preserved communication between the biliary tract and duodenum
   - **Type E:** occlusive injury of the BD at any level from the hepatic bifurcation to the duodenum

DIAGNOSIS

1. Bile leak or injury may be recognized intraoperatively, or diagnosis may be delayed for years.
2. Presenting symptoms and signs of bile leaks
   - Pain
   - Low-grade fever
   - Abdominal tenderness
   - Leukocytosis
   - Minor liver biochemical test elevations
3. Presenting symptoms and signs of major occlusive injuries to BDs
   - Jaundice
   - Pruritus
   - Elevated liver biochemical test levels
   - Cholangitis
4. Imaging studies
   - Nuclear hepatobiliary iminodiacetic acid (HIDA) scan is useful for the diagnosis of a bile leak.
   - Ultrasonography or CT may detect an intraperitoneal bile collection.
   - Benign BD strictures may not result in ductal dilatation on imaging.
   - MRCP can delineate ductal injury; it is the best initial test for delineation of proximal biliary injuries and excluded segments.
   - ERCP is the preferred modality for the diagnosis of major BD injuries.

5. THC may be necessary in certain situations:
   ■ Involvement of the biliary tract above the bifurcation, in which THC can localize the proximal extent and access the injured duct better than ERCP
   ■ Suspicion of an excluded segment of the biliary tract with absent communication between the liver and the distal BD

TREATMENT

1. The goal of therapy for a bile leak is to reduce outflow resistance in the duodenum.

   ■ The procedure of choice is ERCP with stent placement, with or without sphincterotomy.
   ■ The stent does not need to bridge the site of the leak.

2. Percutaneous or operative drainage may be needed for large bile collections.
3. Antibiotics should be administered until the leak is controlled or drained.
4. Surgical treatment
   ■ For major injuries, ligation of the BD and creation of a Roux-en-Y connection between the proximal biliary tree and the jejunum are indicated.
   ■ Smaller injuries may be repaired by suturing the BD over a T-tube.
   ■ Treatment of a complete transection of the BD during surgery by suturing over a T-tube is rarely successful in the long term.
5. Endoscopic therapy of postoperative biliary strictures
   ■ Biliary dilatation and stent placement (multiple plastic stents are preferred) are followed by stent exchanges every 3 to 6 months for at least 1 year.
   ■ Published series differ on the need for balloon dilatation of a stricture before stent placement.
   ■ Good long-term results are achieved in 50% to 80% of patients.
   ■ Endoscopic and surgical treatment have led to similar results in retrospective comparison studies.

Recurrent Pyogenic Cholangitis

OVERVIEW

1. It is characterized by primary intrahepatic stones associated with strictures of the intrahepatic ducts.
2. It is predominantly seen in the Far East and is rare in the United States.
3. Stones are composed mainly of calcium bilirubinate.
4. The syndrome was known previously as Oriental cholangiohepatitis.

PATHOGENESIS

1. The syndrome is associated with bacterial infection of bile.
   ■ Bacterial beta glucuronidases hydrolyze conjugated bilirubin.
   ■ Unconjugated bilirubin binds with calcium and precipitates as calcium bilirubinate, the major constituent of intrahepatic stones.
   ■ Parasitic infections, such as *Ascaris lumbricoides* or *Clonorchis sinensis,* may play a role.
2. It is seen in rural rather than urban areas in endemic countries.
   ■ The low-protein diet prevalent in rural areas decreases biliary glucurolactone, an inhibitor of beta glucuronidase.

■ Endogenous beta glucuronidase activity is enhanced, with further deconjugation of bile that leads to precipitation of calcium bilirubinate.

CLINICAL AND LABORATORY FEATURES

1. It occurs at a younger age than Western gallstone disease.
   ■ It may even occur in young adults and children.

2. Clinical features
   ■ Abdominal pain
   ■ Jaundice
   ■ Infection

3. Laboratory features
   ■ Leukocytosis
   ■ Elevated serum alkaline phosphatase and bilirubin levels
4. Potential consequences
   ■ Liver abscesses (see Chapter 28)
   ■ Atrophy of affected liver segments

DIAGNOSIS

1. Ultrasonography or CT may reveal focal areas of dilated intrahepatic ducts as well as stones.
2. Definitive diagnosis requires ERCP or THC.

TREATMENT

1. Broad-spectrum antibiotics are administered intravenously to treat episodes of acute cholangitis (see earlier).
2. Long-term relief includes surgical options tailored to the individual patient:
   ■ Resection of atrophic hepatic segments (possibly even lobectomy) and diseased ducts draining the affected liver portion
   ■ Anastomosis of jejunum to intrahepatic segments proximal to sites of obstruction
   ■ Creation of permanent access to the BD by means of the skin through which subsequent therapeutic maneuvers may be performed
   ■ Creation of a T-tube tract or loop of jejunum brought to a subcutaneous site to which the BD has been anastomosed
3. Endoscopic therapy
   ■ The proximal location of strictures and stones makes the endoscopic approach difficult.
   ■ ERCP is the first choice for therapeutic intervention, but THC may be necessary because removal of intrahepatic stones by ERCP can be difficult.

Choledochal Cysts

OVERVIEW

1. These anomalies of the biliary tract are characterized by cystic dilatation of variable portions of the intrahepatic and/or extrahepatic ducts.
2. They are more common in Asia than elsewhere.

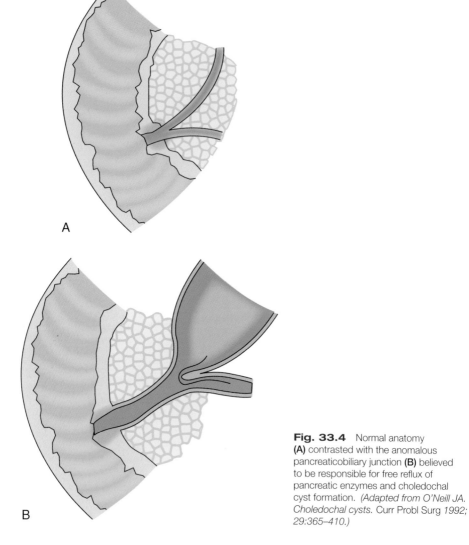

A

B

Fig. 33.4 Normal anatomy **(A)** contrasted with the anomalous pancreaticobiliary junction **(B)** believed to be responsible for free reflux of pancreatic enzymes and choledochal cyst formation. *(Adapted from O'Neill JA. Choledochal cysts.* Curr Probl Surg *1992; 29:365–410.)*

3. The female-to-male ratio is 3:1.
4. They primarily affect children and young adults, but reported age ranges vary greatly.

ETIOLOGY: PROPOSED THEORIES

1. Abnormality in biliary epithelial proliferation when fetal ducts are solid that leads to an abnormally dilated portion proximal to a normal or stenotic distal portion
2. Distal BD stenosis inducing proximal cystic dilatation
3. Intrinsic autonomic dysfunction
   ■ Based on finding deficient postcholinergic neurons in some portions of the cyst wall

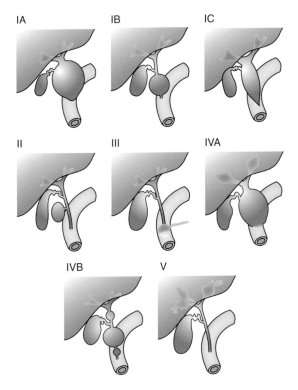

Fig. 33.5 Classification scheme of choledochal cysts suggested by Todani *et al* in 1977 (See text). *(From Savader SJ, Benenati JF, Venbrux AC, et al. Choledochal cysts: classification and cholangiographic appearance. AJR Am J Roentgenol 1991; 156:328.)*

4. Anomalous pancreaticobiliary junction (Fig. 33.4)
   - May result in lack of normal SO function and reflux of pancreatic enzymes into BDs, thus inducing progressive damage and dilatation
   - Common in type I cysts, but not in types II, III, and V cysts (see the next section)

CLASSIFICATION BY TODANI *ET AL* (1977): THE MOST COMMONLY USED SYSTEM (Fig. 33.5)

- Type I: dilatation of the extrahepatic duct alone; the most common type
- Type II: diverticulum of the extrahepatic BD
- Type III: choledochocele, involving only the intraduodenal duct
- Type IVA: multiple extrahepatic and intrahepatic cysts
- Type IVB: multiple extrahepatic cysts only
- Type V: single or multiple intrahepatic cysts (Caroli's disease)

CLINICAL FEATURES

1. Right upper quadrant pain
2. Jaundice
   - Often the sole symptom in infants
3. Palpable abdominal mass
4. Fever
5. Epigastric or diffuse abdominal pain if pancreatitis is present

DIAGNOSIS

1. Ultrasonography or CT may reveal or suggest the diagnosis; MRCP is emerging as a diagnostic modality.
2. Direct cholangiography by ERCP or THC is usually diagnostic.
   - It is also important for classification and planning therapy.
3. THC is best for delineating and potentially draining the proximal biliary ducts.
4. ERCP enables evaluation of the pancreatic duct and the pancreatic-biliary junction.
   - It often reveals an anomalous junction, especially in type I cysts.
   - MRCP obviates the need for ERCP in many cases.

COMPLICATIONS

1. Stone formation within cysts
2. Cholangitis and liver abscesses
3. Acute pancreatitis, with or without stones
   - This is most common with a choledochocele (type III cyst).
4. Secondary biliary cirrhosis
5. Carcinoma
   - It usually occurs within cysts.
   - A significant risk exists after nonresectional surgery.
   - Primary cyst excision reduces the cancer risk markedly but not completely.
   - A preoperative diagnosis of cancer is rare.
   - It has a poor prognosis because of extensive spread.
6. Portal hypertension
7. Cyst rupture with bile peritonitis

TREATMENT

1. Medical management is associated with high morbidity and mortality.
2. Simple drainage is inadequate.
3. Cyst excision and reconstruction of the biliary tree comprise the treatment of choice.
4. **Type I and type II cysts**
   - Excision is followed by reconstruction of the biliary tree with a Roux-en-Y hepaticojejunostomy.
   - Reports have noted success with a laparoscopic approach.
5. **Type III cysts** (choledochoceles)
   - Endoscopic sphincterotomy may be definitive therapy.
6. **Type IV cysts**
   - Excision of the extrahepatic cyst, partial resection of intrahepatic cysts when present, and hepaticojejunostomy are performed.
   - Predominant involvement of the left lobe in type IVA disease may necessitate left hepatic lobectomy.
7. **Type V cysts** (Caroli's disease)
   - Partial hepatectomy is performed for localized disease.
   - Roux-en-Y hepaticojejunostomy with placement of transhepatic stents is performed for diffuse disease.
   - Recurrent stones and strictures are treated with percutaneous techniques.
   - Liver transplantation may be required for severe diffuse disease.

FURTHER READING

Fan ST, Lai EC, Mok FP, et al. Early treatment of acute biliary pancreatitis by endoscopic papillotomy. *N Engl J Med* 1993; 328:228–232.

Filip M, Saftoiu A, Popescu C, et al. Postcholecystectomy syndrome: an algorithmic approach. *J Gastrointestin Liver Dis* 2009; 18:67–71.

Folsch UR, Nitsche R, Ludtke R, et al. Early ERCP and papillotomy compared with conservative treatment for acute biliary pancreatitis: the German Study Group on Acute Biliary Pancreatitis. *N Engl J Med* 1997; 336:237–242.

Freeman ML. Pancreatic stents for prevention of post-endoscopic retrograde cholangiopancreatography pancreatitis. *Clin Gastroenterol Hepatol* 2007; 5:1354–1365.

Freeman ML, Nelson DB, Sherman S, et al. Complications of endoscopic biliary sphincterotomy. *N Engl J Med* 1996; 335:909–918.

Jablonska B, Lampe P. Iatrogenic bile duct injuries: etiology, diagnosis and management. *World J Gastroenterol* 2009; 15:4097–4104.

Neoptolemos JP, Carr-Locke DL, London NJ, et al. Controlled trial of urgent endoscopic retrograde cholangiopancreatography and endoscopic sphincterotomy versus conservative treatment for acute pancreatitis due to gallstones. *Lancet* 1988; 2:979–983.

Nguyen T, Powell A, Daugherty T. Recurrent pyogenic cholangitis. *Dig Dis Sci* 2009; 55:8–10.

Petrov MS, Savides TJ. Systematic review of endoscopic ultrasonography versus endoscopic retrograde cholangiopancreatography for suspected choledocholithiasis. *Br J Surg* 2009; 96:967–974.

Petrov MS, van Santvoort HC, Besselink MG, et al. Early endoscopic retrograde cholangiopancreatography versus conservative management in acute biliary pancreatitis without cholangitis: a meta-analysis of randomized trials. *Ann Surg* 2008; 247:250–257.

Soreide K, Korner H, Havnen J, Soreide JA. Bile duct cysts in adults. *Br J Surg* 2004; 91:1538–1548.

Strasberg SM, Hertl M, Soper NJ. An analysis of the problem of biliary injury during laparoscopic cholecystectomy. *J Am Coll Surg* 1995; 180:101–125.

Todani T, Watanabe Y, Narusue M, et al. Congenital bile duct cysts: classification, operative procedures, and review of thirty-seven cases including cancer arising from choledochal cyst. *Am J Surg* 1977; 134:263–269.

Toouli J. Sphincter of Oddi: function, dysfunction, and its management. *J Gastroenterol Hepatol* 2009; 24(Suppl 3):S57–S62.

Williams EJ, Green J, Beckingham I, et al. Guidelines on the management of common bile duct stones (CBDS). *Gut* 2008; 57:1004–1021.

CHAPTER 34

Tumors of the biliary tract

Keith D. Lillemoe, MD, FACS ■ Michael G. House, MD

Benign Tumors of the Gallbladder

PSEUDOPOLYPS (CHOLESTEROL POLYPS)

1. The most commonly observed polypoid lesion of the gallbladder; accounts for approximately 50% of such lesions
2. Not a true neoplasm, but rather cholesterol-filled projections of gallbladder mucosa protruding into the lumen
3. Usually less than 1 cm in size; visualized on gallbladder imaging studies (ultrasonography, oral cholecystography) as nonmobile filling defects
4. Usually asymptomatic unless associated with gallstones
5. No malignant potential

ADENOMYOSIS

1. Consists of a thickened gallbladder muscular layer with Rokitansky-Aschoff sinuses
2. **Three types: fundal** (most common), appearing as a hemispheric lesion with a central dimple; **segmental**, consisting of an annular stricture; or **diffuse**, involving the entire gallbladder

3. May manifest as muscular hypertrophy secondary to gallbladder dysmotility; therefore, symptoms are relieved by cholecystectomy
4. May be associated with carcinoma of the gallbladder

ADENOMAS

1. True neoplastic epithelial tumors of the gallbladder mucosa
2. Usually manifest as solitary, nonmobile filling defects seen on gallbladder ultrasonography or oral cholecystography
3. Premalignant, with carcinoma in situ found in larger polyps
4. Unlikely to play a major role in the pathogenesis of most gallbladder cancers

TREATMENT

1. Because the histology of polypoid lesions of the gallbladder cannot be determined non-operatively by current methods, patients with polyps larger than 1 cm should undergo cholecystectomy.
2. Polyps up to 1 cm in size, regardless of total number, should be followed by repeat imaging studies every 3 to 6 months.
3. Any patient with biliary symptoms and a gallbladder polyp should undergo cholecystectomy.

Benign Tumors of the Bile Duct

1. These are much less common than benign gallbladder tumors.
2. Histologic types
   - Papillomas
   - Adenomas
   - Cystadenomas: tumors with inner layers of mucin-secreting epithelium, mesenchymal stroma, and an outer layer of hyalinized fibrous tissue
3. They may be solitary or multiple.
4. Symptoms are usually caused by bile duct obstruction, which results in intermittent jaundice or cholangitis.
5. The diagnosis can usually be made by magnetic resonance, endoscopic retrograde, or percutaneous transhepatic cholangiography.
6. Treatment consists of surgical resection of the bile duct, most commonly with reconstruction by hepaticojejunostomy.
7. Both benign cystadenomas and multiple papillomatosis of the bile duct can be associated with a high rate of local recurrence if complete resection is not accomplished.

Carcinoma of the Gallbladder

INCIDENCE

1. Carcinoma of the gallbladder is the most common biliary tract malignancy and the fifth most common gastrointestinal cancer (3% to 4% of gastrointestinal tumors).
2. The incidence has increased as the population has aged. Currently, 6000 to 7000 new cases are diagnosed each year (2.5 cases per 100,000 population).

3. The female-to-male ratio is 3:1.
4. The usual age of onset is the sixth or seventh decade of life.
5. An increased incidence is seen in southwestern Native Americans, Native Alaskans, Mexicans, and Hispanics living in the United States and in residents of northern Japan, Israel, and Chile.
6. A much lower incidence is seen in African Americans and residents of India, Nigeria, and Singapore.

ETIOLOGY

Risk factors for gallbladder carcinoma:
- Gallstones/chronic cholecystitis
- Choledochal cysts
- Anomalous pancreatobiliary duct junction
- Carcinogens
- Estrogens
- Chronic typhoid infection
- Porcelain gallbladder
- Gallbladder polyps

1. Gallstones/chronic cholecystitis
   - Gallstones are present in more than 90% of patients with gallbladder carcinoma; conversely, only 1% of patients with gallstones have gallbladder carcinoma.
   - Larger stones (>3 cm) are associated with a 10-fold higher risk of gallbladder cancer compared with smaller stones.
   - The role of gallstones in the development of gallbladder cancer is likely related to chronic inflammation.
   - Gallstone composition does not seem to affect pathogenesis.
2. Choledochal cysts (see Chapter 33)
   - Choledochal cysts are associated with carcinomas throughout the biliary tract including the gallbladder.
   - The risk of biliary carcinoma increases with age.
   - The risk may be related to an association with an anomalous pancreaticobiliary duct junction, which is frequently seen with choledochal cysts.
   - Surgical removal of choledochal (and gallbladder) cysts is recommended to prevent further reflux of bile and stasis and to eliminate the cancer risk.
3. Anomalous pancreaticobiliary duct junction
   - The long common channel of the pancreatic and common bile duct (type 3B anomaly) appears to be associated with a significantly increased risk of gallbladder cancer.
   - Reflux of pancreatic juice into the biliary tree and bile stasis is the proposed mechanism.
4. Carcinogens
   - Industrial exposure: rubber industry
   - Animal studies: azotoluene, nitrosamines
5. Estrogens: This epidemiologic association may simply be related to the associated increased incidence of gallstones.
6. *Salmonella typhi* infection: This is likely related to chronic irritation and inflammation.
7. Gallbladder wall calcification: Diffuse calcification of the gallbladder wall (porcelain gallbladder) was formerly an indication for cholecystectomy because of the risk of cancer even in asymptomatic patients. More recent studies have suggested that this risk had been

overestimated and is likely less than 5%. Calcification of the gallbladder mucosa is associated with a higher incidence of gallbladder cancer.

8. Gallbladder polyps
   - Adenomas and adenomyosis have clear premalignant potential.
   - Cholecystectomy is indicated for any polyp larger than 1 cm (see earlier).

PATHOLOGY AND STAGING

1. Histologic type
   a. Adenocarcinoma: 90%
      - Scirrhous (90%): infiltrating, desmoplastic, obliterating gallbladder lumen, invading liver
      - Papillary (5%): polypoid, slow growing, late to metastasize
      - Colloid (5%): soft, gelatinous, mucinous tumors filling the gallbladder
   b. Anaplastic: 5%
   c. Squamous (adenosquamous): 2%
   d. Miscellaneous types: 3%
2. Routes of spread
   a. Spread occurs primarily by local extension, typically for fundus-based tumors.
   b. Lymphatic drainage is to the adjacent lymph node basins first—cystic duct, pericholedochal, and hilar lymph nodes (N1). Secondary basins include the retropancreatic, celiac axis, and periaortic nodes (N2).
   c. The veins of the gallbladder drain directly into the liver parenchyma and to branches of the portal vein of segments V and IVB of the liver.
   d. Direct invasion of adjacent structures including the common hepatic duct, duodenum, and colon occurs.
   e. Dissemination occurs to the liver or peritoneal surface.
3. **Staging** (Table 34.1)

TABLE 34.1 ■ **American Joint Commission on Cancer (tumor, node, metastasis [TMN]) staging: summary for carcinoma of the gallbladder**

Stage 0	Carcinoma in situ (T0)
Stage I (T1N0M0)	Tumor invades lamina propria (T1a) or muscular layer (T1b)
Stage II (T2N0M0)	Tumor invades perimuscular connective tissue; no extension beyond serosa or into liver (T2)
Stage IIIA (T3N0M0)	Tumor perforates the serosa (visceral peritoneum) and/or directly invades the liver and/or one other adjacent organ, such as stomach, duodenum, colon, pancreas, or extrahepatic bile ducts (T3); no lymph node involvement
Stage IIIB (T1–3N1M0)	T1–3 with positive nodes confined to the hepatic hilus including nodes along the bile duct, hepatic artery, portal vein, and cystic duct (N1)
Stage IVA (T4N0M0)	Tumor invades main portal vein or hepatic artery or invades two or more extrahepatic organs (T4); no lymph node involvement
Stage IVB (any T, any N, M1 or any T N2M0 or T4N1M0)	Any T with distant metastases (M1); any T with lymph node metastases to celiac, periduodenal, peripancreatic, and/or superior mesenteric lymph nodes (N2); T4 with N1 nodes

Adapted from Edge S, Byrd D, Compton C, et al. AJCC Cancer Staging Manual, 7th ed. New York: Springer-Verlag, 2010.

CLINICAL FEATURES

1. Symptoms (frequency)
   - Abdominal pain (80%): usually of less than 1 month's duration and difficult to distinguish from symptoms of acute cholecystitis or biliary pain
   - Nausea and vomiting (50%)
   - Weight loss (40%)
   - Jaundice (30% to 40%): usually a poor prognostic finding for fundus-based cancers
   - Incidental finding at cholecystectomy for gallstones (10% to 20%; incidental cancers found in 1% of cholecystectomies for symptomatic gallstones)
2. Physical findings: usually indicate advanced disease
   - Right upper quadrant mass
   - Hepatomegaly
   - Jaundice

DIAGNOSIS AND PREOPERATIVE STAGING

1. Laboratory tests
   - Abnormal liver biochemical test levels when tumor or periportal lymphadenopathy is associated with biliary obstruction
   - No reliable tumor marker, including carcinoembryonic antigen (CEA) and carbohydrate antigen 19-9 (CA19-9)
2. Radiologic studies
   a. Ultrasonography
      - Sensitivity of 75% to 80%
      - Findings:
        – Complex mass filling the gallbladder lumen
        – Gallbladder wall thickening
        – Polypoid gallbladder mass
        – Gallstones
        – Normal in up to 10% of patients
   b. Computed tomography (CT)
      - Findings are similar to those of ultrasonography with respect to gallbladder wall thickening or mass.
      - CT defines the extent of disease better than ultrasonography; it demonstrates liver or adjacent organ invasion, liver metastases, lymph node involvement, vascular invasion, and biliary obstruction.
   c. Magnetic resonance imaging (MRI)
      - Magnetic resonance cholangiopancreatography (MRCP) provides a single noninvasive imaging modality that allows complete assessment of the hepatic parenchyma, biliary tree, vasculature, and lymph nodes.
   d. Endoscopic ultrasonography (EUS) aids in determining the extent of local invasion and nodal involvement.
   e. Cholangiography
      - Endoscopic retrograde cholangiopancreatography (ERCP) or percutaneous transhepatic cholangiography (THC) is indicated in patients with clinical evidence of biliary obstruction.
      - The typical cholangiographic appearance is a long stricture of the mid portion of the bile duct usually below the hepatic duct bifurcation.

- Endoscopic or percutaneous stents can be placed for preoperative biliary decompression, to aid in surgical management, or to provide long-term palliation.
  f. Positron emission tomography (PET) lacks sensitivity and is not part of the routine evaluation.
3. Preoperative biopsy and cytologic findings
   - Percutaneous or EUS-guided fine-needle biopsy for histologic or cytologic analysis can be performed in large tumors that appear unresectable.
   - Bile duct or bile cytologic specimens or brushings have a low diagnostic yield.
   - No indication exists to pursue a preoperative tissue diagnosis in patients who are considered candidates for surgical resection.

TREATMENT

1. Nonoperative palliation
   - This is indicated in patients in whom preoperative evaluation reveals extensive local or metastatic disease that precludes resection (stage IVA or B disease).
   - Obstructive jaundice can be palliated with either a Silastic or metallic endoprosthesis or internal-external transhepatic silastic stents; Silastic stents must be changed at 2- to 3-month intervals.
   - Pain, if significant, can be managed with oral narcotics or a percutaneous or EUS-guided celiac axis block.
2. Surgical management
   a. Incidental discovery of gallbladder carcinoma at laparoscopic cholecystectomy
      - With the widespread use of laparoscopic cholecystectomy for symptomatic gallstones, many gallbladder cancers are first encountered in this setting.
      - Laparoscopic cholecystectomy is contraindicated if gallbladder carcinoma is suspected preoperatively.
      - If gallbladder carcinoma is recognized at the time of laparoscopic cholecystectomy, the operation should be converted to an open procedure for resection.
      - If gallbladder carcinoma is recognized pathologically after laparoscopic cholecystectomy, management is dictated by the histologic findings.
        – If carcinoma is limited to the lamina propria of the gallbladder wall and has a negative cystic duct margin (pathologic stage T1a), cholecystectomy is adequate.
        – If carcinoma penetrates into the muscular layer (pathologic stage T1b), consideration should be given to an extended cholecystectomy (similar to that for pathologic stage T2).
        – If carcinoma penetrates into the perimuscular connective tissue (pathologic stage T2), the patient should undergo repeat exploration and partial central hepatectomy including liver segments IVB and V plus regional periportal lymph node dissection and excision of the cystic duct stump.
        – Laparoscopic port site excision is no longer advocated because port site disease typically indicates diffuse peritoneal seeding.
   b. Surgical management of suspected gallbladder carcinoma
      - The resectability rates for gallbladder carcinoma range from 15% to 30%.
      - If the tumor is confined to the lamina propria or muscular layer (pathologic stage T1), simple cholecystectomy is adequate resection in most cases.
      - If the tumor penetrates the gallbladder wall, resection includes the gallbladder, segment V, and the anterior portion of segment IV of the liver and a lymph node dissection, including hilar, choledochal, and retropancreatic nodes.
      - Japanese investigators have advocated more aggressive resection including combined hepatic resection and pancreaticoduodenectomy.

■ Postoperative morbidity and mortality rates are directly related to the extent of resection (Table 34.2).

3. Adjuvant therapy following resection
   ■ A high frequency of distant recurrence supports the need for systemic adjuvant therapy.
   ■ Limited randomized prospective trials are available.
   ■ One prospective randomized phase III trial of adjuvant chemotherapy with 5-fluorouracil and mitomycin C versus surgery alone found that the 5-year survival was significantly better in the adjuvant group (26%) than the control group (14%). The respective 5-year disease-free survival rates were 20.3% and 11.6%.

4. Treatment of unresectable disease
   ■ Modern chemotherapy (gemcitabine and platinum-based agents) is associated with response rates of approximately 20%.
   ■ Radiation therapy, including external beam and intraoperative radiation therapy and brachytherapy, has not been shown consistently to improve survival significantly.

PROGNOSIS

1. Because of the late stage of presentation, the overall 5-year survival rate is less than 10%, with a median survival of 6 months.
2. Survival depends on the stage of tumor:
   ■ Patients with stage I tumors have a 5-year survival rate approaching 100% following simple or extended cholecystectomy.
   ■ Patients with stage II tumors treated with extended cholecystectomy may have a 60% to 80% 5-year survival rate.
   ■ Patients with stage III tumors treated with extended resection have 3- and 5-year survival rates of 60% to 80% and 25%, respectively.
   ■ The median survival in patients with unresectable stage IV disease is only 2 to 3 months.
   ■ Long-term survival after curative resection as a second procedure (following an inadequate first operation) is no different from that after a single procedure.

Carcinoma of the Bile Duct (Cholangiocarcinoma)

INCIDENCE

■ Approximately 25% of hepatobiliary cancers
■ Incidence in the United States of 1.0 per 100,000 population per year

TABLE 34.2 ■ **Morbidity and mortality rates for resection of gallbladder carcinoma**

Resection	Overall morbidity rate (%)	30-day mortality rate (%)
Cholecystectomy	10–15	2
Extended cholecystectomy with central hepatectomy	20–25	<5
Major hepatectomy	45–55	5–10
Hepatopancreaticoduodenectomy	50–65	15–20

- 3000 to 4000 new cases per year in the United States
- Male-to-female ratio of 1.3:1
- Age range of 50 to 70 years

RISK FACTORS

Strong Association
- Caroli's disease
- Choledochal cyst
- Clonorchiasis
- Hepatolithiasis
- Primary sclerosing cholangitis
- Ulcerative colitis
- Thorotrast exposure

Possible Association
- Asbestos
- Dioxin (Agent Orange)
- Isoniazid
- Methyldopa
- Oral contraceptives
- Polychlorinated biphenyls
- Radionucleotides

1. Caroli's disease and choledochal cysts (see Chapter 33)
   a. The reported incidence of cholangiocarcinoma in patients with cystic abnormalities of the biliary tract ranges from 2.5% to 28%.
   b. Patients with cystic lesions of the bile duct tend to develop cholangiocarcinoma 2 to 3 decades younger than patients with sporadic cholangiocarcinoma.
   c. In more than 75% of patients with cholangiocarcinomas associated with choledochal cysts, symptoms first appear in adulthood.
   d. Factors that may account for the development of cholangiocarcinoma in patients with cystic disease of the biliary tract include the following:
      - Reflux of pancreatic exocrine secretions as a result of an anomalous pancreatobiliary duct junction
      - Bile stasis
      - Chronic inflammation and bacterial infection within the cyst
      - Stone formation within the cyst
2. *Clonorchis sinensis* (liver fluke) infection (see Chapter 29)
   - This is common in Asia and is associated with ingestion of raw fish.
   - The adult trematode resides in the intrahepatic and, less commonly, extrahepatic bile ducts, can obstruct biliary flow, and can cause periductal fibrosis, hyperplasia, stricture, and stone formation.
   - *Opisthorchis viverrini* is another liver fluke associated with cholangiocarcinoma.
3. Hepatolithiasis (recurrent pyogenic cholangitis) (see Chapter 33)
   - Cholangiocarcinoma develops in 5% to 10% of patients with hepatolithiasis.
   - Bile stasis, bactibilia, and cystic dilatation may all be associated with this increased risk.
   - Cholelithiasis is seen in up to one third of patients with and without cholangiocarcinoma; therefore, gallbladder stones are not considered a risk factor for cholangiocarcinoma in this setting.

4. Primary sclerosing cholangitis (see Chapter 15)
   - Unrecognized cholangiocarcinoma is found in up to 40% of autopsies in patients dying with and 10% of patients undergoing liver transplantation for primary sclerosing cholangitis.
   - Cholangiocarcinoma in patients with primary sclerosing cholangitis is often manifested by rapid clinical deterioration and progressive jaundice.
   - The prognosis in patients with cholangiocarcinoma and primary sclerosing cholangitis is poor, with a median survival of less than 1 year.
5. Ulcerative colitis
   - The incidence of cholangiocarcinoma in patients with ulcerative colitis ranges from 0.14% to 1.4%, 400 to 1000 times that of the general population.
   - Cholangiocarcinoma develops 20 years earlier in patients with ulcerative colitis than in others.
   - Patients with cholangiocarcinoma and ulcerative colitis tend to have pancolonic involvement and a long duration of disease.
   - The risk of cholangiocarcinoma does not appear to be affected by proctocolectomy.
6. Thorotrast (thorium dioxide)
   - This radiocontrast agent used several decades ago emits alpha particles and, when injected intravenously, is retained in the reticuloendothelial system for life.
   - Cholangiocarcinoma may develop after a mean latent period of 35 years.

PATHOLOGY AND STAGING

1. Histologic type
   - Adenocarcinoma accounts for more than 95% of cases.
   - Rare histologic types include squamous and mucoepidermoid carcinomas, cystadenocarcinomas, carcinoid tumors, and leiomyosarcomas.
   - Histologic types of adenocarcinoma include nodular-sclerosing (most common), scirrhous, diffusely infiltrating, and papillary (often multifocal).
2. Location (Table 34.3)
3. Route of spread
   - Spread occurs most commonly (70%) by direct invasion of the adjacent liver, portal vein, hepatic artery, pancreas, or duodenum.
   - Liver and peritoneal metastases occur in up to 50% of patients.
   - Regional lymph nodes are involved in 75% to 80% of patients.
4. Staging (Table 34.4)

CLINICAL FEATURES

1. Symptoms
   - Jaundice: the most common presenting symptom and present in more than 90% of patients

---

TABLE 34.3 ■ **Frequency of cholangiocarcinoma at various locations (%)**

Intrahepatic biliary tract	5–10
Hepatic duct bifurcation	40–60
Distal bile duct (intrapancreatic)	20–30
Diffuse/multifocal	7–13

TABLE 34.4 ■ **American Joint Commission on Cancer (tumor, node, metastasis [TMN]) staging: summary for cholangiocarcinoma**

Stage 0	Carcinoma in situ
Stage I (T1N0M0)	Tumor confined to bile duct wall (T1)
Stage II (T2a or 2b N0M0)	Tumor invades beyond bile duct wall (T2a); tumor invades liver parenchyma (T2b)
Stage IIIA (T3N0M0)	Tumor invades unilateral branches of portal vein or hepatic artery (T3); no lymph node involvement
Stage IIIB (T1–3N1M0)	T1–3 with regional lymph node metastases
Stage IVA (T4N0–1M0)	Tumor invades main portal vein or branches bilaterally or common hepatic artery; or second-order biliary radicles bilaterally; or second-order biliary radicles with contralateral portal vein or hepatic artery involvement
Stage IVB (Any T N2M0 or any T any NM1)	Any T with periaortic, pericaval, superior mesenteric, or celiac lymph node metastases (N2) or with distant metastasis (M1)

Adapted from Edge S, Byrd D, Compton C, et al. AJCC Cancer Staging Manual, 7th ed. New York: Springer-Verlag, 2010.

- Pruritus
- Weight loss
- Abdominal pain: vague, nonspecific, and mild and sometimes the only symptom in patients with proximal tumors located above the hepatic bifurcation
- Cholangitis (uncommon)
2. Physical findings
   - Jaundice
   - Hepatomegaly
   - Palpable gallbladder: only with distal bile duct cancers

DIAGNOSIS AND PREOPERATIVE EVALUATION

1. Laboratory tests
   - Abnormal liver biochemical test levels include increased serum bilirubin and alkaline phosphatase levels.
   - The prothrombin time is prolonged in patients with long-standing biliary obstruction.
2. Tumor markers
   - Serum CEA, alpha fetoprotein, and CA19–9 individually are of limited value.
3. Radiologic studies
   a. Ultrasonography and CT
      - Findings with hilar tumors are a dilated intrahepatic biliary tract, a contracted gallbladder, liver atrophy, and a normal extrahepatic biliary tract and pancreas.
      - Findings with distal tumors are a dilated intrahepatic and extrahepatic biliary tract with a distended gallbladder.
      - Hilar adenopathy and portal vein patency should be assessed.
      - Distant lymph node sites (N2 disease) should be assessed.
   b. MRI and MRCP
      - These techniques can usually identify the primary tumor, level of biliary radicle involvement, patency of hilar vascular structures, nodal or distal metastases, and lobar atrophy.

- They are more valuable than invasive cholangiography for revealing obstructed and isolated ducts; biliary instrumentation and risk of infection are avoided.
  c. Cholangiography
  - Either ERCP or percutaneous THC should be performed to define the location and extent of the tumor.
  - THC is preferred for proximal biliary tumors because this technique better defines the proximal extent of the tumor.
  - The cholangiographic appearance can predict resectability in proximal cholangiocarcinoma (positive predictive value of 60%).
  - Percutaneous or endoscopic placement of biliary catheters should be planned to permit adequate drainage of the liver remnant following operative resection of hilar cancers.
  - Either ERCP or THC is appropriate for distal bile duct cancers.
  d. PET may detect small tumors, advanced regional lymph node disease, or distant metastases.
  e. Preoperative biopsy and cytologic findings
  - A tissue diagnosis to rule out malignancy is necessary in patients considered for nonoperative management of presumably benign strictures or in those with primary sclerosing cholangitis who are being considered for liver transplantation.
  - Bile cytology demonstrates malignant cells in 30% of cases of cholangiocarcinoma.
  - Cytologic brushings performed either percutaneously or endoscopically yield positive results in 40% to 50% of patients; results improve with multiple attempts; cytologic molecular markers (e.g., fluorescence in situ hybridization [FISH] analysis) may increase detection rates.
  - Percutaneous fine-needle aspiration or cholangioscopic biopsies may increase the diagnostic yield to 67%.

TREATMENT

1. Nonoperative palliation
   - This is indicated in patients with extensive local or metastatic disease that precludes resection (if determined preoperatively).
   - Obstructive jaundice can be palliated with either Silastic or metallic endoprostheses or internal-external Silastic stents; Silastic stents must be changed at 2- to 3-month intervals.
   - In patients with proximal (hilar) cholangiocarcinoma, percutaneous bilateral access is usually necessary.
   - Death is usually the result of recurrent biliary sepsis and liver abscess, which occur as tumor extension occludes proximal bile duct radicles.
2. Surgical palliation
   a. Surgical exploration for attempted resection is indicated in all good-risk patients not determined to have unresectable disease by preoperative staging.
   b. Patients with disseminated disease or extensive tumor involvement of the porta hepatis should undergo minimal intervention.
      - Preoperative biliary catheters should be left in place for palliation of jaundice.
      - Cholecystectomy should be performed to prevent the development of acute cholecystitis.
   c. Surgical approaches for palliation of locally unresectable cholangiocarcinoma:
      - Proximal tumors: operative dilatation of the tumor with placement of Silastic stents and a Roux-en-Y choledochojejunostomy, or a segment III bypass to the left hepatic duct using a Roux-en-Y limb of jejunum
      - Distal tumors: hepaticojejunostomy and gastrojejunostomy

TABLE 34.5 ■ **Morbidity and mortality rates for resection of cholangiocarcinoma**

	Overall morbidity rate (%)	30-day mortality rate (%)
Hepatic bifurcation resection and reconstruction	25–40	<5
Hepatic bifurcation resection, reconstruction, and hepatic lobectomy	40–65	5–15

3. Surgical resection
   a. The approach to intrahepatic cholangiocarcinoma is similar to that for hepatocellular carcinoma, with a standard hepatic resection (see Chapter 27).
   b. Perihilar cholangiocarcinomas require local resection of the hepatic duct above the level of the hepatic duct bifurcation to achieve a microscopically negative margin, including hepatic resection as indicated, with reconstruction performed to a Roux-en-Y jejunal limb; hepatoduodenal lymphadenectomy should be performed.
      ■ Many surgeons advocate routine resection of the caudate lobe (segment I) of the liver for cancers involving the left hepatic duct.
      ■ The addition of a major hepatic resection significantly increases perioperative morbidity and mortality.
      ■ Liver transplantation offers the advantage of resection of all structures potentially involved by tumor even in locally advanced disease. The 5-year survival rate is less than 30%, and the rate of tumor recurrence is 50%. Aggressive neoadjuvant protocols have been developed, including high-dose chemotherapy plus external beam radiation and brachytherapy followed by liver transplantation (Mayo protocol); reported results have been favorable in properly selected patients from the Mayo Clinic series, but the comparison groups were quite disparate. Therefore, liver transplantation cannot be considered standard therapy for hilar cholangiocarcinoma.
   c. Table 34.5 shows the morbidity and mortality rates for hepatic bifurcation resection and reconstruction with and without hepatic lobectomy.
   d. Distal cholangiocarcinomas require pancreaticoduodenectomy (perioperative mortality rate less than 4%, morbidity rate 30% to 40%).
4. Adjuvant therapy following resection
   ■ No randomized, prospective trials are available.
   ■ To date, no single chemotherapeutic agent or combination of agents, with or without radiation, has been shown to be of clear benefit in reducing locoregional recurrence.
   ■ In the absence of prospective data, most groups advocate adjuvant chemotherapy and/or radiation therapy for resected distal cholangiocarcinomas based on the results of prospective trials for resectable pancreatic carcinoma.
5. Treatment of unresectable disease: Randomized controlled trials have shown an overall survival benefit of 4 months with combination chemotherapy (gemcitabine plus cisplatin).

PROGNOSIS

1. Intrahepatic cholangiocarcinoma
   ■ This usually manifests at an advanced stage (only 15% to 20% resectability rate).
   ■ Resectable: The 3-year survival rate is 45% to 60%; median survival is 18 to 30 months.
   ■ Unresectable: Median survival is 7 months.

TABLE 34.6 ■ **Management of perihilar cholangiocarcinoma and outcomes (%)**

Liver resection required	75–100
Margin of resection negative after surgery	50–80
5-yr survival:	
If margin of resection is negative	30–50
If margin of resection is positive	0–10

2. Perihilar cholangiocarcinoma (Table 34.6)
Factors adversely influencing survival include positive surgical margin, low preoperative serum albumin level, and postoperative sepsis.
  a. Unresectable (determined at surgery)
    ■ Median survival of 8 months
    ■ 1-year survival rate of 27%
    ■ 2-year survival rate of 6%
  b. Unresectable (determined preoperatively)
    ■ median survival of 5 months
    ■ 1-year survival rate of 25%
    ■ 2-year survival rate of 5%
3. Distal cholangiocarcinoma
  ■ This has the best resectability rate (>50%).
  ■ When resectable, median survival is 24 months; overall survival rates at 1, 3, and 5 years are 70%, 50%, and 25% to 40%, respectively.
  ■ Factors adversely influencing survival following resection are positive lymph node status and poor tumor differentiation.
  ■ When the tumor is unresectable, median survival is 8 months.

FURTHER READING

Aljiffry M, Walsh M, Molinari M, et al. Advances in diagnosis, treatment and palliation of cholangiocarcinoma: 1990–2009. *World J Gastroenterol* 2009; 15:4240–4262.

Burke ED, Jarnigan WR, Hochwald SN, et al. Hilar cholangiocarcinoma: patterns of spread, the importance of hepatic resection for curative operation, and a presurgical clinical staging system. *Ann Surg* 1998; 228:385–394.

Cho C, Ito F, Rikkers L, et al. Hilar cholangiocarcinoma: current management. *Ann Surg* 2009; 250: 210–218.

Fong Y, Jarnigan W, Blumgart L. Gallbladder cancer: comparison of patients presenting initially for definitive operation with those presenting after prior noncurative intervention. *Ann Surg* 2000; 232:557–569.

Ito F, Agni R, Rettammel RJ, et al. Resection of hilar cholangiocarcinoma: concomitant liver resection decreases hepatic recurrence. *Ann Surg* 2008; 248:273–279.

Jarnigan WR, Fong Y, DeMatteo RP, et al. Staging, respectability, and outcome in 225 patients with hilar cholangiocarcinoma. *Ann Surg* 2001; 234:239–251.

Nakeeb A, Pitt HA, Sohn TA, et al. Cholangiocarcinoma: a spectrum of intrahepatic, perihilar, and distal tumors. *Ann Surg* 1996; 224:463–475.

Rea DJ, Heimbach JK, Rosen CB, et al. Liver transplantation with neoadjuvant chemoradiation is more effective than resection for hilar cholangiocarcinoma. *Ann Surg* 2005; 242:451–458.

Rea DJ, Munoz-Juarez M, Farnell MB, et al. Major hepatic resection for hilar cholangiocarcinoma: analysis of 46 patients. *Arch Surg* 2004; 139:514–523.

Shih SP, Schulick RD, Cameron JL, et al. Gallbladder cancer: the role of laparoscopy and radical resection. *Ann Surg* 2007; 245:893–901.

Takada T, Amano H, Yasuda H, et al. Is postoperative adjuvant chemotherapy useful for gallbladder carcinoma? A phase III multicenter prospective randomized controlled trial in patients with resected pancreaticobiliary carcinoma. *Cancer* 2002; 95:1685–1695.

Vauthey JN, Pawlik TM, Abdalla EK, et al. Is extended hepatectomy for hepatobiliary malignancy justified? *Ann Surg* 2004; 239:722–730.

INDEX

The letter *t* indicates a table, *b* indicates a box, and *f* indicates a figure.